Current Progress in Stem Cells Research

Current Progress in Stem Cells Research

Editor: Sarah Rowe

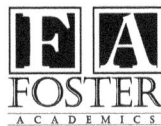

FA
FOSTER
ACADEMICS

www.fosteracademics.com

www.fosteracademics.com

FA
FOSTER
ACADEMICS

Cataloging-in-Publication Data

Current progress in stem cells research / edited by Sarah Rowe.
    p. cm.
Includes bibliographical references and index.
ISBN 978-1-63242-902-5
1. Stem cells. 2. Stem cells--Research. I. Rowe, Sarah.
QH588.S83 C87 2020
616.027 74--dc23

Foster Academics,
118-35 Queens Blvd., Suite 400,
Forest Hills, NY 11375, USA

ISBN 978-1-63242-902-5 (Hardback)

Contents

Preface... VII

Chapter 1   *In vitro* **study of the role of thrombin in platelet rich plasma (PRP)**
preparation: utility for gel formation and impact in growth factors release 1
Huber SC, Cunha JL, Montalvão SAL, da Silva LQ, Paffaro AU, da Silva FAR,
Rodrigues BL, Lana JFSD and Annichino-Bizzacchi JM

Chapter 2   **Cathepsin K Localizes to Equine Bone *In Vivo* and Inhibits Bone Marrow Stem**
and Progenitor Cells Differentiation *In Vitro* 9
Hussein H, Boyaka P, Dulin J, Russell D, Smanik L, Azab M and Bertone AL

Chapter 3   **New Trends in Heart Regeneration** 18
Kochegarov A and Lemanski LF

Chapter 4   **The Adaptability of Somatic Stem Cells** 26
Tweedell KS

Chapter 5   **Mouse iPSC generated with porcine reprogramming factors as a model for**
studying the effects of non-silenced heterologous transgenes on pluripotency 37
Petkov SG, Glage S and Niemann H

Chapter 6   **Epigallocatechin Gallate Inhibits Mouse Mesenchymal Stem Cell Differentiation**
to Adipogenic Lineage 46
Chani B, Puri V, Sobti RC and Puri S

Chapter 7   **Neural stem/progenitor cells maintained *in vitro* under different culture**
conditions alter differentiation capacity of monocytes to generate dendritic cells 55
Lupatov AYu, Poltavtseva RA, Bystrykh OA, Yarygin KN and Sukhikh GT

Chapter 8   **Safety and Feasibility of Autologous Mesenchymal Stem Cell Transplantation in**
Chronic Stroke in Indian patients 63
Bhasin A, Kumaran SS, Bhatia R, Mohanty S and Srivastava MVP

Chapter 9   **Increased motility of mesenchymal stem cells is correlated with inhibition of**
stimulated peripheral blood mononuclear cells *in vitro* 69
Bertolo A, Pavlicek D, Gemperli A, Baur M, Pötzel T and Stoyanov J

Chapter 10   **Randomized controlled trial comparing hyaluronic acid, platelet-rich plasma and**
the combination of both in the treatment of mild and moderate osteoarthritis
of the knee 82
Lana JFSD, Weglein A, Sampson S, Vicente EF, Huber SC, Souza CV, Ambach MA,
Vincent H, Urban-Paffaro A, Onodera CMK, Annichino-Bizzacchi JM,
Santana MHA and Belangero WD

Chapter 11   **Oct4B, CD90, and CD73 are upregulated in bladder tissue following electro-resection of the bladder** 92
Takeuchi T, Tonooka A, Okuno Y, Hattori-Kato M and Mikami K

Chapter 12   **StemRegenin 1 selectively promotes expansion of Multipotent Hematopoietic Progenitors derived from Human Embryonic Stem Cells** 98
Tao L, Togarrati PP, Choi KD and Suknuntha K

Chapter 13   **Mesenchymal stem cells-seeded bio-ceramic construct for bone regeneration in large critical-size bone defect in rabbit** 103
Maiti SK, Ninu AR, Sangeetha P, Mathew DD, Tamilmahan P, Kritaniya D, Kumar N and Hescheler J

Chapter 14   **The Effect of Pro-Neurogenic Gene Expression on Adult Subventricular Zone Precursor Cell Recruitment and Fate Determination After Excitotoxic Brain Injury** 116
Jones KS and Connor BJ

Chapter 15   **Comparing the *in vivo* and *in vitro* effects of hypoxia (3% O₂) on directly derived cells from murine cardiac explants versus murine cardiosphere derived cells** 127
Amirrasouli MM and Shamsara M

Chapter 16   **Long Term Study of Protective Mechanisms of Human Adipose Derived Mesenchymal Stem Cells on Cisplatin Induced Kidney injury in Sprague-Dawley Rats** 137
Elhusseini FM, Saad M-AAA, Anber N, Elghannam D, Sobh M-A, Alsaied A, El-dusoky S, Sheashaa H, Abdel-Ghaffar H and Sobh MA

Chapter 17   **Re-Defining Stem Cell-Cardiomyocyte Interactions: Focusing on the Paracrine Effector Approach** 150
Mahapatra S, Martin D and Gallicano GI

Chapter 18   **Proliferation, migration and differentiation potential of human mesenchymal progenitor cells derived from osteoarthritic subchondral cancellous bone** 167
Krüger JP, Enz A, Hondke S, Wichelhaus A, Endres M and Mittlmeier T

Chapter 19   **Cardiomyogenic Heterogeneity of Clonal Subpopulations of Human Bone Marrow Mesenchymal Stem Cells** 175
Tripathy NK, Rizvi SHM, Singh SP, Garikpati VNS and Nityanand S

Chapter 20   **Generation of dopamine neuronal-like cells from induced neural precursors derived from adult human cells by non-viral expression of lineage factors** 182
Playne R, Jones KS and Connor B

Permissions

List of Contributors

Index

Preface

Stem cells are the cells with the unique ability to differentiate into specialized cell types. The bone marrow, blood and adipose tissue are the three known accessible sources of adult stem cells in humans. Such adult stem cells are of use in various medical therapies for the treatment and prevention of diseases or conditions. Bone marrow transplant is the most common stem-cell therapy. Research is being done to apply stem-cell treatments for the management of neurodegenerative diseases, heart disease, diabetes, etc. Alternative sources of stem cells and innovative techniques for generating organoids using stem cells are being explored. These will enable the understanding of organogenesis, human development and modeling of human diseases. This book aims to shed light on some of the unexplored aspects of stem cells and the recent researches in this field. The various advancements in stem cell therapy are glanced at and their applications as well as ramifications are looked at in detail. Coherent flow of topics, student-friendly language and extensive use of examples make this book an invaluable source of knowledge.

The researches compiled throughout the book are authentic and of high quality, combining several disciplines and from very diverse regions from around the world. Drawing on the contributions of many researchers from diverse countries, the book's objective is to provide the readers with the latest achievements in the area of research. This book will surely be a source of knowledge to all interested and researching the field.

In the end, I would like to express my deep sense of gratitude to all the authors for meeting the set deadlines in completing and submitting their research chapters. I would also like to thank the publisher for the support offered to us throughout the course of the book. Finally, I extend my sincere thanks to my family for being a constant source of inspiration and encouragement.

Editor

In vitro study of the role of thrombin in platelet rich plasma (PRP) preparation: utility for gel formation and impact in growth factors release

Huber SC[1], Cunha JL[1], Montalvão SAL[1], da Silva LQ[1], Paffaro AU[1], da Silva FAR[1], Rodrigues BL[1], Lana JFSD[1], Annichino-Bizzacchi JM[1]

Introduction: The use of PRP has been studied for different fields, with promising results in regenerative medicine. Until now, there is no study in the literature evaluating thrombin levels in serum, used as autologous thrombin preparation. Therefore, in the present study we evaluated the role played by different thrombin concentrations in PRP and the impact in the release of growth factors. Also, different activators for PRP gel formation were evaluated. **Methods:** Thrombin levels were measured in different autologous preparations: serum, L-PRP (PRP rich in leukocytes) and T-PRP (thrombin produced through PRP added calcium gluconate). L-PRP was prepared according to the literature, with platelets and leukocytes being quantified. The effect of autologous thrombin associated or not with calcium in PRP gel was determined by measuring the time of gel formation. The relationship between thrombin concentration and release of growth factors was determined by growth factors (PDGF-AA, VEGF and EGF) multiplex analysis. **Results:** A similar concentration of thrombin was observed in serum, L-PRP and T-PRP (8.13 nM, 8.63 nM and 7.56 nM, respectively) with a high variation between individuals (CV%: 35.07, 43 and 58.42, respectively). T-PRP and serum with calcium chloride showed similar results in time to promote gel formation. The increase of thrombin concentrations (2.66, 8 and 24 nM) did not promote an increase in growth factor release. **Conclusions:** The technique of using serum as a thrombin source proved to be the most efficient and reproducible for promoting PRP gel formation, with some advantages when compared to other activation methods, as this technique is easier and quicker with no need of consuming part of PRP. Noteworthy, PRP activation using different thrombin concentrations did not promote a higher release of growth factors, appearing not to be necessary when PRP is used as a suspension.

Key Words: Platelet Rich Plasma, Thrombin, gel, Leukocytes, Growth factor

Introduction

Platelet rich plasma (PRP) is defined as a concentrate preparation that increases between 4 to 9 folds the basal number of platelets, in reduced plasma volume[1]. Platelets contain over 1100 proteins including growth factors, messengers of the immune system, enzymes, enzyme inhibitors and other bioactive compounds. These factors can improve tissue repair by diverse mechanisms including regulation of inflammation, angiogenesis, synthesis and remodeling of new tissues[2, 3]. For these reasons, PRP has been used in different fields: odontology[4], plastic surgery[5], orthopedics[6], wound healing[7] and aesthetics[8] with promising results. However, biomolecules are known to be quickly released from PRP, losing their activity in a short period of time which could represent a challenge in clinical practice[9].

PRP preparations have been used since 1970s, however they become popular in 1990s. Since then, different protocols emerged to prepare PRP including commercial systems[10]. Despite the promising results published by different research groups, the heterogeneity of protocols for PRP preparation available, render the evaluation of a consistent therapeutic effect quite difficult. *In vitro* studies evidenced that the different methodologies used in the preparation of PRP can affect biological aspects and clinical effects, which depend on several variables, particularly platelet and growth factor concentration, presence or absence of leukocytes and the type of activation[2].

PRP is usually prepared by double centrifugation of anticoagulated blood. The first spin is to separate red blood cells and plasma; the second spin is to concentrate platelets. Despite the existing PRP standardization proposals, there is no consensus regarding centrifugation force or duration. This absence of a standard PRP preparation inhibits any comparisons of treatment efficacy obtained by different research groups. The inclusion or not of leukocytes is also widely discussed in the literature. PRP with leukocytes (L-PRP) presents different biologic activity, which could modify the therapeutic effect[11].

Another important issue is the activation for growth factor release. This activation can be induced by bovine or autologous thrombin, calcium chloride, collagen, freeze & thaw cycles and mechanical trauma. Collagen and thrombin activate platelets by different mechanisms. For the activation of platelets by collagen, they must first adhere to collagen and then became active by it through a second receptor. This kind of platelet activation may require a lengthier mechanism than the cleavage process of thrombin-mediated platelet activation[12]. Park and collaborators demonstrated that thrombin is a strong agonist for induction of PRP cytokines and growth factors release when compared to ADP + calcium or collagen[13]. Once PRP activation is achieved, a fibrin network begins to form with a rapid growth factor release during the first hour, continuing to release cytokines and growth factors from their mRNA for at least another 7 days[14, 15].

Author Names in full: Stephany Cares Huber[1], José Luiz Rosenberis Cunha Júnior[1], Silmara Montalvão[1], Letícia Queiroz da Silva[1], Aline Urban Paffaro[1], Francesca Aparecida Ramos da Silva[1], Bruno Lima Rodrigues[1], José Fabio Santos Duarte Lana[1], Joyce Maria Annichinno-Bizzacchi[1]

[1] *Hemocentro, Haemostasis Laboratory, State University of Campinas UNICAMP, Brazil.*

There is no consensus in the literature regarding the choice of the best activator and whether PRP should be used with or without activation in clinical practice. The most common activation method included a single amount of thrombin in association with calcium chloride. However, different sources and procedures to obtain thrombin can also interfere with the PRP therapeutic effect. Bovine thrombin may present adverse reactions including hemorrhage, thrombosis, and immune reaction, thus, autologous thrombin has been preferred to avoid this clinical complication. Autologous thrombin can be obtained from serum samples or by using calcium gluconate to clot PRP (T-PRP)[16]. In this context, autologous serum, which is simple to obtain, could represent a promising source of thrombin, however this source has not been investigated in practice. Therefore, the impact of thrombin and other PRP activators should be investigated, which led us in the present study to evaluate the role of thrombin in PRP preparations in terms of time for gel formation and of growth factor release.

Material and Methods

Subjects

Forty-two healthy individuals (30 female: 12 male), with mean age of 32.5 years and SD± 9.36 were included. None of the donators had taken any medication that could interfere with hematological parameters. The local Ethic Committee approved data collection and all procedures were in accordance with the ethical standards and with the Helsinki Declaration.

Autologous preparations

Preparation of L-PRP

For each volunteer, peripheral blood was collected by venous puncture in eight vacuum tubes: six 8.5 ml ACD tubes, one EDTA and one tube without anticoagulant (BD Vacutainer). L-PRP preparation was performed according to Amable's methodology[10]; the first spin at 300 g for 5 minutes and the second spin at 700 g for 17 minutes. The buffy-coat rich with leukocytes (L-PRP) was collected from all tubes. At the end of the double spin the top layer plasma was characterized as platelet poor plasma (PPP - 80% volume) and the lower layer was the PRP (20% volume). Platelet counts were carried out in whole blood and PRP samples with Siemens Advia120 and Advia2120i hematology analyzers.

T-PRP

T-PRP was prepared by a modified protocol described by Franco et al.[16]; 1.5 mL of L-PRP were mixed with 0.5 mL of 10% calcium gluconate, and incubated for 15 minutes in a 37 °C water bath. After L-PRP clotting, the tubes were centrifuged at 800 g for 10 minutes, and the supernatant was separated.

Serum

Serum was collected by venous puncture into a tube without anticoagulant and centrifuged at 1260 g for 10 minutes.

Autologous thrombin assessment

We determined thrombin concentration in L-PRP, T-PRP and serum. Thrombin concentration was measured through fluorogenic assay, conducted with an enzyme-specific fluorogenic substrate (FluCa Reagent, Thrombinoscope), and a standard curve of purified

exogenous thrombin (Thrombin Calibrator, Thrombinoscope).

Thrombin generation test (TGT) with CAT Calibrated Automate Thrombogram (CAT) Thrombinoscope (Fluoroskan ascent Thermo was performed in order to investigate the presence and the ability t generate thrombin of the thrombin precursor in the same samples.

Assessment of PRP Gel Formation

L-PRP gel formation was analyzed using thrombin preparation and/or calcium in 12x75 mm polystyrene tubes (Table 1). Nin healthy volunteers were used to produce L-PRP, and the thrombi concentrations were evaluated by fluorogenic assay of T-PRP an serum of each sample. Activators were mixed with each L-PRP in final reaction volume of 200 μL. The tubes were then incubated a room temperature, without agitation. The time required for ge formation was considered as the period between the addition of th activator and the beginning of fibrin formation, as an indire measure of time for PRP gel formation. This protocol is standardize and broadly used for coagulation tests as described by Kitchen an collaborators, and Clinical and Laboratory Standards Institute (CLS) guideline[17, 18].

Table 1: Activators tested for gel formation

Combination	Type of activator	Description
1	T-PRP	Thrombin produced from PRP with Calcium Gluconate 0.5%
2	Serum	Thrombin produced with autologous serum
3	Serum + 0.5% $CaCl_2$	Thrombin produced with autologous serum with 0.5% $CaCl_2$
4	Serum + Calcium Gluconate ($C_{12}H_{22}CaO_{14}$) 0.5%	Thrombin produced with autologous serum with 0.5% $C_{12}H_{22}CaO_{14}$
5	Calcium Chloride ($CaCl_2$) 0.5%	Only with 0.5% $CaCl_2$ without thrombin
6	Calcium Chloride ($CaCl_2$) 2.5%	Only with 2.5% $CaCl_2$ without thrombin
7	Calcium Gluconate ($C_{12}H_{22}CaO_{14}$) 0.5%	Only with 0.5% $C_{12}H_{22}CaO_{14}$ without thrombin
8	Calcium Gluconate ($C_{12}H_{22}CaO_{14}$) 2.5%	Only with 2.5% $C_{12}H_{22}CaO_{14}$ without thrombin

Method to concentrate thrombin for analysis of growth factor releas

Growth factors released from L-PRP were evaluated using thrombi obtained from a modified methodology previously described b Saxena et al.[19]. Thrombin had a concentration of 121 nM, measure through fluorogenic assay, conducted with an enzyme-specifi fluorogenic substrate (FluCa Reagent, Thrombinoscope), and standard curve of purified exogenous thrombin (Thrombi Calibrator, Thrombinoscope).

Quantitative measurement of growth factors released from L-PRP using different thrombin concentrations

The aim of this analysis was to verify whether different thrombin concentrations (0, 2.66, 8 and 24 nM) could interfere with the release of the growth factors. The growth factors evaluated were: platelet derived growth factor (PDGF-AA), epidermal growth factor (EGF) and vascular endothelial growth factor (VEGF) measured through multiplex analysis – Luminex (Milipore). To this end, L-PRP samples were normalized at a concentration of 1200×10^3 platelets/ μl, diluted in PPP and activated with different thrombin concentrations as previously described. The activated samples were incubated in a water bath at 37°C for one hour. Posteriorly, it used two different protocols to evaluate the release of growth factors: 1) The samples were then treated with 3 cycles of nitrogen to dissolve the clot, as described by Matsui and Tabata[20], and 2) The samples were centrifuged at 200g for 5 minutes and the supernatant was used, as described in manufacturer procedures The protocols of Luminex were carried out following the manufacturer's instructions.

Statistical analysis

Variables were tested to verify the normality using the Shapiro-Wilk test. As the variables did not have a normal distribution, Friedman test with Dunn's post-test were used for all comparisons. Spearman's rank correlation coefficient test was used for the correlation tests. The GraphPad Prism 5.0 software was used and $p < 0.05$ was considered significant.

Results

PRP characterization

The methodology for PRP preparation was able to recover high concentrations of platelets (PLT) and white blood cells (WBC) as shown in Figure 1 (A and B). The figure evidenced the mean and standard error (SE) of basal PLT and WBC and the recovery in the L-PRP of the donators. The mean of platelet concentration in L-PRP was 1912×10^3 cells/μl, which represents 7.1 folds higher from the basal number (270.4); The mean of white blood cells in L-PRP was 9.8×10^3 cells/μl, which represents 1.5 folds higher from the basal number (2.3). The mean of red blood cells (RBC) in L-PRP was 0.2289×10^6 cells/μl SE ± 0.026

Preparation of autologous thrombin depends on the method and on inter-individual variability

In order to assess the amount of thrombin in the different types of preparations, all analyses were performed in the same individual sample for serum, L-PRP and T-PRP. No statistically significant difference was observed (p= 0.4363) between different preparations, and the mean thrombin concentrations were 8.63 nM in L-PRP, 8.13 nM in serum and 7.56 nM in T-PRP (Figure 2A). The coefficient of variation (CV %) of thrombin level for L-PRP, serum and T-PRP were 43.0 %, 35.07%, 58.24%, respectively. The serum samples showed a lower CV % when compared to other methods

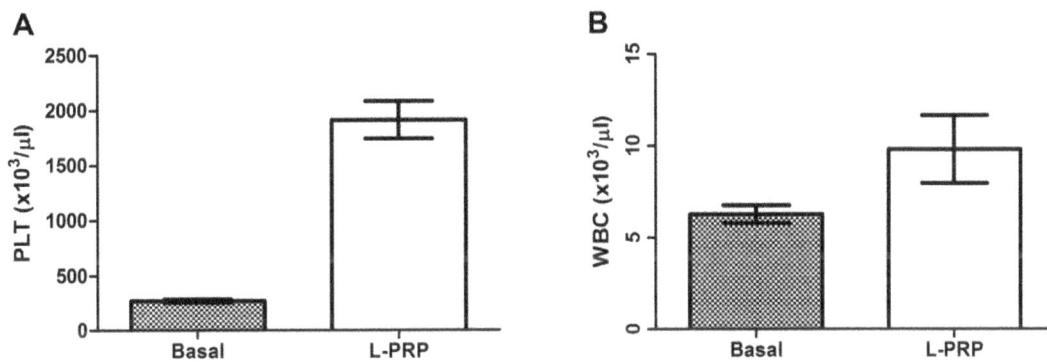

Figure 1: Graphic showing the platelet number of basal and L-PRP (A) and recovery of white blood cells in L-PRP relative to basal number (B), N= 9

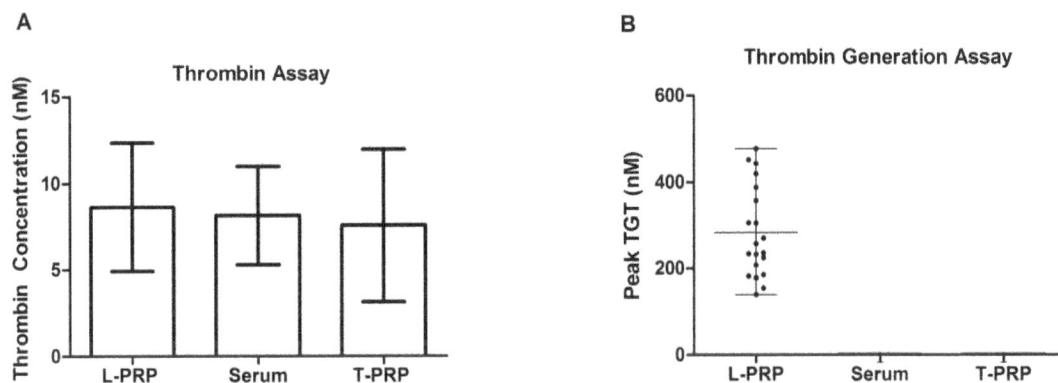

Figure 2: Graphic showing mean of thrombin concentration (A) and peak of thrombin generation by flurogenic assay in PRP, Serum and T-PRP among 20 healthy individuals (B). Mean concentration of thrombin 8.63 ± 3.73 nM in L-PRP, 8.13 ± 2.85 nM in serum and 7.56 ± 4.40 nM in T-PRP

A

Thrombin Assay

B

Correlation analysis

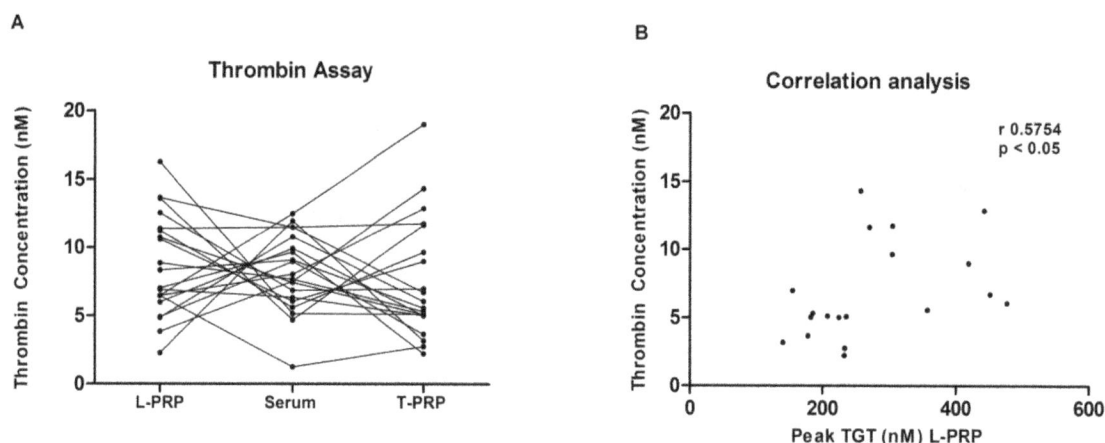

Figure 3: *Graphic showing the inter and intra individual variation of thrombin levels in plasma and serum from 20 healthy individuals (A) and showing a significant correlation between thrombin concentration in L-PRP and peak of thrombin generation by thrombin generation test (TGT) (B), r= 0.5754 p< 0.05*

Despite of the similar results between the mean of thrombin, no intra-individual trend line was observed, i.e. individuals with high amounts of thrombin in PRP did not show higher amounts of thrombin in T-PRP or serum. The intra-individual CV varied from 1.62 to 91.68% (Figure 3A).

As expected, the TGT test revealed the presence of thrombin precursors only in the L-PRP samples (Figure 2B). TGT results observed in L-PRP presented a statistically significant correlation with the thrombin concentrations measured in L-PRP samples (r=0.575, p<0.05) as demonstrated in Figure 3B.

Serum and T-PRP presented a similar period required for PRP gel formation

The time required for L-PRP fibrin formation varied from 1.5 to approximately 22 minutes, except for serum alone and calcium chloride 2.5% which did not promote fibrin clot. T-PRP showed significantly shorter time when compared to all uses of calcium alone (calcium chloride / gluconate) (p<0.05), as evidenced in Figure 4. Serum used in association of 0.5% calcium chloride (CaCl2) or 0.5% gluconate showed significantly shorter time in relation of calcium gluconate 0.5% ($C_{12}H_{22}CaO_{14}$) (p<0.05) (Figure 4).

The means (± Standard Deviation) of the time (in minutes) for fibrin formation of all activators were: T-PRP: 1.52 ± 0.45, Serum + 0.5% Calcium Gluconate ($C_{12}H_{22}CaO_{14}$): 7.98 ± 4.91, Serum + 0.5% Calcium Chloride (CaCl2): 7.49 ± 3.38, Calcium Chloride 0.5% (CaCl2): 13.92 ± 3.02, Calcium Gluconate 0.5% ($C_{12}H_{22}CaO_{14}$): 22.01 ± 7.00, Calcium Gluconate 2.5% ($C_{12}H_{22}CaO_{14}$): 15.42 ± 4.02, as showed in Figure 4.

In order to standardize the procedure above, the thrombin concentrations were evaluated in all nine individuals that were used in this experiment. The mean and coefficient of variation of thrombin concentration in serum and T-PRP were 6.1 nM (CV% 46.5) and 4.8 nM (CV% 69.4), respectively.

Growth factor release did not vary according to different thrombin concentrations

Three thrombin concentrations (2.66, 8 and 24 nM) were evaluated

for promoting platelet activation and PDGF-AA, EGF and VEGF release. The aim was to identify a correlation between thrombin levels and growth factor release. For this experiment 9 L-PRP were prepared from different healthy individuals, and the platelet number was standardized to 1200×10^3 platelets/ µl. No difference was observed between protocols 1 (with nitrogen cycles) and 2 (centrifugation) in the release of growth factors according different thrombin concentrations, as evidenced in the Figure 5 (A and B).

The mean and standard deviation for level of growth factors released in protocol 1 were: EGF 599.3 pg/mL ± 241.9 for 0 nM, 504.3 pg/mL ± 247.3 for 2.66 nM, 519.4 pg/mL ± 202.9 for 8 nM and 538.8 pg/mL ± 208.2 for 24 nM. VEGF 1426 pg/mL ± 1711 for 0 nM, 1840 pg/mL ± 2379 for 2.66, 1328 pg/mL ± 1715 for 8nM and 1136 pg/mL ± 1295 for 24 nM. PDGF-AA 126789 pg/mL ± 219745 for 0 nM, 43122 pg/mL ± 22307 for 2.66 nM, 43820 pg/mL ±16927 for 8 nM, 40531 pg/mL ±10676 for 24 nM.

For the protocol 2 (with centrifugation), the mean and standard deviation for level of growth factors released were: EGF 23258 pg/mL ± 44544 for 0 nM, 104629 pg/mL ± 133511 for 2.66 nM, 41070 pg/mL ± 63675 for 8 nM and 38075 pg/mL ± 71324 for 24 nM. VEGF 13492 pg/mL ± 26127 for 0 nM, 53950 pg/mL ± 81493 for 2.66, 45926 pg/mL ± 103653 for 8nM and 30599 pg/mL ± 61828 for 24 nM. PDGF-AA 32262 pg/mL ± 47399 for 0 nM, 36343 pg/mL ± 16821 for 2.66 nM, 23028 pg/mL ± 22064 for 8 nM, 19046 pg/mL ±16676 for 24 nM.

It was observed that the concentrations of growth factors released using the protocol 2 (centrifugation) presents, in general, higher values compared with the release promoted by protocol 1 (nitrogen cycles). This difference was significant only in EGF values in the concentration of 2.66 and 8 nM (p<0.0001).

As shown in Figure 5, for all thrombin concentrations and protocols used, the levels of growth factors released were similar, evidencing that the concentration of thrombin did not interfere with the release of growth factors in the protocols tested by this study (p>0.05).

Discussion

In this study, we evaluated the influence of thrombin in PRP

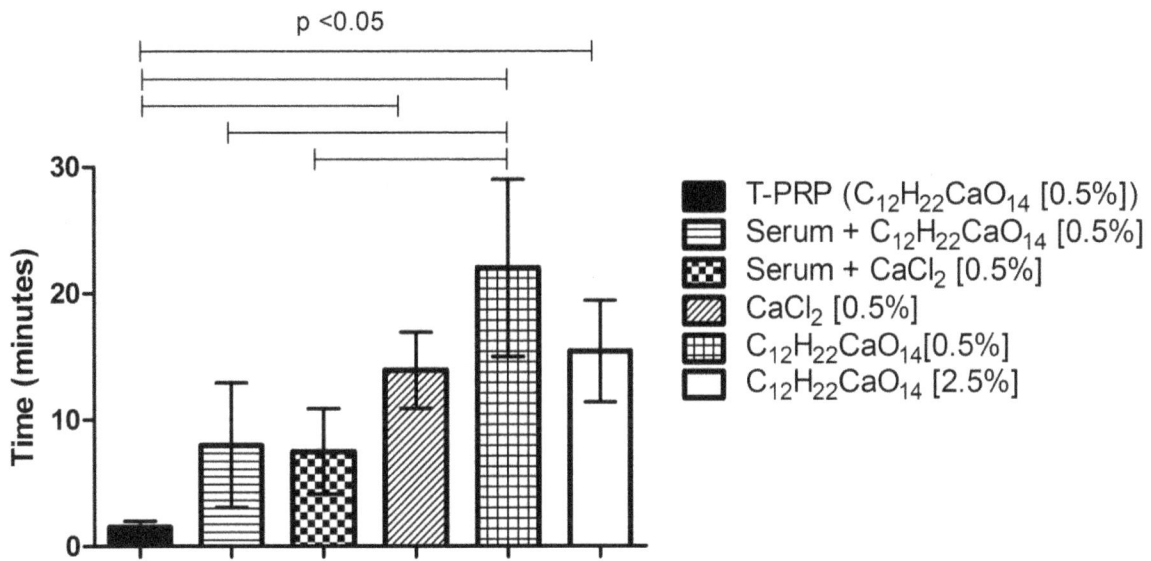

Figure 4: *Graphic showing the mean time that different activators took to form the fibrin clot. The use of serum alone and calcium chloride [2.5%] did not induce clot formation until 30 minutes tested; N=9*

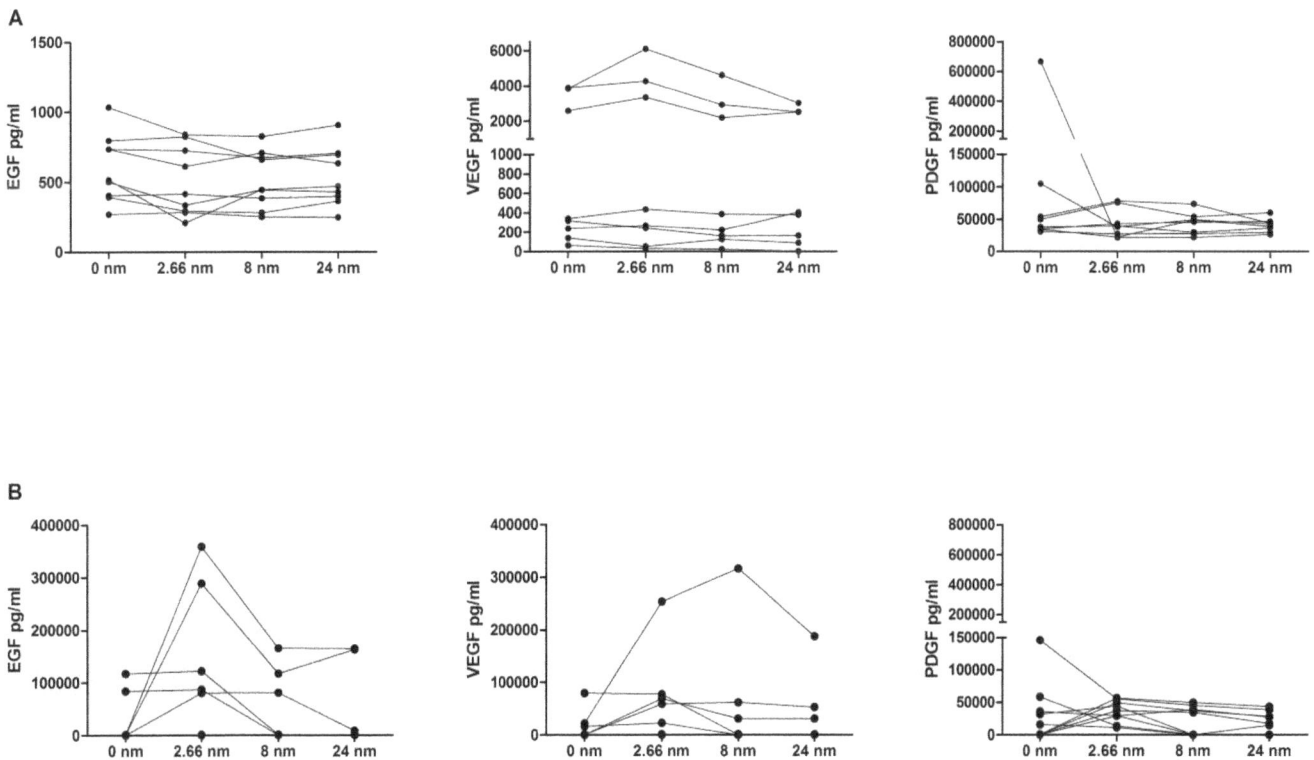

Figure 5: *Graphic showing levels of growth factors measured in L-PRP normalized to 1200 x 10³ platelets/ µl through Multiplex assay according different concentrations of thrombin. A) Protocol 1, using nitrogen cycles; B) Protocol 2, using centrifugation. p> 0.05 in all analysis.*

preparations. The main aspects investigated were the time for gel formation and the growth factor release. The levels of autologous thrombin were first assessed in serum, L-PRP and T-PRP in the same individual sample, in order to compare and identify the highest thrombin level. Thrombin levels were also evaluated in serum, as this could represent a simple and easy autologous thrombin source. L-PRP was used as basal sample. Unexpectedly, we demonstrated similar levels of thrombin in all preparations. It is well known that thrombin is consumed during fibrin clot formation, and we hypothesized that no thrombin would be present in the serum samples. Our results probably presented residual thrombin formed during serum preparation. *In vitro* residual thrombin had previously been described by Weiner in an assay to evaluate indirect antithrombin activity in serum samples[21]. Otherwise, we also did not expect to detect thrombin in L-PRP, as these samples were anticoagulated. These results are probably due to pre-analytical variables that promote tissue factor release and the activation of coagulation before ACD is mixed to the blood.

An interesting analysis was the capacity of thrombin generation evaluated in L-PRP, serum and T-PRP samples. As expected, precursor thrombin proteins were present only in L-PRP samples. This confirms that all autologous thrombin measured in the serum and T-PRP samples were residual, resulting from the manipulation of the samples. Furthermore, L-PRP thrombin concentration showed a correlation with precursor thrombin proteins levels demonstrated by TGT, this means that when the detection of residual thrombin was high, higher was the capacity of thrombin generation.

Despite the similar mean of thrombin level between serum, T-PRP and L-PRP, a high inter and intra individual variability was observed. Serum presented the lowest inter individual CV. This variability may interfere in clinical practice and is in accordance with our experience, as we have observed a large difference in the period required for platelet gel formation between individual samples. Jo and collaborators showed a similar period required for platelet gel formation with calcium gluconate used singly[22]. Our results evidenced that a synergism of thrombin and calcium ions is needed to obtain platelet gel in a short period of time. When each one was evaluated individually, clotting time with calcium alone was close to four folds higher and with serum alone, there was no gel formation.

Regarding this difference in the time required for platelet gel formation, we hypothesized that thrombin levels could interfere in this process and in the release of growth factors from platelets. For this reason, growth factor release was studied for different thrombin concentrations. There is no discussion in the literature regarding the minimum autologous thrombin levels required for the PRP growth factor release. Unexpectedly, we demonstrated through our experiments that the release of growth factors did not increase with higher thrombin concentrations. Actually, we showed that higher concentrations of thrombin yielded a more consistent clot, which was difficult to dissolve with nitrogen.

The use of serum as a source of autologous thrombin achieved good results in growth factor release and in promoting gel formation. In addition, the use of serum samples to obtain autologous thrombin introduces some practical benefits, as no laboratory treatment was required, thus consuming less preparation time, and presenting higher reproducibility. Indeed, according to our results, PRP used as a suspension requires no activation as the levels of growth factor release were similar in both activated and non-activated samples. Probably in this situation, the application of PRP *in vivo* would be activated when exposed to collagen, elastin, and other proteins.

Amable and collaborators used a mathematical formula to evaluate thrombin levels in 1×10^6 platelet concentration, in order to compare

the results with other studies. In their study, PRP was activated with 9 nM of thrombin after an incubation of 16 hours[10]. The levels of growth factors released were close to 8500 pg/ml of PDGF-AA and 500 pg/ml of EGF. When these levels were compared with our results we demonstrated that EGF levels were very similar (mean of 519.4 ± 202.9 pg/ml) when using the same thrombin concentration, however, the PDGF-AA levels were much higher in our study (43820 ± 16927) using the protocol 1. In order to evaluate if the protocols may change the levels of growth factors release, we performed the protocol 2 without nitrogen cycles, and the results were even higher. We believe that the all the procedures to evaluate the release of growth factors have some technical limitations which lead to a variability of the results.

Anitua *et al.*, described the kinetics of growth factor release in platelet clots rich in growth factors (PRGF) activated with 10% $CaCl_2$ up to 8 days of incubation, and in L-PRP after 24 hours of activation[23]. The clots were evaluated with scanning electron microscopy (SEM) in order to evaluate fibrin formation. The weakness of this study is the small number of samples (n=3) and the presentation of the data, in percentage or log, which does not enable comparison with other studies. In 2015, Anitua *et al.*, published another study evaluating the kinetics of other growth factors release (PDGF-AB, transforming growth factor (TGF-β1), VEGF, hepatocyte growth factor (HGF), insulin-like growth factor (IGF-I), EGF) and interleukins (IL-1β and IL-16) in PRGF and L-PRP clots from 3 donators activated with CaCL2 during 8 days[24]. When compared to our results we found a similar result regarding VEGF, during the first hour, however, the EGF levels were higher in our study (mean of 599 pg/ml - not treated). These high levels could be attributed to the difference in activation (calcium and thrombin) and the nitrogen cycles, used to dissolve the clot and release all the growth factor inside the clot, therefore increasing the concentrations. As expected, pro-inflammatory cytokines were significantly higher in L- PRP during all the period of *in vitro* experiment (8 days).

Martineau *et al.*, also studied the kinetics of growth factors release (VEGF, PDGF-BB, TGF-β1) according to different concentrations of thrombin and calcium, and demonstrated similar results when compared to our experiments[25]. Indeed, as we observed in our study, VEGF and EGF did not have a significant increase in the release regarding the concentration of activators.

Finally, a practical result of our study was showing the advantages in using serum with calcium instead of T-PRP to activate platelets for gel formation, as this is an easy, quick, low cost and reproducible method, with no laboratory handling and no consuming of PRP. According to our study, no thrombin activation is required for platelet suspension, as the release of the growth factors PDGF-AA, EGF and VEGF is the same with and without the presence of thrombin.

Conclusion

Residual levels of thrombin were detected in serum, T-PRP and autologous thrombin preparations. Serum proved to be the most reproducible technique to activate PRP for gel formation and presented some advantages when compared to other activation methods, such as the easier and faster preparation and the lack of necessity of using part of PRP. Therefore, autologous thrombin can conveniently be prepared from serum samples and be useful for gel preparation. However, the activation with different thrombin concentrations does not show a correlation with release of the growth factors PDGF-AA, VEGF and VEGF, suggesting that no activation is required when using a platelet suspension.

References

1. Marx RE. Platelet-rich plasma: evidence to support its use. J Oral Maxillofac Surg. 2004;62(4):489-96.
2. Andia I, Abate M. Platelet-rich plasma: underlying biology and clinical correlates. Regen Med. 2013;8(5):645-58.
3. Arnoczky SP, Sheibani-Rad S. The basic science of platelet-rich plasma (PRP): what clinicians need to know. Sports Med Arthrosc. 2013;21(4):180-5.
4. Albanese A, Licata ME, Polizzi B, Campisi G. Platelet-rich plasma (PRP) in dental and oral surgery: from the wound healing to bone regeneration. Immun Ageing. 2013;10(1):23.
5. Cervelli V, Bocchini I, Di Pasquali C, De Angelis B, Cervelli G, Curcio CB, Orlandi A, Scioli MG, Tati E, Delogu P, Gentile P. P.R.L. platelet rich lipotransfert: our experience and current state of art in the combined use of fat and PRP. Biomed Res Int. 2013;2013:434191.
6. Scarpone M, Rabago D, Snell E, Demeo P, Ruppert K, Pritchard P, Arbogast G, Wilson JJ, Balzano JF. Effectiveness of Platelet-rich Plasma Injection for Rotator Cuff Tendinopathy: A Prospective Open-label Study. Glob Adv Health Med. 2013;2(2):26-31..
7. Carter MJ, Fylling CP, Parnell LK. Use of platelet rich plasma gel on wound healing: a systematic review and meta-analysis. Eplasty. 2011;11:e38.
8. Cervelli V, Garcovich S, Bielli A, Cervelli G, Curcio BC, Scioli MG, Orlandi A, Gentile P. The effect of autologous activated platelet rich plasma (AA-PRP) injection on pattern hair loss: clinical and histomorphometric evaluation. Biomed Res Int. 2014;2014:760709.
9. Kutlu B, Aydin RST, Akman AC, Gumusderelioglu M, Nohutcu RM. Platelet-rich plasma-loaded chitosan scaffolds: preparation and growth factor release kinetics. J Biomed Mater Res B Appl Biomater. 2013;101(1):28-35.
10. Amable PR, Carias RB, Teixeira MV, da Cruz Pacheco I, Corrêa do Amaral RJ, Granjeiro JM, Borojevic R. Platelet-rich plasma preparation for regenerative medicine: optimization and quantification of cytokines and growth factors. Stem Cell Res Ther. 2013;4(3):67.
11. Perez AG, Lana JF, Rodrigues AA, Luzo AC, Belangero WD, Santana MH. Relevant aspects of centrifugation step in the preparation of platelet-rich plasma. ISRN Hematol. 2014; 2014: 176060.
12. Brass LF. Thrombin and platelet activation. Chest. 2003;124(3 Suppl):18S-25S.
13. Park HB,Yang JH and Chung KW. Characterization of the cytokine profile of platelet rich plasma (PRP) and PRP-induced cell proliferation and migration: Upregulation of matrix metalloproteinase-1 and -9 un HaCat cells. Korean J Hematol. 2011;46(4):265-73.
14. Liao HT, Marra KG, Rubin JP. Application of platelet-rich plasma and platelet-rich fibrin in fat grafting: basic science and literature review. Tissue Eng Part B Rev. 2014;20(4):267-76.
15. Senzel L, Gnatenko DV, Bahou WF. The platelet proteome. Curr Opin Hematol. 2009;16(5):329-33.
16. Franco D, Franco T, Schettino AM, Filho JM, Vendramin FS. Protocol for obtaining platelet-rich plasma (PRP), platelet-poor plasma (PPP), and thrombin for autologous use. Aesthetic Plast Surg. 2012;36(5):1254-9.
17. Kitchen S, McCraw A, Echenagucia M. Diagnosis of Hemophilia and other bleeding disorders - A laboratory manual. World Federation of Hemophilia 2010; 2° ed: 1-144.
18. Clinical and Laboratory Standards Institute (CLSI) guideline. One-stage prothrombin time (PT) test and activated partial thromboplastin time (APTT) test; approved guideline H47-HA2 2008; 28(20).
19. Saxena S, Jain P, Shukla J. Preparation of two component Fibrin Glue and its clinical evaluation in skin grafts and flaps. Indian J Plast Surg 2003;36 (1):14-7.
20. Matsui M, Tabata Y. Enhanced angiogenesis by multiple relase of platelet-rich plasma contents and basic fibroblats growth factor from gelatin hydrogels. Acta Biomater. 2012;8(5):1792-801.
21. Weiner M. Residual serum thrombin activity. Clin Chem. 1958;4(4):271-7.
22. Jo CH, Roh YH, Kim JE, Shin S, Yoon KS. Optimizing platelet-rich plasma gel formation by varying time and gravitational forces during centrifugation. J Oral Implantol. 2013;39(5):525-32.
23. Anitua E, Zalduendo MM, Alkhraisat MH, Orive G. Release kinetics of platelet-derived and plasma- derived growth factors from autologous plasma tich in growth factors. Ann Anat. 2013;195(5):461-6.
24. Anitua E, Zalduendo MM, Prado R, Alkhraisat H, Orive G. Morphogen and proinflammatory cytokine release kinetics from PRGF-endoret fibrin scaffolds: evaluation of the effect of leukocyte inclusion. J Biomed Mater Res A. 2015;103(3):1011-20.
25. Martineau I, Lacoste E, Gagnon G. Effects of calcium and thrombin on growth factor release from platelet concentrates: Kinetics and regulation of endothelial cell proliferation. Biomaterials. 2004;25(18):4489-502.

Abbreviations

PRP	:	Platelet Rich Plasma
L-PRP	:	Platelet Rich Plasma enriched with Leukocytes
T-PRP	:	Thrombin produced through Platelet Rich Plasma
PDGF	:	Platelet Derived Growth Factor
VEGF	:	Vascular Endothelial Growth Factor
EGF	:	Epidermal Growth Factor
CV	:	Coefficient of Variation
SD	:	Standard Deviation
ACD	:	Acid Citrate Dextrose anticoagulant
PPP	:	Platelet Poor Plasma
CAT	:	Calibrated Automated Thrombin
PLT	:	Platelets
WBC	:	White Blood Cells
TGT	:	Thrombin Generation Test
PRGF	:	Platelet Clot Rich in Growth Factors
CaCl2	:	Calcium Chloride
SEM	:	Scanning Electron Microscopy
TGF-β1	:	Transforming Growth Factor
HGF	:	Hepatocyte Growth Factor
IGF	:	Insulin-like Growth Factor

Potential Conflicts of Interests

None

Acknowledgements

The authors would like to thank FAPESP and CNPq for their financial support.

Corresponding Author

Stephany Cares Huber, Rua Carlos Chagas 480 - Hemocentro de Campinas – Cidade Universitária Zeferino Vaz – Campinas – SP - Brazil - CEP 13083-878; Email: stephany_huber@yahoo.com.br; Alternative email: ste.crimson@yahoo.com.br

Cathepsin K Localizes to Equine Bone *In Vivo* and Inhibits Bone Marrow Stem and Progenitor Cells Differentiation *In Vitro*

Hussein H[1], Boyaka P[2], Dulin J[1], Russell D[2], Smanik L[1], Azab M[1], Bertone AL[1,2]

Abstract

Selective inhibition of Cathepsin K (CatK) has a promising therapeutic potential for diseases associated with bone loss and osseous inflammation, such as osteoarthritis, periodontitis, and osteoporosis. In horses, stress-related bone injuries are common and accompanied by bone pain and inflammation resulting in excessive bone resorption and periostitis. VEL-0230 is a highly selective inhibitor of CatK that significantly decreased bone resorption and increased bone formation biomarkers. The goal of this study was to demonstrate the presence of CatK in equine bone and a simultaneous influence on the bone marrow cellular components including function and differentiation. Our objectives were: 1) to investigate the tissue localization of CatK protein in equine bone using immunohistochemistry, and 2) to determine the effect of CatK inhibition on osteoclastogenic, chondrogenic and osteogenic differentiation potential of equine stem and progenitor cells *in vitro* using histochemical staining and differentiation-related gene expression analyses. Bone biopsies, harvested from the tuber coxae and proximal phalanx of six healthy horses, were processed for immunostaining against CatK. Sternal bone marrow aspirates were cultured in 0, 1, 10, or 100 μM of VEL-0230 and subsequent staining scoring and gene expression analyses performed. All cells morphologically characterized as osteoclasts and moderate number of active bone lining osteoblasts stained positive for CatK. Histochemical staining and gene expression analyses revealed a significant increase in the osteoclastogenic, chondrogenic and osteogenic differentiation potential of equine bone marrow cells, which was VEL-0230-concentration dependent for the latter two. These results suggested that CatK inhibition may have anabolic effects on bone and cartilage regeneration that may be explained as a feedback response to CatK depletion. In conclusion, the use of CatK inhibition to reduce inflammation and associated bone resorption in equine osseous disorders may offer advantages to other therapeutics that would require further study.

Key Words: Osteoblast, Osteoclast, Chondrocyte, Osteoporosis, Bone resorption

Introduction

Cathepsin K (CatK) has become a major therapeutic target for the treatment of bone loss from osteoporosis[1], with potential for use in other diseases associated with bone resorption. The discovery of CatK, the predominant collagenase expressed in osteoclasts (OC), has revealed the significance of its inhibition of bone resorption *via* suppression of osteoclast activity. Multiple CatK inhibitors have been developed and have shown variable success in clinical trials to increase bone density and decrease pain[2-4]. Inhibitors of CatK, such as Odanacatib and VEL-0230/NC-2300, block the entire activity of CatK and can interfere with other signaling pathways known to be under the influence of CatK such as the innate immune response and inflammation[4-7]. We have investigated the pharmacokinetics of a potent CatK inhibitor, VEL-0230, in healthy exercising horses for future therapeutic application in equine patients with osteo-inflammatory conditions[8]. Cathepsin K inhibition ameliorated the inflammatory response of equine bone marrow mononuclear cells stimulated by Toll like receptors (TLR) -4 and TLR-9 ligands *in vitro* along with evidence of suppressed bone resorption and increased bone formation *in vivo* due to repeated VEL-0230 administration in healthy exercising horses[9,10]. The precise role of CatK in the immune system is unclear and maybe attributed, in part, to the location and tight integration between the bone and bone marrow. The latter constitutes the body reserve for immune, stem and progenitor cells.

Significant levels of CatK expression have been detected in osteoclasts, synovium, and chondrocytes of human and animal tissues[11-14]. One study has also demonstrated significant CatK expression in osteocytes and osteoblasts of human decalcified bone sections[15]. Similarly, expression levels of CatK were detected in equine *ex-vivo* cartilage tissue and in osteoclast-like cells generated *in vitro*[16,17]. However, CatK expression pattern in equine bone has not been studied, and may be relevant to equine bone and inflammatory diseases. Equine bone marrow serves as a source of mononuclear cells, growth factors and stem and progenitor cells. It has been used clinically to promote repair of musculoskeletal tissues including ligaments, tendons and articular cartilage regeneration[18-20]. Stem and progenitor cells differentiation has been found to share many pathways and common molecular regulatory factors with the immune system[21-24]. Hence, we hypothesized that CatK inhibition *in vitro*, using VEL-0230 in concentrations similar to the ones which suppressed inflammation in stimulated equine bone marrow nucleated cells[9], would significantly alter the

Author Names in full: Hayam Hussein[1], Prosper Boyaka[2], Jennifer Dulin[1], Duncan Russell[2], Lauren Smanik[1], Mohamed Azab[1], Alicia L. Bertone[1,2]

[1]Department of Veterinary Clinical Sciences, College of Veterinary Medicine, The Ohio State University, Columbus, OH, USA; [2]Department of Veterinary Biosciences, College of Veterinary Medicine, The Ohio State University, Columbus, OH, USA.

differentiation potential of equine stem and progenitor cells along the three main cell lineage of the skeletal system, which may provide relevance into the effect of VEL-0230 on bone. Our study aimed, firstly, to investigate the tissue localization of CatK protein in equine bone using immunohistochemistry and subsequent histomorphologic analysis. The second aim of this study was to determine the effect of CatK inhibition on osteoclastogenic, chondrogenic, and osteogenic differentiation *in vitro* using histochemical stains and differentiation-related gene expression analyses. For the second aim, osteoclastogenic, chondrogenic, and osteogenic induced cells were processed for tartrate-resistant acid phosphatase (TRAP), toluidine blue, von Kossa and alizarin red S staining, respectively and subsequent staining scoring was performed. Furthermore, quantitative real time polymerase chain reaction (qRT-PCR) was performed to quantify relative gene expression associated with osteoclastogenic differentiation (CatK, Receptor activator of nuclear factor kappa-B ligand [RANKL], TRAP), chondrogenic differentiation (Aggrecan, Collagen 2A, SOX9), and osteogenic differentiation (alkaline phosphatase, osteopontin, Runt-related transcription factor 2 [RUNX2]).

2. Materials And Methods

2.1 Animals

Seven young horses (3-5 years), three females and four males, free from lameness and systemic disease based on physical examination, were used in this study. All experimental protocols were pre-approved by the Institutional Animal Care and Use Committee (IACUC) of the Ohio State University.

2.2 Bone biopsy

Biopsy samples were collected from six of the horses from the Tuber coxae (TC), a non-weight-bearing bone, and the proximal phalanx (P1), a weight-bearing bone, as previously described[10]. Horses were randomly assigned to left or right TC and forelimb P1.

2.3 Immunostaining of bone CatK

Cathepsin K was immunostained in representative sections of formalin-fixed decalcified TC and P1 bone specimens using a standard Biotin/streptavidin horseradish peroxidase method[25]. Paraffin sections were de-waxed through Xylene (Sigma-Aldrich, St. Louis, MO) and descending gradient of ethanol treatments. To reduce nonspecific binding, the tissue samples were treated with the avidin/biotin blocking kit per manufacturer's instructions (SP-2001, Vector Laboratories, Burlingame, CA), followed by three 5 minute washes with Phosphate buffered Saline (PBS). Bone CatK was then immunostained using a pre-validated Rabbit polyclonal CatK antibody (1:50) as a primary antibody (Biorbyt Ltd, Cambridgeshire, UK) with which samples were incubated at 4°C overnight followed by incubation for 30 minutes with biotinylated Goat anti-Rabbit immunoglobulins (Vector Laboratories, UK) as a secondary antibody. Bone samples were developed with a peroxidase substrate solution (NovaRED, Vector Laboratories, Burlingame, CA) for 10 minutes to stain CatK-positive osteoclasts. Slides were washed quickly in PBS to terminate the reaction, taped dry, counterstained with hematoxylin, taped dry, cover-slipped, and allowed to dry in the dark for 2 days. Three regions of interest (ROIs) within the trabecular bone of TC and P1 were analyzed under 200x magnification for determination of total number of osteoclasts, total number of bone lining osteoblasts, CatK-positive osteoclasts, CatK-positive bone lining (endosteal) osteoblasts and bone surface (BS) using Bioquant OSTEO software (Bioquant OSTEO 7.20.10; Bioquant Image Analysis Co.). The staining intensity of CatK-positive osteoclasts and osteoblasts was scored by a blinded evaluator (HH) as following: 0 (no staining), 1 (mild staining), 2 (moderate staining), 3 (marked staining). The average

percentage of CatK-positive osteoclasts was calculated as (CatK-positive OC/total OC). In addition the average number of CatK-positive OC were quantified per bone surface (N.OC/mmBS).

2.4 Bone marrow aspiration and processing for cell differentiation assays

Sternal bone marrow was isolated from seven horses and processed according to the methods previously described[9]. The processed bone marrow concentrates from each horse was cultured in monolayer under four experimental conditions, in triplicate, of 0, 1, 10, or 100 μM of a CatK inhibitor (VEL-0230) (Freestride Therapeutics Inc., MI, USA) in culture media, to select both the adherent cells (bone marrow derived-mesenchymal stromal cells (BMD-MSCs) which were driven down the chondrogenic and osteogenic pathways) or the non-adherent fraction which was driven down the osteoclastogenic pathway.

2.4.1 Osteoclastogenic differentiation and staining assay

An aliquot of fresh concentrated bone marrow was cultured for six hours in 10% FBS supplemented DMEM, at approximately 1×10^7 cells/cm^2 in a 75 cm^2 culture flask, 37°C, 5% CO_2. The non-adherent cells were driven to differentiate into equine osteoclast-like cells (OCLs); separated by centrifugation at 500 g, 4°C for 10 minutes and re-suspended in α-MEM, pH 7.2, supplemented with 10 % (v/v) FBS, 25ngml^{-1} rhM-CSF (R&D Systems), 10ngml^{-1} rhRANKL (R&D Systems), 10^{-8} M 1,25 dihydroxyvitamin D3 (vitamin D3, Affiniti Research Products, UK). Cells were plated at a density of 2.5X10^6 cells cm^2 in collagen-coated six well plates. Half the medium was replaced twice weekly. After 7 days, non-adherent cells were removed by trypsinization for 2 minutes. After 15 minutes of further trypsinization the remaining cells, which were enriched for OCLs, were collected by gentle scraping using a cell scraper and cytospins on poly-Llysine coated slides (Sigma, St Louis, MO) were performed. The cytospin preparations of OCLs were processed for TRAP staining using a commercial acid phosphatase leucocyte kit (Sigma, St Louis, MO) according to the manufacturer's protocol. The number of TRAP-positive multinucleated cells (≥ 3 nuclei) in five representative fields under 200X magnification was counted and averaged to determine the representative number of OCLs for each experimental condition.

2.4.2 Chondrogenic differentiation and staining assay

Bone marrow-derived MSCs, selected by adherence in monolayer culture of processed fresh bone marrow concentrates for up to 3 days, were isolated and differentiated to chondrocytes using Lonza® Poietics TM human mesenchymal stem cell media and modified protocol. Fifteen ml centrifuge tubes were used for chondrogenic induction, with 1×10^6 MSCs/tube to form a pellet. After induction for 21 days, pellets were removed and fixed by incubation in formalin for 24 hours. Formalin-fixed chondrocyte pellets were sectioned and stained for glycosaminoglycan with toluidine blue stain (Fisher scientific, USA) for 30 seconds and then washed briefly in tap water. The degree of cartilaginous extracellular matrix staining (purple color) was scored by a blinded evaluator (HH) in three microscopic fields under 200X magnification as: 0 (no staining), 1 (mild staining; < 30% of the microscopic field), 2 (moderate staining; 30-60%), 3 (marked staining; > 60%).

2.4.3 Osteogenic differentiation and staining assay

A fraction of the BMD-MSCs were differentiated to osteoblasts using Lonza® Poietics TM human mesenchymal stem cell media and modified protocol. A 6-well plate was used for osteogenic induction with 1×10^6 MSCs/well. Basal medium was used for the first 24 hours to allow adherence. Induction medium was changed every

3 days thereafter. The cells were analyzed after 28 days for deposition of calcium phosphate and calcium, in accordance with a von Kossa and alizarin red S staining protocols, respectively. In brief, the wells were washed twice with PBS solution and then fixed in phosphate-buffered 10% formalin for 10 minutes. The monolayers were then processed for von Kossa and alizarin red S staining. For von Kossa staining, cells were serially dehydrated in solutions of ethanol (70%, 95%, and 100%; 2 times for each concentration) and then allowed to air dry. Cells were then serially rehydrated in solutions of ethanol (100%, 95%, and 80%; 2 times for each concentration). Finally, cells were rehydrated in water twice. Silver nitrate solution (2%) was added, and the cells were exposed to sunlight for 20 to 40 minutes. The cells were then rinsed 2 times with water, and 5% sodium thiosulfate was added; cells were allowed to equilibrate for 3 minutes. Cells then were rinsed with water, and acid fuchsin counterstain (5 mL of 1% acid fuchsin with 95 mL of picric acid and 0.25 mL of 12N HCl) was added. After incubation for 5 minutes, the cells were washed with water (2 times), 95% ethanol, and 100% ethanol before image analysis by use of a viewing microscope where mineralized nodules were stained dark brown or black. For Alizarin red S staining, 2% alizarin red S (Sigma) was prepared in distilled water and the pH was adjusted to 4.1–4.3 using 0.5% ammonium hydroxide. Formalin-fixed osteogenic monolayers were washed, and stained with alizarin red S for 10–15 minutes. After removal of unincorporated excess dye with distilled water, the mineralized nodules were labeled as red spots. The degree of mineralized nodules staining with each stain was scored by a blinded evaluator (HH) in three microscopic fields under 20X magnification as following: 0 (no staining), 1 (mild staining; < 30% of the microscopic field), 2 (moderate staining; 30-60%), 3 (marked staining; > 60%).

2.5 Gene expression analyses

Total RNA was isolated using Guanidinium thiocyanate-phenol-chloroform extraction method (TRIzol® and Chlorophorm;

Invitrogen). Complimentary (c) DNA was generated from 1 μg total RNA using High Capacity cDNA Reverse Transcription Kits (Applied Biosystems, Foster City, CA, USA) according to the manufacturer's instructions using MJ Research PTC-150 Thermal Cycler (MJ Research, USA). Relative gene expression analysis was performed using equine-specific custom primers (Primer3 software; Steve Rozen, Helen J. Skaletsky, 1998). Quantification of gene expression relevant to the osteoclastogenic, chondrogenic and osteogenic pathways using qRT-PCR was performed for all experimental conditions of the differentiation assays in a total volume of 50 μl using 96-well microwell plates, an ABI PRISM 7000 sequence detector and SYBR® Green PCR Master Mix (Applied BioSystems). Cycle threshold (Ct) values were obtained for all analyzed genes during log phase of the cycle and expression level was compared between different experimental conditions using 2-ΔΔ Ct. Non-induced cells were used as reference samples and Glyceraldehyde 3-phosphate dehydrogenase (GAPDH) was used as a reference housekeeping gene. Table (1) lists the corresponding forward and reverse nucleotides sequences for the primers used in the qRT-PCR.

2.6 Statistical analysis

The data was graphed as mean with standard deviation (SD), with the exception of the chondrogenic and osteogenic staining score data, which was graphed as median and interquartile range. All data were statistically analyzed using SPSS v.18.0 (IBM Corp., Armonk, NY, USA). Normality within the different variables was investigated using Shapiro-Wilk test. The comparison between the TC and P1 data was performed using paired sample student t test. Comparisons between different CatK inhibitor concentrations were performed using Friedman test for the chondrogenic and osteogenic staining scored data, and the one-way analysis of variance with repeated measures for all other data, followed by Duncan's Multiple Range Test. Significance was determined when $P < 0.05$.

Table 1: The forward and reverse nucleotides sequences for primers used in the q RT-PCR.

	Gene	Primer sequences
Osteoclastogenic differentiation-related genes	CatK	Fwd: 5′CAGAGATTGCCATTCCGTTT3′ Rev: 5′ATAGAATCAGCCCCAGGACA3′
	RANKL	Fwd: 5′CGACATCCCATCAGGTTCCC3′ Rev: 5′ CCCGACCAGTATTTGGTGCT3′
	TRAP	Fwd: 5′CTGGTCTTGAACAGGGACTTG3′ Rev: 5′AGAACGGCATAGGCTTTGTG3′
Chondrogenic differentiation-related genes	Aggrecan	Fwd: 5′TGCACAGACCCCGCCAGCTA3′ Rev: 5′GTCTCTAAACTCAGTCCACG3′
	Collagen 2A	Fwd: 5′ GCTTCCACTTCAGCTATGGA3′ Rev: 5′ TGTTTCGTGCAGCCATCCTT3′
	SOX9	Fwd: 5′CGCCGAAGCTCAGCAAGA3′ Rev: 5′CGCTTCTCGCTCTCGTTCA3′
Osteogenic differentiation-related genes	Alkaline phosphatase	Fwd: 5′TGGGGCTAAGCTCTGGAGTC3′ Rev: 5′ACTGATGTTCCAATCCTGCTCG3′
	Osteopontin	Fwd: 5′CGCAGATCTGAAGACCAGTA3′ Rev: 5′GGAATGCTCACTGGTCTCAT3′
	RUNX2	Fwd: 5′CTCCAACCCACGAATGCACTA3′ Rev: 5′CGGACATACCGAGGGACATG3′
Internal control gene	GAPDH	Fwd: 5′CAACGAATTTGGCTACAGCA3′ Rev: 5′CTGTGAGGAGGGGAGATTCA3′

3. Results

3.1 CatK protein distribution in equine decalcified bone sections

All morphologically characterized osteoclasts stained positive for CatK in both TC and P1 trabecular bone and there was no difference in CatK staining intensity between the two bone types (data not shown). Figure 1A shows a microscopic image of Cathepsin K-positive, multinucleated osteoclasts within the resorption pits. There was a significant increase in the number of CatK-positive osteoclasts per bone surface in the P1 compared to the TC trabecular bone data (Figure 1B). A moderate number of active bone lining osteoblasts stained CatK-positive. The percent of CatK-positive osteoblasts did not differ between trabecular bone of TC and P1, and were 65.4±7.4% and 62.6±6.2% of total bone lining osteoblasts, respectively. Figure 1C shows a microscopic image of CatK-positive osteoblasts. The staining intensity of CatK-positive osteoblasts did not differ between both bone types (data not shown).

3.2 Effect of CatK inhibition on osteoclastogenic potential of equine progenitor cells

The osteoclastogenic-induced cells of all four experimental conditions showed had varying numbers of TRAP-positive multinucleated OCLs (Figure 2A). There was significant increase in the number of TRAP-positive multinucleated OCLs due to CatK inhibition at VEL-0230 concentration of 100 μM compared to the other 3 experimental conditions (Figure 2B). Gene expression

analysis revealed increases in relative CatK and RANKL gene expression at 100 μM concentration, and in relative TRAP gene expression at 10 and 100 μM concentration compared to the 0 concentration of VEL-0230 in culture media (Figure 2C).

3.3 Effect of CatK inhibition on chondrogenic potential of equine BMD-MSCs

The toluidine blue-stained sections of chondrogenic pellets showed production of glycosaminoglycan from chondrocytes (Figure 3A). There was a significant increase in toluidine blue staining score due to CatK inhibition at VEL-0230 concentration of 100 μM (P<0.05), compared to the other concentrations (Figure 3B). There were significant increases in relative Aggrecan, Collagen 2A and SOX9 gene expressions (P<0.05), which were VEL-0230- concentration dependent (Figure 3C).

3.4 Effect of CatK inhibition on osteogenic potential of equine BMD-MSCs

The induced BMD-MSCs formed osteoblasts were stained positive for von Kossa (Figure 4A) and Alizarin Red-S (Figure 4B). There was a significant increase in both von Kossa and Alizarin Red-S staining scores due to CatK inhibition at a VEL-0230 concentration of 10 and 100 μM (P<0.05), compared to the other experimental conditions (Figure 4C). There were significant increases in relative alkaline phosphatase, osteopontin, and RUNX2 gene expressions (P<0.05), which were VEL-0230- concentration dependent (Figure 4D).

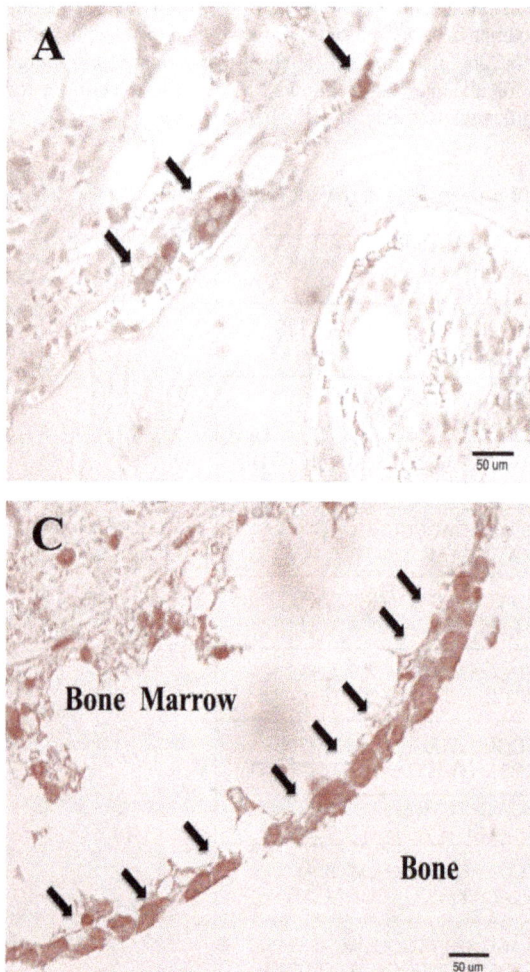

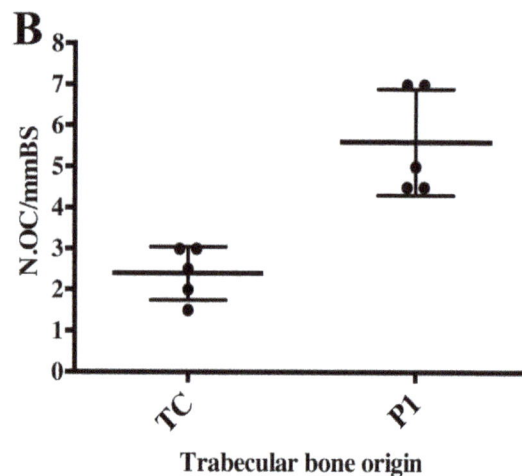

Figure 1 Cathepsin K (CatK) protein distribution in equine decalcified bone sections. There were no differences between tuber coxae (TC) and first phalanx (P1) trabecular bone percent and staining intensity of CatK-positive osteoclasts (OC) and osteoblasts. **A.** A microscopic image of Cathepsin K-positive, multinucleated osteoclasts (black arrows) within the resorption pits in one region of interest. **B.** Mean ± standard deviation of CatK-positive OC per bone surface, showing significant increase in number of CatK-positive OC in trabecular bone of P1 compared to TC (P<0.05). **C.** A microscopic image of CatK-positive osteoblasts (black arrows) in one region of interest.

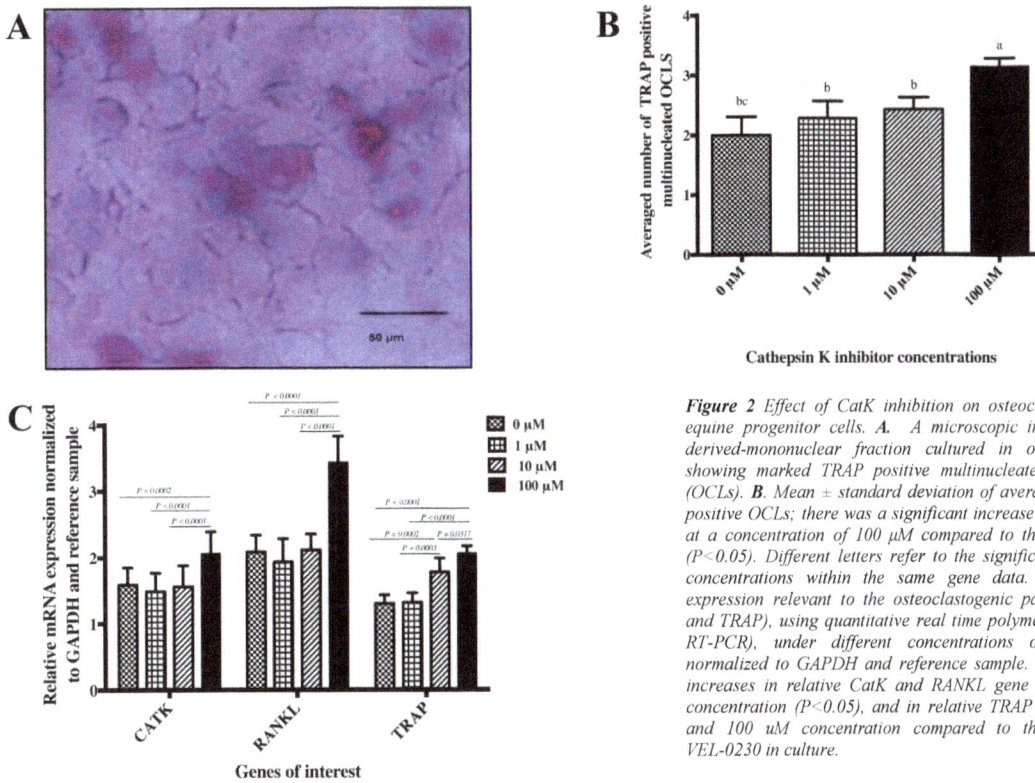

Figure 2 *Effect of CatK inhibition on osteoclastogenic potential of equine progenitor cells.* **A.** *A microscopic image of bone marrow derived-mononuclear fraction cultured in osteoclastogenic media showing marked TRAP positive multinucleated osteoclast-like cells (OCLs).* **B.** *Mean ± standard deviation of averaged number of TRAP-positive OCLs; there was a significant increase due to CatK inhibition at a concentration of 100 μM compared to the other concentrations (P<0.05). Different letters refer to the significance between different concentrations within the same gene data.* **C.** *Analysis of gene expression relevant to the osteoclastogenic pathway (CatK, RANKL and TRAP), using quantitative real time polymerase chain reaction (q RT-PCR), under different concentrations of a CatK inhibitor, normalized to GAPDH and reference sample. There were significant increases in relative CatK and RANKL gene expression at 100 uM concentration (P<0.05), and in relative TRAP gene expression at 10 and 100 uM concentration compared to the 0 concentration of VEL-0230 in culture.*

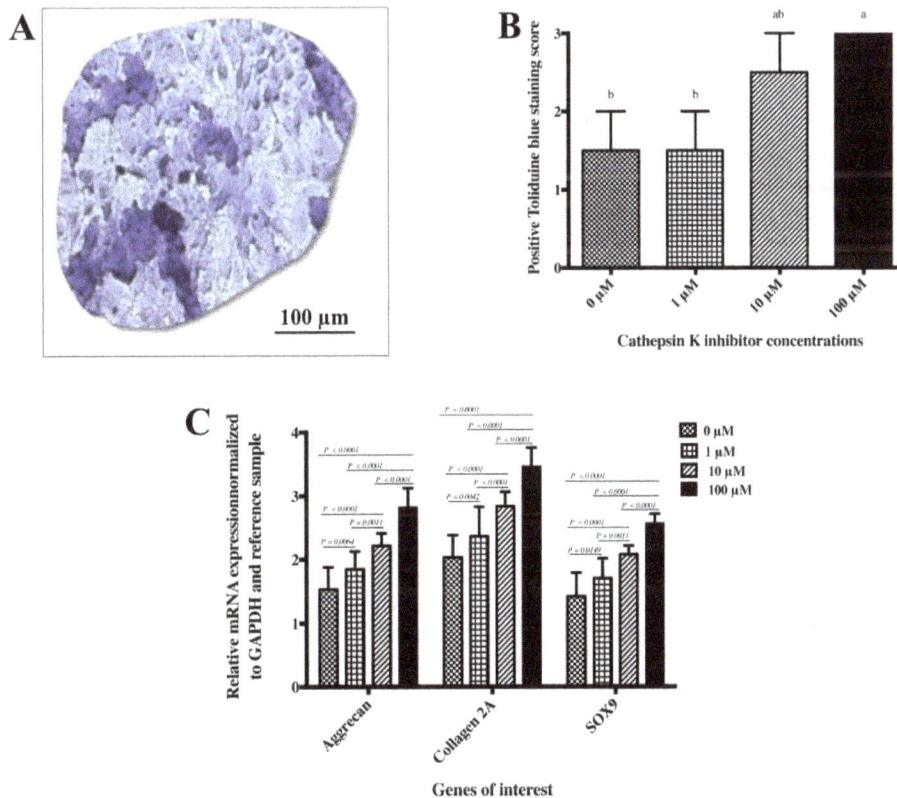

Figure 3 *Effect of CatK inhibition on chondrogenic potential of equine bone marrow-derived mesenchymal stromal cells (BMD-MSCs). A. A microscopic image of toluidine blue staining of a chondrogenic pellet. B. Median with interquartile range of toluidine blue staining score of chondrogenic pellets; there was a significant increase due to CatK inhibition at a concentration of 100 μM compared to the other concentrations (P<0.05). Different letters refer to the significance between different concentrations within the same gene data. C. Analysis of gene expression relevant to the chondrogenic pathway, using qRT-PCR, under different concentrations of a CatK inhibitor, normalized to GAPDH and reference sample. There were significant increases in relative Aggrecan, Collagen 2A and SOX9 gene expressions, which were VEL-0230- concentration dependent (P<0.05).*

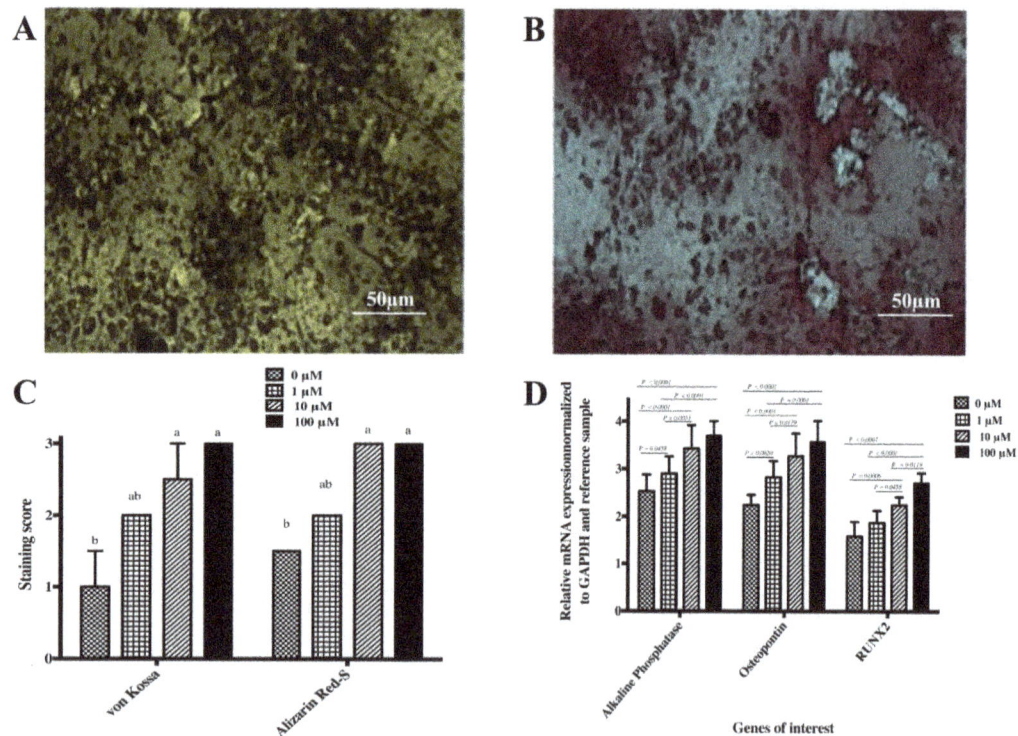

Figure 4 *Effect of CatK inhibition on osteogenic potential of equine BMD-MSCs. Cells were induced to form osteoblast by culturing in osteogenic induction medium for 28 days, followed by staining with von Kossa (A) and Alizarin Red-S (B). C. Median with interquartile range of von Kossa and Alizarin Red-S staining score of induced BMD-MSCs; there was a significant increase due to CatK inhibition at a VEL-0230 concentration of 10 and 100 μM compared to the other concentrations (P<0.05). Different letters refer to the significance between different concentrations within the same gene data. D. Analysis of gene expression relevant to the osteogenic pathway, using qRT-PCR, under different concentrations of a CatK inhibitor, normalized to GAPDH and reference sample. There were significant increases in relative alkaline phosphatase, osteopontin, and RUNX2 gene expressions, which were VEL-0230- concentration dependent (P<0.05).*

4. Discussion

For the first time, we characterized the spatial expression pattern of CatK protein in representative decalcified sections of equine weight-bearing and non-weight-bearing bone. Cathepsin k was abundantly expressed in bone cells; osteoclasts and osteoblasts. Furthermore, we propose a novel regulatory function for CatK in bone marrow stem and progenitor cell differentiation. Besides retaining their differentiation capacities, *ex vivo* selected equine bone marrow stem and progenitor cells had significantly greater osteoclastogenic, chondrogenic and osteogenic differentiation potential under the effect VEL-0230, implying an inhibitory role for CatK. As hypothesized, CatK inhibition using VEL-0230 in concentrations comparable to what suppressed pro-inflammatory cytokines secretion by stimulated equine bone marrow cells in our previous study[9], has significantly altered the differentiation potential of these cells along the three main cell lineage of the skeletal system *in vitro*. Owing to the close relation and tight integration between the immune and skeletal systems, multiple osteoimmunoregulatory molecules have been identified and reviewed[26]. For instance, macrophage colony-stimulating factor (M-CSF), receptor activator of nuclear factor-κB (NF-κB), RANKL, and tumor necrosis factor (TNF)-family cytokine are all examples for such molecules, which are expressed/secreted by immune cells and also regulate osteoclastogenesis. It is possible that CatK could similarly exert such regulatory roles in both immune response and skeletal system cell differentiation *in vivo*. Although limited evidence regarding CatK expression in immune cells such as macrophage and dendritic cells have been established so far[5, 27], possible uptake by those and other immune and differentiating progenitor cells may occur through mechanisms of endocytic recycling which may explain such osteoimmunoregulatory of CatK[28].

All osteoclasts and a moderate number of bone lining osteoblasts stained positive for CatK indicating abundance in bone and potential for influence on bone turnover in horses. While there were no differences in CatK staining intensity and percent CatK-positive cells of total cells between tuber coxae non-weight-bearing bone and first phalanx weight-bearing bone, there was a significantly greater number of osteoclasts per weight-bearing bone surface compared to the non weight-bearing bone. This is presumably due to the fact that weight bearing is an important factor influencing bone remodelling including the osteoclastic bone resorption phase in which CatK would play an important role[29]. Cathepsin K is the main collagenolytic proteinase secreted by osteoclasts in the bone-resorbing state[4]. Although it has long been thought that osteoclasts are the only source of CatK, CatK expression was detected in other cell types in health and disease conditions[11-14, 16, 30, 31]. In this study, a relatively great percent of bone lining osteoblasts of healthy horses showed marked expression of CatK similar to what have been reported in human bone[15] and did explain in part the bone resorption activity of osteoblast-like cells that have been revealed in a previous report[32]. There is a continuous need for optimization of current and future anti-resorptive medications to minimize potential adverse effect on bone formation and promote dual bone antiresorptive anabolic effect[33]. Hence, the previous findings of our study highlighted the need for more research regarding the potential effect of different CatK inhibitors on bone formation and osteoblast function.

The results of the current study revealed increased osteoclastogenic, chondrogenic and osteogenic differentiation potential of equine bone marrow derived stem and progenitor cells in contact with CatK inhibitor. The increase in the osteoclastogenic differentiation potential was only noted at the greatest concentration of VEL-0230 in culture media. Previous data has reported elevated levels of osteoclastogenesis in CatK-deficient mice possibly as a positive feedback of impaired bone resorption[34]. It is possible that a positive feedback loop could initiate osteoclastogenesis to compensate for the loss of CatK activity and the pause in bone resorption, the later which was not investigated in our study. While these data may suggest that CatK inhibition, as an antiresorptive therapeutic approach, may be overridden by the up-regulation of osteoclastogenesis, the clinical relevance of such outcome might be influenced by effects on the primary osteoclast progenitor cell population *in vivo* and also the therapeutic drug dose. In the current study, VEL-0230 was used *in vitro* in concentrations greater than the maximum plasma concentration achieved *in vivo* after drug administration in our previous studies. VEL-0230 was used in a mass concentration of 0.3 µg/ml of culture media to achieve the lowest molar concentration of 1µM. However, the maximum plasma concentration of VEL-0230 did not exceed 0.1µg/ml, achieved using an oral dose regimen of 4mg/kg of body weight q7 days in healthy exercising horses, and by which resulted in a marked decline in bone resorption without altering the number of osteoclasts as confirmed by TRAP staining of bone biopsies and subsequent analysis[8, 10].

Cathepsin K inhibition *in vitro* significantly up-regulated the differentiation potential of BMD-MSCs towards the chondrogenic and osteogenic pathways in a VEL-0230-concentration dependent manner, implying a causal relationship. These data may provide relevance into the clinical efficacy of CatK inhibition on bone and cartilage and suggest potential anabolic effects of this particular antiresorptive approach on bone and cartilage regeneration. It has been concluded that osteoclast specific CatK deletion stimulates S1P-dependent bone formation[35]. The coupling between bone resorption and formation has been established and could account, in part, for the lack of, or decrease in, osteoblastic activity due to other anti-resorptive administration[36]. However, our previous research using repeated VEL-0230 dosing in horses did reveal a significant increase in bone formation biomarkers [10] and agreed with other research utilizing different CatK inhibitors, which reported maintained or increased bone formation due to therapeutic inhibition of CatK[37-40].

Our current study provided important findings and additional data for the therapeutic inhibition of CatK, which may be relevant to the clinical use of VEL-0230 in horses. Bisphosphonates, a major antiresorptive class of drugs, have gained popularity in veterinary medicine with wide range of therapeutic applications in equine musculoskeletal disorders that are associate with increased bone resorption/inflammation[41]. However, multiple reports have elucidated the off-target effect of bisphosphonates administration and *in vitro* cell culture treatment on osteoclastogenesis as well as motility, viability and osteogenic differentiation of osteoblast progenitors, which in turn resulted in over suppression of bone turnover and formation, leading to osteonecrosis[42-45].

Conclusion

We concluded that the use of CatK inhibition over other current systemic, local, or regional treatments to moderate bone resorption and inflammation in equine osseous disorders would not be anticipated to interfere with the stem and progenitor cells regenerative and differentiation capacities and may offer advantages that would require further study.

Referemces

1. Mukherjee K, Chattopadhyay N. Pharmacological inhibition of cathepsin K: A promising novel approach for postmenopausal osteoporosis therapy. Biochem. Pharmacol.2016;117:10-9.

2. Russell RGG, Tsoumpra MK, Lawson MA, Chantry AD, Ebetino FH, Pazianas M. Antiresorptives. The Duration and Safety of Osteoporosis Treatment: Springer; 2016; 17-36.

3. McDougall J, Schuelert N, Bowyer J. Cathepsin K inhibition reduces CTXII levels and joint pain in the guinea pig model of spontaneous osteoarthritis. Osteoarthr. Cartil.2010;18(10):1355-7.

4. Svelander L, Erlandsson-Harris H, Astner L, Grabowska U, Klareskog L, Lindstrom E, Hewitt E. Inhibition of cathepsin K reduces bone erosion, cartilage degradation and inflammation evoked by collagen-induced arthritis in mice. Eur. J. Pharmacol.2009;613(1):155-62.

5. Asagiri M, Hirai T, Kunigami T, Kamano S, Gober H-J, Okamoto K, Nishikawa K, Latz E, Golenbock DT, Aoki K. Cathepsin K-dependent toll-like receptor 9 signaling revealed in experimental arthritis. Science2008;319(5863):624-7.

6. Hao L, Chen J, Zhu Z, Reddy MS, Mountz JD, Chen W, Li Y-P. Odanacatib, a cathepsin K-Specific inhibitor, inhibits inflammation and bone loss caused by periodontal diseases. J. Periodontol.2015;86(8):972-83.

7. Hirai T, Kanda T, Sato K, Takaishi M, Nakajima K, Yamamoto M, Kamijima R, DiGiovanni J, Sano S. Cathepsin K is involved in development of psoriasis-like skin lesions through TLR-dependent Th17 activation. J. Immun. 2013;190(9):4805-11.

8. Hussein H, Ishihara A, Menendez M, Bertone A. Pharmacokinetics and bone resorption evaluation of a novel Cathepsin K inhibitor (VEL-0230) in healthy adult horses. J. Vet. Pharmacol. Ther.2014;37(6):556-64.

9. Hussein H, Boyaka P, Dulin J, Bertone A. Cathepsin K inhibition renders equine bone marrow nucleated cells hypo-responsive to LPS and unmethylated CpG stimulation in vitro. Comp. Immunol. Microbiol. Infect. Dis.2016;45:40-7.

10. Hussein H, Dulin J, Smanik L, Drost W, Russell D, Wellman M, Bertone A. Repeated oral administration of a cathepsin K inhibitor significantly suppresses bone resorption in exercising horses with evidence of increased bone formation and maintained bone turnover. J Vet Pharmacol Ther. 2017;40(4):327-334.

11. Drake FH, Dodds RA, James IE, Connor JR, Debouck C, Richardson S, Lee-Rykaczewski E, Coleman L, Rieman D, Barthlow R. Cathepsin K, but not cathepsins B, L, or S, is abundantly expressed in human osteoclasts. J. Biol. Chem.1996;271(21):12511-6.

12. Hummel KM, Petrow P, Franz J, Müller-Ladner U, Aicher W, Gay R, Brömme D, Gay S. Cysteine proteinase cathepsin K mRNA is expressed in synovium of patients with rheumatoid arthritis and is detected at sites of synovial bone destruction. J rheumat. 1998;25(10):1887-94.

13. Muir P, Schamberger GM, Manley PA, Hao Z. Localization of Cathepsin K and Tartrate - Resistant Acid Phosphatase in Synovium and Cranial Cruciate Ligament in Dogs with Cruciate Disease. Vet. Surg.2005;34(3):239-46.

14. Uusitalo H, Hiltunen A, Söderström M, Aro H, Vuorio E. Expression of cathepsins B, H, K, L, and S and matrix metalloproteinases 9 and 13 during chondrocyte hypertrophy and endochondral ossification in mouse fracture callus. Calcif. Tissue Int.2000;67(5):382-90.

15. Mandelin J, Hukkanen M, Li T-F, Korhonen M, Liljeström M, Sillat T, Hanemaaijer R, Salo J, Santavirta S, Konttinen YT. Human osteoblasts produce cathepsin K. Bone 2006;38(6):769-77.

16. Vinardell T, Dejica V, Poole A, Mort J, Richard H, Laverty S. Evidence to suggest that cathepsin K degrades articular cartilage in naturally occurring equine osteoarthritis. Osteoarthritis Cartilage 2009;17(3):375-83.

17. Gray A, Davies M, Jeffcott L. Localisation and activity of cathepsins K and B in equine osteoclasts. Res. Vet. Sci.2002;72(2):95-103.

18. Fortier LA, Potter HG, Rickey EJ, Schnabel LV, Foo LF, Chong LR, Stokol T, Cheetham J, Nixon AJ. Concentrated bone marrow aspirate improves full-thickness cartilage repair compared with microfracture in the equine model. J Bone & Joint Surg. 2010;92(10):1927-37.

19. Godwin E, Young N, Dudhia J, Beamish I, Smith R. Implantation of bone marrow-derived mesenchymal stem cells demonstrates improved outcome in horses with overstrain injury of the superficial digital flexor tendon. Equine Vet. J.2012;44(1):25-32.

20. Herthel DJ, editor. Enhanced suspensory ligament healing in horses by stem cells and other bone marrow components. AA proceedings; 2001.

21. Tidball JG, Villalta SA. Regulatory interactions between mu and the immune system during muscle regeneration. Amer Physi. Reg., Integ. and Comp. Phys.2010;298(5):R1173-R87.

22. Liu Y, Wang L, Kikuiri T, Akiyama K, Chen C, Xu X, Yang Chen W, Wang S, Shi S. Mesenchymal stem cell-based tis regeneration is governed by recipient T lymphocytes via IF [gamma] and TNF-[alpha]. Nat. Med.2011;17(12):1594-601.

23. Mourkioti F, Rosenthal N. IGF-1, inflammation and stem ce interactions during muscle regeneration. Tre Immunol.2005;26(10):535-42.

24. Sotiropoulou PA, Perez SA, Gritzapis AD, Baxevanis C Papamichail M. Interactions between human mesenchymal s cells and natural killer cells. Stem Cells2006;24(1):74-85.

25. Bratthauer GL. The Avidin–Biotin Complex (ABC) Method Other Avidin–Biotin Binding Methods. Immunocytochem methods and protocols2010:257-70.

26. Takayanagi H. Osteoimmunology: shared mechanisms crosstalk between the immune and bone systems. Nat. Rev. Imm 2007;7(4):292-304.

27. Bühling F, Reisenauer A, Gerber A, Krüger S, Weber E, Bröm D, Roessner A, Ansorge S, Welte T, Röcken C. Cathepsin K marker of macrophage differentiation? J path. 2001;195(3):375-8

28. Grant BD, Donaldson JG. Pathways and mechanisms of endoc recycling. Nature reviews Molecular cell biology 2009;10(9):5 608.

29. Vico L, Collet P, Guignandon A, Lafage-Proust M-H, Thomas Rehailia M, Alexandre C. Effects of long-term micrograv exposure on cancellous and cortical weight-bearing bones cosmonauts. The Lancet2000;355(9215):1607-11.

30. Sukhova GK, Shi G-P, Simon DI, Chapman HA, Libby Expression of the elastolytic cathepsins S and K in human athero and regulation of their production in smooth muscle cells. J. C Invest.1998;102(3):576.

31. Bühling F, Waldburg N, Gerber A, Häckel C, Krüger S, Reinh D, Brömme D, Weber E, Ansorge S, Welte T. Cathepsin expression in human lung. Cellular Peptidases in Imm Functions and Diseases 2: Springer; 2002. p. 281-6.

32. Mulari M, Qu Q, Härkönen P, Väänänen H. Osteoblast-like c complete osteoclastic bone resorption and form new minerali bone matrix in vitro. Calcif. Tissue Int.2004;75(3):253-61.

33. Karsdal MA, Qvist P, Christiansen C, Tanko LB. Optimis antiresorptive therapies in postmenopausal women. Dr 2006;66(15):1909-18.

34. Kiviranta R, Morko J, Alatalo SL, NicAmhlaoibh R, Ristel Laitala-Leinonen T, Vuorio E. Impaired bone resorption

cathepsin K-deficient mice is partially compensated for enhanced osteoclastogenesis and increased expression of ot proteases via an increased RANKL/OPG ratio. B 2005;36(1):159-72.

35. Lotinun S, Kiviranta R, Matsubara T, Alzate JA, Neff L, Lüth A, Koskivirta I, Kleuser B, Vacher J, Vuorio E. Osteoclast-specific cathepsin K deletion stimulates S1P-dependent bone formation. The J. clin.invest. 2013;123(2):666-81.

36. Hochberg MC, Greenspan S, Wasnich RD, Miller P, Thompson DE, Ross PD. Changes in bone density and turnover explain the reductions in incidence of nonvertebral fractures that occur during treatment with antiresorptive agents. J of Clinical Endocr. & Met. 2002;87(4):1586-92.

37. Xiang A, Kanematsu M, Kumar S, Yamashita D, Kaise T, Kikkawa H, Asano S, Kinoshita M. Changes in micro-CT 3D bone parameters reflect effects of a potent cathepsin K inhibitor (SB-553484) on bone resorption and cortical bone formation in ovariectomized mice. Bone 2007;40(5):1231-7.

38. Jerome C, Missbach M, Gamse R. Balicatib, a cathepsin K inhibitor, stimulates periosteal bone formation in monkeys. Osteoporos. Int.2011;22(12):3001-11.

39. Pennypacker BL, Chen CM, Zheng H, Shih MS, Samadfam R, Duong LT. Inhibition of Cathepsin K Increases Modeling-Based Bone Formation, and Improves Cortical Dimension and Strength in Adult Ovariectomized Monkeys. J. Bone Miner. Res. 2014;29(8):1847-58.

40. Schaller S, Henriksen K, Sveigaard C, Heegaard AM, Hélix N, Stahlhut M, Ovejero MC, Johansen JV, Solberg H, Andersen TL. The chloride channel inhibitor NS3736 prevents bone resorption in ovariectomized rats without changing bone formation. J. Bone Miner. Res.2004;19(7):1144-53.

41. Soto SA, Barbará AC. Bisphosphonates: pharmacology and clinical approach to their use in equine osteoarticular diseases. J. Equ. Vet. Sci. 2014;34(6):727-37.

42. Bartl R, Frisch B, von Tresckow E, Bartl C. Bisphosphonates in medical practice: actions-side effects-indications-strategies: Springer Science & Business Media; 2007.

43. Piccione M, Durgam S, Stewart M. Impact of Bisphosphonate on Osteoprogenitor Cell Differentiation. Enliven: J Stem Cells Regen Med2016;3(2):003.

44. Acil Y, Möller B, Niehoff P, Rachko K, Gassling V, Wiltfang J, Simon M. The cytotoxic effects of three different bisphosphonates in-vitro on human gingival fibroblasts, osteoblasts and osteogenic sarcoma cells. J. Cranio-Maxillofacial Surg.2012;40(8):e229-e35.

45. Hughes D, MacDonald B, Russell R, Gowen M. Inhibition of osteoclast-like cell formation by bisphosphonates in long-term cultures of human bone marrow. J. Clin. Invest.1989;83(6):1930.

Abbreviations

CatK:	Cathepsin K
OC:	Osteoclast
TLR:	Toll like receptors
TRAP:	Tartrate-resistant acid phosphatase
qRT-PCR:	quantitative real time polymerase chain reaction
RANKL:	Receptor activator of nuclear factor kappa-B ligand
RUNX2:	Runt-related transcription factor 2
TC:	Tuber coxae
P1:	Proximal phalanx
ROIs:	Regions of interest
BS:	Bone surface
BMD-MSCs:	Bone marrow derived-mesenchymal stromal cells
OCLs:	Osteoclast-like cells
Ct:	Cycle threshold
GAPDH:	Glyceraldehyde 3-phosphate dehydrogenase
SD:	Standard deviation
M-CSF:	Macrophage colony-stimulating factor
TNF:	Tumor necrosis factor

Potential Conflicts of Interests

None

Acknowledgements

The authors thank FreeStride Therapeutics, USA, for the generous supply of VEL-0230. This study was supported by the Trueman Endowment at the College of Veterinary Medicine and a PhD Scholarship for Dr. Hussein from the Egyptian Ministry of Higher Education.

* This work was presented as a poster at The 9th Annual Translational to Clinical (T2C) Regenerative Medicine Wound Care Conference, Columbus, OH, USA, May 2016.

Corresponding Author

Alicia Bertone, Address: Veterinary Medical Academic Building 1900 Coffey Rd., Room 325, Columbus, OH 43210 USA; Email: Bertone.1@osu.edu

3

New Trends in Heart Regeneration

Kochegarov A[1], Lemanski LF[1]

Abstract

In this review, we focus on new approaches that could lead to the regeneration of heart muscle and the restoration of cardiac muscle function derived from newly-formed cardiomyocytes. Various strategies for the production of cardiomyocytes from embryonic stem cells, induced pluripotent stem cells, adult bone marrow stem cells and cardiac spheres from human heart biopsies are described. Pathological conditions which lead to atherosclerosis and coronary artery disease often are followed by myocardial infarction causing myocardial cell death. After cell death, there is very little self-regeneration of the cardiac muscle tissue, which is replaced by non-contractile connective tissue, thus weakening the ability of the heart muscle to contract fully and leading to heart failure. A number of experimental research approaches to stimulate heart muscle regeneration with the hope of regaining normal or near normal heart function in the damaged heart muscle have been attempted. Some of these very interesting studies have used a variety of stem cell types in combination with potential cardiogenic differentiation factors in an attempt to promote differentiation of new cardiac muscle for possible future use in the clinical treatment of patients who have suffered heart muscle damage from acute myocardial infarctions or related cardiovascular diseases. Although progress has been made in recent years relative to promoting the differentiation of cardiac muscle tissue from non-muscle cells, much work remains to be done for this technology to be used routinely in translational clinical medicine to treat patients with damaged heart muscle tissue and return such individuals to pre-heart-attack activity levels.

Key Words: Cardiac muscle regeneration, Embryonic stem cells, MicroRNAs, Adult stem cells, Mesenchymal stem cells, Induced pluripotent stem cells

Introduction

Atherosclerosis is a pathological condition resulting in the narrowing of blood vessels due to an accumulation of atherosclerotic plaques between the smooth muscle and endothelial layer leading to acute myocardial infarction with major damage to the cardiac muscle and even death to the individual. These plaques consist of lipids, calcium deposits, cellular debris and so-called foam cells. Molecular and cellular mechanisms for the origin(s) of atherosclerosis are not well understood. LDL (Low-density lipoprotein) accumulation in blood vessels that can be associated with age-related diseases such as diabetes are thought to be a primary step in the origin of atherosclerosis.

Currently, many researchers favor an inflammatory hypothesis in which LDL accumulation and its oxidation triggers an inflammatory response recruiting monocytes to the area and converting these cells into macrophages[1,2]. Macrophages engulf oxidized LDL and become foam cells, containing large droplets of lipid (lipid-loaded macrophages) that resemble foam in appearance in the atherosclerotic plaques[3]. When these lipid loaded macrophages die, they release their contents into the spaces between the vascular endothelium and smooth muscle layer creating a lipid core[3]. The other cells deposit fibers along the internal endothelial lining of blood vessels. Blood platelets can attach to the atherosclerotic plaques creating a blood clot that blocks or severely reduces the blood supply to, for example, the heart muscle and without blood, the myocardium is deprived of

oxygen causing damage or death to the cardiac cells. Restoring blood flow to the heart after a myocardial infarction (MI) may cause even further damage of the muscle due to oxidative stress, known as reperfusion injury. Once the heart muscle has been damaged, very little repair or regeneration takes place to form functional new cardiac muscle.

Biomedical scientists and physicians have been working for more than 50 years to find ways to repair the heart muscle following a heart attack. Although a number of medications and procedures have been developed to provide significant improvements in heart function, none to date have provided a means to actually regenerate the damaged cardiac muscle and return the patients to pre-heart-attack activity levels. A major problem in heart regeneration after a myocardial infarction is that cardiomyocytes die and are replaced by non-contracting fibrous scar tissue rather than new cardiac muscle cells. This supports function of the damaged heart temporarily, but in the long term, it weakens the organ's ability to contract normally and increases the risk of a further heart attack. This is the major reason why myocardial infarctions are a leading killer around the world. Currently, the only option for a severely failing heart is organ transplantation and recently-developed heart-assist devices. Since the early 2000s, scientists have been trying to use pluripotent stem cells to grow new muscle in damaged hearts. Stem cells can produce multiple cell lineages in the body; the hope is that they will be able to generate new cardiomyocytes. However, earlier enthusiasm for using stem cell therapy to accomplish heart regeneration has declined because, to date, stem cells that show reliable cardiac lineage markers

Author Names in full: Andrei Kochegarov[1],Larry F Lemanski[1]

[1]Department of Biological and Environmental Sciences, Texas A&M University-Commerce, Commerce, Texas, USA

have not met with major success in clinical trials using stem cell therapy. In spite of the clinical difficulties, multiple approaches and strategies continue to be investigated to regenerate injured heart tissue. These basic science approaches include studies on small molecules, microRNA treatment and stem cell differentiation in laboratory settings (summarized with reference citations in Table 1).

1. Cardiomyocyte proliferation

A significant obstacle for self-regeneration of damaged heart tissue is the inability of adult cardiomyocytes to proliferate. In mammals, cardiomyocytes decrease their ability to proliferate during late embryonic development and almost completely lose this proliferation ability a few days after birth. The other obstacle for cardiomyocyte proliferation is the lack of fusion of cardiomyocytes in a functional (but not anatomical) syncytium. The use of tissue scaffolds and tissue engineering may be useful in a functional and formal structure[4-7]. Originally, therapy with stem cells involved the simple injection of derived cardiomyocytes into the site of injury. Although this approach has shown promise in some experiments, many researchers noted some drawbacks such as low cellular retention and low engraftment rate of injected cells. To overcome these problems alternate approaches were developed, such as construction of biomimetic scaffolds using synthetic and natural materials and decellularized tissue scaffolds in the site of injury. These scaffolds provide places for the attachment and mechanical support of differentiated cardiomyocytes. The permanent scaffolds should be designed to meet many requirements including integration with cells inside the heart, electrical conduction, diffusion of oxygen and nutrients, and should stimulate cardiac differentiation and not cause an immune reaction. Biodegradable scaffolds are presumed to degrade over time, but are replaced with cardiomyocytes and extracellular matrix. One of the most advanced and promising approaches is to inject, together with

cells, self-assembling peptide nanofibers, which rapidly self-assemble into a 3D nanofibril net on which the cells can grow[8].

In the mid-gestation prenatal developmental period, the labeling index of new DNA synthesis was found to be 33% in 12 day in utero embryos; however, at birth, DNA synthesis in neonatal mice was estimated to be 2%, and at 4-6 days postnatally, the DNA synthesis had increased to 10%[9]. This increase takes place without cytokinesis, causing binucleation, multinucleation and polyploidisation of cardiac myocytes, without increases in cell numbers. During normal mouse heart development, cardiomyocyte proliferation virtually stops by post-natal day 7, coinciding with a significant reduction of heart muscle differentiation. DNA synthesis in adult mouse heart, normal or injured, has been found to be extremely low at 0.0005% of the cells[10].

In the human heart, apparently related to levels of development and aging, cardiomyocyte turnover is higher at age 10 (2% per year), decreases by age 25 (1% per year) and further decreases at age 75 (0.45% per year)[11]. The source of new cardiomyocytes in humans is still not known. One hypothesis suggests that adult cardiomyocytes or a subpopulation of them, are able to proliferate at a very low rate. Recent animal studies conclude that cardiac stem cells contribute little to the proliferation of cardiomyocytes in adult mammals[12]. Alternatively, it has been proposed that cardiac progenitor cells or cardiac adult stem cells exist and proliferate in mature mammalian hearts[13,14]. This hypothesis is supported by localizing and isolating cardiac stem-cell-like progenitor cells in mammalian heart tissue[15]. However, the natural rate of cardiomyocyte proliferation is not adequate to replenish myocardial cell loss after myocardial infarction. There are published studies that suggest several potentially promising ways to stimulate heart regeneration as listed below in Table 1:

Table 1 Approaches to stimulate heart regeneration

Approaches to stimulate cardiomyocyte proliferation/differentiation	Results	References
Delivery of Follistatin-Like-Protein 1 (FSTL1) to the infarcted heart using a collagen patch	Activated cardiomyocyte proliferation in border zone resulting in regeneration of injured heart	Wei et al., 2015[16]
Multiple human micro RNA: miRNAs: miR-1825, miR-199a, miR-99a, miR-548c, miR-23b and others	Cardiomyocyte proliferation in vitro is promoted by adding these microRNAs	Pandey et al., 2015[18]
miRNA-204	Cardiomyocyte proliferation in vitro and in vivo is enhanced	Liang et al., 2015[19]
miR-410 and miR-495	Expression of miR-410 and miR-495 stimulates cardiomyocyte DNA synthesis and cell division of cardiomyocytes	Clark et al., 2015[21]
ESC-derived exosomes	Stimulates and activates repair mechanisms of heart tissue after myocardial infarction in vivo	Kishore, et al., 2016[23] Khan et al., 2015[24]
Induction of active ErbB2 (receptor of NRG1)	Promotes cardiac muscle cell division and dedifferentiation in vivo	D'Uva et al., 2015[28]
Neuregulin-1	Stimulates cardiac regeneration by cardiomyocyte protection (38%) and proliferation (62%) in vivo in both mouse and human	Polizzotti et al., 2015[29]
Acidic fibroblast growth factor (FGF1) and neuregulin-1 (NRG1)	Stimulates cardiac regeneration and cardiomyocyte proliferation in a rat myocardial infarction model	Formiga et al., 2014[30]
Use of RNAs in tissue cultured cells	Non-muscle stem cells express cardiac specific troponin-T and show cardiomyocyte morphologies in culture	Kochegarov et al., 2015[55,56]
Use of tissue scaffolds and tissue engineering strategies	Provide structural matrix scaffolds on which new cardiac cells can grow when stimulated by growth factors for cardiomyocytes	Boffito et al., 2014[4] Tallawi et al., 2015[5] Wang et al., 2013[6] Alrefai et al., 2015[7] Davis et al., 2005[8]

Follistatin-Like-Protein 1 (FSTL1) is an epicardium-secreted factor that appears to have a cardioprotective role by activation of vascular remodeling and proliferation of cardiomyocytes. FSTL1 is a glycoprotein from the follistatin family that often accumulates in heart muscle cells, vascular cells, and fibroblasts; its expression is activated after ischemic and infarction injuries. In previous research, it was shown that FSTL1 increases cardiomyocyte survival and angiogenesis in infarcted areas of the heart. Recent research by Wei et al.,[16] suggests that FSTL1 also stimulates cardiomyocyte proliferation[16]. In fact, in a series of experiments, FSTL1 protein was delivered using collagen patches loaded with FSTL1 as depicted in Figure 1. Application of patches loaded with the FSTL1 protein to the heart after myocardial infarction, significantly improved the survival of myocytes, attenuated fibrosis, increased the number of vessels in injured areas and stimulated cardiomyocyte proliferation in the border zone of the heart infarct. Proliferating cardiomyocytes were present mostly in the border zone, presumably because this zone has a continuous blood supply. In the definitive infarcted area, proliferating cardiomyocytes were much reduced[16]. Thus, epicardial delivery of FSTL1 through collagen patch delivery significantly improved heart regeneration by activating cardiomyocyte proliferation.

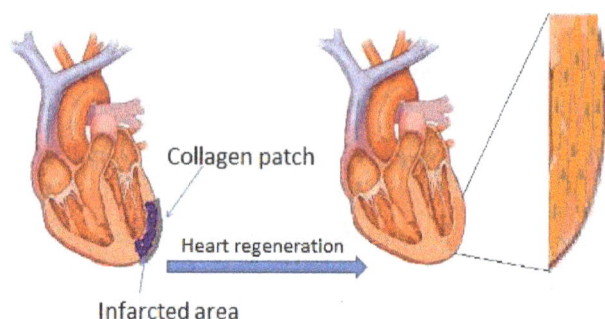

Figure 1. *Diagramatic representation of delivery of Follistatin-Like-Protein 1 (FSTL1) to the infarcted area of a heart using a collagen patch.*

Multiple microRNAs have been reported as being promising for promoting cardiac muscle regeneration by causing a stimulation of cardiomyocyte proliferation and differentiation. MicroRNAs play a significant role in the regulation of gene expression as well as in modifications at the post-transcriptional level. Experiments by Chen et al.,[17] show that transgenic overexpression of miR-17-92 in cardiomyocytes causes cardiomyocyte proliferation in adult hearts. Notably, combinations of miR-590, miR-199a, and the miR-17-92 induce mouse cardiomyocyte proliferation both in vitro and in vivo[17]. Moreover, overexpression of miR-17-92 in adult cardiomyocytes protects cardiac muscle tissue from injuries induced by infarction. To date, the most potent microRNAs that appear to induce cardiomyocyte proliferation in tissue culture experiments have been human miR-1825, miR-199a-3p, miR-99a-5p, miR-548c-3p and miR-23b-3p[18]. MiRNA-204 overexpression stimulates cardiomyocyte proliferation in neonatal and adult rat cardiomyocytes in vitro[18]. In these experiments, miRNA-204 seems to upregulate cyclins through inhibition of the JARID2 signaling system (Cyclin A, Cyclin B, Cyclin D2, Cyclin E, CDC2) and appears to be responsible for progression of the cell cycle and proliferation[19]. Another very promising approach was described recently for the delivery of neuregulin into infarcted heart tissue using biodegradable microparticles made of polylactic glycolic acid and polyethylene glycol[20]. Using this approach, microparticles loaded with neuregulin degrade up to 12 weeks, slowly releasing the active compound. This material also was shown to be resistant to phagocytosis by macrophages and other immune cells which is important for targeted delivery. Technically, these microparticles can be applied to infarcted hearts as a spray with biodegradable glue.

In other studies, overexpression of miR-410 and miR-495 results in robust neonatal cardiomyocyte proliferation[21]. The miRNAs together with other regulating cardiogenic factors appear to be synthesized by endothelial cells, cardiac stem cells, fibroblasts and other cells. Moreover, these factors are shuttled via extracellular vesicles (exosomes) into cardiomyocytes where they regulate cardiogenesis during development and regeneration[22]. ESC-derived exosomes provide novel delivery tools to shuttle factors from ES cells to stimulate and activate repair mechanisms after myocardial infarction[23]. In another recent study, mouse ESC-derived exosomes enhanced a cardiac proliferative response, vascular angiogenesis, cardiomyocyte survival, and reduced fibrotic scar formation after myocardial infarction. Studies of exosome active factors revealed a significant presence of miR290-295 and miR-294[24]. Small organic molecules also can be used to activate cardiomyocyte proliferation. In previous experiments, the administration of 2, 3, 5, 4'-tetrahydroxystilbene-2-O-β-d-glucoside (THSG) have shown protection of in vivo heart muscle tissue from ischemic injuries of rat cardiac stem cells (CSC) in culture and an increased expression of cardiac specific markers for stem cells in vitro[25].

Neuregulin-1 (NRG1) growth factor induces the growth and differentiation of many types of cells including epithelial, glial, neuronal, and skeletal muscle cells. NRG1 also was found to be an important factor in heart development, because mice with mutations in NRG1 or with loss of two receptors for this factor (ErbB2 and ErbB4), die from a lack of differentiation of normal heart muscle[26]. Neuregulin-1 (NRG1) may induce heart regeneration through the proliferation and survival of stem cells as summarized in Figure 2. Very recently, Yutzey et al., have suggested that Neuregulin-1 administration may promote cardiac regeneration[27]. Activation of a signaling mechanism by Neuregulin-1 through its receptor ErbB2 has been shown to induce proliferation of quiescent cardiomyocytes and trigger cardiomyocyte proliferation after myocardial infarction[28-30]. Based on other studies, the Hyppo/Yap pathway is believed to participate in regulating organ size during development, although the mechanism(s) controlling organ size in adults is not known[31]. Recently, approaches to inhibit the Hyppo pathway by microRNAs have been proposed as a stimulant of cardiac proliferation[32].

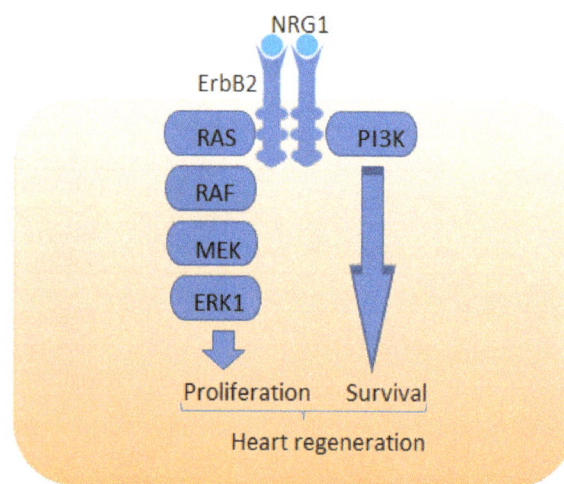

Figure 2. *Neuregulin-1 (NRG1) appears to induce heart regeneration through the activation of proliferation and survival of stem cells.*

2. Cell-Based Therapy for Heart Failure

2.1 Bone marrow

Bone marrow has been found to have various cell types, including three types of stem cells: 1. hematopoietic stem cells (HSC); 2. mesenchymal stem cells (MSC); and 3. endothelial progenitor cells (EPCs). The stem cells from bone marrow are often termed bone marrow mononuclear cells (BM-MNC). Recent studies suggest that unfractionated BM-MNCs consist of a mixed population of hematopoietic cells, including monocytes and lymphocytes, hematopoietic cells and mesenchymal cells. Studies in animal models of the ischemic myocardium indicate that mononuclear bone marrow stem cells implanted into the heart improve angiogenesis, left ventricular function and cardiac muscle perfusion[33]. Currently, autologous bone marrow stem cell transplants are considered safe to use as a treatment to improve post-myocardial infarction hearts in humans[34]. From 2002 to 2010, the first stem-cell-based clinical trials for AMI (acute myocardial infarction) with transplanted heterogeneous adult BM-MNC showed a significant decrease in infarction size and an overall improved myocardial oxygen uptake resulting in a statistically significant 15% reduction of inpatient mortality[35].

2.2 Mesenchymal stem cells (MSC)

Mesenchymal stem cells obtained from bone marrow are multipotent stem cells with fibroblast-like morphologies. Mesenchymal stem cells are separated from other bone-marrow cells based on their adhesive properties. Mesenchymal stem cells adhere to plastic tissue culture plates within 24 to 48 hours, while red blood cells and hematopoetic progenitor cells (HCS) from bone marrow do not; thus, all cells that attach to the tissue culture dishes during this time, have been reported by Tondreau et al.[36] to be pure MSC.

MSC readily differentiate into osteoblasts and chondrocytes as well as adipocytes, skeletal muscle myocytes/myotubes and pancreatic islet cells. The differentiation of MSC into cardiomyocytes also has been known for a long time and recent experiments confirm that these cells express cardiac specific markers for cardiomyocytes. Moreover, grafted MSC-derived cardiomyocyes have been observed at the site of transplantation[37,38]; proliferation of endogenous cardiomyocytes were noted after MSC treatment[39]. In vivo studies in other laboratories did not observe the engraftment of MSCs in murine infarcted hearts several weeks after acute MI[40], and survival of the engrafted MSC was only about 2%, with no evidence of cardiomyocyte differentiation in these cells[41]. Currently, most MSC described for in vivo studies report that the engrafted MSC die within two weeks of transplantation with little or no direct cardiac differentiation[41,42]. These observations have led to the idea that MSC transplantation into an infarcted heart may promote heart regeneration without incorporation of the MSC into the myocardium; rather paracrine factors (cytokines and growth factors) stimulate cardiomyocyte proliferation and neovascularization of the infarcted areas resulting in myocardial regeneration[43]. Cardiosphere-derived cells described in Section 2.3 may use a similar mechanism to MSC as summarized in Figure 3.

The first clinical trials of MSC were completed in 1995 when MSC were injected into patients' hearts to test the safety of the treatment. Since then, numerous experiments have been conducted which show a statistically significant improvement of 7% in myocardial regeneration and cardiac function in animal models after human MSC treatment[44]. Interestingly, it was shown that treatment with MSC can retard natural heart senescence and increase the life span in rodents by 22%[45,46]. Although initially MSC were derived from bone marrow, more recently it has been found that MSC reside in and can be isolated from multiple adult tissues in the body such as dental pulp,

umbilical cord blood, uterus, adipose tissue, peripheral blood, fallopian tubes, fetal liver, lung, etc. Thus, there are potentially numerous options for retrieving immune-compatible MSC from the body of a prospective patient for potential use in the treatment of heart failure/myocardial damage in that same patient.

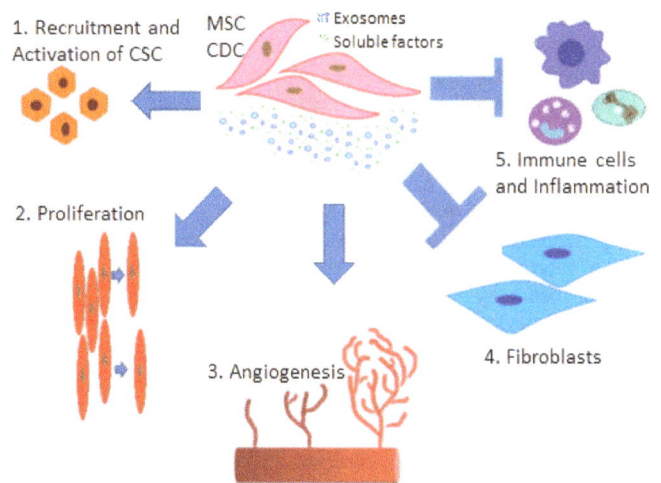

Figure 3. *A model for a possible paracrine mechanism of how MSC (mesenchymal stem cells) and CDC (cardiosphere-derived cells) promote heart regeneration via the secretion of exosomes (extracellular vesicles) and soluble factors by: 1. Recruitment and activation of cardiac stem cells (CSC), 2. Proliferation of cardiomyocytes in situ, 3. Angiogenesis and neovascularization, 4. Inhibition of fibrosis. 5. Inhibition of inflammation.*

2.3 Cardiosphere-Derived Cells (CDC)

Cardiosphere-derived cells (CDC) as described here are those cells isolated from myocardial biopsy specimens of patients undergoing heart surgery. The heart fragments from these biopsies are cultured on fibronectin-coated Petri plates. After a few days in culture, the biopsied heart cells form into a monolayer over which smaller, rounded cells migrate. These small rounded cells appear to be of cardiogenic lineages and can be retrieved by enzymatic treatment followed by replating on poly-d-lysine-coated culture dishes using cardiac growth medium. The cells that remain adherent to the poly-d-lysine–coated dishes after several days in culture are discarded, while the free floating "cardiospheres" are placed on fibronectin-coated culture dishes and grown into a monolayer[46,47]. Experiments performed by Marban's group demonstrated that cardiospheres and CDC express antigenic properties of stem cells, as well as cardiac contractile proteins and proteins related to cardiac electrophysiology[48]. Cardiac-derived cells injected into the myocardial infarct border zones appear to integrate into the heart wall and end up in the infarct zone. At three weeks post-injection, the healthy living myocardium in the infarct zone is significantly larger in the CDC-treated hearts[48]. To date, cell therapy with CDC has proven to be effective in repairing damaged human myocardial tissue. At this point, however, the source of the new heart muscle tissue per se and the mechanisms underlying its formation remain unknown. These new cardiomyocytes may have come from residual adult cardiac stem cells that were already present in the recipient heart muscle tissue and stimulated to form from the effects of paracrine factors resulting from the presence of the CDC (Figure 3). Scientists propose that CDC may localize to the area of the infarct and release factors which stimulate the heart to repair itself, ultimately reducing infarction size and fibrotic scar tissue and promoting growth of the heart muscle. After several weeks, the CDC clear from the heart without apparent side effects. Many investigators now think that these cells, as with bone marrow-derived cells, show minimal long-term engraftment or cardiac differentiation and instead work principally through paracrine signaling pathways[44].

2.4 Adipose-derived stem cells

Adipose-derived stem cells were found in adipose tissue and have recently attracted substantial attention as a source of stem cells with multiple potentials to differentiate into cartilage, vascular and muscle tissues including cardiomyocytes. These cells can be harvested easily from subcutaneous adipose tissue under local anesthesia by a procedure known as lipoaspiration. Adipose-derived stem cells are adult stem cells that morphologically resemble mesenchymal cells from bone marrow, which is why they are sometimes called adipose-derived mesenchymal cells. Different approaches for the differentiation of adipose-derived stem cells into cardiomyocytes have been reported, including treatment of permeabilized adipose-derived stem cells by a nuclear and cytoplasmic extract from rat cardiomyocytes[49]. Interestingly, these cells were able to differentiate spontaneously when grafted into the myocardium without any preliminary treatment[50]. Expression of multiple cardiomyocyte-specific markers also was reported including sarcomeric α-actinin, desmin and cardiac troponin I[49]. The other distinct characteristics of cardiomyocytes that were observed in differentiating adipose-derived stem cells are appearance of sarcomeric striations, multinucleation and formation of beating cells, that all strongly argue for functional differentiation into cardiac myocytes of the adipose-derived stem cells[49].

2.5 Embryonic Stem Cells and Induced Pluripotent Stem Cells

Initial attempts at the differentiation of human embryonic stem cells (hESC) were started as soon as the first hESC cell line was derived in 1998 at the University of Wisconsin. It is now known that hESC are derived from the pluripotent inner cell mass of early blastocyst embryos. They have active telomerase and can rebuild shortening chromosome ends, and therefore, are considered to be immortal. Under selected conditions in cell culture, ESC are able to differentiate into multiple cell types. Early approaches resulting in spontanous differentiation resulted in a very low cardiomyocyte output (5-10%). Current approaches for inducing cardiomyocyte differentiation in culture routinely use activin A in combination with bone morphogenetic protein 4 (BMP4)[51]. In another protocol, BMP2 (bone morphogenic protein 2), TGFβ (transforming growth factor) and TNFα (tumor necrosis factor)[52] were used to induce cardiac differentiation of hESC in culture. Others have reported that activation of the receptor for tyrosine-protein kinase, erbB-4 pathway by growth factors, neuregulins-2 and heparin-binding EGF-like growth factor, significantly enhance cardiac differentiation[52]. Some micro-RNAs induce cardiomyocyte proliferation, as well as differentiation of hESC and iPSC. MiR-499 (myomiR family) was reported to enhance differentiation of definitive myocardial cells from human cardiac progenitor cells and hESC[53,54].

In our laboratory, we use the approach of combining the formation of embryoid bodies followed by treatment with a new form of MiR-499 that increases cardiomyocyte output up to 70-80% as determined by the expression of cardiac-specific troponin-T and tropomyosin[55]. In addition, we have discovered a new cardiac -inducing RNA (CIR) that also significantly enhances cardiac differentiation from mESC and human iPSC; this RNA does not belong to the micro-RNA family, but rather appears to be part of RNA coding genes[56]. In our earlier studies, computer analyses of RNA secondary structures show significant similarities to a previously discovered myofibril-inducing RNA (MIR) described in salamander, that also promotes nonmuscle cells to differentiate into cardiac muscle in salamander hearts as well as mouse and human stem cells[57,58].

One of the problems that has been reported is that the retention rate of ESC in heart grafts is very low and the engrafted ESC do not appear to survive in the heart for prolonged periods[59]. The amount of detectable engrafted cells becomes very low after 2-3 weeks transplantation[60,61]. From this observation, many researchers have concluded that the majority of benefit for heart regeneration after MI is likely via paracrine effects of the cell[62]. This problem potentially may have another consequence; if engrafted cells do not stay at the place of engraftment, but are swept away by blood flow or by some other cellular movement/migratory mechanism and end up residing in other organs, they could contribute to tumor/cancer development. To help resolve this issue, researchers have invented a "pro-survival cocktail", including IGF1 (100 ng ml^{-1}) and cyclosporine A (0.2 mM), that helps to enhance retention and survival of engrafted cells after transplantation into the recipient heart[61].

Another potential problem with using hESC to generate cardiac tissue is the problem that allogenic cells will require life-long immunosuppression therapy. This problem may be resolved with cardiomyocytes differentiated from a patient's own iPSC that presumably are completely immune autologous. In spite of these potential concerns, there are multiple reports of successful differentiation of grafted iPSC that form into functional cardiomycytes in hearts of different species contributing to heart regeneration after myocardial infarction[62,63]. It seems likely that increased success may result from using inbred lines of a given species which have genetically similar allopathic strains with reduced immunogenic reactions to the transplanted cells. Using iPSC derived from the same animal (or same human patient) should eliminate totally the immunocompatability problem in these kinds of procedures.

Other concerns have been expressed relative to those approaches used to induce potentially transplanted pluripotent cells with virus vectors for cell de-differentiation; if such viruses cause disease or cancer, integration into a recipient's genome or transformation of healthy cells into cancer cells would be a major medical problem. This problem now may be able to be resolved by using de-differentiated iPSC formed with non-viral vectors. Human iPSC are functionally similar to human embryonic stem cells, in that they express the same markers of pluripotency. Molecular mechanisms of cardiomyocyte differentiation remain unknown; thus, approaches used for differentiation are currently rather empirical. Considering the similarities in differentiation properties between hESC and iPSC, their differentiation into cardiomyocytes logically would seem to be able to use similar approaches. Clearly, further experimentation using in vitro and in vivo approaches will be required to determine the best ways to accomplish the induced differentiation of pluripotent stem cells to form into normal functioning cardiac muscle tissue in vivo. Once accomplished, this technology would lead to the regeneration of cardiac muscle in patients who have suffered from heart damage due to heart attacks or other disease processes such that these patients could fully recover and return to pre-heart-attack activity levels again.

Summary

Numerous studies have been completed on heart development with respect to finding ways to regenerate functional cardiac muscle tissue after myocardial damage has resulted from acute myocardial infarction (AMI) or related cardiac disease processes. Although a variety of approaches have been used to stimulate nonmuscle tissues/cells to differentiate into cardiac lineages in vitro and in vivo with variable levels of success, reliable and reproducible clinical protocols to regenerate new healthy heart muscle tissue to treat human patients after myocardial infarction or other disease processes have yet to be achieved. It has been well known that heart disease is the leading cause of death, accounting for over 8,500,000 individuals every year worldwide. Also, every year millions of people have heart attacks (acute myocardial infarctions) and survive. Since human cardiac tissue does not regenerate significantly following injury, many of these survivors' physical activities, quality of life and independence are impaired. The development of new regenerative medical technologies through continued research in replacing damaged cardiac muscle tissue using stem cells and/or growth factors hold great promise for future cures of the many people around the world affected by cardiac disease. Being able to define the mechanism(s) directing and regulating the differentiation of nonmuscle cells (e.g., induced pluripotent stem cells) to form into vigorously and rhythmically contracting cardiac muscle tissue would represent a major breakthrough in modern medicine and biology. Moreover, being able to convert nonmuscle stem cells from a given patient for use in the repair of damaged heart or other tissues in that same patient promises to provide an immunologically compatible cure for heart and other diseases with tremendous medical, humanitarian and economic benefits to our society and to the world.

References

1. Sparrow, CP, Olszewski, J. Cellular oxidation of low density lipoprotein is caused by thiol production in media containing transition metal ions. J Lipid Res. 1993:34 (7):1219–28.
2. Ross R. Atherosclerosis — An inflammatory disease. N Engl J Med. 1999:340 (2):115–26.
3. Moore KJ, Sheedy FJ, Fisher EA. Macrophages in atherosclerosis: a dynamic balance. Nat Rev Immunol. 2013;13(10):709-21.
4. Boffito M, Sartori S, Ciardelli G. Polymeric scaffolds for cardiac tissue engineering: requirements and fabrication technologies. Polym Int 2014; 63:2–11.
5. Tallawi M, Rosellini E, Barbani N, Cascone MG, Rai R, Saint-Pierre G, Boccaccini AR. Strategies for the chemical and biological functionalization of scaffolds for cardiac tissue engineering: a review. J R Soc Interface. 2015;12(108):20150254.
6. Wang B, Wang G, To F, Butler JR, Claude A, McLaughlin RM, Williams LN, de Jongh Curry AL, Liao J. Myocardial scaffold-based cardiac tissue engineering: application of coordinated mechanical and electrical stimulations. Langmuir. 2013;29(35):11109-17.
7. Alrefai MT, Murali D, Paul A, Ridwan KM, Connell JM, Shum-Tim D. Cardiac tissue engineering and regeneration using cell-based therapy. Stem Cells Cloning. 2015:8:81-101.
8. Davis ME, Motion JP, Narmoneva DA, Takahashi T, Hakuno D, Kamm RD, Zhang S, Lee RT. Injectable self-assembling peptide nanofibers create intramyocardial microenvironments for endothelial cells. Circulation. 2005;111(4):442–50
9. Soonpaa MH, Kim KK, Pajak L, Franklin M, Field LJ. Cardiomyocyte DNA synthesis and binucleation during murine development. Am J Physiol. 1996;271(5 Pt 2):H2183-9.
10. Soonpaa MH, Field LJ. Assessment of cardiomyocyte DNA synthesis in normal and injured adult mouse hearts. Am J Physiol. 1997 ;272(1 Pt 2):H220-6.
11. Bergmann O, Bhardwaj RD, Bernard S, Zdunek S, Barnabé-Heider F, Walsh S, Zupicich J, Alkass K, Buchholz BA, Druid H, Jovinge S, Frisén J. Evidence for cardiomyocyte renewal in humans. Science. 2009;324(5923):98-102.
12. Senyo SE, Steinhauser ML, Pizzimenti CL, Yang VK, Cai L, Wang M, Wu TD, Guerquin-Kern JL, Lechene CP, Lee RT. Mammalian heart renewal by pre-existing cardiomyocytes. Nature. 2013;493(7432):433-6.
13. Hsieh PC, Segers VF, Davis ME, MacGillivray C, Gannon J, Molkentin JD, Robbins J, Lee RT. Evidence from a genetic fate-mapping study that stem cells refresh adult mammalian cardiomyocytes after injury. Nat Med. 2007;13(8):970-4.
14. Valiente-Alandi I, Albo-Castellanos C, Herrero D, Arza E, Garcia-Gomez M, Segovia JC, Capecchi M, Bernad A. Cardiac Bmi1(+) cells contribute to myocardial renewal in the murine adult heart. Stem Cell Res Ther. 2015;6:205.
15. Ghazizadeh Z, Vahdat S, Fattahi F, Fonoudi H, Omrani G, Gholampour M, Aghdami N. Isolation and characterization of cardiogenic, stem-like cardiac precursors from heart samples of patients with congenital heart disease. Life Sci. 2015;137:105-15.
16. Wei K, Serpooshan V, Hurtado C, Diez-Cuñado M, Zhao M, Maruyama S, Zhu W, Fajardo G, Noseda M, Nakamura K, Tian X, Liu Q, Wang A, Matsuura Y, Bushway P, Cai W, Savchenko A, Mahmoudi M, Schneider MD, van den Hoff MJ, Butte MJ, Yang PC, Walsh K, Zhou B, Bernstein D, Mercola M, Ruiz-Lozano P. Epicardial FSTL1 reconstitution regenerates the adult mammalian heart. Nature. 2015;525(7570):479-85.
17. Chen J, Huang ZP, Seok HY, Ding J, Kataoka M, Zhang Z, Hu X, Wang G, Lin Z, Wang S, Pu WT, Liao R, Wang DZ. Mir-17-92 cluster is required for and sufficient to induce cardiomyocyte proliferation in postnatal and adult hearts. Circ Res. 2013 ;112(12):1557-66.
18. Pandey R, Ahmed RPH. MicroRNAs inducing proliferation of quiescent adult cardiomyocytes. Cardiovasc Regen Med. 2015;2(1). pii:e519.
19. Liang D, Li J, Wu Y, Zhen L, Li C, Qi M, Wang L, Deng F, Huang J, Fei L, Liu Y, Ma X, Yu Z, Zhang Y, Chen YH. miRNA-204 drives cardiomyocyte proliferation via targeting Jarid2. Int J Cardiol. 2015;201:38-48.
20. Pascual-Gil S, Simón-Yarza T, Garbayo E, Prosper F, Blanco-Prieto MJ. Tracking the in vivo release of bioactive NRG from PLGA and PEG–PLGA microparticles in infarcted hearts. J Controlled Release. 2015; 220(Pt A): 388-396.
21. Clark AL, Naya FJ. MicroRNAs in the myocyte enhancer factor 2 (MEF2)-regulated Gtl2-Dio3 noncoding RNA locus promote cardiomyocyte proliferation by targeting the transcriptional coactivator Cited2. J Biol Chem. 2015;290(38):23162-72.
22. Das S, Halushka MK. Extracellular vesicle microRNA transfer in cardiovascular disease. Cardiovasc Pathol. 2015;24(4):199-206.
23. Kishore R, Khan M. More than tiny sacks: Stem cell exosomes as cell-free modality for cardiac repair. Circ Res. 2016;118(2):330-43.
24. Khan M, Nickoloff E, Abramova T, Johnson J, Verma SK, Krishnamurthy P, Mackie AR, Vaughan E, Garikipati VN, Benedict C, Ramirez V, Lambers E, Ito A, Gao E, Misener S, Luongo T, Elrod J, Qin G, Houser SR, Koch WJ, Kishore R. Embryonic stem cell-derived exosomes promote endogenous repair mechanisms and enhance cardiac function following myocardial infarction. Circ Res. 2015;117(1):52-64.
25. Song F, Zhao J, Hua F, Nian L, Zhou XX, Yang Q, Xie YH, Tang HF, Sun JY, Wang SW. Proliferation of rat cardiac stem cells is induced by 2, 3, 5, 4'-tetrahydroxystilbene-2-O-β-D-glucoside in vitro. Life Sci. 2015;132:68-76.
26. Zhao YY, Sawyer DR, Baliga RR, Opel DJ, Han X, Marchionni MA, Kelly RA. Neuregulins promote survival and growth of cardiac myocytes. Persistence of ErbB2 and ErbB4 expression in neonatal and adult ventricular myocytes. J Biol Chem. 1998;273(17):10261-9.
27. Yutzey KE. Regenerative biology: Neuregulin 1 makes heart muscle. Nature. 2015;520(7548):445-6.
28. D'Uva G, Aharonov A, Lauriola M, Kain D, Yahalom-Ronen Y, Carvalho S, Weisinger K, Bassat E, Rajchman D, Yifa O, Lysenko M, Konfino T, Hegesh J, Brenner O, Neeman M, Yarden Y, Leor J, Sarig R, Harvey RP, Tzahor E. ErbB2 triggers mammalian heart regeneration by promoting cardiomyocyte dedifferentiation and proliferation. Nat Cell Biol. 2015;17(5):627-38.
29. Polizzotti BD, Ganapathy B, Walsh S, Choudhury S, Ammanamanchi N, Bennett DG, dos Remedios CG, Haubner BJ, Penninger JM, Kühn B. Neuregulin stimulation of cardiomyocyte regeneration in mice and human myocardium reveals a therapeutic window. Sci Transl Med. 2015;7(281):281ra45.
30. Formiga FR, Pelacho B, Garbayo E, Imbuluzqueta I, Díaz-Herráez P, Abizanda G, Gavira JJ, Simón-Yarza T, Albiasu E, Tamayo E, Prósper F, Blanco-Prieto MJ. Controlled delivery of fibroblast growth factor-1 and neuregulin-1 from biodegradable microparticles promotes cardiac repair in a rat myocardial infarction model through activation of endogenous regeneration. J Control Release. 2014;173:132-9.

31. Lin Z, Pu WT. Harnessing Hippo in the heart: Hippo/Yap signaling and applications to heart regeneration and rejuvenation. Stem Cell Res. 2014;13(3 Pt B):571-81.

32. Tian Y, Liu Y, Wang T, Zhou N, Kong J, Chen L, Snitow M, Morley M, Li D, Petrenko N, Zhou S, Lu M, Gao E, Koch WJ, Stewart KM, Morrisey EE. A microRNA-Hippo pathway that promotes cardiomyocyte proliferation and cardiac regeneration in mice. Sci Transl Med. 2015;7(279):279ra38.

33. Waksman R, Baffour R. Bone marrow and bone marrow derived mononuclear stem cells therapy for the chronically ischemic myocardium. Cardiovasc Radiat Med. 2003;4(3):164-8.

34. Nuri MM, Hafeez S. Autologous bone marrow stem cell transplant in acute myocardial infarction.J Pak Med Assoc 2012;62(1):2-6.

35. Strauer BE, Steinhoff G. 10 years of intracoronary and intramyocardial bone marrow stem cell therapy of the heart: from the methodological origin to clinical practice. J Am Coll Cardiol. 2011;58(11):1095-104.

36. Tondreau T, Lagneaux L, Dejeneffe M, Delforge A, Massy M, Mortier C, Bron D. Isolation of BM mesenchymal stem cells by plastic adhesion or negative selection: phenotype, proliferation kinetics and differentiation potential. Cytotherapy 2004. 6(4):372–379.

37. Konstantinou D, Lei M, Xia Z, Kanamarlapudi V. Growth factors mediated differentiation of mesenchymal stem cells to cardiac polymicrotissue using hanging drop and bioreactor. Cell Biol Int. 2015;39(4):502-7.

38. Hafez P, Jose S, Chowdhury SR, Ng MH, Ruszymah BH, Abdul Rahman Mohd R. Cardiomyogenic differentiation of human sternal bone marrow mesenchymal stem cells using a combination of basic fibroblast growth factor and hydrocortisone. Cell Biol Int. 2016 ;40(1):55-64.

39. Hatzistergos KE, Quevedo H, Oskouei BN, Hu Q, Feigenbaum GS, Margitich IS, Mazhari R, Boyle AJ, Zambrano JP, Rodriguez JE, Dulce R, Pattany PM, Valdes D, Revilla C, Heldman AW, McNiece I, Hare JM. Bone marrow mesenchymal stem cells stimulate cardiac stem cell proliferation and differentiation. Circ Res. 2010;107(7):913-22.

40. Iso Y, Spees JL, Serrano C, Bakondi B, Pochampally R, Song YH, Sobel BE, Delafontaine P, Prockop DJ. Multipotent human stromal cells improve cardiac function after myocardial infarction in mice without long-term engraftment. Biochem Biophys Res Commun. 2007;354(3):700-6.

41. Leiker M, Suzuki G, Iyer VS, Canty JM Jr, Lee T. Assessment of a nuclear affinity labeling method for tracking implanted mesenchymal stem cells. Cell Transplant. 2008;17(8):911-22.

42. Murry CE, Palpant NJ, MacLellan WR. Cardiopoiesis in motion: primed mesenchymal stem cells for ischemic cardiomyopathy. J Am Coll Cardiol. 2013;61(23):2339-40.

43. Gallina C, Turinetto V, Giachino C. A new paradigm in cardiac regeneration: The mesenchymal stem cell secretome. Stem Cells Int. 2015;2015:765846.

44. Chimenti I, Smith RR, Li TS, Gerstenblith G, Messina E, Giacomello A, Marbán E. Relative roles of direct regeneration versus paracrine effects of human cardiosphere-derived cells transplanted into infarcted mice. Circ Res. 2010;106(5):971-80.

45. Zhang M, Liu D, Li S, Chang L, Zhang Y, Liu R, Sun F, Duan W, Du W, Wu Y, Zhao T, Xu C, Lu Y. Bone marrow mesenchymal stem cell transplantation retards the natural senescence of rat hearts. Stem Cells Transl Med. 2015;4(5):494-502.

46. Mansilla E, Roque G, Sosa YE, Tarditti A, Goya RG. A rat treated with mesenchymal stem cells lives to 44 months of age. Rejuvenation Res. 2016;19(4):318-21.

47. Messina E, De Angelis L, Frati G, Morrone S, Chimenti S, Fiordaliso F, Salio M, Battaglia M, Latronico MV, Coletta M, Vivarelli E, Frati L, Cossu G, Giacomello A. Isolation and expansion of adult cardiac stem cells from human and murine heart. Circ Res. 2004;95(9):911-21.

48. Smith RR, Barile L, Cho HC, Leppo MK, Hare JM, Messina E, Giacomello A, Abraham MR, Marbán E. Regenerative potential of cardiosphere-derived cells expanded from percutaneous endomyocardial biopsy specimens. Circulation. 2007;115(7):896-908.

49. Gaustad KG, Boquest AC, Anderson BE, Gerdes AM, Collas P. Differentiation of human adipose tissue stem cells using extracts of rat cardiomyocytes. Biochem Biophys Res Commun. 2004;314(2):420-7.

50. Strem BM1, Zhu M, Alfonso Z, Daniels EJ, Schreiber R, Beygui R, MacLellan WR, Hedrick MH, Fraser JK. Expression of cardiomyocytic markers on adipose tissue-derived cells in a murine model of acute myocardial injury. Cytotherapy. 2005;7(3):282-91.

51. Chong JJ, Yang X, Don CW, Minami E, Liu YW, Weyers JJ, Mahoney WM, Van Biber B, Cook SM, Palpant NJ, Gantz JA, Fugate JA, Muskheli V, Gough GM, Vogel KW, Astley CA, Hotchkiss CE, Baldessari A, Pabon L, Reinecke H, Gill EA, Nelson V, Kiem HP, Laflamme MA, Murry CE. Human embryonic-stem-cell-derived cardiomyocytes regenerate non-human primate hearts. Nature. 2014;510(7504):273-7

52. Hamidi S, Letourneur D, Aid-Launais R, Di Stefano A, Vainchenker W, Norol F, Le Visage C. Fucoidan promotes early step of cardiac differentiation from human embryonic stem cells and long-term maintenance of beating areas. Tissue Eng Part A. 2014;20(7-8):1285-94.

53. Sluijter JP, van Mil A, van Vliet P, Metz CH, Liu J, Doevendans PA, Goumans MJ. MicroRNA-1 and -499 regulate differentiation and proliferation in human-derived cardiomyocyte progenitor cells. Arterioscler Thromb Vasc Biol. 2010;30(4):859-68.

54. Wilson KD, Hu S, Venkatasubrahmanyam S, Fu JD, Sun N, Abilez OJ, Baugh JJ, Jia F, Ghosh Z, Li RA, Butte AJ, Wu JC. Dynamic microRNA expression programs during cardiac differentiation of human embryonic stem cells: role for miR-499. Circ Cardiovasc Genet. 2010;3(5):426-35.

55. Kochegarov A, Moses-Arms A, Hanna M, Lemanski LF. Micro RNA-499c induces the differentiation of stem cells into cardiomyocytes. International Archives of Medicine. 2015; 8(58).

56. Kochegarov A, Moses-Arms A, Lemanski LF. A fetal human heart cardiac-inducing RNA (CIR) promotes the differentiation of stem cells into cardiomyocytes. In Vitro Cell Dev Biol Anim. 2015;51(7):739-48.

57. Moses-Arms A, Kochegarov A, Arms J, Burlbaw S, Lian W, Meyer J, Lemanski LF. Identification of a human mitochondrial RNA that promotes tropomyosin synthesis and myocardial differentiation. In Vitro Cell Dev Biol Anim. 2015;51(3):273-80.

58. Zhang C, Jia P, Huang X, Sferrazza GF, Athauda G, Achary MP, Wang J, Lemanski SL, Dube DK, Lemanski LF. Myofibril-inducing RNA (MIR) is essential for tropomyosin expression and myofibrillogenesis in axolotl hearts. J Biomed Sci. 2009;16:81.

59. Ye J, Gaur M, Zhang Y, Sievers RE, Woods BJ, Aurigui J, Bernstein HS, Yeghiazarians Y. Treatment with hESC-derived myocardial precursors improves cardiac function after a myocardial infarction. PLoS One. 2015;10(7):e0131123.

60. van Laake LW, Passier R, den Ouden K, Schreurs C, Monshouwer-Kloots J, Ward-van Oostwaard D, van Echteld CJ, Doevendans PA, Mummery CL. Improvement of mouse cardiac function by hESC-derived cardiomyocytes correlates with vascularity but not graft size. Stem Cell Res. 2009;3(2-3):106-12.

61. Yeghiazarians Y, Gaur M, Zhang Y, Sievers RE, Ritner C, Prasad M, Boyle A, Bernstein HS. Myocardial improvement with human embryonic stem cell-derived cardiomyocytes enriched by p38MAPK inhibition. Cytotherapy. 2012;14(2):223-31.

62. Ye L, Chang YH, Xiong Q, Zhang P, Zhang L, Somasundaram P, Lepley M, Swingen C, Su L, Wendel JS, Guo J, Jang A, Rosenbush D, Greder L, Dutton JR, Zhang J, Kamp TJ, Kaufman DS, Ge Y, Zhang J. Cardiac repair in a porcine model of acute myocardial infarction with human induced pluripotent stem cell-derived cardiovascular cells. Cell Stem Cell. 2014;15(6):750-61.

63. Wendel JS, Ye L, Tao R, Zhang J, Zhang J, Kamp TJ, Tranquillo RT. Functional effects of a tissue-engineered cardiac patch from human induced pluripotent stem cell-derived cardiomyocytes in a rat infarct model. Stem Cells Transl Med. 2015;4(11):1324-32.

Abbreviations

AMI:	Acute myocardial infarction
BM-MNC:	Bone marrow mononuclear cells
BMP2:	Bone morphogenic protein 2
BMP4:	Bone morphogenetic protein 4
CDC:	Cardiosphere-derived cells
CSC:	Cardiac stem cells
EGF:	Epidermal growth factor
EPCs:	Endothelial progenitor cells
ESC:	Embryonic stem cells
FGF1:	Acidic fibroblast growth factor
FSTL1:	Follistatin-like protein 1
hESC:	Human embryonic stem cells
IGF1:	Inhibiting growth factor
iPSC:	Induced pluripotent stem cells
LDL:	Low-density lipoprotein
mESC:	Mouse embryonic stem cells
MI:	Myocardial infarction
MSC:	Mesenchymal stem cells
NRG1:	Neuregulin-1
TGFβ:	Transforming growth factor
TNFα:	Tumor necrosis factor

Potential Conflicts of Interests

None

Acknowledgments

We are grateful to Ms Mallory Dennie and Ms Sharon L Lemanski for excellent secretarial support during the preparation of the manuscript.

The current affiliation for Dr. Kochegarov is: Dr. Andrei Kochegarov, UCLA Peds-Neonatology, Box 951752, A-3-375, Los Angel California, 90095-1752, USA. E-mail: aKochegarov@mednet.ucla.edu

Grants

National Institutes of Health, Bethesda, Maryland 20892, USA; National Science Foundation, Arlington, Virginia 22230, USA; American Heart Association, Dallas, Texas 75231, USA; Chancellor's Research Initiative, Texas A&M University System, College Station, TX 77840, USA awarded to Dr. Lemanski.

Corresponding Author

Lemanski, Larry F, Department of Biological and Environmental Sciences, Texas A&M University-Commerce, PO Box ? Commerce, Texas, 75429, USA; E-mail: Larry.Lemanski@tamuc.edu;

4

The Adaptability of Somatic Stem Cells

Tweedell KS[1]

Cell and tissue specific somatic stem cells develop as dynamic populations of precursor cells to discrete tissue and organ differentiation during embryonic and fetal stages and their potential evolves with development. Some of their progeny are sequestered into separate cell niches of tissues as adult somatic stem cells at various times during organ development and differentiation These are diverse cell populations of stem and progenitor cells that respond to homeostatic needs for cell and tissue maintenance and the cycling of differentiated cells for physiological/endocrinological changes. Nominally, multipotent stem cells in one or more niches follow specific lineages of differentiation that can be followed by diverse markers of differentiation. The activation of precursors appears to be stochastic and results in a population of heterogeneous progenitor cells. When variations in the functional need of the tissue or organ occurs, the progenitor cells exhibit flexibility in their differentiation capacity. Regulation of the progenitors is the result of signals from the stem cell niche that can cause adaptive changes in the behavior or function of the stem -progenitor cell lineage. A possible mechanism may be alteration in the differentiation capacity of the resident or introduced cells. Certain quiescent stem cells also serve as a potential cell reservoir for trauma induced cell regeneration through adaptive changes in differentiation of stem cells, progenitor cells and differentiated cells. If the stem-progenitor cell population is normally depleted or destroyed by trauma, differentiated cells from the niche microenvironment can restore the specific stem potency which suggests the process of dedifferentiation.

Key Words: Somatic stem cell; Adaptation; Dedifferentiation; Plasticity; Niche

Adult somatic stem cells (SSCs) are self-renewing groups of cells in tissues and organs that can produce specific lineages of precursor cells leading to differentiated cell progeny. They are retained from organogenesis throughout life for cell maintenance, repair and regeneration[1]. During differentiation SSCs are established in unique cell/ECM niches. Niches are tissue specific sites *in vivo* consisting of differentiated cells that modulate stem cells. The niche histological composition varies extensively in different tissues but often includes stromal cells, extracellular matrix, blood vessels, neurons and tissue related precursor differentiated cells[2]. The stem cell population is often a mixture of quiescent stem cells (or active stem cells) and progenitor cells in various levels of differentiation. The surrounding niche cells regulate stem and progenitor cells and serve both as a specific topographical and functional site[3, 4, 5]. SSCs are often multipotent and their lineage leads to uni-potent progenitors for terminal differentiated cells. Activated stem cells divide symmetrically to produce identical cells for self-renewal. Alternatively, an asymmetric cell division produces a reserve stem cell and a cytoplasmic partitioned progenitor cell committed to a specific pathway. Where there is a cyclic demand for somatic cell renewal, short lived, intermediate transit amplifying (TA) cells proliferate extensively before differentiation into adult cells[4,5]. The resident population of diverse progenitors is possibly recruited and selected for their developmental potential to meet a specific function. The niche modulates stem cell function needed to maintain physiological needs for homeostasis and organismic variations in growth, maturation, reproduction and senescence that can alter stem/progenitor behavior[6]. Stem cells and their progeny within the niche may also be transient rather than fixed and adaptable to unusual conditions during tissue homeostasis or trauma

that affects or depletes the cell population[7]. Studies on quiescent stem cells indicate they are maintained by epigenetic, transcriptional and post-transcriptional controls[8]. Self-renewing stem cells are maintained by niche derived signals such as Wnt found in multiple mammalian tissues[9]. While developmental determination of the stem cells from the quiescent state to active renewing stem and progenitor cells follows a directional lineage, there are indications that the identity of the stem cell states is fluid and exhibits plasticity[10]. The co-existence of quiescent and active stem cells has been described[11] and the interconversion of quiescent and active cells is bi-directional[12]. The concept of a stem cell as a discrete entity is evolving into that of a biological function with a degree of plasticity[13]. The functionality of stem cells has been broadened to include undifferentiated cells, facultative cells and differentiated cells[14]. A key feature of these changes in cell fate is differentiation. It is possible that the degree of differentiation can be manipulated both within a specific lineage and between niches, during normal or abnormal needs for repair. Several SSC systems are examined here for the multiple controlling factors that enable the natural progression of differentiation in the stem cell lineage and for evidence that the determined cells are adaptable possibly by dedifferentiation.

Cell Specific Stem Cells

1. Hematopoietic Stem Cells

In the adult mammal a number of separate stem cells are found in the bone marrow. A well characterized and utilized stem cell is that responsible for hematopoiesis, the hematopoietic stem cell (HSC).

Author Names in full: Kenyon S. Tweedell[1]

[1]*Department of Biological Sciences, University of Notre Dame, Notre Dame IN 46556 USA.*

HSCs are found in the endosteal and perivascular regions of the bone marrow of the adult mammal and are precursors to blood cell components consisting of the lymphoid progenitors of the immune system and myeloid precursors to the multiple blood cell phenotypes. The process of hematopoiesis has its roots in embryonic and fetal stages, first occurring in the yolk sac, an area of the aorta-gonad mesonephros (AGM) then the placenta and next the fetal liver. Several signaling pathways occur including, Notch 1, regulated by a transcription of Runx1, and the CDX-HOX pathway. The interpretation of HSCs colonization is in a state of flux and evidence has implicated the fetal liver as their origin. One view has HSCs of the liver entering the adult bone marrow, a second states that they are seeded in both sites at the same time but direct tracking has not been demonstrated[15]. The fetal liver is the first tissue from which HSCs have been purified. In the fetal/adult bone marrow, the HSC niche is associated with trabecular bone closely linked to adherent osteoblasts. The niche is viewed as a mixture of HSCs, progenitor cells and stromal cells embedded in a well vascularized extracellular matrix (ECM). Adhesion to the osteoblasts is by a nuclear-cadherin/beta-catenin complex.

Alternate HSC niches in the bone marrow are in perivascular sites proximal to the endothelium[6]. The Wnt/beta catenin and Notch-Delta pathways drive the adult HSC lineages. There are many molecular similarities between the fetal and adult HSC stem cells that were analyzed by DNA analysis using bioinformatics and hybridization techniques that outlines the complete molecular phenotype of the HSC[16].

Many primitive HSCs are quiescent or reserved, used for homeostasis or in response to injury while others are active cycling stem cells that replenish the rapid turnover of blood cells. The migration of HSCs from the fetal mouse niche in the liver into the adult bone marrow niche results in dramatic changes from an active proliferating state into a quiescent mode. It has been postulated that separate quiescent and active populations of HSCs coexist in the bone marrow[15] and they are regulated as they migrate into each of them[11]. Studies with the chemokine CXCL12 (a protein that regulates the immune response and HSC migration) indicate that HSCs and progenitors are located in perivascular niches while lymphoid progenitors exist in endosteal niches[17]. A specific HSC marker has been found in mice, ESAM (endothelial cell selective adhesion molecule) that is retained for life. It is also expressed in human CD34+ cells recovered from human cord blood[18]. Supporting cells in the bone marrow niche, osteoblasts and osteoclasts, mesenchymal progenitors and vascular (reticular) cells, regulate the homeostasis and activation of these stem cells[15]. HSCs are identified initially by the detection of cell surface markers that express antigenic clusters of differentiation (CDs). Those found in animals often differ from CDs in the human although there are some that are conserved with murine animals. In addition, there is often overlap with those found in other tissues. As self-renewal of stem cells ceases, progenitors form, differentiate and the CDs expressed also changes. In the human, the CD34+is the primary clinical marker for HSC/progenitors. It is often expressed with the lineage antigen (Lin-) in combination with CD38+, CD45, CD90, CD133 along with Tie (angiopoietin-receptor) and c-kit (tyrosine kinase KIT)[19].

A compendium of phenotypes in the HSC lineage through successive levels of differentiation to the ten terminal differentiated blood cells has been described for both murine animals and the human. The catalog of CDs differs in either species but the individual phenotypes between the replicating stem cells and the first multipotent progenitor is remarkably similar within each species. The self renewal of mouse HSCs expresses a phenotype of Lin-, c-kit, Flk2-. CD34 and Slamf1- (receptors for HSC stem and early progenitors). The human cell array shows CD38-, CD90+ and CD45RA- plus CD34+ and Lin-. Two

surface markers, CD34 and Lin- are conserved in the two species and their presence extends from the activated stem and progenitor lineage to the final restricted progenitors for terminal differentiated cells [20]. Normal HSCs has been found in various niches from bone to cord blood. CD44 is involved in adhesion of cells to the ECM by hyaluron and is a receptor for the cytokine osteopontin (Opn) in the bone marrow. CD 90 is related to stem cell quiescence and CD 123 serves stem cell differentiation [20] (Table 1).

Another parameter of HC stem cell specificity are signaling molecular pathways whose function is to enable HSC renewal as well as promoting differentiation lineages. The canonical Wnt pathway promotes the emergence of HSCs from the mesodermal endothelium of the dorsal aorta during early development. Niche cells communicate with their stem cell components through individual clusters of signaling molecular pathways. Another link (Tie receptor/angiopoietin 1) regulates HSC adhesion and promotes quiescence while (Opn) from osteoblast cells down regulates HSC proliferation. Niche osteoblasts also express an N-cadherin/β-catenin complex thought to mediate attachment of HSCs in their niche. A proposed Wnt signal-nuclear β-catenin sequence regulates HSC proliferation while c-Myc interaction with Notch signals appears to regulate HSC differentiation[6]. In the adult, quiescent stem cells in the endosteal zone are maintained by inhibitory signals such as BMP, OPN and sFRP1. Active stem cells in the central zone are stimulated by Wnt, fibroblast growth factor (FGF) and SDF1 (stromal derived epidermal factor) pathways from endothelial cells, megakaryocytes and reticular cells[11].

The local niche environment may accomplish stem cell maintenance of HSC's with cell-cell contact or at a distance[19]. The effect of niche influence on resident HSC stem cells is extensive. Murine granulocyte macrophage cytokines can instruct the hematopoietic lineage[21]. The stem cell factor (SCF), is produced by perivascular mesenchymal cells and endothelial cells that maintain HSC's in both embryonic and adult tissues. This is a key perivascular niche that provides multiple cell types during homeostasis[22]. When the stem cell population is depleted, newly introduced stem cells behave as the original cells[19], an attribute found in developing organ primordia and shared by the blastemal cells in the regenerating vertebrate limb [23].

It had been generally held that a common pluripotent primitive stem cell produces two lines of multipotent stem cells, progenitors to the lymphoid immune system cells and the other forms myeloid stem cells, with eight precursors to a multiple blood cell lineage[15]. The original concept predicted a long term lineage sequence of oligo-potent progenitors into unipotent progenitors. The classical view that multipotent HSCs produce multipotent progenitors for the separate common myeloid progenitor (CMP) and lymphoid lineages has been modified for both the murine fetal liver and adult bone marrow[24].

The niche of the fetal mouse liver contains HSC stem cells and associated pericytes that express Nestin and a neural/glial antigen 2 (NGA2) when both cells are in a high proliferation state[25]. With continued development, the cells move into a HSC niche of the adult bone marrow where the HSCs and pericytes evolve into a quiescent state. Concomitantly, two studies have provided evidence that multipotent common myeloid progenitors follow a different differentiation sequence in the fetal mouse niche compared to the adult niche. Single cell culture assays[26] showed the presence of oligopotent cells in the fetal niche that do not exist in the definitive adult state. This view was substantiated in a second investigation[27] with single-cell transcriptome analysis of 2700 myeloid progenitors in the mouse. The analysis failed to detect any type of CMP cells with multipotent progenitor ability in the adult.

Table 1: Somatic stem cell constituent markers and pathways

SOMATIC STEM CELL CONSTITUENT MARKERS   **PATHWAYS**

Stem Cell	State: STAGE	Quiescent	Active	Progenitors - Differentiation	Components	Func
HSC	Develop.	CHD7[39]	CXCL-12[15,17] SCF [22]		Wnt,FGF,SDF-1[11] Notch1, RunX, CDX-HOX, PGE2[15]	Q A
	Adult	BMP,OPN, FRP1[11]	SCF, SCA1+, CD34-,LIN,Flk2, Slamf1-, ckit[20] H: Lin-,CD34, CD45RA-,CD38-,CD 90[20]	Sca 1+, Flk2, c-kit, Lin -, Slamf1+, CD27+, CD34+[20] IL7RA+[19] ESAM[18] NG2, Nestin[25] H: Lin, c-kit, IL3RA, Cd10+.CD38, CD45RA, CD90, CD334+, CD123,Tie.[19,20]	OPN, BMP,FRP[11] Wnt/N/beta catenin,c-myc Notch[6] Wnt, FGF, SDF-1[11] Wnt/beta catenin ,Notch, Delta ll 1[15]	Q A Df
NSC/ NCC	Develop.			Sox2, Pax6,Nestin, GFAP GLT-1,CBP, BLBP, Vimentin[29,30]	Wnt/catenin. SHH, BMP, RA,FGF [35]	Df
	Adult	CHD7[39]		GLAST,CBP,GFAP,BLBP,GLT1,TGF, FGF, RA,TN-.C,RC-1,2,Nestin,Vimentin.,GS, Pdgf [30,34,35,40]	Notch/delta ll1,Wnt, Jag.1, Ephrin B[37,38] Wnt/.catenin,SHH,TGAF,TFG,PDGF,EGFR[40,42,45]	Q Df
PrSC	Develop.		Lgr4[49,58]	Lgr4, Lin-, Scz1+, CD49[49,58]		A
	Adult			ckit, CD44, CD133, CD117[51] CD 138, CD49f, K5, K8, K14,K18, PSA[56] H CD133, TROP 2,CD44, CD49f[53,54]	Alpha 6 Integrin[50] . Wnt, Notch/Delta, Jagged1, SHH[57,58] H: alpha/beta integrin[53]	Df
MaSC	Develop.			K14,K19 [61,62]	Wnt	Df
	Neonatal			K5,K8,K14+,K19+,EGRF[62,63,65]		Df
	Adult	Laminin1[61]		K5, K8, K14+, K19+, lin-, CD24, CD29+ CD29-,CD49f+ [61,62,65]	Notch/Jag. 1, Wnt, Integrins, EGFR, E,P cadherins[63,67]	Q
	Pregnancy			K8, K14,K18,CD24,CD29[65]	Wnt, Notch/Delta, SHH, HOX,FGF,TGF,p Cadherin[67]	Df
	Lactation			K14, K18, p63, β-casein[64]		Df
ISC	Develop.	LRC[74]		Lgr5	Wnt,SHH,Hox,FGF,TGF[69]	Df
	Adult	Bmi1 H2B[78,79,83] Lgr5[12,73]	Lgr5[12,74,77,83], Bmi1, Hopx, Sox9 mTert,Lrig1[79,82]	Lgr5, Delta ll1, Bmi1 [82]	Notch/Delta 1[80,82] Wnt-, Wnt+, Wnt+/catenin, EGFR[83]	Q,A Df

H: human, Q: quiescent, A: Active, Df. Differentiation. [xx]: Reference

Rather, the HSC compartment produces individual unipotent progenitors for all myeloid, erythroid and megakaryocyte progeny. Intermediate oligopotent precursors are replaced by individual unipotent progenitors for lymphoid progenitors, T and B lymphocytes and natural killer cells. HSCs evolve with a sequence of developmental sites as they age. While stem and progenitor cells follow a specific lineage, their function may vary as dictated by cell regulatory components in separate osteoblast and vascular niches. HSCs are viewed as groups of related cells, with varying potential, controlled by transcription factors and input from separate, adjoining cellular niches. The active population of HSCs maintains the cycling blood cells while the quiescent population responds to acute cell loss[18].

2. Neural Stem Cells

In mammals, morphogenetic and cellular changes in the embryonic neural tube form the primitive forebrain (telencephalon) mid-brain and hind-brain. Neurogenesis is initiated in the ventricular zone of the brain wall when concurrent changes in cell shape and migration are associated with the formation of embryonic neuroepithelial (NE) cells, the source of primary neural stem cells in the developing brain that are multipotent progenitors to neurons and glial cells[28]. Early symmetrical divisions of the proliferating embryonic NE cells express specific neural cell markers, Sox2, Pax6 and the production of Nestin (an intermediate filament protein) and a glial fibrillary acetic protein (GFAP) marker[29]. Early on, NE cells along the subventricular zone (SVZ) produce progenitors to neurons followed by asymmetric divisions leading to more restricted progenitors of radial glial (RG) cells that multiply and eventually replace all NE cells[30]. The RG cells also exhibit characteristics of astroglial cells, a glutamate transporter (GLT1), Ca+ binding protein (CBP), GFAP, vimentin and a brain lipid binding protein (BLPP)[30]. Cre recombinase (Cre-lox) mapping demonstrated that these NE cells are the source of neural stem cells (NSCs) since they can form both neurons and radial glial cells (RF) in the embryo[31].In the developing brain, RG cells form astrocytes but also form neurons. From these observations, a unified cell continuum of stem cell formation, from the embryo to the adult, was proposed resulting in a neuroepithelial-radial glia-astrocyte lineage[32]. Embryonic neurogenesis in the cortex proceeds by asymmetric division that produces an RG cell and a neuron progenitor or indirectly through one or two divisions of intermediate progenitor cells for neurons in the ventricular zone (VZ). Heterogeneous neurons which differ according to their locality or their developmental stage are controlled by activation of an extensive range of transcription factors. Furthermore, the RG cells produce separate intermediate progenitor cells that generate either neurons or astrocytes during embryonic development and in the adult[33,34].

In the neonatal stage, RG cells continue to produce neurons and oligodendrocytes via intermediate progenitor cells. A sub-population of RG cells, known as B cells, convert into astrocytes in the (SVZ). These are the source of NSCs in the adult and generate neural intermediate progenitor cells that culminate in neuroblasts (precursor neurons). The RG cells express astroglial markers: GLASt, BLBP, Tenascin C (TN-C),GFAP, Nestin, Vimentin, RC1,2. Other astrocyte-like neural stem cells, originally derived from embryonic RG cells also have glial cell properties[34]. These adult astrocyte-like NSCs appear to be pre-determined for a specific neuronal or glial fate[35]. In the post- natal rodent brain the radial glia-astrocyte stem cell sequence yields neurons, ependymal cells and astrocytes in two niches of the adult brain One region is located in the brain wall adjacent to the lateral ventricles of the forebrain, the sub-ventricular zone (V-SVZ), that ultimately generates olfactory bulb interneurons. A second is found in the subgranular zone (SGZ) the dentate gyrus of the brain

hippocampus[29,34]. Neural intermediate progenitor cells generate diverse neurons and intermediate glial progenitor cells form heterogeneous oligodendrocytes[34,35]. Other evidence has indicated that similar niches exist in circum-ventricular organs (CVOs) along the ventricular midline and in novel niches along the 3rd and 4th ventricles in the adult[36]. See Table I and Abbreviation List.

Components of the neural stem cell niche promote quiescence and insure stem cell identity. Neural stem cells in the SVZ niche depend upon direct cell to cell contact with endothelial cells of the vascular niche. Two proteins, endothelial ephrin B2 and Jagged 1 prevent the production of mitogens that inhibit differentiation[37]. Adult mouse quiescent NSCs in the subventricular zone are also reinforced by the induction of the Notch ligand Delta-like 1 (Delta ll 1) signaling pathway in activated NSCs, presumably by feedback on the reserve stem cells[38]. In the hippocampus a chromatin remodeling factor, chromo-domain-helicase-DNA binding protein 7 (CHD7), represses the transcription of several positive regulators of cell cycle induction[39]. Stem cell activation leads to their repression allowing stem cell renewal and neurogenesis of adult neurons and glial cells (astrocytes and oligodendrocytes)[40]. The diversity of the neural stem cell populations found in adult neural niches reflects the plasticity of the NSCs. They consist of sequential cell stages, Type B1 astrocytes (radial astrocytes), that develop Type C transit amplifying cells (intermediate progenitors) which divide to form Type A granule cells (neuroblasts), precursors of differentiated neurons[29,40-43]. There are three different compartments (domains) of the adult V-SVZ niche which allow for regulation of stem cell function during homeostasis, cell regeneration and aging[42]. The ventricular chamber is lined with multi-ciliated ependymal cells (B1) in the first domain (DI). Moving inward into the ventricular wall, domain II (DII), B1 astrocyte cells form transit amplifying "C" cells that divide to form A cells (neuroblasts). In the third innermost zone (DIII), B1 cells are in communication with blood vessels via extended cell processes [40,43]. A variety of growth factors, ligands and signaling pathways appear to regulate B1 cells and progenitor cells behavior in all three domains[42]. Many soluble factors (TGFs, IGFs, PDGFs, BMPs, Wnt, SHH) and retinoic acid are found in the cerebral spinal fluid (CSF) that can affect cell proliferation, neurogenesis and oligodendrogenesis [40,42,43]. The ependymal cells secret noggin which enhances progenitor cells and neuroblast formation[42]. Other factors are released from blood and endothelial cells. Notch signaling is viewed as bidirectional between niche cells, stem cells and their progeny during homeostasis and regeneration[40]. For example, neurotransmitters from serotoninergic axons appear to regulate interactions between B1 cells, progenitor cells and newly formed neuroblasts [43].

In the SGV of the brain hippocampus a different niche compartment has been described with multiple pathways for radial cell development[42]. Three similar domains of radial astrocytes (RA) are located within the dentate gyrus, DI, a subgranular zone adjacent to blood vessels, DII, a granular zone where RAs interact with their progeny and DIII, an inner molecular zone that exposes RA cell extensions to neuronal networks. Since the gyrus lacks a ventricle, Domain I in the gyrus is the Hilus, a deep region of intermediate progenitor cells (IPC) and blood vessels. Here, factors from blood vessels, endothelial cells and RA cells stimulate RA type 1 cells to form intermediate progenitor cells (IPCs) that migrate into the upper granular zone. Domain II consists of the RA cell bodies that are anchored with a primary cilium in the hilus along with a mixed lineage of IPCs (type 1 and 2) and granule (type 3) cells. When mature, granule cells become anchored by an axon into the Hilus and apically send dendrites into the inner molecular layer of domain III.

The RA cell bodies also extend projections into the molecular layer forming dense branches of mossy fiber axons. In domain II there is cell-cell interaction between NSCs, their progeny and granules cells and their behavior is regulated by various neuro-transmitters such as (GABA). Domain III is an inner molecular layer of other glial cells, axons and synaptic terminals. The two neurogenic niches of neural stem cells harbor B1 astrocytes in the SVZ and radial astrocytes in the SGZ. The functions of quiescence, cell proliferation and progenitor differentiation appears to be regulated by specific cell to cell interaction with their progeny and soluble factors from blood vessels, the ventricular fluid and neuronal interchange that provide alternative avenues for niche regulation. The multiple signaling pathways remain to be identified in vivo and may cross regulate on the same cell[42]. These and other biophysical properties of the dynamic niches control neural stem cell function during homeostasis, and regeneration[40,43] and neurogenesis in both SVZ and SGV declines with age[42].

3. Neural Crest Precursors

Other neural stem cell derivatives originate from the neural crest cells (NCC), a cache of pluripotent migratory stem cells that arise from the lateral margins of the embryonic brain and spinal cord. They form the sensory and motor neurons, ganglia of the peripheral and enteric nervous system, glial cells, melanocytes, endocrine cells and diverse types of mesenchyme cells. Another small subset of stromal cells originating from NC cells express the protein Nestin and also contribute to the maintenance of HSCs[22]. Early experiments by Le Douarin et al. on chick-embryo/quail – adult chimeras indicated that NCC differentiate into a specific type of glial cell that is dependent upon the microenvironment where they develop[44]. Another quality of differentiated cells from the NCC lineage is their plasticity in the adult. The differentiation of glial cells and melanocytes can be reversed when the cells are returned to an intermediate precursor. A reciprocal conversion between glial cells and melanocytes occurs by dedifferentiation into a multipotent progenitor[44]. The most widely distributed glial cells are Schwann cells that surround axons with myelin throughout the body. In the adult, Schwann cells are also found to dedifferentiate into stem-like cells in response to injury, reverting to a precursor state that promotes new axon regeneration and re-myelination of injured neurons[45]. Adult Schwann cells may act upon perivascular smooth muscle and invade the bone marrow hematopoietic stem cell niche, secreting a transforming growth factor-beta that keeps the stem cells quiescent[45]. The wide spread glial plasticity between cell and tissue interactions of NCCs and non-NC derivatives of perivascular muscle, bone marrow and mesentery during development, injury and malignancy implicates NCC stem cell-like cells in diseases and neoplasia. The behavior and defects in NCCs or their interactions with its environment may help in the etiology of several diseases[46]. For example, Schwann cells will dedifferentiate in diseases such as leprosy, caused by Myobacteriium leprae. This disease causes Schwann cells to dedifferentiate, lose their glial identity and transform into highly migratory "stem cell-like cells". The Schwann cell precursors can then differentiate into new cells in vivo.

4. Prostate gland stem cells

The primordium of the prostate gland arises from an interaction of embryonic endodermal buds that develop multiple solid rod branches within a mesenchyme capsular cell mass. Androgen production ultimately controls epithelial morphogenesis of the solid tubular rods and buds which leads to duct formation within the buds followed by epithelial cell differentiation into basal cells and secretory luminal cells that face the duct lumen. Rare neuroendocrine cells in the layer, extend from the basement membrane between the luminal cells.

An early prediction of prostate stem cells (PrSC) was obtained when dissociated prostate epithelial cells and embryonic urogenital sinus mesenchyme fragments were derived from murine embryonic or adult donors and implanted into the kidney subcapsular space or implanted intra-muscularly in adult mice. Prostatic branching tubules were regenerated in the implants along with prostate cell markers[48]. Later, prostate tissue cells in a basal phenotype, identified as stem cells by the antigenic profile Lin- (mixed lineage marker), SCA1+(stem cell protein antigen) and CD 49f were isolated by FACS and cultivated in vitro. When combined with inductive stroma and implanted into the sub-capsule of the kidney or into the skin of immune-deficient mice, they regenerated tubules with an outer basal layer, an inner luminal layer and neuro-endocrine cells[49].

Other isolations with in vitro cultivation of prostate cells utilized a variety of generic stem cell markers, and putative specific prostate stem cell combinations. Purified cells from the proximal duct with SCA-1 (stem cell protein antigen) that often co-expressed alpha 6 integrin were most effective in restoring the prostate[50]. Single cell isolates from the proximal urethra also expressed stem cell receptors (Lin(-) SCA-1+, c-kit, CDs 44, 133). They and a PC marker CD 117, can generate secretion –producing prostate tissue in vivo[51]. These studies of prostate basal cell and luminal cells resulted in regeneration of secretory prostate cells when implanted in vivo. The prostate stem cell niches were located in the basal cell layer, proximal to the urethra[52] and in the tip of proximal prostatic ducts[50,51]. In the human prostate, a subset of basal cells expressing alpha2/beta 1 integrin, a prostate cell surface marker and CD133 would produce prostate-like acini when transplanted into immune-compromised mice[53]. Similarly, a subpopulation of human prostate basal epithelial cells, expressing (Trop2), CD44 and CD49f, formed self-renewing prostaspheres in vitro that were implanted along with rat urogenital sinus mesenchyme into immunocompromised mice. Tubular structures formed in the implants that differentiated into discrete basal and luminal cells in vivo[54].

Based on the murine and human data Goldstein proposed a prostate epithelial hierarchy where basal stem cells produce a multipotent progenitor that generates all three types of epithelial cells[55]. During post-natal development, lineage tracing experiments on the prostate epithelium of mice verified that basal multipotent stem cells (intermediate cells) do differentiate into three main lineages. Basal cells expressed keratin (K), K5 and K14 along with a common transcription factor, p63, whereas luminal or secretory cells expressed K8 and K18 plus an androgen receptor, a prostate-specific antigen and prostate acid phosphatase and thirdly, neuroendocrine cells produced synaptophysin, chromogranin A and neuropeptides. Both unipotent basal progenitors and unipotent luminal progenitors were also present[56]. During homeostasis in the adult there is a shift from multipotent progenitors to separate unipotent basal and luminal cell progenitors as stem cell sources. Induction of prostate cell regeneration also results from activation of unipotent stem cell progenitors[56].

When prostaspheres and an in vivo prostate reconstitution assay were combined, the Wnt pathway induces Sc-1+, CD49f + basal/ stem cell proliferation. Up regulation of target genes led to an increase in K5+, K8+, p63+ prostate progenitor cells. Induction of Notch signaling in prostate progenitors inhibits their proliferation and normal morpho-genesis. The opposing roles of Wnt/ Notch signals is attributed to modulation of Notch by Wnt signaling[57]. Early development of the prostate gland (which is post-natal in rodents) in Lin-/Sca1+/CD49f+ basal stem cells, is associated with the expression of of Lgr4 (a G-protein coupled receptor) that occurs prior to any lineage differentiation in the neonatal gland. Yet, continued morphogenesis and differentiation is regulated by LGr4 expression. Notch and sonic hedgehog (SHH) pathways are key targets in prostate stem cells and progenitors, both promoting morphogenesis and early differentiation. Lgr4 expression modulates both cell proliferation and differentiation through Wnt/ßcatenin signaling. Induction of Wnt signaling in basal stem cells down regulates Notch and blocks proliferation and morphogenesis of acini but induction of Notch in progenitors inhibits their proliferation. The inactivation or ablation of Lgdr4 down loads both Notch 1 and SHH expression and also blocks both morphogenesis and differentiation. It appears that Wnt modulation of Notch regulates proliferation and maintenance of epithelial progenitors[58]. Based on the multiple stem cell-progenitor involvement in prostate homeostasis and regeneration, it has been hypothesized that any progenitor cell can produce cells leading to differentiated secretory luminal cells. Moreover, the oncogenic transformation of these precursor cells is the basis for the genotypic variation and degree of malignancy found in prostatic cancer[59].

5. Mammary Gland Stem Cells

Development of the mammary gland has primordial origins analogous to that of the prostate gland. Ectodermal cells forms primary solid cellular buds that subsequently branch within external mesenchymal tissue. At the fetal-neonatal stage two hollow chambers exist, a multi-branched terminal lobular unit and a basal terminal end chamber. The mammary gland epithelium becomes organized into a layer of luminal-alveolar secretory cells and a layer of basal myoepithelial (MEP) cells that interact with the ECM. The basal epithelial cells are controlled by the beta1-integrin gene and these cells regulate the growth and differentiation of the luminal secretory cells[60]. Evidence of a multipotent mammary stem cell, capable of producing the entire mammary branching network was provided by single cell isolations from 8 week old mice. A subpopulation of cells isolated by FACS, were identified by Lin, CD29hi, CD24+ markers. A majority of these cells expressed the myoepithelial cytokeratin 14 (K14) marker. Double sorted Lin-, CD29hi, CD24+ cells were recovered, marked with a LacZ transgene, cultivated into buds in vitro and then transplanted into mammary gland fat pads where 6/102 recipients developed ductal structures of both luminal and myoepithelial cells. Further differentiation of lobulo-alveolar components occurred when transplants were made into adults during pregnancy and parturition. A separate cell population expressed the luminal cell marker, K18 and additional analysis indicated their cell progeny had a luminal cell fate when exposed to lactogenic conditions. The single cell isolates of self-replicating, multipotent stem cells, were defined as mammary gland stem cells (MaSCs)[61].

The human breast stem cell hierarchy changes as gland development proceeds and increases in complexity from the fetal -neonatal stage, into the adult gland and during pregnancy. These cells are identified by different cell surface markers, CD24, CD29, CD44, CD49f and EpCAM. The developmental sequence can be followed by changes in cytokeratin staining (K). In the early fetus, luminal and basal cell lineages are established that are double negative for K14 and K19 markers. At the neonatal stage, multipotent progenitors, K14+, K19+ are produced by ductal/lobular cell and myoepithelial cells. In the adult, multipotent progenitor cells are recognized by keratin markers for two types of ductal lobular cells and a basal/myoepithelial cells [62].

The basal epithelium appears to be the source of MaSCs, progenitor cells and differentiated basal cells. Isolation of basal cells from the mammary gland using Lin-, CD24+. CD29hi from virgin mice

identified multipotent MaSCs with a more specific cell marker, a transmembrane endothelial protein C receptor (EPCR) for a Wnt target in the mammary gland from "Matrigel" cell cultures. Upon transplantation, these cells regenerated mammary gland components and also acted a multipotent stem cells in physiological lineage tracing with a knock-in allele of the EPCR receptor[63]. Another parameter of MaSC adaptation appears during mammary gland lactation. Based on the recovery of breast stem cells from human breast milk and analysis by extensive in vitro testing looking for the expression of human embryonic stem cell (hESCs) transcription factors. A proposed lineage from a common multipotent stem cell, CD49f, is the source for generating separate branches of luminal or myoepithelial progenitors. The luminal progenitor develops into ductal cells (K 19) or an alveolar luminal cell progenitor (K18). During lactation, the latter differentiates into a novel K18/ß- casein, an a-lactalbumin secretory cell. Myoepithelial cells (K14) originate from separate progenitors[64]. Progenitors of the mammary gland are frequently modified due to the cyclic nature of the mammary gland during each menstrual (estrus) cycle. Evidence from genetic lineage studies indicates that the stem cell identity varies from the fetal to neo-natal, during homeostasis and pregnancy[64]. As a result, there is a special relationship between the adult basal stem cells and their micro-environmental niche that separates them from neonatal stem cells.

A group of lineage tracing experiments and clonal analysis of the mouse mammary gland were performed in situ, under physiological conditions, on embryonic, adult and pregnancy phases of the mammary glands. Using keratin gene derived K14, yellow fluorescent proteins (YFP+) cells it was confirmed that all mammary gland epithelial lineages were derived from multipotent K14 expressing progenitors which included myo-epithelial and luminal cells during embryonic development. At the beginning of puberty and during homeostasis, it was found that two types of lineage restricted cells differentiated into either myoepithelial or liminal cell lineages. In vivo experiments based on immune-staining indicated that cells during puberty and in adult virgin mice which expressed K-14, were limited to myoepithelial cells. This continued into adult life and during multiple pregnancies. No K-14 expressing cells contributed to the luminal lineage during their expansion at puberty. In contrast, K-8/YFP+ expressing stem cells were limited to the luminal cell lineage during puberty, adult gland homeostasis and continued through 3 consecutive cycles of pregnancy and lactation. These separate, long lived, unipotent stem cells also demonstrated massive expansion during pregnancy[65]. New investigations on the in situ in changes of the mouse mammary gland utilized a multicolored Cre reporter gene and observations by 3D confocal imaging, combined with specific markers and immuno-staining in several transgenic mice that allowed in vivo identification of both stem cells and progenitors[66]. The contribution of progenitor cells at different stages during development and the adult was determined by producing transgenic strains specific to basal and luminal lineages, using green fluorescent protein (GFP) linked-to a reverse tetracycline transcriptional activator (tTA) and an internal ribosome entry site, (GFP-rTIR). The transcription factor Elf5, from a signature gene for mouse and human alveolar tissue differentiation, was employed. FACs analysis showed that the Elf5-GFP was confined to the luminal layer but not the basal/MaSC cell population in pubertal and adult mammary glands. Tracing luminal progenitor cells in vivo indicated they induced alveologenesis which expanded during puberty. The basal cell population of MaSCs and myoepithelial followed with keratin K5 and FACS analysis using GFP showed they were confined to myoepithelial cells. Bipotent K5 expressing cells cells were tracked and found during morphogenesis, puberty and homeostasis in the adult. The fate of restricted luminal progenitors utilized the same triple-transgenic mice combined with floxed multicolored (confetti) reporter alleles. Elf5-labeled cells contribute to alveolar cells in pregnancy and about 60% of them express 2-4 fluorescent proteins. The data promoted a common basal cell precursor, a bipotent mammary gland stem cell, which yielded both myoepithelial and luminal cells. These bipotent stem cells were active during morphogenesis, homeostasis in the adult mouse, and physiological changes during pregnancy and lactation. The lineage of the unique progenitor cells supports a model that states cell replenishment is initiated by MaSCs and continued by long lived unipotent progenitors[66].

Several signaling pathways control mammary stem cell development, particularly progenitor cells that maintain homeostasis. Niche-derived mammary gland proteins and ECM molecules were found to specify bipotent human progenitor cells[67]. Cell cultures of human progenitor cells indicated the niche maintained quiescence, the progenitor state and directed differentiation toward myoepithelial and luminal stages. Progenitor cell fate occurred through integrin signaling along with Notch, EGFR and both E- and P-cadherins. It was concluded that the regulation does not dictate pre-determined programs but the niche imposes specific behavior upon them. *In vivo* analysis indicated Laminin 1 maintains quiescent cells. The Notch ligand, Jagged 1 imposed the K14+/K19 progenitor phenotypes and with P- cadherin selected the K14+/K19+ phenotype in the MEP cells[67]. The mammary stem cell niche can also modulate the differentiation response of other unrelated stem cell hierarchies when they are transplanted into the mammary niche that further reflects their plasticity (see discussion)[68]. This niche regulatory function also parallels the regulatory role of the early regeneration blastema on introduced foreign primordia[23] and the reactivation of ectopic cells in a vacant Drosophila niche[20]. Yet, the neoplastic conversion of mammary stem cells as potential cancer cell precursors provides a parallel to lineage studies on developing mammary cells. An antibody study on human breast cell origin found that normal epithelial K19+ luminal cells from the breast are localized in >95% of human breast carcinomas[62].

6. *Intestinal Stem Cells*

The mucosal lining of the small intestine in the late embryo consists of a continuous epithelium, along the intestinal lumen, that develops multiple finger-like projections of villi separated by crypts between their bases. In the crypt, the epithelium forms crypt based columnar cells (CBC) and by the late embryo/early post-natal period, the crypts have stem cells and progenitor cells along with Paneth cells at the crypt bottom. Gut development forms by an interaction of the Wnt canonical signaling pathway and the TGF-ß superfamily pathway along with FGF, hedgehog (SSH) & Hox proteins that control cell division and fate[69]. Proliferating cells in the embryonic crypt of mice are polyclonal, i.e. biparental, but early in postnatal life, cloned pools of adult stem cells result from asymmetric cell divisions. In the human adult, the intestinal crypts may also contain multipotent, self renewing stem cells capable of replacing millions of cells every few days. Adult homeostasis was postulated as regulation of stem cells and their progeny by niche derived signals, signaling pathways, transcription and growth factors that direct their fate[69,70]. An early study by Cheng and Leblond[71] showed that the CBC cells, dispersed between Paneth cells, were long lived, self-renewing multipotent intestinal stem cells (ISCs) that maintain homeostasis of the differentiated cell types found along the entire villus epithelium. These terminal cells are enterocytes, goblet cells, entero-endocrine cells, tuft cells and M cells[72]. The cyclic replacement of the differentiated cells along the villi begins by cell amplification of

progenitor transit amplifying (TA) cells in the crypt niche. The TA cells cycle into differentiated lineages as they migrate up the villus to replenish the differentiated cells in the epithelium. The existing absorptive, secretory and hormonal cells are replaced every 4 to 5 days after they undergo apoptosis and escalate into the intestinal lumen. Paneth cells remain in the crypt base where they produce an anti-microbial substance, nurture the ISCs and are replaced by transient cell precursors[73]. The marker gene for CBC cells, Lgr5+ (Leucine G protein receptor) identified the CBC cells as the active intestinal stem cells (ISC) in the crypt[74]. Activation of a Lac Z reporter gene showed that all cell types of the villus epithelium appearing in the ribbon of cells produced from the Lgr5+ marked gene in the CBC cells, were invariably in contact with Paneth cells [75].

Yet, other observations by Potten *et al.*[76] on chimeric mouse embryos proposed a stem cell model where active ISCs were located in the number +4 cell position from the crypt base, on the villus above the Paneth cells. They were identified as DNA (thymidine) label retaining (LRCs) that cycle every 4 hours. It was postulated that the +4 cells are a subset of LRCs, quiescent reserve DNA label retaining cells (LRCs) which are transient precursors of Paneth cells. When the ISC pool is depleted the LRCs can dedifferentiate into Lrg5+ ICS cells[73]. The quiescent and active stem cell subpopulations have separate functions, Lgr5+ for the former and Lgr5- in the latter[12]. They occupy separate yet adjoining niche locations[77]. A definitive lineage tracing of the +4 stem cells employed a marker, Bmi1, a proto- oncogene, which identified reserve, slow cycling stem cells that differed from the active cells[78]. The two stem cell populations showed an interconversion, based on the exchange of Hopx, a homeobox protein reported as specific marker for 4+ cells[79].

6.1 Cell regeneration and plasticity

Following crypt damage, the quiescent Paneth cell precursors can revert back to Lgr5+ stem cells for stem cell replacement and regeneration and thus serve as reserve stem cells. They demonstrated the plasticity of intestinal stem cells[73]. A new probe of the quiescent stem cells came from the induction of histone H2B labeled by yellow fluorescent protein (YFP) that labeled all crypt cells, except Paneth cells. After pulse, chase and dilution of cell division, labeled LRCs in the crypt base were identified by markers for entero-endocrine cells, (Lgr5+) CBC and +4 cells, including Paneth cells. The quiescent +4 cells were also genetically marked with histone H2B using a duel split Cre recombinase fusion, then followed in vivo. This marking separated the non-dividing Paneth cells from all the other cell types. After irradiation induced damage the same LRC cells became self-renewing, multipotent stem cells. The quiescent cells are progenitor-like, capable of reverting to the stem cell state[79]. Further support was found in a study of the TA cells at the +5 position that were identified as secretory multipotent progenitor cells. These cells expressed the Notch ligand, Delta-like (Dll1) and by lineage tracing, they could generate clones of goblet cells, entero-endocrine cells, Paneth cells and tuft cells. When exposed to irradiation injury that destroyed the CBC stem cells, the DLL1+ cells became Lgr5+, CBC stem cells, another measure of adaptability[80,81]. These observations indicate the intestinal crypt contains several populations of reserve stem cells. The plasticity of these reserve progenitors is regulated by the stem cell niche that produces the necessary signals to direct the committed progenitors back into multipotent adult stem cells. In an acute injury, the Lgr5 cells are lost but the Paneth cells and +4 cells are intact. The surviving +4 cells reserve stem cells restore the Lgr5+ stem cell pool for epithelial cell renewal via a TA population that generates a population of Paneth precursor cells which ultimately differentiate into Paneth cells[81]. A model of crypt dynamics with *in vivo* experimentation was presented to analyze the dynamics of ISCs during homeostasis, regenerative repair and tumorigenesis[82]. They noted that active CBC stem cells and +4 quiescent stem cells express functional and molecular markers. Also, CBC stem cells and differentiated entero-endocrine cells high on the villus express Sox9 and EGFP, verifying their connection. Stem cells at the +4 position have been further identified by immuno-staining and lineage tracing (Bmi1, Lrigl, mTert and Hopx), which indicated they are long lived, slow cycling, can be activated by injury, and can repopulate the CBC pool. Also, two intestinal cell markers, Bmi1 and mTert (mouse teleomerase reverse transcriptase) have identified that there are functionally distinct populations. Lgr5 marks active ISCs that are regulated by Wnt, while Bmi1 marks quiescent ISCs that do not respond to Wnt regulation[83]

Summary

Adult somatic stem cells are tissue-specific quiescent or active self-renewing reserve cells that exist in microenvironmental cellular niches. The activated stem cells are accompanied by precursor progenitor cells in various degrees of specialization for terminal differentiated cells. Components of the niche modulates the stem and precursor cell functions. This continuum of cells nominally serves to regenerate cells for tissue/organ homeostasis and exhibits considerable multipotency that decreases as differentiation progresses to the final specialized cell. This plasticity is often attributed to the active recruitment of particular progenitor cells for specific needs. Another view is that individual populations of the stem cell lineage can produce a functional plasticity through modulation of their differentiation by dedifferentiation or transdifferentiation[13]. Rather than a unique catalog of cells, it has been proposed that variations in the stem cell lineage might be achieved transiently . Evidence indicates that the niche does not always elect predetermination of the stem cell lineage but individual signaling imposes specific behavior on them[67]. A second aspect is stem cell response to damage produced by trauma. One proposal is the presence of facultative stem cells, a subset of daughter cells that can revert to stem cells for damage control[84]. It is possible that modulation of differentiation can occur in regeneration of both normal stem cell lineage and trauma induced events. The active selection of poised progenitor cells by the niche is likely the avenue for normal homeostasis, but temporary demands from physiological changes could trigger a rapid replenishment of the stem cell lineage through modulation of the differentiated state. This is illustrated in the niche imposed changes in the behavior of MaSCs during pregnancy and lactation that were not the result of pre-determination[67]. Other stem cells elicit a default response. For example, when HSC cells are depleted, newly introduced differentiated cells behave as the original stem cells[20]. When the neural stem cell pool is depleted, glial cells and melanocytes dedifferentiate into an intermediate bipotent progenitor[44]. After depletion of intestinal stem cells, the label retaining cells can dedifferentiate into Lgr5 intestinal cells[79]. In response to injury, differentiated Schwann cells can dedifferentiate into stem-like cells [45]. Similarly, after destruction of the stem cell population from trauma, the stem cells may be replaced by differentiated osteoblasts from the niche which would evoke their de-differentiation[22]. Following destruction of the crypt columnar cells, the Notch ligand expressing cells become Lgr5+ CBC stem cells[80,81]. After damage to the intestinal crypt, the Paneth cells can also revert to Lgr5 cells[72]. Evidence suggests that there are functionally different quiescent and active stem cells in the intestine. The Bmi1 quiescent cells respond to

injury for regeneration, whereas the Lgr5 population acts during homeostasis[83]. The regulatory potential of the niche also affects differentiation of cells from stem cells of different cell lineages[68]. Neural stem cells are modified to those of the mammary gland after transplantation into the mammary crypt[85]. Similarly, the mammary niche can redirect the cell fate of spermatogenic cells[86]. Both examples illustrate the regulatory power of the niche to produce adaptive changes in differentiation of the stem cell lineage.

References

1. Slack JM. Origin of stem cells in organogenesis. Science. 2008;322(5907):1498-501.
2. Jones DL, Wagers AJ. No place like home: anatomy and function of the stem cell niche. Nat Rev Mol Cell Biol. 2008;9(1):11-21.
3. Spradling A, Drummond-Barbosa D, Kai T. Stem cells find their niche. Nature.2001;414(6859):98-104.
4. Sell S. Stem cell origin of cancer and differentiation therapy. Crit Rev Oncol Hematol. 2004 ;51(1):1-28.
5. Scadden DT. The stem-cell niche as an entity of action. Nature. 2006;441(7097):1075-9.
6. Moore KA, Lemischka IR. Stem cells and their niches. Science. 2006;311(5769):1880-5.
7. Tropepe V, Turksen K. The ontogeny of somatic stem cells. Stem Cell Rev. 2012;8(2):548-50.
8. Cheung TH, Rando TA. Molecular regulation of stem cell quiescence. Nat Rev Mol Cell Biol. 2013;14(6):329-40.
9. Clevers H, Loh KM, Nusse R. Stem cell signaling. An integral program for tissue renewal and regeneration: Wnt signaling and stem cell control. Science.2014;346(6205):1248012.
10. Tang DG. Understanding cancer stem cell heterogeneity and plasticity. Cell Res. 2012;22(3):457-72.
11. Li L, Clevers H. Coexistence of quiescent and active adult stem cells in mammals. Science. 2010;327(5965):542-5.
12. Takeda N, Jain R, LeBoeuf MR, Wang Q, Lu MM, Epstein JA. Interconversion between intestinal stem cell populations in distinct niches. Science. 2011;334(6061):1420-4.
13. Blau HM, Brazelton TR, Weimann JM. The evolving concept of a stem cell: entity or function? Cell. 2001;105(7):829-41.
14. Clevers H. STEM CELLS. What is an adult stem cell? Science. 2015;350(6266):1319-20.
15. Orkin SH, Zon LI. Hematopoiesis: an evolving paradigm for stem cell biology.Cell. 2008;132(4):631-44.
16. Phillips RL, Ernst RE, Brunk B, Ivanova N, Mahan MA, Deanehan JK, Moore KA, Overton GC, Lemischka IR. The genetic program of hematopoietic stem cells. Science. 2000;288(5471):1635-40.
17. Ding L, Morrison SJ. Haematopoietic stem cells and early lymphoid progenitors occupy distinct bone marrow niches. Nature. 2013;495(7440):231-5.
18. Yokota T, Oritani K, Butz S, Kokame K, Kincade PW, Miyata T, Vestweber D, Kanakura Y. The endothelial antigen ESAM marks primitive hematopoietic progenitors throughout life in mice. Blood. 2009;113(13):2914-23.
19. Morrison SJ, Spradling AC. Stem cells and niches: mechanisms that promote stem cell maintenance throughout life. Cell. 2008;132(4):598-611.
20. Seita J, Weissman IL. Hematopoietic stem cell: self-renewal versus differentiation. Wiley Interdisc Rev Syst Biol Med. 2010;2(6):640-53.
21. Rieger MA, Hoppe PS, Smejkal BM, Eitelhuber AC, Schroeder T. Hematopoietic cytokines can instruct lineage choice. Science. 2009;325(5937):217-8.
22. Ding L, Saunders TL, Enikolopov G, Morrison SJ. Endothelial and perivascular cells maintain haematopoietic stem cells. Nature. 2012;481(7382):457-62.
23. Tweedell KS. The urodele limb regeneration blastema: the cell potential. ScientificWorldJournal. 2010;10:954-71.
24. Cabezas-Wallscheid N, Trumpp A. STEM CELLS. Potency finds its niches. Science. 2016;351(6269):126-7.
25. Khan JA, Mendelson A, Kunisaki Y, Birbrair A, Kou Y, Arnal-Estapé A, Pinho S, Ciero P, Nakahara F, Ma'ayan A, Bergman A, Merad M, Frenette PS. Fetal liver hematopoietic stem cell niches associate with portal vessels. Science. 2016;351(6269):176-80.

26. Notta F, Zandi S, Takayama N, Dobson S, Gan OI, Wilson G, Kaufmann KB, McLeod J, Laurenti E, Dunant CF, McPherson JD, Stein LD, Dror Y, Dick JE. Distinct routes of lineage development reshape the human blood hierarchy across ontogeny. Science. 2016 Jan 8;351(6269):aab2116.

27. Paul F, Arkin Y, Giladi A, Jaitin DA, Kenigsberg E, Keren-Shaul H, Winter D, Lara-Astiaso D, Gury M, Weiner A, David E, Cohen N, Lauridsen FK, Haas S, Schlitzer A, Mildner A, Ginhoux F, Jung S, Trumpp A, Porse BT, Tanay A, Amit I. Transcriptional Heterogeneity and Lineage Commitment in Myeloid Progenitors. Cell. 2015;163(7):1663-77.

28. Gage FH. Mammalian neural stem cells. Science. 2000;287(5457):1433-8.

29. Doetsch F, Caillé I, Lim DA, García-Verdugo JM, Alvarez-Buylla A.Subventricular zone astrocytes are neural stem cells in the adult mammalian brain. Cell. 1999;97(6):703-16.

30. Götz M, Huttner WB. The cell biology of neurogenesis. Nat Rev Mol Cell Biol. 2005;6(10):777-88.

31. Anthony TE, Klein C, Fishell G, Heintz N. Radial glia serve as neuronal progenitors in all regions of the central nervous system. Neuron. 2004;41(6):881-90.

32. Alvarez-Buylla A, García-Verdugo JM, Tramontin AD. A unified hypothesis on the lineage of neural stem cells. Nat Rev Neurosci. 2001;2(4):287-93.

33. Ihrie RA, Alvarez-Buylla A. Cells in the astroglial lineage are neural stem cells. Cell Tissue Res. 2008;331(1):179-91

34. Kriegstein A, Alvarez-Buylla A. The glial nature of embryonic and adult neural stem cells. Annu Rev Neurosci. 2009;32:149-84.

35. Grabel L. Developmental origin of neural stem cells: the glial cell that could. Stem Cell Rev. 2012;8(2):577-85.

36. Lin R, Iacovitti L. Classic and novel stem cell niches in brain homeostasis and repair. Brain Res. 2015;1628(Pt B):327-42.

37. Ottone C, Krusche B, Whitby A, Clements M, Quadrato G, Pitulescu ME, Adams RH, Parrinello S. Direct cell-cell contact with the vascular niche maintains quiescent neural stem cells. Nat Cell Biol. 2014;16(11):1045-56.

38. Kawaguchi D, Furutachi S, Kawai H, Hozumi K, Gotoh Y. Dll1 maintains quiescence of adult neural stem cells and segregates asymmetrically during mitosis. Nat Commun. 2013;4:1880.

39. 39. Jones KM, Sarić N, Russell JP, Andoniadou CL, Scambler PJ, Basson MA. CHD7 maintains neural stem cell quiescence and prevents premature stem cell depletion in the adult hippocampus. Stem Cells. 2015;33(1):196-210.

40. Silva-Vargas V, Crouch EE, Doetsch F. Adult neural stem cells and their niche: a dynamic duo during homeostasis, regeneration, and aging. Curr Opin Neurobiol. 2013;23(6):935-42.

41. Riquelme PA, Drapeau E, Doetsch F. Brain micro-ecologies: neural stem cell niches in the adult mammalian brain. Philos Trans R Soc Lond B Biol Sci. 2008;363(1489):123-37.

42. Fuentealba LC, Obernier K, Alvarez-Buylla A. Adult neural stem cells bridge their niche. Cell Stem Cell. 2012;10(6):698-708.

43. Tong CK, Chen J, Cebrián-Silla A, Mirzadeh Z, Obernier K, Guinto CD, Tecott LH, García-Verdugo JM, Kriegstein A, Alvarez-Buylla A. Axonal control of the adult neural stem cell niche. Cell Stem Cell. 2014;14(4):500-11.

44. Dupin E, Real C, Glavieux-Pardanaud C, Vaigot P, Le Douarin NM. Reversal of developmental restrictions in neural crest lineages: transition from Schwann cells to glial-melanocytic precursors in vitro. Proc Natl Acad Sci U S A. 2003;100(9):5229-33.

45. Jessen KR, Mirsky R. The origin and development of glial cells in peripheral nerves. Nat Rev Neurosci. 2005;6(9):671-82.

46. Takahashi Y, Sipp D, Enomoto H. Tissue interactions in neural crest cell development and disease. Science. 2013;341(6148):860-3.

47. Masaki T, Qu J, Cholewa-Waclaw J, Burr K, Raaum R, Rambukkana A. Reprogramming adult Schwann cells to stem cell-like cells by leprosy bacilli promotes dissemination of infection. Cell. 2013;152(1-2):51-67.

48. Xin L, Ide H, Kim Y, Dubey P, Witte ON. In vivo regeneration of murine prostate from dissociated cellpopulations of postnatal epithelia and urogenital sinus mesenchyme . Proc Natl Acad Sci U S A. 2003; 100: (Suppl 1) 11896-903.

49. Xin L, Lukacs RU, Lawson DA, Cheng D, Witte ON. Self-renewal and multilineage differentiation in vitro from murine prostate stem cells. Stem Cells. 2007;25(11):2760-9.

50. Burger PE, Xiong X, Coetzee S, Salm SN, Moscatelli D, Goto K, Wilson EL. Sca-1 expression identifies stem cells in the proximal region of prostatic ducts with high capacity to reconstitute prostatic tissue. Proc Natl Acad Sci U S A. 2005;102(20):7180-5.

51. Leong KG, Wang BE, Johnson L, Gao WQ. Generation of a prostate from a single adult stem cell. Nature. 2008;456(7223):804-8.

52. Lawson DA, Xin L, Lukacs RU, Cheng D, Witte ON. Isolation and functional characterization of murine prostate stem cells. Proc Natl Acad Sci U S A. 2007;104(1):181-6.

53. Richardson GD, Robson CN, Lang SH, Neal DE, Maitland NJ, Collins AT. CD133, a novel marker for human prostatic epithelial stem cells. J Cell Sci. 2004;117(Pt 16):3539-45.

54. Garraway IP, Sun W, Tran CP, Perner S, Zhang B, Goldstein AS, Hahm SA, Haider M, Head CS, Reiter RE, Rubin MA, Witte ON. Human prostate sphere-forming cells represent a subset of basal epithelial cells capable of glandular regeneration in vivo. Prostate. 2010;70(5):491-501.

55. Goldstein AS, Stoyanova T, Witte ON. Primitive origins of prostate cancer: in vivo evidence for prostate-regenerating cells and prostate cancer-initiating cells. Mol Oncol. 2010;4(5):385-96.

56. Ousset M, Van Keymeulen A, Bouvencourt G, Sharma N, Achouri Y, Simons BD, Blanpain C. Multipotent and unipotent progenitors contribute to prostate postnatal development. Nat Cell Biol. 2012;14(11):1131-8.

57. Shahi P, Seethammagari MR, Valdez JM, Xin L, Spencer DM. Wnt and Notch pathways have interrelated opposing roles on prostate progenitor cell proliferation and differentiation. Stem Cells. 2011;29(4):678-88.

58. Luo W, Rodriguez M, Valdez JM, Zhu X, Tan K, Li D, Siwko S, Xin L, Liu M. Lgr4 is a key regulator of prostate development and prostate stem cell differentiation. Stem Cells. 2013;31(11):2492-505.

59. Strand DW, Goldstein AS. The many ways to make a luminal cell and a prostate cancer cell. Endocr Relat Cancer. 2015;22(6):T187-97.

60. Faraldo MM, Taddei-De La Hosseraye I, Teulière J, Deugnier MA, Moumen M, Thiery JP, Glukhova MA. [Mammary gland development: Role of basal myoepithelial cells]. J Soc Biol. 2006;200(2):193-8.

61. Petersen OW, Polyak K. Stem cells in the human breast. Cold Spring Harb Perspect Biol. 2010;2(5):a003160.

62. Shackleton M, Vaillant F, Simpson KJ, Stingl J, Smyth GK, Asselin-Labat ML, Wu L, Lindeman GJ, Visvader JE. Generation of a functional mammary gland from a single stem cell. Nature. 2006;439(7072):84-8.

63. Wang D, Cai C, Dong X, Yu QC, Zhang XO, Yang L, Zeng YA. Identification of multipotent mammary stem cells by protein C receptor expression. Nature. 2015;517(7532):81-4.

64. Van Keymeulen A, Rocha AS, Ousset M, Beck B, Bouvencourt G, Rock J, Sharma N, Dekoninck S, Blanpain C. Distinct stem cells contribute to mammary gland development and maintenance. Nature. 2011;479(7372):189-93.

65. Hassiotou F, Beltran A, Chetwynd E, Stuebe AM, Twigger AJ, Metzger P, Trengove N, Lai CT, Filgueira L, Blancafort P, Hartmann PE. Breastmilk is a novel source of stem cells with multilineage differentiation potential. Stem Cells. 2012;30(10):2164-74.

66. Rios AC, Fu NY, Lindeman GJ, Visvader JE. In situ identification of bipotent stem cells in the mammary gland. Nature. 2014;506(7488):322-7.

67. LaBarge MA, Nelson CM, Villadsen R, Fridriksdottir A, Ruth JR, Stampfer MR, Petersen OW, Bissell MJ. Human mammary progenitor cell fate decisions are products of interactions with combinatorial microenvironments. Integr Biol (Camb). 2009;1(1):70-9.

68. LaBarge MA. On stem cells in the human breast. Cold Spring Harb Perspect Biol. 2012;4(5). pii: a013441.

69. Mishra L, Shetty K, Tang Y, Stuart A, Byers SW. The role of TGF-beta and Wnt signaling in gastrointestinal stem cells and cancer. Oncogene. 2005;24(37):5775-89.

70. Medema JP, Vermeulen L. Microenvironmental regulation of stem cells in intestinal homeostasis and cancer. Nature. 2011;474(7351):318-26.

71. Cheng H, Leblond CP. Origin, differentiation and renewal of the four main epithelial cell types in the mouse small intestine. V. Unitarian Theory of the origin of the four epithelial cell types. Am J Anat. 1974;141(4):537-61.

72. Clevers H. The intestinal crypt, a prototype stem cell compartment. Cell. 2013;154(2):274-84.

73. Clevers H, Batlle E. SnapShot: the intestinal crypt. Cell. 2013;152(5):1198-1198.e2.

74. Clevers H. Stem Cells: A unifying theory for the crypt. Nature. 2013;495(7439):53-4.

75. Barker N, van de Wetering M, Clevers H. The intestinal stem cell. Genes Dev. 2008;22(14):1856-64.

76. Potten CS. Extreme sensitivity of some intestinal crypt cells to X and gamma irradiation. Nature. 1977;269(5628):518-21.

77. Li VS, Clevers H. In vitro expansion and transplantation of intestinal crypt stem cells. Gastroenterology. 2012;143(1):30-4.

78. Sangiorgi E, Capecchi MR. Bmi1 is expressed in vivo in intestinal stem cells. Nat Genet. 2008;40(7):915-20.

79. Buczacki SJ, Zecchini HI, Nicholson AM, Russell R, Vermeulen L, Kemp R, Winton DJ. Intestinal label-retaining cells are secretory precursors expressing Lgr5. Nature. 2013;495(7439):65-9.

80. van Es JH, Sato T, van de Wetering M, Lyubimova A, Nee AN, Gregorieff A, Sasaki N, Zeinstra L, van den Born M, Korving J, Martens AC, Barker N, van Oudenaarden A, Clevers H. Dll1+ secretory progenitor cells revert to stem cells upon crypt damage. Nat Cell Biol. 2012;14(10):1099-104.

81. Barker N. Adult intestinal stem cells: critical drivers of epithelial homeostasis and regeneration. Nat Rev Mol Cell Biol. 2014;15(1):19-33.

82. Carulli AJ, Samuelson LC, Schnell S. Unraveling intestinal stem cell behavior with models of crypt dynamics. Integr Biol (Camb). 2014;6(3):243-57.

83. Yan KS, Chia LA, Li X, Ootani A, Su J, Lee JY, Su N, Luo Y, Heilshorn SC, Amieva MR, Sangiorgi E, Capecchi MR, Kuo CJ. The intestinal stem cell markers Bmi1 and Lgr5 identify two functionally distinct populations. Proc Natl Acad Sci U S A. 2012;109(2):466-71.

84. Visvader JE, Clevers H. Tissue-specific designs of stem cell hierarchies. Nat Cell Biol. 2016;18(4):349-55.

85. Booth BW, Mack DL, Androutsellis-Theotokis A, McKay RD, Boulanger CA, Smith GH. The mammary microenvironment alters the differentiation repertoire of neural stem cells. Proc Natl Acad Sci U S A. 2008;105(39):14891-6.

86. Boulanger CA, Mack DL, Booth BW, Smith GH. Interaction with the mammary microenvironment redirects spermatogenic cell fate in vivo. Proc Natl Acad Sci U S A. 2007;104(10):3871-6.

Abbreviation

Ang1	Angiopoietin, vascular growth factor
Bmi1	Proto-oncogene
BMP	Bone morphogenetic protein
c-kit	Receptor for tyrosine kinase
Cre-	Recombinase site specific enzyme for DNA
ECM	Extracellular matrix
EFFR	Epidermal growth factor receptor
FACS	Fluorescence activated cell sorting
FGF	Fibroblast growth factor
GFAP	Glial fibrillary acidic protein
Hox	Transmission factors for axial patterning
Hopx	Homeobox for lethality
IGF	Insulin-like growth factor
LaxZ	Transgene for β galactosidase
Lrg5	Leucine g protein receptor
Lin-	Lineage (negative) antigen
MEP	Myoepithelial cell
Notch	Transmembrane protein signaling pathway
OPN	Osteopontin, bone matrix protein
Pax6	Paired box transcription factor, brain
PDGF	Platlet derived growth factor
Pten	Phosphatase and tensin protein
SHH	Sonic hedgehog signaling pathway
SCA-1	General stem cell antigen
Sox2	Sex determining transcription factor
TGAFβ	Transforming growth factor signaling pathway
Tie	Angiopoietin receptor
Trop2	Trophoblast cell surface glycoprotein
VEGF	Vascular endothelial growth factor
Wnt	Signaling transduction pathway

Potential Conflicts of Interests

None

Corresponding Author

Kenyon S. Tweedell, Department of Biological Sciences, University of Notre Dame, Notre Dame IN 46556 USA;
Email Tweedell.1@nd.edu

5

Mouse iPSC generated with porcine reprogramming factors as a model for studying the effects of non-silenced heterologous transgenes on pluripotency

Petkov SG[1], Glage S[2], Niemann H[3]

Abstract

Mouse somatic cells can be reprogrammed to pluripotency by the ectopic expression of four pluripotency transcription factors, Oct4, Sox2, c-myc, and Klf4. Usually, silencing of the exogenous reprogramming factors is considered to be essential for complete reprogramming and differentiation. In the vast majority of studies, murine pluripotency transcription factor sequences have been used for the reprogramming of mouse fibroblasts to induced pluripotent stem cells (iPSC). The effectiveness of xenogeneic transcription factors in miPSC generation has not yet been investigated in detail. Here, we evaluated transposon-based vectors with four porcine pluripotency factors for their ability to reprogram mouse fetal fibroblasts (MEFs) harboring an Oct4-EGFP reporter construct to pluripotency. Additionally, we examined the effects of the non-silenced heterologous transgenes on the expression levels of key endogenous pluripotency markers and the differentiation capacities of the miPSC. Within 8 days of transfection with porcine reprogramming transcription factors the MEFs acquired typical compact miPSC morphology and upregulated expression of endogenous Oct4 and other critical pluripotency genes. Consequently, the transgenes under the control of the TetO promoter became silenced, while the CAG-controlled constructs were expressed throughout the period of culture. Despite the continuous transgene expression, the CAG-miPSC showed normal morphology and were capable of differentiation into the three primary germ layers *in vitro* and *in vivo*. However, the expression levels of important endogenous pluripotency markers, Klf4, c-myc, Rex1, and Utf1, were significantly lower in CAG-miPSC compared with TetO-miPSC with silenced reprogramming cassettes. Surprisingly, the endogenous Oct4 and Sox2 expression levels were not affected by the residual transgene expression. Our results suggest that porcine reprogramming transcription factors are suitable for production of miPSC, but silencing of the heterologous transgenes may be necessary for complete reprogramming to pluripotency.

Key Words: iPSC; Reprogramming; Silencing

Introduction

The fate of a terminally differentiated somatic cell can be reversed by ectopic expression of pluripotency-related factors, as demonstrated by Takahashi and Yamanaka[1]. In experiments that have since revolutionized the stem cell field, it was demonstrated that elevated expression of only four proteins such as Oct4, Sox2, c-myc, and Klf4 leads to upregulation of endogenous pluripotency transcription factors and ultimately to acquisition of pluripotent characteristics by the reprogrammed cells[2,3]. To underscore the difference to alternative reprogramming methods (e.g. by somatic cell nuclear transfer, cell extracts, etc.), the resulting stem cells have been termed "induced pluripotent stem cells" (iPSC). During the reprogramming process, the balance between the expression levels of the endogenous pluripotency genes and the transgenes is thought to be critical for the success of the reprogramming of somatic cells to iPSC, with the epigenetic silencing of the retroviral transgenes coinciding with the up-regulation of the endogenes[4]. It has been shown that over-expression of Oct4 in mouse embryonic stem cells (mESC) leads to mesodermal differentiation[5], while elevated Sox2 expression causes neuroectodermal specification[6]. Consequently, the net concentration levels of Oct4 and Sox2 in the iPSC would need to

be maintained within a narrow range characteristic for ESC. In support of this hypothesis, it was demonstrated that following upregulation of the corresponding endogenous pluripotency factors, the transgenes became gradually silenced in successfully reprogrammed iPS cells[7,8]. Persisting transgene expression results in perturbations in the reprogramming process, usually leading to partially reprogrammed states (Class I iPSC), as shown by Mikkelsen and co-workers[9]. Residual transgene expression restricted the differentiation capacities of human iPSC[10] and affected epigenetic signatures and gene expression levels of miPSC compared with mESC[11]. Moreover, in a recent report, miPSC produced with transposon-delivered transgenes that were continuously expressed by supplementation with doxycycline (DOX) were reversed to an alternative pluripotency state (F-state), characterized by aberrant colony morphology and dependency on the continuous transgene expression for their maintenance[12].

It has been convincingly demonstrated that the differentiation capacities of murine iPSC lines with constitutive expression of non-silenced reprogramming factors are limited. However, conflicting results were reported by different research groups. The miPSC produced in the first attempts of Takahashi and Yamanaka[1] did not silence the reprogramming factors and were not able to differentiate

Author Names in full: Stoyan G Petkov[1], Silke Glage[2], Heiner Niemann[3]

[1] German Primate Center, Goettingen, Germany, [2] Hannover Medical School, Hannover, Germany, [3] Institute for Farm Animal Genetics (FLI), Neustadt, Germany

and form chimeras. Similarly, transgene-expressing miPSC were unable to differentiate and upon injection into immunodefficient mice formed homogenous tumors, consisting of undifferentiated cells expressing high levels of Oct4[13]. On the other hand, the use of a constitutively expressed reprogramming cassette led to miPSC with normal ESC-like characteristics, which were capable of forming the three primary germ layers in teratomas[14]. However, these cells also exhibited gene expression differences compared with ESC and excision of the loxP-flanked transgenes resulted in miPSC with complete pluripotency characteristics.

While the vast majority of miPSC described in the literature have been generated with murine pluripotency transcription factors, there have been very few reports on the use of transgenes from other species. Only one study has reported the use of human reprogramming factors to successfully reprogram mouse fibroblasts to iPSC[15]. In addition, the silencing of non-murine reprogramming factors as well as the effects of the non-silenced xenogeneic transgenes on the expression of endogenous pluripotency genes and its relationship with differentiation of miPSC have not been yet investigated. Here, we explored the possibility to use porcine transcription factors for the reprogramming of mouse embryonic fibroblasts (MEFs) to pluripotency. Established miPSC lines constitutively expressing the four porcine Yamanaka factors (pOCT4, pSOX2, pc-MYC, and pKLF4) under the control of the ubiquitous CAG promoter were characterized for pluripotency and their differentiation potential together with the expression levels of master pluripotency genes were compared with those of miPSC produced either with a silenced or CRE recombinase-excised reprogramming cassette.

Materials and methods

Unless specified otherwise, the chemicals and kits used in this study were purchased from Sigma-Andrich.

Derivation of mouse fetal fibroblasts for feeder cells and reprogramming

Outbred NMRI mice were purchased from Harlan Laboratories (Horst, Netherlands) and were used to establish MEFs for feeder layers. C57BL/6 mice harboring Oct4-EGFP pluripotency gene reporter (OG2) were kindly provided by Prof. Hans Schoeler (Max-Planck-Institute for Molecular Biomedicine, Muenster, Germany) and were used to generate MEFs for reprogramming to iPSC. For the generation of MEFs, pregnant mice were sacrificed at day 13-13.5 of gestation, fetuses were dissected and the heads, livers, mesonephros, and hearts were removed. The remaining parts, including limb buds and body wall were minced with a scalpel blade, incubated in trypsin/EDTA solution for 20 min at 37°C and disaggregated to single cells and clumps by vigorous pipetting after adding warm culture medium. The culture medium used was high glucose DMEM (Lonza), supplemented with 15% fetal bovine serum (FBS) (Gibco, Lot 41Q2035K), non-essential amino acids (GE Healthcare), sodium pyruvate, 2 mM Glutamine (GE Healthcare), and 0.1 mM 2-mercaptoethanol. Feeder cells were produced by treating MEFs from NMRI mice with 10 µg/ml mitomycin C for 2 hours.

Reprogramming expression vectors

The construction of the Sleeping Beauty (SB) transposon plasmids with either the Tet-On (TetO) promoter (SB-TetO-pOSMK-IRES-Tomato, used together with SB-CMV-rTA-IRES-Neo[r]) or with the constitutive CAG promoter (SB-CAG-pOSMK-IRES-Tomato) for expression of the porcine OCT4, SOX2, c-MYC, and KLF4 have been described previously[16]. To create a CRE-excisable version, the CAG promoter and the polyadenylation signal were amplified using loxP-containing forward or reverse primer, respectively, and these

modified sequences were used to replace the originals by standard DNA cloning techniques, thus generating a loxP-flanked CAG-pOSMK-IRES-Tomato-pA cassette. For efficient integration into MEFs, the plasmid with a hyperactive version of the SB (SB100x) was co-transfected with each of the reprogramming transposons. The SB transposon vector backbone and transposase expression plasmids were provided by Dr. Zoltan Ivics (Paul-Ehrlich-Institute, Langen, Germany).

Mouse iPSC generation and culture

Three different MEF lines from C57BL/6-OG2 mice were electroporated at passages 3-4 with the SB transposon and transposase plasmids as described by Petkov et al. [16] and plated on gelatinized T75 flasks. The cells were cultured in MEFs culture medium for 2-3 days and then were then split 1:3-1:4 to T75 flasks with mitotically inactivated MEF feeders and the medium was supplemented with 1000 U/ml ESGRO murine leukemia inhibitory factor (mLIF) (Millipore). When vectors with the TetO promoter were used, the medium was supplemented with 5 µg/ml DOX. The OCT4-EGFP-positive colonies with ESC-like morphology were manually picked at day 10-11 post-transfection, disaggregated with Trypsin/EDTA, and cultured individually on mytomycin C-inactivated MEFs to establish individual cell lines. The established miPSC were regularly split every 3-4 days at ratio 1:15-1:20 by trypsinization and maintained on fresh feeders in ESGRO medium for over 70 passages. For generation of transgene-free miPSC, the miPSC harboring the "floxed" version of the reprogramming transposon were transfected with SB-CAG-CRE-IRES-Puro[r] vector using Lipofectamine 2000 (Life Sciences) as instructed by the manufacturer and selected with culture medium supplemented with 3 µg/ml puromycin.

Alkaline phosphatase (AP) staining and immunocytochemistry

The cultured were fixed with 4% Formalin solution for 5 min (for AP) or 15 min (antibody staining) and washed with PBS prior to further processing. For AP staining, a solution containing 1 mg/ml Fast Red and 0.4 mg/ml Naphtol-BI-Phosphate in AP-buffer (100 mM NaCl2, 100 mM Tris (pH 9.5), and 50 mM MgCl2) was applied to the fixed wells. The AP-positive cells were discerned by the formation of insoluble red-brown precipitate. The presence of SSEA-1, SSEA-3, SSEA-4, TRA-1-60, and TRA-1-81 expression in miPSC was assessed by incubation with primary antibodies (Thermo; Cat. numbers 41-1200, MA1-020X, 41-4000, 41-1000, 41-1100, respectively), diluted in PBS with 2% Knockout Serum Replacement (KSR) (Invitrogen) at concentration 10 ng/ml for 1 hour, followed by washing with PBS and incubation with the secondary peroxidase - conjugated antibody. For staining of neuronal-like cells, the anti-PGP 9.5 primary antibody (DACO) was used in a similar protocol. The expressed proteins were visualized after incubation with peroxidase substrate from AEC staining kit.

Reverse transcription, PCR, and real-time PCR

For RNA extraction, the miPSC cultures were washed 3 times with Ca- and Mg-free PBS and incubated in the same solution for 15 minutes at 37 degrees C. The miPSC colonies were detached from the feeders by gentle pipetting, collected in a 15 ml centrifuge tube and allowed to settle on the bottom of the tube for 10 min. The supernatant containing single cells (presumably mostly feeder MEFs) was carefully removed, the pellet was re-suspended in PBS and the colonies were pelleted by centrifugation, lysed in TRI reagent (Ambion), and total RNA was extracted as instructed by the manufacturer. Reverse-transcription was carried out with MuLV Reverse Transcriptase (Applied Biosystems). Polymerase chain reaction was performed using 50 ng reverse transcribed RNA per 25 µl reaction volume using Platinum Taq Polymerase (Invitrogen).

Real-time relative quantitative analysis was run on the ABI 7500 Fast System using SYBR Green Master Mix (Applied Biosystems). The primers used for PCR and real-time PCR analysis of endogenous mouse pluripotency markers Oct4, Sox2, Nanog, c-myc, Klf4, Rex1, and Utf1 as well as for the differentiation markers alpha fetoprotein (Afp), Sox17, Gata4, Gata6, cardiac troponin, myosin heavy chain (MHC), nestin, β-III tubulin, and Pax6 are shown in Table S1. The primers used for the amplification of the mouse endogenous pluripotency genes were specific only for the mouse cDNA sequences and did not amplify the pig pOSMK cassette (results not shown). The primers used for the amplification of the pOSMK-IRES-Tomato construct were a forward primer binding at the end of KLF4 and a reverse primer binding to IRES (shown in Table S1). The data from the relative quantitative analysis were analyzed with GeneEx software (bioMCC). Statistically significant differences were determined by Student's t-test performed by the same computer program.

Karyotyping

Three lines each from TetO- and CAG miPSC at passages 58-60 were treated with Demecolcine solution (Sigma, D1925) added at 100 μl/10ml culture medium for 35 min. The cells were harvested by trypsinization, incubated in hypotonic solution (0.28% KCl + 0.25% Na Citrate) for 25 min at 37°C, and fixed in cold (-20°C) methanol: acetic acid (3:1) fixative for 1 hour. Metaphase spreads were produced by dropping 50 μl drops onto glass slides placed at a slight angle over steaming water bath (95°C) and waiting 1 min before removal and air drying. The metaphase spreads were stained with 2% Giemsa solution. The metaphase chromosomes of at least 15 metaphase spreads per cell line were counted to determine whether the cells had normal karyotype.

Embryoid body (EB) formation

Mouse iPSC colonies were separated from the feeder as described above in subsection 2.5, disaggregated to single cells with trypsin, and suspended in basic culture medium without ESGRO. "Hanging drops" were then produced by making 25 μl drops on the inner side of a 10 mm Petri dish lid (containing 2000 cells/drop) and placing the lid back on the dish filled with PBS (to prevent drying of the drops). After 5 days in "hanging drops" culture, the emerging embryoid bodies were plated in gelatin-treated 6-well plates and cultured further for 15 days with changes of the medium every 3-4 days. For neuronal differentiation, the attached EBs were cultured in N2 medium (DMEM/F12 supplemented with sodium pyruvate, amino acids, penicillin-streptomycin, and N2 supplement (Thermo)).

Teratoma formation

Prior to conducting the animal experiments, permission was obtained from the local animal welfare authority (LAVES).

Nude immunodeficient mice were produced by mating outbred NMRI strain parents. A total of 13 nude mice (7 mice/TetO group and 6 mice/CAG group) were injected each with 1 x10^6 putative iPSC derived from reprogramming with the porcine vectors subcutaneously in the right flank. The mice were observed daily for 3 weeks. After reaching the critical size of the tumour (1 cm), the animals were sacrificed. Biopsies were taken for DNA/RNA extraction, and tissues were fixed in neutral buffered 4% formalin not exceeding 48 h, dehydrated (Shandon Hypercenter, XP) and subsequently embedded in paraffin (TES, Medite). Sections (2-3 μm thick, microtome Reichert-Jung 2030), were deparaffinized in xylene and H&E stained according to standard protocols. The morphological evaluation for the presence of the three germ layers (Axioskop 40, Zeiss microscope) was performed by a trained pathologist and representative microphotographs were taken (AxioCam MRc, Zeiss).

Results

Reprogramming to pluripotency

Transfected MEFs cultured on inactivated feeders formed O4-EGFP-positive colonies with typical miPSC-like morphology within 7-8 days post-transfection (Figure 1A, D). A number of granular colonies consisting of round, highly refractory cells were also observed.

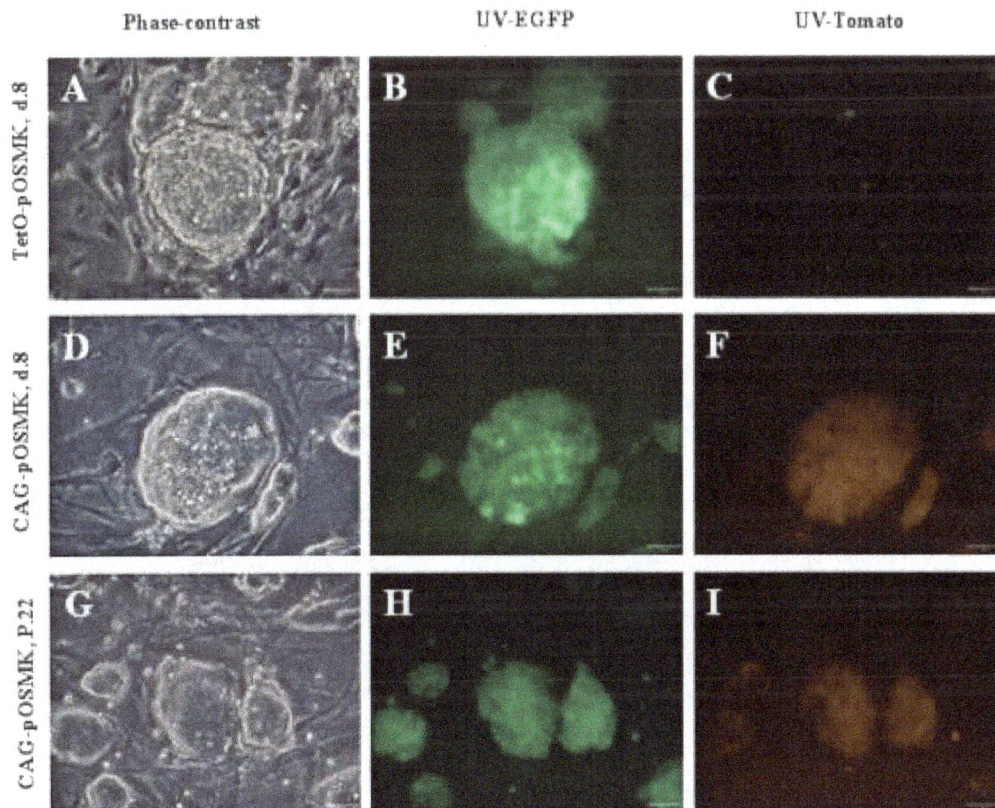

Phase-contrast   UV-EGFP   UV-Tomato

Figure 1. Mouse iPSC generated with Sleeping Beauty transposons carrying porcine reprogramming factors. A) TetO-miPSC at day 8 post-transfection with typical miPSC morphology. B) Oct4-EGFP reporter expression in the colony in image A. C) Silenced pOSMK-IRES-Tomato expression except in some cells in image A. D) CAG-miPSC at day 8 post-transfection. The colony has compact miPSC-like morphology. E) Expression of Oct4-EGFP reporter in the colony shown in image D. F) Expression of non-silenced pOSMK-IRES-Tomato construct in the colony from image D. G) CAG-miPSC at P.22. The colonies maintained compact miPSC morphology. H) Oct4-EGFP reporter expression in the colonies shown in image G. I) Expression of pOSMK-IRES-Tomato in the colonies shown in image G. (All scale bars = 50 μm).

There was no significant difference in the timing of EGFP-positive colony appearance between the different groups where transposons with TetO or CAG were used. In most miPSC colonies produced with the TetO promoter, the Tomato fluorescence (indicating pOSMK transgene expression) disappeared completely from the cells by day 10-11 of primary cultures (Figure 1C), and was no longer detectable in the presence of DOX, indicating successful transgene silencing. The colonies that retained the Tomato fluorescence were not picked. All miPSC produced with CAG promoters retained weak Tomato expression throughout the entire time of culture (>70 passages) (Figure 1 F, I). All of the picked colonies (12 colonies/transfected MEF line) formed clonal lines when cultured in individual wells; however, some TetO-lines showed signs of differentiation after 3-4 passages and were discarded. Five lines from each group were chosen for long-term culture.

Expression of master pluripotency markers

The pluripotency-related surface antigens AP and SSEA-1 were expressed in both groups, while SSEA-3, SSEA-4, TRA-1-61, and TRA-1-80 were not detected (Figure 2). RT-PCR confirmed expression of the endogenous Oct4, Sox2, Nanog, c-myc, Klf4, Rex1, and Utf1 in both CAG- and TetO-miPSC (Figure 3A). Expression of the transgenes was detected only in the CAG group (Figure 3A). To determine whether there was a difference in the expression levels of endogenous pluripotency genes between the CAG and TetO groups, we carried out real-time relative quantitation analysis. While there was no significant difference in the expression of Oct4, Sox2, and Nanog ($P>0.05$), the expression levels of c-myc, Klf4, Rex1, and Utf1 were significantly higher in the TetO group compared with the CAG-miPSC ($p<0.05$) (Figure 3B). When the pOSMK cassette was removed from the CAG group by CRE expression, there was no significant change in the expression levels of the endogenous pluripotency genes ($p>0.05$), except for Utf1, which was up-regulated in the CRE-treated cells ($p<0.01$) (Figure 3C).

Karyotyping

Each of the 6 examined miPSC lines had 20 chromosome pairs and no aberrations from the normal diploid karyotype

were found (Figure S1).

In vitro and in vivo differentiation

The cells from both experimental groups formed EBs within 5 days of differentiation culture in "hanging drops". Upon attachment on gelatin-treated plastic surfaces, the cells expanded and spontaneously differentiated into epithelial-like cells (Figure 4A, endoderm), neuronal-like cells that reacted positively with the anti-PGP 9.5 antibody (Figure 4A, ectoderm), and rhythmically contracting cardiac myocytes (Figure 4A, mesoderm; Video S1). The expression of differentiation markers Afp, Sox17, Gata4, Gata6, MHC, troponin, nestin, β-III tubulin, and Pax6 in EB was confirmed by RT-PCR (Figure 4B).

When injected into immunodefficient mice, 3/7 (43%) mice injected with cells from the TetO group and 6/6 (100%) mice injected with miPSC from the CAG group formed teratomas within 3 weeks post-injection. Histological analysis of the teratomas revealed presence of the three germ layers in teratomas produced with miPSC from both the TetO and CAG groups (Fig. 5). We also visually examined fresh biopsies for the presence of EGFP fluorescence as indication of undifferentiated cells and found EGFP-positive cells in one of the CAG-miPSC-derived teratomas. The expression levels of key endogenous pluripotency genes, the pOSMK transgenes, and main differentiation markers were compared between miPSC from the CAG group and the teratomas by real-time relative quantitative analysis. As expected, Oct4, Nanog, Rex1, and Utf1 were significantly down-regulated, while differentiation markers Afp, Sox17, Gata4, Gata6, Pax6, and Nestin were significantly up-regulated in teratomas (all $p<0.01$) (Fig. 6). There was no significant difference in the expression levels of Sox2 and Klf4, while c-myc was significantly higher expressed in teratomas ($P<0.05$). These results were similar to the TetO group, except for c-myc, which did not show a significant difference (results not shown). Expression of the reprogramming pOSMK cassette could still be detected in two teratomas generated with CAG-miPSC, but the expression levels were low, as suggested by real-time PCR threshold values higher than 33, so relative quantitative analysis could not be reliably completed.

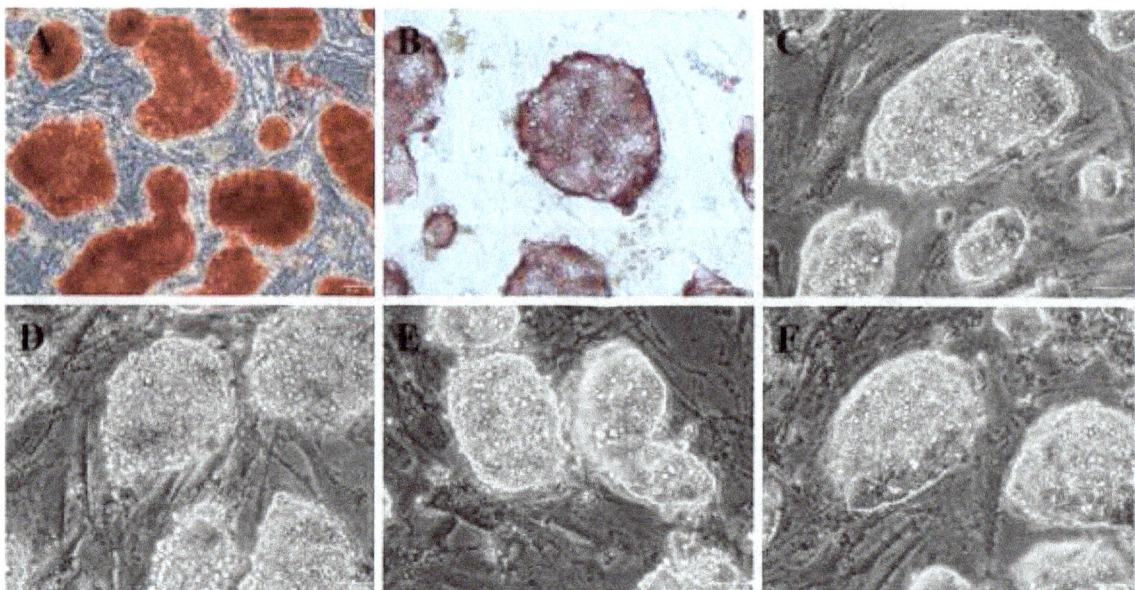

Figure 2. Expression of surface pluripotency markers in CAG-miPSC at P. 22. A) AP. B) SSEA-1. C) SSEA-3. D) SSEA-4 E) TRA-1-60. F) TRA-1-81. (Scale bars = 50 μm).

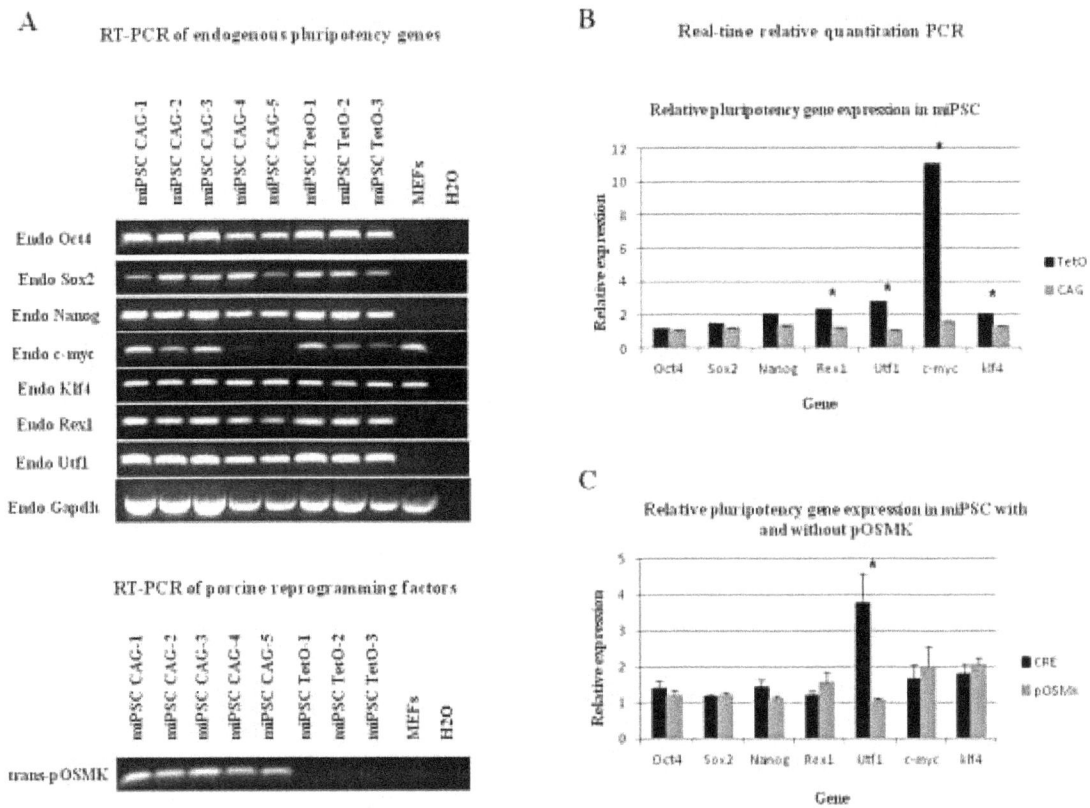

Figure 3. Gene expression in miPSC produced with porcine reprogramming factors. A) RT-PCR analysis of major endogenous pluripotency genes and transgenes in miPSC. B) Real-time relative quantitative analysis of expression level differences between TetO- and CAG-miPSC. C) Real-time relative quantitative analysis of expression level differences between miPSC with CRE-excised and still expressed transgenes. Statistically significant differences (p< 0.05) are indicated with asterisks.

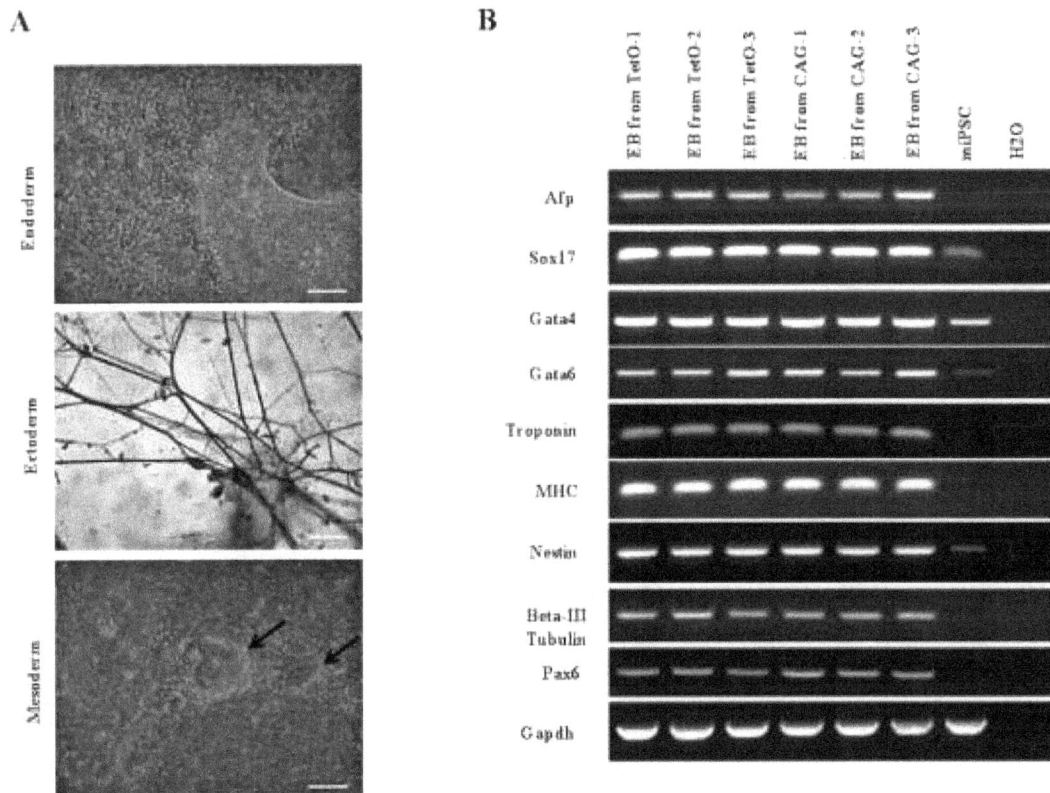

Figure 4. In vitro and in vivo differentiation of miPSC produced with porcine reprogramming factors. A) In vitro differentiation of CAG-miPSC: epithelial-like cells (endoderm) (scale bar = 50 mm), neuronal-like cells positive for PGP 9.5 (ectoderm) (scale bar = 20 mm), and spontaneously contracting cardiac myocytes (mesoderm), indicated with arrows (scale bar = 50 mm). (For additional data on cardiomyocyte contraction, see Supplementary Video 1). B) Expression of differentiation markers in EB outgrowths by RT-PCR.

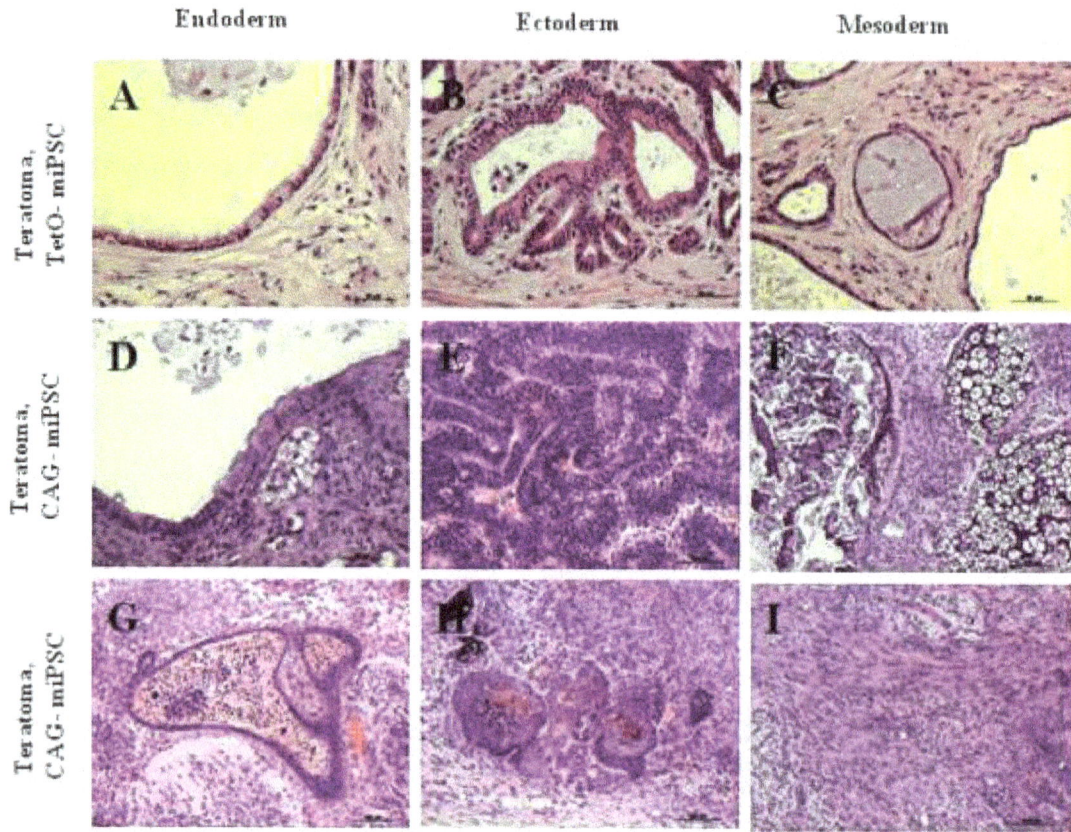

Figure 5. *In vivo differentiation of miPSC in teratomas. TetO-miPSC injected into nude mice formed ciliated epithelium with mucous- producing cells (A), neuronal tubes (B), and connective tissue (C) (scale bars = 50 μm). CAG-miPSC differentiated into ciliated epithelium (D), neural tubes (E), cartilage and bone (F), epithelial cysts (G), keratinized epithelium (H), and connective tissue (I). (Scale bars = 100 μm).*

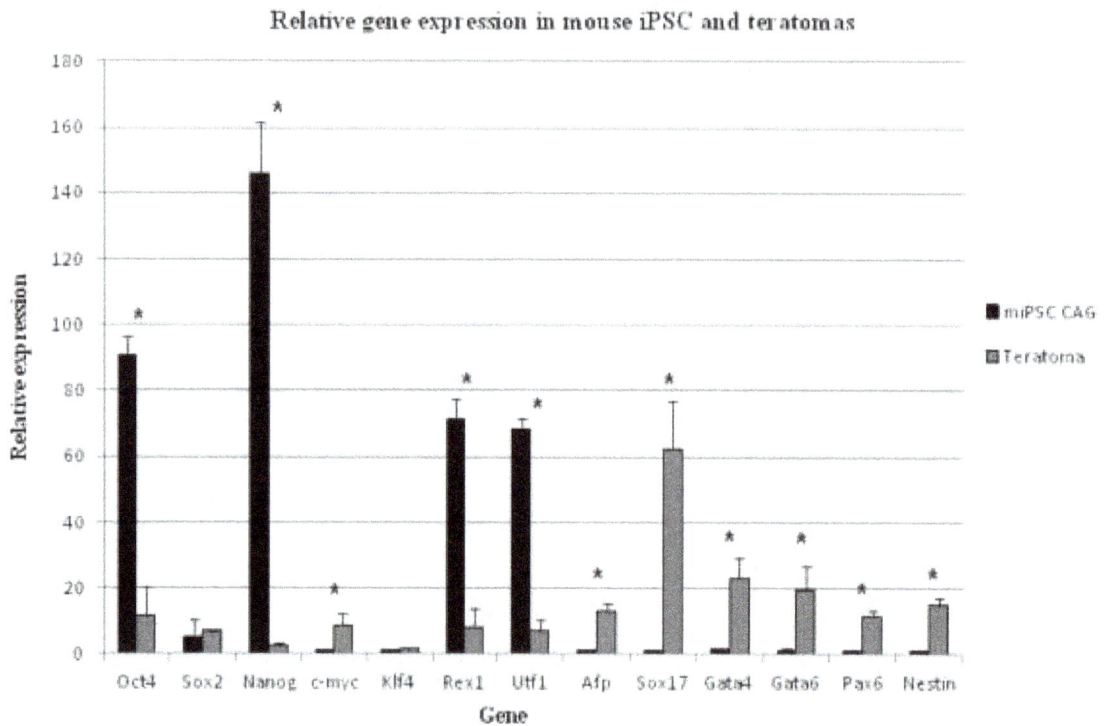

Figure 6. *Real-time relative quantitation analysis of gene expression in CAG-miPSC and teratomas. Statistically significant differences are indicated with asterisks.*

Discussion

Here, we investigated whether four porcine reprogramming transcription factors were able to successfully reprogram MEFs to pluripotency. The amino acid sequences for Oct4, Sox2, c-myc, and Klf4 are evolutionary highly conserved, although not fully identical between mouse and pig (88%, 98%, 93%, and 94%, respectively; amino acid sequence alignments are shown on Figure S2). Thus, it was necessary to confirm that the porcine proteins can in fact reprogram somatic cells across species. As expected, the MEFs changed proliferation and morphology and upregulated endogenous OCT4 expression, as demonstrated by the presence of EGFP fluorescence and subsequently confirmed by RT-PCR. The picked colonies proliferated robustly and established cell lines with typical compact miPSC morphology and expression of key pluripotency markers such as AP, SSEA-1, Oct4, Sox2, Nanog, Klf4, Rex1, and Utf1. At the same time, the TetO-promoter-controlled transgenes were silenced, even in the presence of DOX. This result is in contrast with other reports, where transposon-delivered transgenes were not silenced by the reprogrammed cells if the culture medium was continuously supplemented with DOX[12, 17]. A possible explanation for our results is that the porcine transgenes are more efficiently recognized and silenced by the miPSC. Silencing of the reprogramming transcription factors has been described as an essential prerequisite for successful reprogramming[2, 7- 9]. Thus, porcine reprogramming factors may be useful for the production of miPSC, particularly where significant nucleotide sequence differences between the transgenes and the endogenous pluripotency genes are desired.

Another interesting question of this study was whether the mouse cells would balance the expression levels of key endogenous pluripotency genes with the non-silenced porcine transgenes. We obtained cell lines with silenced (TetO-regulated) and non-silenced (CAG-regulated) reprogramming cassettes, which enabled us to address this question by comparing the expression levels of endogenous pluripotency genes between the two groups. Surprisingly, we found no significant differences in the expression levels of endogenous mouse Oct4 and Sox2 between the cells with silenced vs. expressed transgenes. Additionally, the expression levels of these genes did not change even after the transgenes were removed by expression of CRE recombinase. These results suggest that the porcine transgenes did not participate in the regulation of endogenous Oct4 and Sox2 expression after the initial induction. Moreover, none of the cells from the CAG-group showed any signs of differentiation that would be expected from elevated total Oct4 and Sox2 expression levels. A possible explanation for this outcome could be the very low expression levels of the transgenes, as suggested by our real-time PCR analysis. Another possibility is that the specifying signals ensuing from elevated total Oct4 and Sox2 levels had balanced each other, preventing differentiation into any of the germ layers. On the other hand, the expression levels of the endogenous c-myc, Klf4, Rex1, and Utf1 were significantly lower in cell lines with non-silenced transgenes compared with the TetO group. Excision of the reprogramming cassette by CRE-recombinase resulted in significant upregulation of Utf1, but failed to upregulate the rest.

Despite the deviations in the expression of important pluripotency markers, the cell lines with residual expression of the four Yamanaka factors were capable of differentiation into derivatives of the three primary germ layers *in vitro* and *in vivo* (by forming fully differentiated teratomas) similar to the TetO- group. When we examined the expression levels of pluripotency and differentiation-related genes in teratomas and iPSC lines, we found that, as expected, the pluripotency markers were down-regulated while the differentiation markers were up-regulated, suggesting normal differentiation process in the CAG-iPSC.

Unlike the miPSC in an alternative state of pluripotency (F-state) described recently[12], our miPSC lines with non-silenced reprogramming factors have compact ES-like morphology and do not depend on the expression of the transgenes for their maintenance; therefore, they do not necessarily fall into an alternative pluripotency state category. Nevertheless, it has been shown that even subtle aberrations in miPSC with residual transgene expression could impair the full developmental competency of miPSC[11, 14]. The lower expression of important pluripotency markers such as Rex1, Utf1, and Klf4 in CAG-miPSC suggests that this may also apply for miPSC produced with non-silenced porcine transcription factors. In future work, the cells will be tested for chimera formation to ascertain whether they are fully competent iPSC.

Conclusions

In conclusion, we successfully established miPSC using four porcine reprogramming transcription factors and examined the effects of the non-silenced transgenes on the expression levels of key endogenous pluripotency markers. The residual expression of the transgenes affected expression levels of important pluripotency genes such as c-myc, Klf4, Rex1, and Utf1. These results suggest that porcine pluripotency transcription factors are suitable for reprogramming of mouse somatic cells to pluripotency, but epigenetic silencing of the xenogeneic transgenes may be necessary for complete acquisition of pluripotency.

References

1. Takahashi K. and Yamanaka S. Induction of pluripotent stem cells from mouse embryonic and adult fibroblast cultures by defined factors. Cell 2006; 126(4): 663-76.

2. Okita K, Ichisaka T, Yamanaka S. Generation of germline-competent induced pluripotent stem cells. Nature 2007; 448: 313-7.

3. Takahashi K, Tanabe K, Ohnuki M, Narita M, Ichisaka T, Tomoda K, Yamanaka S. Induction of pluripotent stem cells from adult human fibroblasts by defined factors. Cell 2007; 131(5): 861-72.

4. Hotta A and Ellis J. Retroviral Vector Silencing During iPS Cell Induction: An Epigenetic Beacon that Signals Distinct Pluripotent States. J Cell Bioch. 2008; 105(4): 940–8.

5. Niwa H, Miyazaki J, Smith A. Quantitative expression of Oct-3/4 defines differentiation, dedifferentiation or self-renewal of ES cells. Nat Genet 2000; 24(4): 372–6.

6. Kopp J, Ormsbee B, Desler M, Rizzino A. Small increases in the level of Sox2 trigger the differentiation of mouse embryonic stem cells. Stem Cells 2008; 26(4): 903-11.

7. Papapetrou E, Tomishima M, Chambers S, Mica Y, Reed E, Menon J, Tabar V, Mo Q, Studer L, Sadelain M. Stoichiometric and temporal requirements of Oct4, Sox2, Klf4, and c-Myc expression for efficient human iPSC induction and differentiation. 2009; 106(31): 12759-64.

8. Wernig M, Meissner A, Foreman R, Brambrink T, Ku M, Hochedlinger K, Bernstein BE, Jaenish R. In vitro reprogramming of fibroblasts into a pluripotent ES-cell-like state. Nature 2007; 448(7151): 318–24.

9. Mikkelsen T, Hanna J, Zhang X, Ku M, Wernig M, Schorderet P, Bernstein BE, Jaenish R, Lander ES, Meissner A. Dissecting direct reprogramming through integrative genomic analysis. Nature 2008; 454(7200): 49-55.

10. Ramos-Mejía V, Montes R, Bueno C, Ayllón V, Real P, Rodríguez R, Menendez P. Residual expression of the reprogramming factors prevents differentiation of iPSC generated from human fibroblasts and cord blood CD34+ progenitors. PLoS One 2012; 7(4): e35824.

11. Sommer C, Christodoulou C, Gianotti-Sommer A, Shen S, Sailaja B, Hezroni H, Spira A, Meshorer E, Kotton DN, Mostoslavsky G. Residual expression of reprogramming factors affects the transcriptional program and epigenetic signatures of induced pluripotent stem cells. PLoS One 2012; 7(12): e51711.

12. Tonge PD, Corso AJ, Monetti C, Hussein SM, Puri MS, Michael IP, Li M, Lee DS, Mar JC, Cloonan N, Wood DL, Gauthier ME, Korn O, Clancy JL, Preiss T, Grimmond SM, Shin JY, Seo JS, Wells CA, Rogers IM, Nagy A. Divergent reprogramming routes lead to alternative stem-cell states. Nature 2014; 516(7530), 192-7.

13. Brambrink T, Foreman R, Welstead G, Lengner C, Wernig M, Suh H, Jaenish R. Sequential expression of pluripotency markers during direct reprogramming of mouse somatic cells. Cell Stem Cell 2008; 2(2): 151–9.

14. Sommer CA, Sommer AG, Longmire TA, Christodoulou C, Thomas DD, Gostissa M, Alt FW, Murphy GJ, Kotton DN, Mostoslavsky G. Excision of reprogramming transgenes improves the differentiation potential of iPS cells generated with a single excisable vector. Stem Cells 2010; 28(1): 64-74.

15. Talluri T, Kumar D, Glage S, Garrels W, Ivics Z, Debowski K, Behr R, Kues W. Non-viral reprogramming of fibroblasts into induced pluripotent stem cells by Sleeping Beauty and piggyBac transposons. Bioch Bioph Res Com. 2014; 450(1), 581–7.

16. Petkov S, Hyttel P, Niemann H. The choice of expression vector promoter is an important factor in the reprogramming of porcine fibroblasts into induced pluripotent cells. Cell Repr. 2013; 15(1): 1-8.

17. Woltjen K, Michael IP, Mohseni P, Desai R, Mileikovsky M, Hämäläinen R, Cowling R, Wang W, Liu P, Gertsenstein M, Kaji K, Sung HK, Nagy A. PiggyBac transposition reprograms fibroblasts to induced pluripotent stem cells. Nature 2009; 458(7239): 766–70.

Abbreviations

Afp:	Alpha-fetoprotein
AP:	Alkaline Phosphatase
CAG:	Synthetic Promoter containing the (C) cytomegalovirus early enhancer element, (A) the promoter, the first exon and the first intron of chicken beta-actin gene, and (G) the splice acceptor of the rabbit beta-globin gene
DMEM:	Dulbecco's Modified Eagle's Medium
DOX:	Doxycycline
EGFP:	Enhanced Green Fluorescent Protein
FBS:	Fetal Bovine Serum
iPSC:	Induced Pluripotent Stem Cells
mESC:	Mouse Embryonic Stem Cells
Klf4:	Kruppel-Like Factor 4
MEFs:	Mouse Embryonic Fibroblasts
MHC:	Myosin Heavy Chain
Oct4:	POU Domain, Class 5, Transcription Factor 1
Pax6:	Paired Box Protein 6
PBS:	Phosphate-Buffered Saline
PCR:	Polymerase Chain Reaction
RT:	Reverse Transcription
SB:	Sleeping Beauty Transposon/Transposase
Sox2:	SRY (sex determining region Y)-box 2
Sox17:	SRY (sex determining region Y)-box 17
c-myc:	V-Myc Avian Myelocytomatosis Viral Oncogene Homolog
UTF1:	Undifferentiated Embryonic Cell Transcription Factor 1

Potential Conflicts of Interests

None

Acknowledgments

Dr. Wilfried Kues (Institute of Farm Animal Genetics, Friedrich-Loeffler-Institute, Mariensee, Neustadt, Germany) for the injection of the immunodefficient mice. Dr. Hans Schoeler (Max-Planck-Institute for Molecular Biomedicine, Muenster, Germany) for providing the OG2 reporter mice. Dr. Zoltan Ivics (Paul-Ehrlich Institute, Langen, Germany) for providing the SB transposon backbone and the SB transposase expression plasmid. Dr. Poul Hyttel (University of Copenhagen, Copenhagen, Denmark) for allowing us to use and modify the transposon plasmid which was generated by Dr. Stoyan Petkov in his laboratory.

Sponsor / Grants

German Research Foundation (Deutsche Forschungsgemeinschaft), Grant Ni 256/ 32-1.

Additional Information

Supplementary Information accompanies this article. Supplementary figures, Video and table are linked to the online version of the article.

Corresponding Authors

1. Stoyan Petkov, German Primate Center, Kellnerweg 4,37077 Göttingen, Germany; Email: spetkov@dpz.eu
2. Heiner Niemann, Institute for Farm Animal Genetics, Friedrich-Loeffler-Institute, Hoeltystrasse 10, 31535 Neustadt am Ruebenberge, Germany; Email: heiner.niemann@fli.bund.de

6

Epigallocatechin Gallate Inhibits Mouse Mesenchymal Stem Cell Differentiation to Adipogenic Lineage

Chani B[1], Puri V[2], Sobti RC[3], Puri S[1]

Epigallocatechin gallate (EGCG) is a major component of green tea polyphenols having a potent anti-oxidant potential. Besides inhibiting the growth of many cancer cell types and inducing proliferation and differentiation in keratinocytes, it has been shown to promote reduction of body fat. The fact that mesenchymal stem cells (MSCs) have ability to self-renew and differentiate into the cells of mesodermal lineages, such as fat and bone, it is, thus, possible that EGCG may directly be involved in affecting fat metabolism through its effect on mesenchymal stem cells. Hence, with this aim, the present study was designed to determine the effect of EGCG on mouse mesenchymal stem cells, C3H10T1/2 cells differentiation into adipocytes. To understand this process, the cells were incubated with varying concentrations of EGCG (1 μM, 5 μM, 10 μM, 50 μM) in the presence and /or absence of adipogenic medium for 9 days. The results demonstrated that, EGCG inhibited the cells proliferation, migration and also prevented their differentiation to adipogenic lineage. These effects were analyzed through the inhibition of wound healing activity, reduction in Oil red O stained cells, together with decrease in the expression of Adipisin gene following EGCG treatment. These observations thus demonstrated anti-adipogenic effect of EGCG with a possibility of its role in the therapeutic intervention of obesity.

Key Words: Epigallocatechin gallate, Pluripotency, Mesenchymal stem cell, C3H10T1/2 cells

Introduction

Obesity is characterized by the over-accumulation of fat in the adipose tissue. It is generally considered as a big risk factor for diabetes, hypertension, heart disease and numerous other pathological conditions. Genetic as well as environmental factors are implicated in the genesis of obesity[1].The obese state develops by deposition of increased number of adipocytes via mitogenesis and differentiation processes[2]. Adipocytes store excess energy, but when overloaded they become resistant to insulin, which compromises their ability to accumulate lipids and facilitates alterations in structure and metabolism in remote tissues, such as pancreas, liver and muscles[3-5]. Excessive oxidation in adipose cells is common and triggers cellular stress[6, 7]. So it is conceivable that anti-oxidant and/or anti-inflammatory therapies that act on adipose tissue may have potential benefits in the amelioration of obesity-related diseases. Numerous studies on low-toxicity natural products like Genistein, conjugated Linoleic acid (CLA), Docosahexaenoic acid, Epigallocatechin Gallate, Quercetin, Resveratrol and Ajoene have shown their effects on adipocytes during stage specific development. These polyphenols, thus, classify themselves as one of the strategy for preventing obesity and treating related metabolic disorders.

In the present study, potential of EGCG, a potent polyphenol, was employed to study its effects on mesenchymal stem cell differentiation into adipocytes. EGCG is the most abundant ingredient, comprising approximately 50% (w/w) of the total catechins in green tea. It has been shown to reduce the incidence of cancer[8-10], collagen-induced arthritis[11],

neurodegenerative diseases[12] and diabetes[13]. Furthermore, EGCG has also been reported to reduce body weight and body fat [14]. When injected into rats, EGCG reduces their food uptake, lipid absorption, blood triacylglycerol (TAG), cholesterol and leptin levels, and stimulates energy expenditure, fat oxidation, high-density lipoprotein levels and fecal lipid excretion[14-15]. It also reduces cell number and TAG content during the differentiation of pre-adipocytes suggesting that EGCG regulates the mitogenic, endocrine and metabolic functions of adipocytes[14, 16].

The mesenchymal stem cells (MSCs) besides being suggested as a better model system to study the fat metabolism also possess a key characteristic of being immunologically well tolerated and hence serve as an attractive candidate for regenerative medicine. However, none of the studies have targeted EGCG's anti-adipocytic effect on MSCs. MSCs are a heterogeneous population of plastic-adherent, fibroblast-like cells, which in culture have ability to self-renew and differentiate into mesodermal and non-mesodermal derived tissues[17-19]. Advancements in understanding tissue specific differentiation of MSCs in conjunction with global genomic and proteomic profiling of MSCs have not only provided insights into their biology, but also made MSCs-based clinical trials a reality for treating various debilitating diseases and genetic disorders. The C3H10T1/2 cell line constitutes a reliable MSC model cell system for the study of stem cell differentiation[20, 21]. Therefore, the present study was designed to analyze the effects of EGCG on the mouse mesenchymal cell line C3H10T1/2 differentiation, employing adipogenesis as a paradigm.

Author Names in full: Baldeep Chani[1], Veena Puri[2], Ranbir Chander Sobti [3], Sanjeev Puri[1]

[1]Centre for Stem Cell & Tissue Engineering; [2]Systems Biology & Bioinformatics; [3]Biotechnology Department; [4]Biotechnology branch, University Institute of Engineering & Technology, Panjab University, Chandigarh, India

Materials and Methods

Cell culture

The mouse mesenchymal stem cell line (C3H10T1/2) was maintained in growth medium DMEM (with high glucose content), supplemented with 10% FBS (heat inactivated), 100 U penicillin, and 100 µg/ml streptomycin. All the experiments were performed using third passaged cells. The cells were plated at a concentration of 1.5×10^6 cells per well of the six well plate in the above mentioned growth medium and kept in an incubator maintained at 37 °C in the atmosphere of air and CO_2 (5%). All the experiments were performed 24 h post establishing the cells in culture and designated this time as 0-day of culture.

Viability based on continuous growth studies

Varying amounts of EGCG (1µM, 5 µM, 10 µM and 50 µM) were used to study the growth of EGCG cells through microscopic assessment of the morphology of C3H10T1/2 cell line. For this, 24 h post establishment the cells (1.5×10^6 cells/well of a six well plate) were treated at the above mentioned concentrations and observed under phase contrast microscope for any morphological characterization.

Cell migration (Scratch assay) as an indicator of cellular proliferation

Wound healing assay was performed as a measure of cell migration capacity and cell division following treatment of the cells with varying concentrations of EGCG (1µM, 5µM). For this, the cells were scratched off leaving a continuous gap of ~1cm broad across the wells of six well plates. The markings were placed so as to obtain same area for the microscopic comparison. The time taken by the cells to migrate in the area of scratch followed by filling of the wound (gap) was used as a measure of the proliferation potential of the EGCG.

Cell counting

Cells were seeded into 6-well plate and treated with 1 µM, 5µM EGCG. On the day of counting, cells were rinsed twice with 37°C sterile PBS and trypsinized, centrifuged at 4,000 rpm for 5 minutes. The supernatant was discarded and then cells were counted with the help of haemocytometer.

Regulation of adipogenic differentiation by EGCG

The cells were seeded in six-well plates at a density of 1.5×10^5 cells/well. Two days after reaching ~80 % confluence stage (day 0), the C3H10T1/2 cells were treated with 1µg/ml insulin, 0.25 µM dexamethasone, 0.5 mM 3-isobutyl-1-methylxanthine (adipogenic differentiation-induction medium) for 9 days. The differentiation maintenance medium was changed once in two days until the cells were harvested. To test EGCG effects on adipogenesis, EGCG at a concentration of 1 µM was added to the differentiation induction medium until the cells were harvested. The regulatory effect on adipogenic differentiation by EGCG was analyzed by staining of the cells with Oil red O, while for the molecular characterization the effect on adipogenic marker gene Adipsin was analyzed as per the following:

Oil red O (ORO) staining

Briefly, the C3H10T½ cells were seeded in six-well plates at a density of 1.5×10^5 cells/well. Two days after reaching ~80 % confluency (day 0), the cells were treated with adipogenic differentiation medium in the presence or absence of EGCG as per the protocol mentioned above. For the staining purpose, the cells were fixed for a period of 5 min with 10% formalin followed by washing with 60% isopropanol. The cells were then incubated with Oil red O solution for 1 hour at room temperature and then were rinsed with water. Stained cells were visualized microscopically and observations recorded.

TAG quantification

The cells were fixed and stained using same method as mentioned above. The cells were then washed with water. The stained triglyceride droplets were extracted for 10 minutes with 1 ml isopropanol and the absorbance was read at 510 nm. The triglyceride content is standardized by triolein.

RT- PCR analysis

Total RNA of C3H10T1/2 cells under different experimental conditions were extracted by Trizol method (Invitrogen) according to the manufacturer's instructions. Specific PCR amplification procedures were carried employing forward and reverse primers of Adipsin (422 bp) (Forward 5'- ATG GTA TGA TGT GCA GAG TGT AG -3'; Reverse 5'- CAC ACA TCA TGT TAA TGG TGA C -3'), Glyceraldehyde 3-Phospho- dehydrogenase (150 bp) (Forward 5'-TCT TGG CTA CAC TGA GGA C-3'; Reverse 5'-TGT TGC TGT AGC CGT ATT CA-3'). The amplified products were analyzed on 0.6 % agarose gels.

Statistical analysis

Statistical analysis was done using Student's t-test. It was used to examine the differences between the control, EGCG-treated groups. Results were expressed as means ± S.E.M. of values from at least three independent experiments in triplicate determinations. Statistical significance was represented with an asterisk for p-value < 0.05.

Results

Effects of EGCG on cell viability

In the present study, EGCG was used to evaluate its anti-adipogenic differentiation potential in mesenchymal stem cell line, C3H10T1/2. The preliminary study was planned to discern the growth viability of these cells to the varying concentrations of EGCG (1 µM, 5 µM, 10 µM and 50µM). As shown in figure 1, twenty four hours post treatment, the lower two concentrations of EGCG i.e. 1 µM, (Figure 1b) 5 µM (Figure 1c) were well tolerated by these cells and the cells showed normal fibroblast like morphology along with retaining the same growth pattern as compared to control cells (Figure 1a). The cells remained adhered as flat evenly placed monolayers and the nuclei were evenly spaced as described by Reznikoff et al (1973)[22]. The higher concentrations of EGCG 10 µM (Figure 1d) and 50 µM (Figure 1e) were found to be toxic to the cells as these cells showed altered morphology with many showing apoptotic alterations viz. cell shrinking (black arrow), detachment (white arrow) (Figure 1 d & e). Further, it was also observed that cells remained viable and continue to grow at both the 1 µM and 5 µM concentrations of EGCG for 3 days (Figure 1 g & h), and even after till 9th days (data not shown) in culture.

Effects of EGCG on cells migration ability

Having observed that the low concentrations of EGCG are well tolerated, its effect on the cell behavior was characterized. For this EGCG's effect on cell migration (indirect proliferation) was studied employing scratch assay.

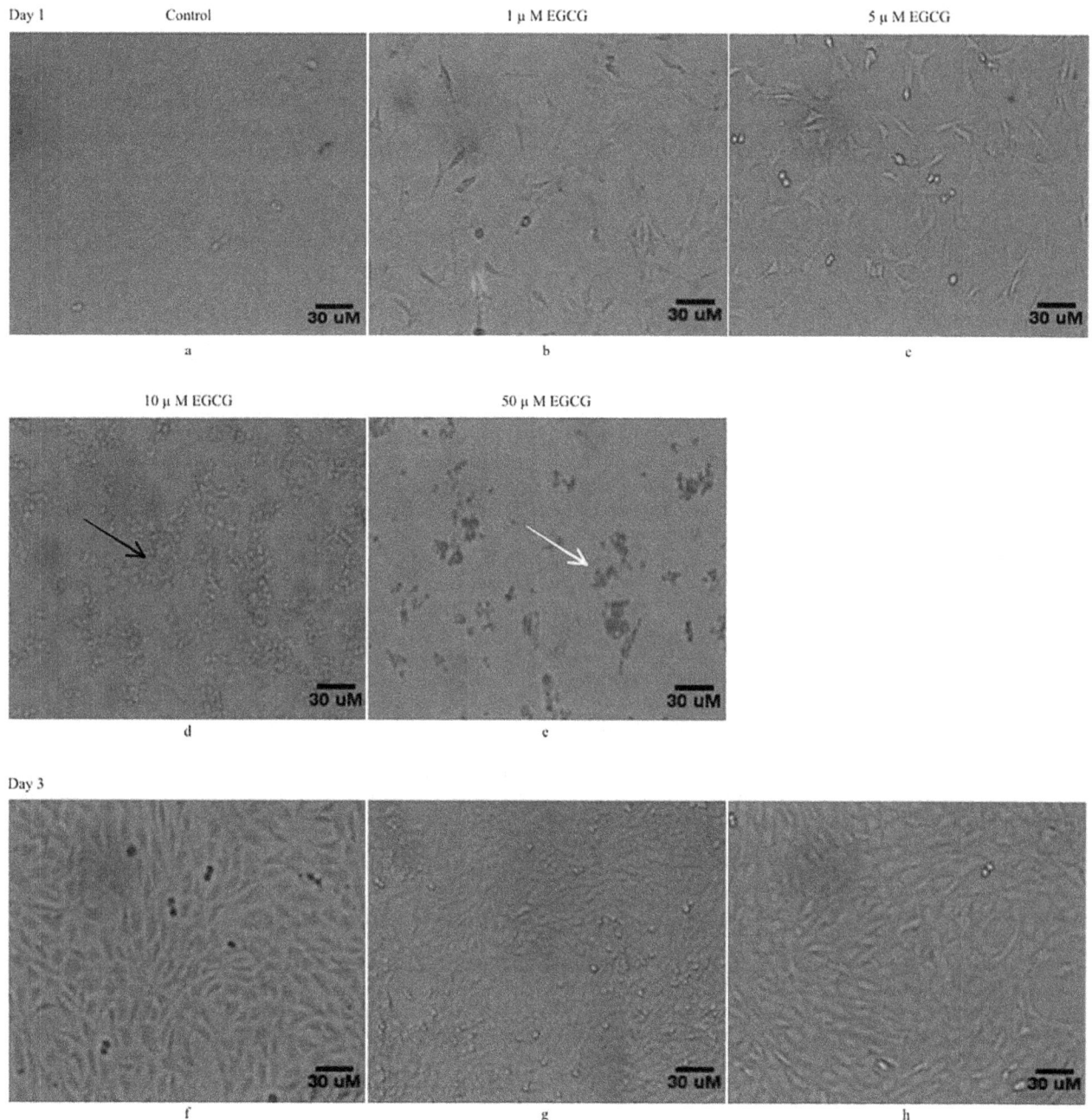

Figure 1: *Low concentrations of EGCG treatment maintains for the cell viability: C3H10T1/2 cells were exposed to different concentrations of EGCG i.e. 1µM, 5µM 10µM, and 50µM EGCG. The morphology of the cells was observed under phase contrast microscopy (100 x). Photomicrographs a), b), c), d), & e) represents control cells, cells treated with1 µM, 5 µM, 10µM, & 50µM EGCG, respectively at day1 while f), g), & h) represent control cells and cells treated with 1 µM and 5 µM EGCG, respectively at day 3. Where ever shown, the black arrows represent cells undergoing shrinkage and white arrows represent cell detachment indicating toxicity to the cells. Since, the concentrations of EGCG at 1µM, 5µM are well tolerated by cells, these were allowed to grow continuously till day 3 (Figure g & h) without producing any toxicity in comparison to control cells (Figure f).*

Confluent monolayer cells were scratched (~1cm) 24 h post establishment and were washed with PBS to remove any suspended cells. The day of scratch was marked as day 0, following the scratch, the cells were then treated with two different EGCG concentrations i.e.1 µM and 5 µM. The migration of the cells in scratched area was assessed by phase contrast microscopy at 24 hours post scratch (day 1). As the scratch produced remained uneven, a 1 cm area was marked within the scratched area to enumerate the extent of the cell migration. As shown in figure 2 a, b & c, the scratched area was devoid of any cellular structure following scratch (day 0). Twenty four hours after the scratch (day1), the cells in control well (compare Figure 2a versus 2d) quickly migrated and filled majority of the scratched area. On the other hand, the cells exposed to

EGCG whether at 1 µM (Figure 2e) or at 5 µM (Figure 2f) were very slow to migrate to the scratched area as compared to cells in the cells in control well (Figure 2d). Further, the concentration of 5µM of EGCG was, found to be rather more effective (Figure 2f) in preventing the cell migration as compared to 1µM of EGCG (Figure 2e). Since the cell migration is also a proxy to cell proliferation, it is imperative to suggest that EGCG shows a inhibitory potential on mesenchymal stem cell proliferation. In order to further reiterate these observations, cell counting assay was performed. For this 20,000 cells were seeded in 6-well plate. After 24 hours, the medium was replaced by fresh growth medium containing 1µM and 5µM concentrations of EGCG while the cells in control group received growth medium only.

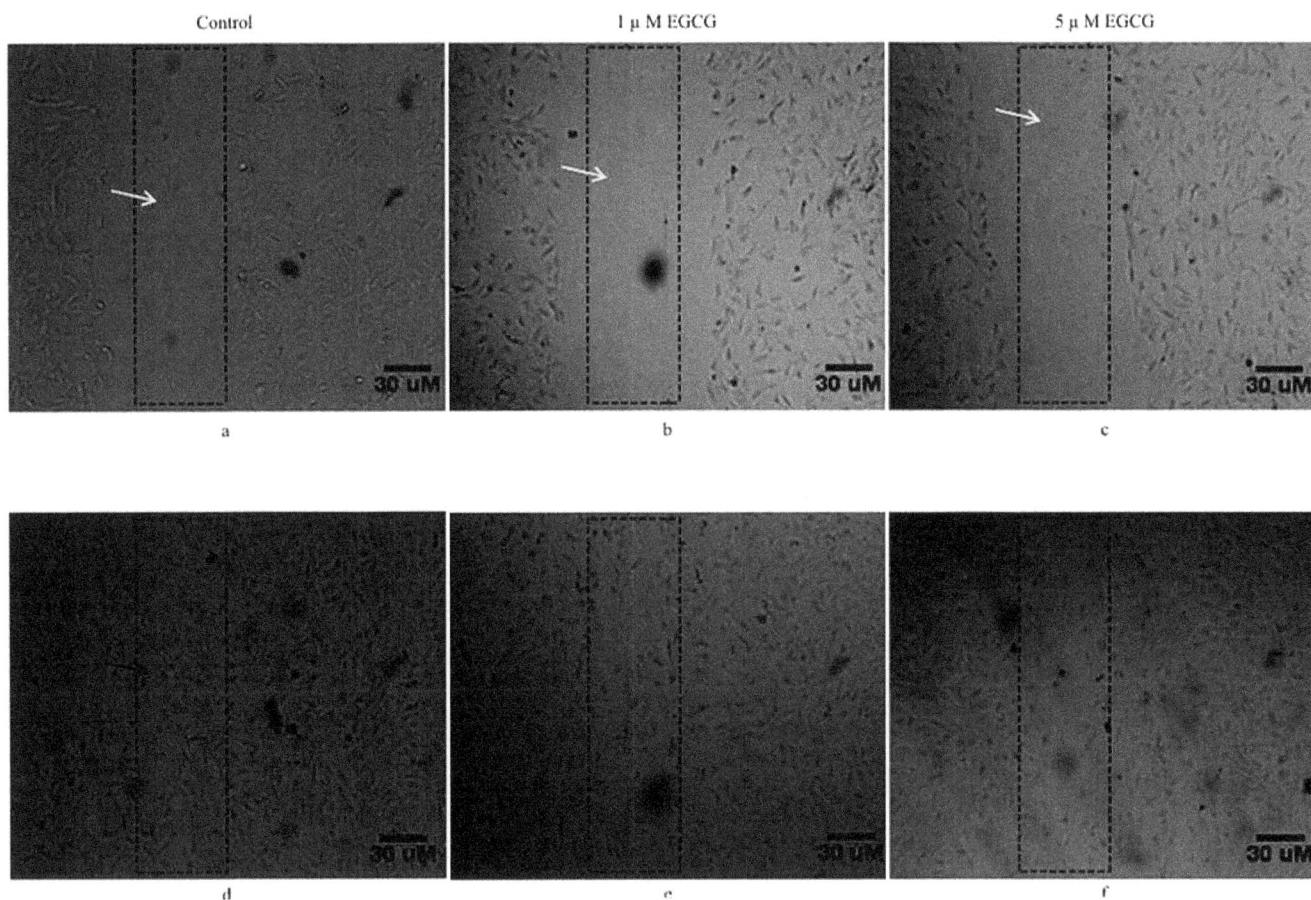

Figure 2: *EGCG inhibits Cell Migration (Scratch assay). The cell migration (indirect proliferation) was studied following addition of 1µM and 5µM EGCG to the cells following scratch in the C3H10T1/2 cells. The effect of EGCG on cell migration was recorded at different time points. The photomicrographs a), b), & c) represent images taken at 0 hour (immediately after scratching) and those in d), e), & f) represent images after 24 hours after scratching. Photomicrograph of control (d) show the wound closure by C3H10T1/2 cells after 24 hours. As can be seen from photomicrographs e, f, the EGCG at 1µM and 5µM concentrations inhibited cell migration and prevented filling of the scratched area. White arrow represents scratched area, black arrow represents cell migration.*

The cells were trypsinized 24 h post EGCG treatment and were quantified. As shown in figure 3, the total count of the cells in control wells was found to be ~ 5.5±0.01 x10^4 (repeated in triplicate), the EGCG treatment interfered with the growth activity and both at 1µM and 5µM concentrations of EGCG the cell count was found to be ~ 4.5±0.2 x10^4 and ~ 3.3±0.1 x10^4, respectively.

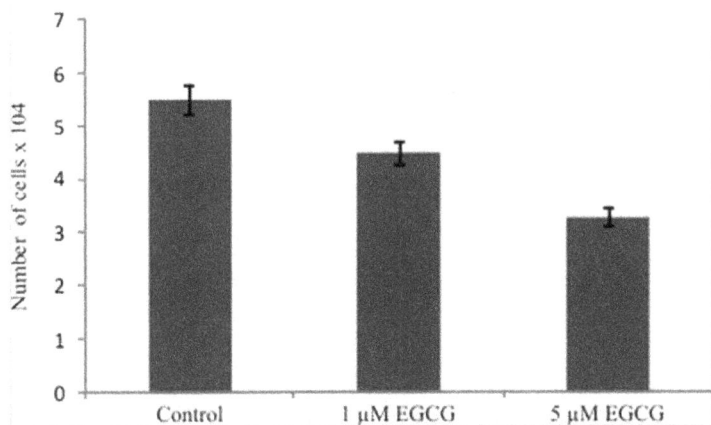

Figure 3: EGCG treatment reduces stem cells number. Effect of EGCG on the total cell number was analyzed by growing C3H10T1/2 cells in the presence of 1 µM or 5 µM EGCG. About 20,000 cells were plated in six well plate. Twenty four hours following treatment the cells from control and EGCG treated cells were trypsinized and counted. At both the concentrations of EGCG the cell numbers were found to be significantly reduced as compared to control cells. The values represent mean ± SEM for three independent experiments.

Effects of EGCG on Adipogenesis

Having observed the cells behavior to EGCG, the differentiation potential of EGCG on C3H10T1/2 mesenchymal stem cells was analyzed. Adipogenesis was used as a differentiation paradigm. The cells were treated with adipogenic differentiation induction medium (DIM) cocktail either alone (Figure 4b1) or in combination with EGCG 1µM (Figure 4c1). Any changes in the cells morphology, under phase contrast microscope, were followed continuously for a period of nine days. The comparison of cellular morphology among control (Figure 4a1-a4), DIM (Figure 4b1-b4) as well as DIM plus EGCG (Figure 4c1-c4) treated cells in photo-micrographs showed that within in three days of treatments the cells underwent changes in the morphology marked by increase in size (black arrows) and appearance of small vacuolar (oil lobules, white arrows) structures specifically in DIM treated cells (Figure 4b2). The size of these oil like droplets in the cells increased continuously till the 9th day post treatment. The EGCG addition to these DIM treated cells though did not vary the cells morphology (black arrows) drastically but certainly prevented the formation of these vacuolar structures (Figure 4c2-c4).

Such an inhibitory ability of EGCG on Adipogenesis was further validated by microscopic images of treated C3H10T1/2 cells captured after Oil red O staining (Figure 5c) in comparison to DIM treated cells (Figure 5b) and by measuring the triglyceride

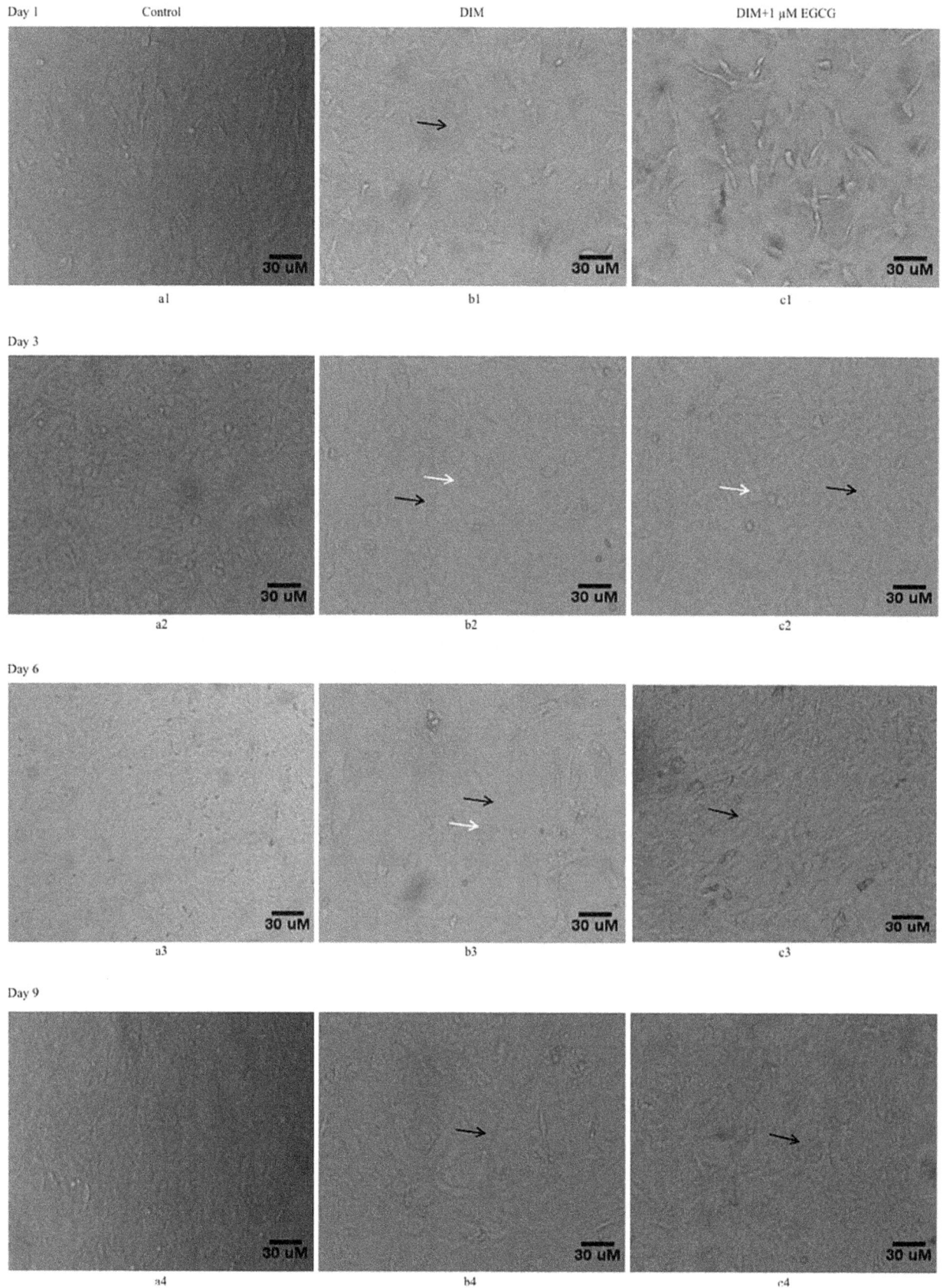

Figure 4: EGCG exposure prevented changes in differentiating C3H10T1/2 cellular morphology. *The differentiating adipocytes possess special morphology which was observed in the C3H10T1/2 mesenchymal stem cells when exposed to adipogenic differentiation cocktail (DIM). These cells were then followed for 9 days in culture. The effect of 1μM EGCG and on C3H10T1/2 morphology (Adipogenic) following DIM as analyzed through phase contrast microscopy (100 x). Photomicrographs a1), a2), a3), a4) represents control cells, b1), b2), b3), b4) represent cells treated with DIM, and the images c1), c2), c3), c4) represent cells treated with 1 μM EGCG along with DIM. At day 6th and 9th morphology of the cells treated with DIM (Figure b3, b4) changed with respect to control cells and they appeared more globular (black arrow) with vacuoles (white arrow) as compared to morphology shown by control untreated cells (Figure a3, a4). The EGCG treatment to the DIM exposed cells prevented the changes in the cells morphology with significant reduction in the globular looking cells harboring vacuoles as seen in the cells exposed to DIM (Figure c3, c4).*

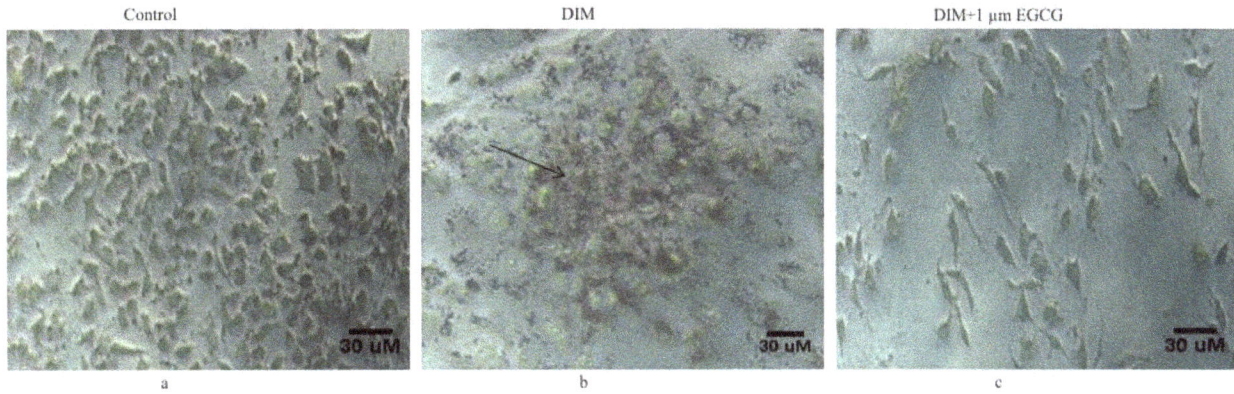

Figure 5: EGCG prevented lipid accumulation in differentiating C3H10T1/2 cells: The lipid accumulation in the cells undergoing adipogenic differentiation was analyzed by Oil red O staining following EGCG treatment. Photomicrographs a), b) & c) represented control cells, cells treated with DIM & cells treated with DIM along with 1 μM EGCG, respectively. Black arrow represents red stained lipids. As can be seen the EGCG prevented C3H10T1/2 cells differentiation to adipogenic lineage.

content through spectrometric analysis (510 nm) of the extracted Red stain color by isopropanol for 10 min from the stained cells (Figure 6). The values are expressed as a percentage with respect to the positive control (cells treated with DIM alone). Addition of EGCG to DIM treated cells produced approximately 40% reduction in the red stained cells in comparison to the cells treated with DIM alone (Figure 6). These observations thus suggested that EGCG function as anti-adipogenic agent by preventing mesenchymal stem cell differentiation.

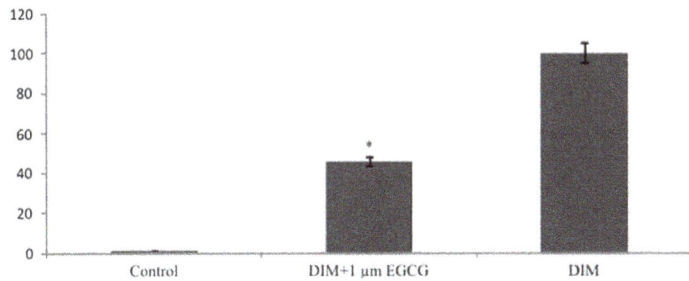

Figure 6: Inhibition of Triglyceride content in adipogenic differentiating C3H10T1/2 cells by EGCG. Since the red stain of Oil red O is indicative of the triglyceride content, its levels were observed by taking absorbance at 510 nm. The EGCG treatment to the DIM exposed cells significantly reduced the absorbance of the extracted red color in comparison to the Cells exposed to DIM only. The values represent mean ± SEM for three independent experiments.

Effects of EGCG on adipsin expression

To understand the molecular event involved in such an anti-adipogenic role of EGCG, the expression levels of adipsin, a marker for adipocytic differentiation was analyzed. The total RNA was isolated and reverse transcribed from control, DIM and DIM plus EGCG treated cells at day 9th following the treatments followed by PCR amplification employing primers specific to adipsin gene. The electrophoretogram of the amplified product from control (lane-1, Figure 7a), DIM treated (lane-4, Figure 7a) and DIM plus EGCG treated (lane-3, Figure 7a) demonstrated that DIM treatment produced amplification of a product corresponding to molecular size of ~422 bp which remained under expressed in control cells (lane-1, Figure 7a) and cells treated with EGCG alone (lane-2, Figure 7a). The EGCG addition to DIM treated cells produced ~ two fold reduction in the expression of adipsin in comparison to DIM treatment alone, albeit

its levels remained more to adipocytes.than the control (Figure 7 a & b). These observations thus further reiterated that EGCG possessed the anti-adipogenic potential and inhibited the adipogenic differentiation of mesenchymal stem cells in culture.

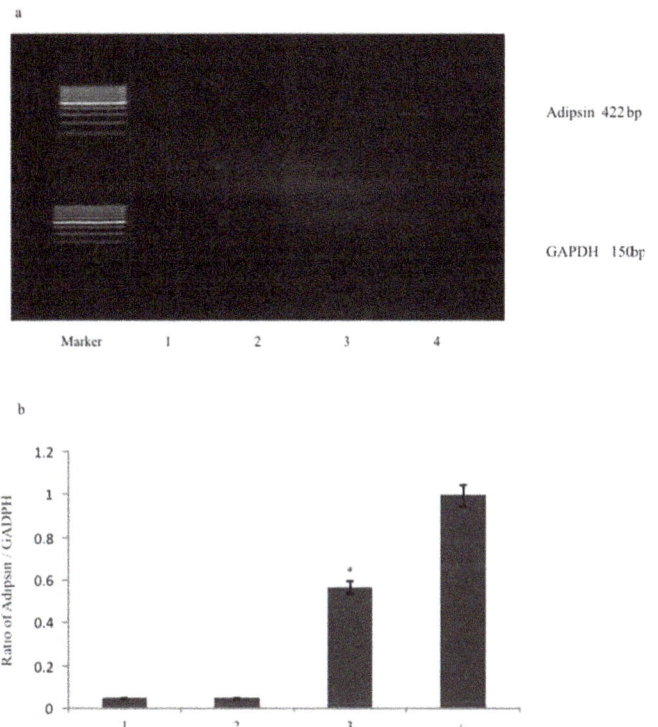

Figure 7: a) EGCG down regulated the adipsin gene expression: RT-PCR analysis of adipsin, glyceraldehydes 3-Phosphate dehydrogenase gene was analyzed in control, DIM treated and DIM Plus EGCG treated cells. The lane-1 represents electrophoretogram of the amplified product (422 bp) from control (without treatment) cells, lane-2 represents EGCG treated cells, lane-3 represents amplified product following DIM and 1μM EGCG treatment and the lane-4 represented the amplification of a product following DIM treatment. It was observed that EGCG treatment down regulated the expression of adipsin in the cells undergoing adipogenesis. (Compare Lane 3 with lane 4). b) The densitometric analysis of amplified adipsin product was analyzed and it was observed that EGCG treatment significantly reduced the expression of adipsin gene expression. The graph represented densitometric analysis of adipsin relative to GADPH. The values represent mean ± SEM of three independent experiments (n=3).

Discussion

In the present study we investigated the effects of Epigallocatechin Gallate on adipogenic differentiation of the mesenchymal stem cells. The observations of the present study demonstrated that EGCG inhibited the lipid accumulation in the mesenchymal stem cells destined to differentiate in adipocytic cells following exposure to adipogenic differentiation medium. Besides its anti-adipogenic role, EGCG also prevented cell migration, an indirect marker for the cell proliferation[23]. Whether this anti-proliferative effects is akin to anti-adipogenic character of EGCG though warrants further study, but flurry of information lend support to this association. Based on the known pre-adipocyte murine cell culture models viz. 3T3-L1, 3T3-F442A and Ob17, it is known that upon reaching confluency and growth arrest, the opportunistic re-entry to cell cycle through hormonal induction led these pre-adipocytic cells to go through multiple cycles of post-confluence mitosis, called mitotic clonal expansion (MCE)[24]. It is rather a basic regimen of terminal adipocyte differentiation. As shown in the present study the inhibition of staining, restrained cell migration together with reduction in total cell number, by EGCG, advocates for its ability to prevent C3H10T1/2 mesenchymal stem cells differentiation into adipocytic lineage following hormonal cocktail exposure (Insulin, dexmethasone, 3-isobutyl-1-methylxanthine). This cocktail is known to induce adipogenesis in various cell lines, including C3H10T1/2 cells[25]. Adipsin a marker gene for differentiation is expressed at high levels in adipose tissue and is a regulator of lipid accumulation in adipocytes[26]. Results of present study demonstrated down regulation of adipsin expression in EGCG treated cells as compared to cells treated with differentiation hormonal cocktail. These observations though preliminary certainly points towards maintaining stem cell pluripotency and also provided a sound framework to assess the stem cell behavior (proliferation and differentiation) when treated with green tea polyphenol EGCG. Moreover, Tang *et al* (2003)[24] demonstrated that preventing the entry into S phase in 3T3-L1 cells during MCE completely hampered the process ensuing adipogenesis. Similar, observations by Kuri-Harcuch and Marsch-Moreno (1983)[27] demonstrating direct relation between the inhibition of DNA synthesis in 3T3-F442A cells and prevention of the formation of fat cells further corroborated the observations of the present study. Earlier studies have shown that EGCG besides inhibiting the differentiation of pre-adipocytic cells also brings about wide range of biological functions like anti-oxidant, anti-cancer, anti-angiogensis[28]. Previous reports describing growth arrest and differentiation of exponentially growing keratinocytes indicated that a dose of 50 μM and 100 μM of EGCG increased the conversion of undifferentiated kertainocytes into corneocytes with concomitant decreased cell proliferation[29, 30]. This represents an important step in cells behavior to EGCG treatment. However, this certainly does not seem to be the universality, as in the present study concentration of 10 μM, 50 μM were found to be rather toxic to mesenchymal stem cells C3H10T1/2. Whereas, lower doses of EGCG 1 μM and 5 μM were sufficient reduce the proliferation of mesenchymal cells in a dose dependent manner. EGCG also reduced the migration of C3H10T1/2 cells as observed through scratch assay. Multitudinous reports[31, 32] providing support to the fact that EGCG inhibits the proliferation and migratory behavior of proliferating cells further lend credibility to the observations of the present study. A growing body of work suggests that stem cells and cancer cell seems to posses some common molecular mechanisms (genomic/epigenomic/nongenomic) for retaining their characteristics off course deciding controlled or deregulated proliferation[33,34]. The inhibition of proliferation (migration in scratch area) of stem cells by EGCG may plausibly target similar molecular events as observed in cancer cells. These observations are also corroborated by the fact that EGCG treatment reduced the cell count significantly further suggesting that EGCG might be regulating cell proliferation which is an important character for long term maintenance of cell pleuripotency. Together with ability of EGCG to suppress the adipogenesis of MSC, as seen in the present study, it seems that EGCG may function as two-edged sword whereby besides anti-proliferative action, it also reduces adipogenesis. The anti-obesity role of EGCG further gets corroboration from recent studies[34, 35] though the precise mechanism remains elusive. Present results showed that EGCG inhibited the differentiation of C3H10T1/2 cell lines and so it can be used as drug supplement for controlling the obesity which is responsible for associated diseases like diabetes and heart problems. Thus, it is possible that as in pre-adipocytic cells, the EGCG treatment to mesenchymal stem cells also follows such a paradigm to inhibit the Adipogenesis. The inhibition of adipsin gene expression, by EGCG thus prevents the mesenchymal stem cell differentiation induced by adipogenic differentiation cocktail. Beside this reduction in the expression of adipsin, a parallel reduction in the lipid accumulation in the differentiating mesenchymal stem cells was also notified.

Based on these observations, it is pertinent to claim that EGCG, an important flavonoid of green tea, possesses the ability to limit the mesenchymal stem cells differentiation to adipogenic lineage. This may provide a rational approach towards developing EGCG as a multifaceted molecule for the intervention of obesity related disorders, including carcinogenesis.

References

1. Lee WJ, Koh EH, Won JC, Kim MS, Park JY, Lee KU. Obesity: the role of hypothalamic AMP-activated protein kinase in body weight regulation. Int J Biochem Cell Biol. 2005;37(11):2254-9.

2. Liao S, Kao YH, Hiipakka RA. Green tea: biochemical and biological basis for health benefits. Vitam Horm. 2001;62:1-94.

3. Yu YH, Zhu H. Chronological changes in metabolism and functions of cultured adipocytes: a hypothesis for cell aging in mature adipocytes. Am J Physiol Endocrinol Metab. 2004;286(3):E402-10.

4. Jernås M, Palming J, Sjöholm K, Jennische E, Svensson PA, Gabrielsson BG, Levin M, Sjögren A, Rudemo M, Lystig TC, Carlsson B, Carlsson LM, Lönn M. Separation of human adipocytes by size: hypertrophic fat cells display distinct gene expression. FASEB J. 2006;20(9):1540-2.

5. Rull A, Camps J, Alonso-Villaverde C, Joven J. Insulin resistance, inflammation, and obesity: role of monocyte chemoattractant protein-1 (or CCL2) in the regulation of metabolism. Mediators Inflamm. 2010;2010. pii: 326580.

6. Furukawa S, Fujita T, Shimabukuro M, Iwaki M, Yamada Y, Nakajima Y, Nakayama O, Makishima M, Matsuda M, Shimomura I. Increased oxidative stress in obesity and its impact on metabolic syndrome. J Clin Invest. 2004;114(12):1752-61.

7. Yeop Han C, Kargi AY, Omer M, Chan CK, Wabitsch M, O'Brien KD, Wight TN, Chait A. Differential effect of saturated and unsaturated free fatty acids on the generation of monocyte adhesion and chemotactic factors by adipocytes: dissociation of adipocyte hypertrophy from inflammation. Diabetes. 2010;59(2):386-96.

8. Mitscher LA, Jung M, Shankel D, Dou JH, Steele L, Pillai SP. Chemoprotection: a review of the potential therapeutic antioxidant properties of green tea (Camellia sinensis) and certain of its constituents. Med Res Rev. 1997;17(4):327-65.

9. Ahmad N, Mukhtar H. Green tea polyphenols and cancer: biologic mechanisms and practical implications. Nutr Rev. 1999;57(3):78-83.

10. Lin JK, Liang YC, Lin-Shiau SY. Cancer chemoprevention by tea polyphenols through mitotic signal transduction blockade. Biochem Pharmacol. 1999;58(6):911-5.

11. Haqqi TM, Anthony DD, Gupta S, Ahmad N, Lee MS, Kumar GK, Mukhtar H. Prevention of collagen-induced arthritis in mice by a polyphenolic fraction from green tea. Proc Natl Acad Sci U S A. 1999;96(8):4524-9.

12. Mandel S, Youdim MB. Catechin polyphenols: neurodegeneration and neuroprotection in neurodegenerative diseases. Free Radic Biol Med. 2004;37(3):304-17.

13. Song EK, Hur H, Han MK. Epigallocatechin gallate prevents autoimmune diabetes induced by multiple low doses of streptozotocin in mice. Arch Pharm Res. 2003;26(7):559-63.

14. Kao YH, Hiipakka RA, Liao S. Modulation of endocrine systems and food intake by green tea epigallocatechin gallate. Endocrinology. 2000;141(3):980-7.

15. Dulloo AG, Duret C, Rohrer D, Girardier L, Mensi N, Fathi M, Chantre P, Vandermander J. Efficacy of a green tea extract rich in catechin polyphenols and caffeine in increasing 24-h energy expenditure and fat oxidation in humans. Am J Clin Nutr. 1999;70(6):1040-5.

16. Kim H, Hiraishi A, Tsuchiya K, Sakamoto K. (-) Epigallocatechin gallate suppresses the differentiation of 3T3-L1 preadipocytes through transcription factors FoxO1 and SREBP1c. Cytotechnology. 2010;62(3):245-55.

17. Friedenstein AJ, Chailakhjan RK, Lalykina KS. The development of fibroblast colonies in monolayer cultures of guinea-pig bone marrow and spleen cells. Cell Tissue Kinet. 1970;3(4):393-403.

18. Pittenger MF, Mackay AM, Beck SC, Jaiswal RK, Douglas R, Mosca JD, Moorman MA, Simonetti DW, Craig S, Marshak DR. Multilineage potential of adult human mesenchymal stem cells. Science. 1999;284(5411):143-7.

19. Izadpanah R, Trygg C, Patel B, Kriedt C, Dufour J, Gimble JM, Bunnell BA. Biologic properties of mesenchymal stem cells derived from bone marrow and adipose tissue. J Cell Biochem. 2006;99(5):1285-97.

20. Bowers RR, Kim JW, Otto TC, Lane MD. Stable stem cell commitment to the adipocyte lineage by inhibition of DNA methylation: role of the BMP-4 gene. Proc Natl Acad Sci U S A. 2006;103(35):13022-7.

21. Huang H, Song TJ, Li X, Hu L, He Q, Liu M, Lane MD, Tang QQ. BMP signaling pathway is required for commitment of C3H10T1/2 pluripotent stem cells to the adipocyte lineage. Proc Natl Acad Sci U S A. 2009;106(31):12670-5.

22. Reznikoff CA, Brankow DW, Heidelberger C. Establishment and characterization of a cloned line of C3H mouse embryo cells sensitive to postconfluence inhibition of division. Cancer Res. 1973;33(12):3231-8.

23. Punathil T, Tollefsbol TO, Katiyar SK. EGCG inhibits mammary cancer cell migration through inhibition of nitric oxide synthase and guanylate cyclase. Biochem Biophys Res Commun. 2008;375(1):162-7.

24. Tang QQ, Otto TC, Lane MD. Mitotic clonal expansion: a synchronous process required for adipogenesis. Proc Natl Acad Sci U S A. 2003;100(1):44-9.

25. Pantoja C, Huff JT, Yamamoto KR. Glucocorticoid signaling defines a novel commitment state during adipogenesis in vitro. Mol Biol Cell. 2008;19(10):4032-41.

26. White RT, Damm D, Hancock N, Rosen BS, Lowell BB, Usher P, Flier JS, Spiegelman BM. Human adipsin is identical to complement factor D and is expressed at high levels in adipose tissue. J Biol Chem. 1992;267(13):9210-3.

27. Kuri-Harcuch W, Marsch-Moreno M. DNA synthesis and cell division related to adipose differentiation of 3T3 cells. J Cell Physiol. 1983;114(1):39-44.

28. Singh M, Singh N. Curcumin counteracts the proliferative effect of estradiol and induces apoptosis in cervical cancer cells. Mol Cell Biochem. 2011;347(1-2):1-11.

29. Balasubramanian S, Efimova T, Eckert RL. Green tea polyphenol stimulates a Ras, MEKK1, MEK3, and p38 cascade to increase activator protein 1 factor-dependent involucrin gene expression in normal human keratinocytes. J Biol Chem. 2002;277(3):1828-36.

30. Hsu S, Lewis J, Singh B, Schoenlein P, Osaki T, Athar M, Porter AG, Schuster G. Green tea polyphenol targets the mitochondria in tumor cells inducing caspase 3-dependent apoptosis. Anticancer Res. 2003;23(2B):1533-9.

31. De Amicis F, Russo A, Avena P, Santoro M, Vivacqua A, Bonofiglio D, Mauro L, Aquila S, Tramontano D, Fuqua SA, Andò S. In vitro mechanism for downregulation of ER-α expression by epigallocatechin gallate in ER+/PR+ human breast cancer cells. Mol Nutr Food Res. 2013;57(5):840-53.

32. Braicu C, Gherman CD, Irimie A, Berindan-Neagoe I. Epigallocatechin-3-Gallate (EGCG) inhibits cell proliferation and migratory behaviour of triple negative breast cancer cells. J Nanosci Nanotechnol. 2013;13(1):632-7.

33. Taipale J, Beachy PA. The Hedgehog and Wnt signalling pathways in cancer. Nature. 2001;411(6835):349-54.

34. Huo JS, Baylin SB, Zambidis ET. Cancer-like epigenetic derangements of human pluripotent stem cells and their impact on applications in regeneration and repair. Curr Opin Genet Dev. 2014;28:43-9.

35. Klaus S, Pültz S, Thöne-Reineke C, Wolfram S. Epigallocatechin gallate attenuates diet-induced obesity in mice by decreasing energy absorption and increasing fat oxidation. Int J Obes (Lond). 2005;29(6):615-23.

Abbreviations

CLA	:	Conjugated Linoleic acid
DIM	:	Differentiation induction medium
DMEM	:	Dulbecco's Modified Essential Medium
EGCG	:	Epigallocatechin Gallate
FBS	:	Fetal bovine serum
MSC	:	Mesenchymal Stem Cell
ORO	:	Oil red O
PBS	:	Phosphate buffered saline
RNA	:	Ribonucleic acid
RT-PCR	:	Reverse transcription-polymerase chain reaction
TAG	:	Triacylglycerol

Potential Conflicts of Interests

None

Sponsors/Grants

This work is funded by Council of Scientific and Industrial Research (CSIR), New Delhi, India, Department of Science and Technology PURSE Grant to Center for Stem cell and Tissue Engineering, Panjab University Chandigarh, India. The funders had no role in study design, data collection and analysis, decision to publish, or preparation of the manuscript.

Corresponding Author

Sanjeev Puri, Coordinator, Stem Cell & Tissue Engineering, Biotechnology, UIET, Panjab University Chandigarh, Sector-14, India, Pin code-160014; E-mail: s_puri@pu.ac.in;spuri_1111@yahoo.com

7

Neural stem/progenitor cells maintained *in vitro* under different culture conditions alter differentiation capacity of monocytes to generate dendritic cells

Lupatov AYu[1], Poltavtseva RA[2], Bystrykh OA[2], Yarygin KN[1], Sukhikh GT[2].

Abstract

Cell therapy of the nervous system disorders using neural stem/progenitor cells (NSPCs) proved its efficacy in preclinical and pilot clinical studies. The mechanisms of the beneficial effects of NSPCs transplantation include replacement of damaged cells, paracrine activation of the regeneration, and immunomodulation. Detailed assessment of NSPCs-induced immunomodulation can contribute to better control of autoimmune reactions and inflammation in patients with neurodegenerative diseases. Interactions of NSPCs with dendritic cells (DCs), the key players in the induction of the immune system response to antigens are of particular interest. Here, we demonstrate that co-culturing of monocytes with NSPCs obtained and grown utilizing serum-containing medium instead of growth factor-containing serum-free medium, results in total suppression of monocyte differentiation into DCs. The effect is similar to the action of mesenchymal stem cells (MSCs). No significant effect on DCs maturation was observed. Cultures of NSPCs set up and maintained in serum-free medium have no influence on monocyte differentiation and DCs maturation. Therefore, the effects of NSPCs upon DC differentiation from monocytes strongly depend on culture conditions, whereas the molecular marker expression patterns are similar in both types of NSPCs cultures. In broader prospective, it means that cells with almost identical phenotypes can display opposite immunological properties depending upon culture conditions. It should be taken into account when developing NSPCs-based cell products for regenerative medicine.

Key Words: Neural stem cells, Neural progenitor cells, Immunomodulation, Dendritic cells, Cell therapy

Introduction

Allogeneic NSPCs have great potential as prospective therapeutic agents, due to low immunogenicity[1, 2] and the ability to stimulate restoration of the nervous tissue via paracrine mechanisms[3]. Moreover, it has been suggested that NSPCs, like MSCs, can suppress certain immunological reactions[4, 5]. *In vivo* data and co-culture experiments demonstrated NSPCs' capability to inhibit a number of immunological processes including proliferation and activation of T-cells in response to CNS-derived antigens or non-specific polyclonal stimuli[6, 7], as well as pro-inflammatory signal molecule expression[8]. They are also able to reduce the number of memory cells and to increase the amount of IL-4 and IL-10 secreting CD4 positive T-cells[7]. NSPCs strongly suppress inflammation in the experimental autoimmune encephalomyelitis model[5, 9]. Immunomodulation is probably the main mechanism of the healing effects of NSPCs transplantation in neuroinflammatory and autoimmune neurodegenerative diseases. In some cases, NSPCs may exert their action at the peripheral lymphoid organs level, without even entering the central nervous system[7,9].

Dendritic cells (DCs) are a crucially important type of immune cells contributing to the development of the immune response to autologous and foreign antigens by efficient antigen capture, processing and presenting to lymphocytes. The advent of functionally active DCs includes two stages. At the first stage differentiation of CD34 positive bone marrow precursors or circulating monocytes delivers immature DCs exhibiting high phagocytic activity. Their interaction with lymphocytes not only fails to induce immune response, but can initiate the lymphocytes' anergy or tolerance to antigens[10]. In the presence of the factors of inflammation, immature DCs enter the second, maturation stage including the reduction of phagocytic activity[11,12], enhancement of the expression of the major histocompatibility complex (MHC) and co-stimulation molecules, and the onset of the expression of chemokine receptors guiding DCs' migration towards the lymphatic nodes[13]. In the lymphatic nodes, DCs initiate immune responses by presenting antigens to lymphocytes. Importantly, DCs are a commonly recognized target for negative immunoregulation by MSCs derived from different tissues[14, 15]. To the contrary, the effects of NSPCs on DCs' differentiation and maturation have not been fully disclosed.

Usually, NSPC cultures are established and maintained using serum-free media supplemented with the epidermal growth factor to keep the cells undifferentiated[16]. Nevertheless, every NSPC culture is a mix of cells at varying differentiation stages. Variability of NSPC culture composition may depend upon the source of cell material and the conditions during culture initiation and maintenance. The presented study shows that substitution of growth factors in the NSCP culture medium for fetal calf serum (FCS) can alter the *in vitro* effects of NSPCs upon DCs differentiation suggesting change of some of their *in vivo* immunomodulation properties.

Author Names in full: Alexey Yu Lupatov[1], Rimma A Poltavtseva[2], Oxana A Bystrykh[2], Konstantin N Yarygin[1], Gennady T Sukhikh[2]

[1]Institute of Biomedical Chemistry, Moscow, Russia, [2]Research Center of Obstetrics, Gynecology and Perinatology, Moscow, Russia

Materials and methods

Cell cultures

NSPC cultures were initiated as described elsewhere[17] from cells of the neocortical portions of the brain of non-viable fetuses at 9-10 weeks of gestation obtained after therapeutic abortions in full accordance with the national regulations after getting patient's written consent. The work protocols were approved by the Research Center of Obstetrics, Gynecology and Perinatology (Moscow, Russia) ethical committee.

Serum-containing culture medium comprised DMEM/F12 (Gibco), 15 mM Hepes, 2 mM L-glutamine, 10% FCS (HyClone), and antibiotic-antimicotic solution (Gibco). In the serum-free medium FCS was substituted for the epidermal growth factor (EGF) – 20 ng/ml, basic fibroblast growth factor (FGF-2) – 20 ng/ml (both from ProSpec), heparin – 8 ug/ml, and N-2 supplement (Gibco). After more than 1/3 of neurospheres exceeded 250 um diameter, cell aggregates were destroyed by repetitive pipetting. Bone marrow MSC cultures were set up as described earlier[18].

Twenty four hours before setting up the NSPCs co-culture with monocytes, neurospheres were disaggregated and issuing cells transferred to a 24-well plate (Corning) and maintained at 37°C and 5% CO_2 in 0.5 ml DMEM/F12 medium with 10% FCS. The following day, plated-NSPCs were treated with 10 μg/ml Mitomycin C (Sigma-Aldrich) for 2 hours and washed thrice with Hanks' solution before the addition of monocytes. Monocytes were obtained by the immunomagnetic separation of mononuclear cells utilizing Dynabeads® Untouched™ Human Monocytes Kit (Invitrogen). The mononuclear cells were isolated from the peripheral blood by Ficoll gradient centrifugation for 30 min at 400g. Blood samples were collected from healthy donors in the Research Center of Obstetrics, Gynecology and Perinatology (Moscow, Russia) in accordance with the national regulations. Isolated monocytes were suspended in RPMI-1640 medium (Gibco) supplemented with 5% heat inactivated FCS, 50 μg/ml gentamycin and 2 mM HEPES (Stem Cells) and transferred to the wells with probed cells in the amount of 2×10^5 cells per well. Monocyte differentiation was induced with 80 ng/ml granulocyte macrophage colony-stimulating factor (GM-CSF) and 50 ng/ml interleukine-4 (IL-4) (both from ProSpec). After 4 days the cells were suspended and monocyte differentiation evaluated by flow cytometry.

To study NSPCs' effects on the DCs maturation DCs were first obtained by monocyte differentiation in 25 cm² culture flasks (Corning) in the presence of GM-CSF and IL-4. In 4 days, DCs were transferred to 24-well plates in the amount of 2×10^5 cells per well. The wells were pre-seeded with NSPCs as described above. Besides GM-CSF and IL-4, the co-culture medium was supplemented with 1 μg/ml bacterial lipopolysaccharide (LPS; sigma-Aldrich) or 20 ng/ml tumor necrosis factor alfa (TNF-a; Prospec) and 1 μg/ml prostaglandin E2 (PGE2; sigma-aldrich). After 3 days DCs maturity was evaluated by flow cytometry.

Immunocytochemistry

For immunocytochemical analysis neurospheres were fixed on glass slides with paraformaldehyde; monoclonal antibodies (MoAbs, Abcam) against markers of NSPCs differentiation were added, followed by anti-species secondary antibodies (Chemicon) labeled with Rodamine or FITC. Visualization was carried out with Zeiss Axiovert 200M microscope utilizing confocal and epifluorescence regimens.

Flow cytometry

For flow cytometry analysis cells were immunostained with fluorochrome-conjugated MoAbs (BD Bioscience) against specific cellular markers. In the case of intracellular staining Cytofix/Cytoperm™ solution (BD Bioscience) was used. Fluorescence intensity and light scattering were measured with FACS-Aria flow cytometer/cell sorter (BD Bioscience).

Results

We studied 3 cultures set up and grown in serum-free medium (designated as Cn, where "n" is the autopsy number) and 4 cultures maintained in FCS-containing medium (denoted Sn). C235 and S235 cultures were raised from the same autopsy sample (Table 1).

Neurospheres maintained in FSC-containing medium looked similar to "classic" neurospheres grown in serum-free conditions (Figure 1A), although they were harder to disaggregate. If the amount of culture medium allowed free flotation of neurospheres, only a small fraction of them adhered to plastic and initiated adhesive cultures of NSPCs. Adhesive NSPCs formed clusters consisting either of cells with fibroblast-like morphology (Figure 1B), or cells with thin long processes forming web-like structures (Figure 1C), probably revealing initial stages of glial and neuronal differentiation, respectively. Both "C" and "S" type of neurospheres expressed early neuroblast marker βIII-tubulin. They also were positive for glial fibrillary acidic protein (GFAP), an intermediate filament protein typically expressed in astroglia (Figure 1D,E). Like "classic" neurospheres, neurospheres obtained and cultured in the presence of FCS, included cells positive for nestin, a type VI intermediate filament protein of the neuroectoderm and nerve tube neuroepithelium, as well as vimentin, another intermediate filament protein expressed in neural and reactive astrocytes precursor cells (Figure 1E). Nestin and vimentin expression was also observed during NSPCs transfer into the adhesive state (Figure 1F). A quantitative analysis of disaggregated neurospheres by flow cytometry revealed a slight increase in the expression of GFAP in cells cultured in the presence of FCS (Figure 1G). Therefore, marker expression analysis demonstrated close similarity between cellular composition of neurospheres maintained in medium with FCS and "classic" neurospheres from "C" type cultures.

Table 1. NSPCs cultures studied.

Culture	Presence of FBS in culture medium	Days in culture prior to co-cultivation with monocytes	Passage number
C56	no	48	5
C69	no	36	4
C235	no	12; 52	0; 6
S235	yes	12; 52	0; 6
S163	yes	62	7
S164	yes	51	5
S170	yes	38	4

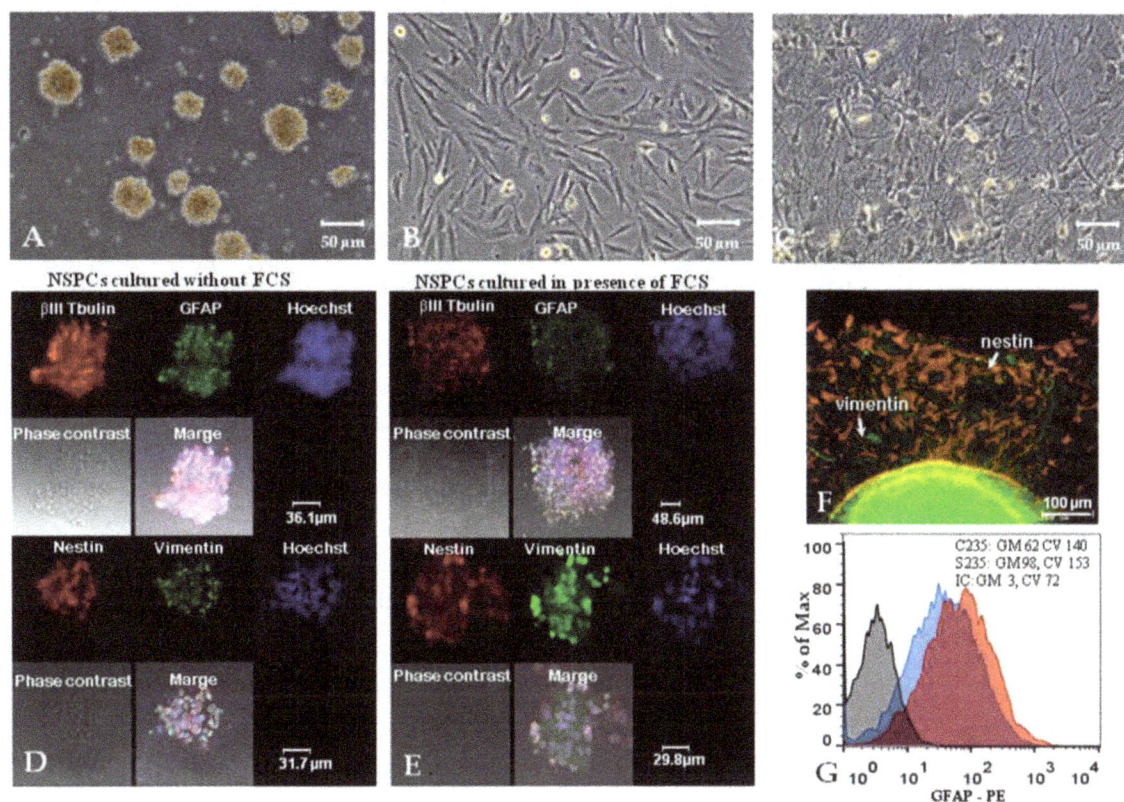

Figure 1. Neural stem/progenitor cells (NSPCs) isolated and maintained in the presence of fetal calf serum (FCS) demonstrate similarities to "classic" NSPCs grown in serum-free medium.

(A-C) Phase contrast microscopy of S170 culture in FCS-containing medium: neurospheres (A); fibroblast-like cells (B) and web-like structures (C) formed by NSPCs. (D-E) Expression of βIII Tubulin, glial fibrillary acidic protein (GFAP), nestin and vimentin by NSPCs maintained as neurospheres in serum free (D) or FCS-containing (E) medium, confocal microscopy of C235 (serum-free medium) and S235 (FCS-containing medium) cultures. (F) Expression of nestin (red) and vimentin (green) by cells relocating from neurospheres to plastic-adherent state in S170 culture grown in FCS-containing medium, fluorescent microscopy. (G) Flow cytometry analysis of GFAP expression: C235 (serum-free medium) culture– blue curve, S235 (FCS-containing medium) culture– red curve, isotype control (IC) – grey curve. Geometric means (GM) and coefficients of variation (CV) are displayed in the upper right corner.

We compared the ability of NSPCs from "S" and "C" cultures to modulate the process of monocyte differentiation to DCs. NSPCs were transferred to adhesive state and co-cultivated with peripheral blood monocytes isolated from healthy donors. Bone marrow MSCs-monocyte co-culture was used as control. Differentiation of monocytes was initiated by the addition of GM-CSF and IL-4. After 4 days in co-culture, cells were suspended, double-stained with fluorochrome-conjugated MoAbs against monocyte marker CD14 and DCs marker CD1a, and cell suspension was analyzed by flow cytometry. Differentiation efficacy was estimated by assessing the ratios of the numbers of cells expressing CD14 or CD1a. NSPCs from "S" cultures established and maintained in medium with FCS effectively blocked DC differentiation from monocytes (Figure 2 A,B), while NPSCs from "C" cultures grown under "classic" serum-free conditions had no influence on DC differentiation (Figure 2C,D). This cannot be explained by the variability of the properties of cells derived from different donors, because S235 and C235 cultures prepared from the same tissue sample produced different effects (Figure 2B, D). Importantly, S235 and C235 cultures were also tested immediately after neurosphere formation, before the first passaging and at that early stage they did not affect the differentiation of DCs (result not shown). The summary of the results for all tested cultures is presented in Figure 2E. The inhibitory action of NSPCs from "S" cultures was dose-dependent and similar to the effect of bone marrow MSCs.

Flow cytometry analysis of CD83 and HLA-DR expression in all cultures presented in Table 1, demonstrated that co-culturing of immature DCs with NSPCs did not significantly alter their LPS-

(Figure 3) or TNFα-PGE2-induced maturation irrespective of what, "S" or "C", type of NSPCs culture was examined. However, in some experiments, we detected moderate decrease in CD 83 expression within the CD 83 positive subpopulation (Figure 3C) or reduction of the quantity of cells with high for HLA-DR expression (Figure 3D).

In order to compare "C" and "S" cultures with respect to the types of cells they are composed of, C235 and S235 cultures derived from the same autopsy sample were stained with fluorochrome-conjugated MoAbs against a number of surface markers and analyzed by flow cytometry (Figure 4). Neither C235, nor S235 cells expressed differentiating neuroblasts and epithelial cells marker CD24 or markers of hematopoietic cells including CD34, the most common hematopoetic stem cell marker. Both types of cultures displayed relatively low staining with the antibody against CD133 stem cell marker. Since MSCs actively suppress DCs differentiation from monocytes, we estimated the likelihood of NSPCs conversion to MSCs-like phenotype in serum-containing medium and found it implausible, since we failed to find any cells positive for MSCs-associated CD104 (endoglin) or CD54 (ICAM-1) among S235 cells. CD90 (Thy-1), a glycoprotein present in the plasma membranes of both MSCs and neurons was weakly expressed only by C235 NSPCs suggesting their readiness for neurogenic differentiation. Unlike C235, S235 culture contained a small subset of cells expressing CD44 and an even smaller subpopulation of cells positive for CD73. Though the assortment of cell types present in NSPC cultures grown in the presence or absence of FCS may be slightly different, the difference seems too small to define NSPCs' suppressive effects on the immune system.

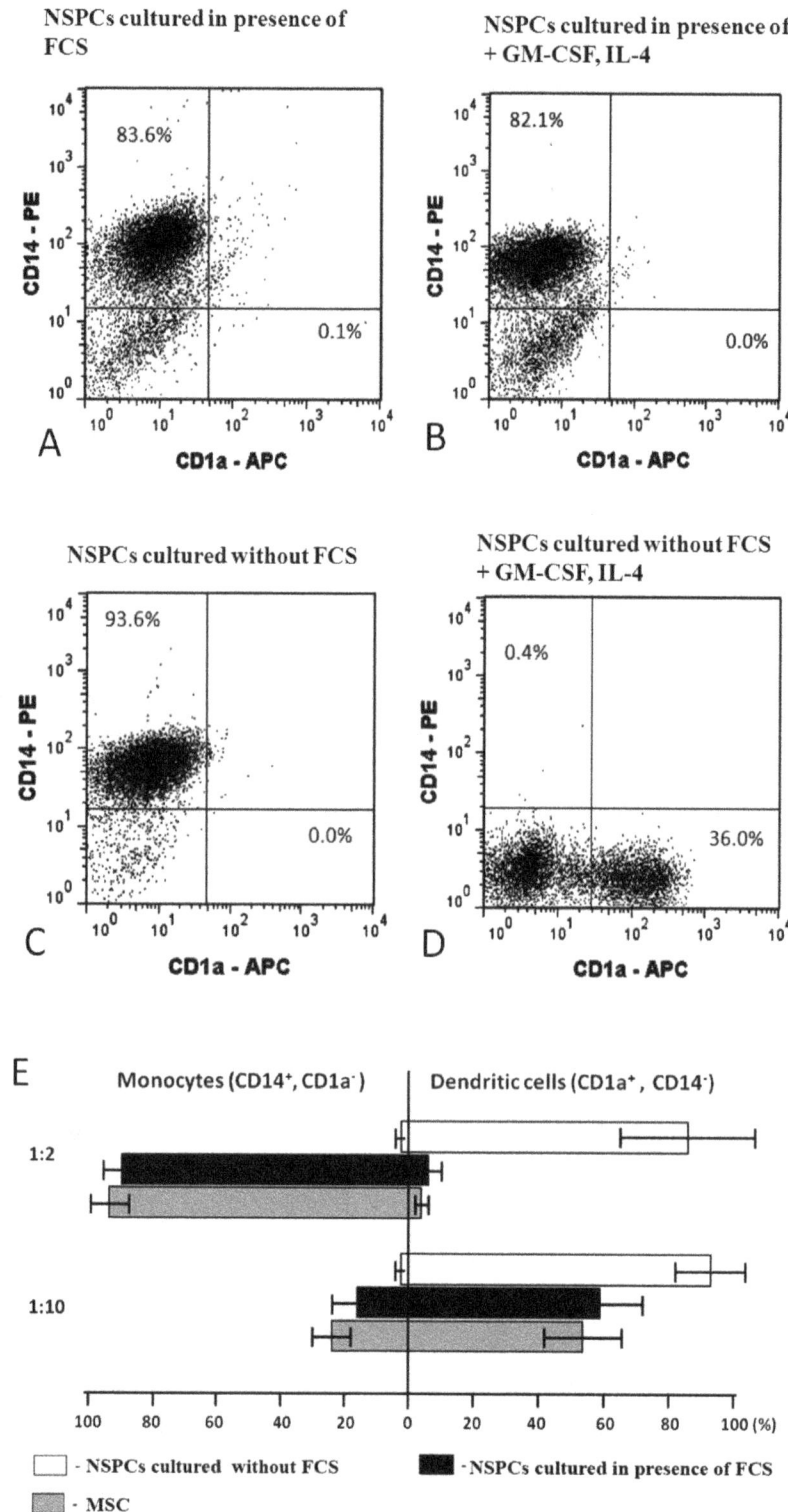

Figure 2. Effects of neural stem/progenitor cells (NSPCs) grown with or without fetal calf serum (FCS) upon differentiation of dendritic cells (DCs) from monocytes.

Co-cultivation of NSPCs from FCS-containing S235 culture (A, B) or FCS-free C235 culture (C, D) with monocytes at 1:2 NSPC/monocyte ratio in the absence (A, C) or presence (B, D) of differentiation factors: granulocyte macrophage colony-stimulating factor (GM-CSF) and interleukine-4 (IL-4). After 4 days in co-culture the cells were suspended, double stained with fluorescent monoclonal antibodies (MoAbs) against monocyte marker CD14 and DC marker CD1a and analyzed by flow cytometry. (E) Combined data for 3 "C" type (serum-free medium) cultures and 4 "S" type (FCS-containing medium) NSPCs cultures. Co-cultures with mesenchymal stem cells (MSCs) were used as positive control. Left-side columns: relative percentage of remaining monocytes calculated by formula: C/M×100% (C – percentage of CD14 positive monocytes in co-culture, M - percentage of CD14 positive monocytes in co-culture without GM-CSF and IL-4); right-side columns: relative percentage of emerging DCs calculated by formula: C/M×100% (C – percentage of CD1a positive DCs in co-culture, M - percentage of CD1a positive DCs in monoculture). Ratios of effector cells and monocytes in the co-culture well shown on the left. Percentages of both monocytes and DCs significantly differ between serum-free NSPCs cultures and FCS-containing NSPCs cultures. Mann Whitney statistical test was used to test for statistical significance, P < 0.05).

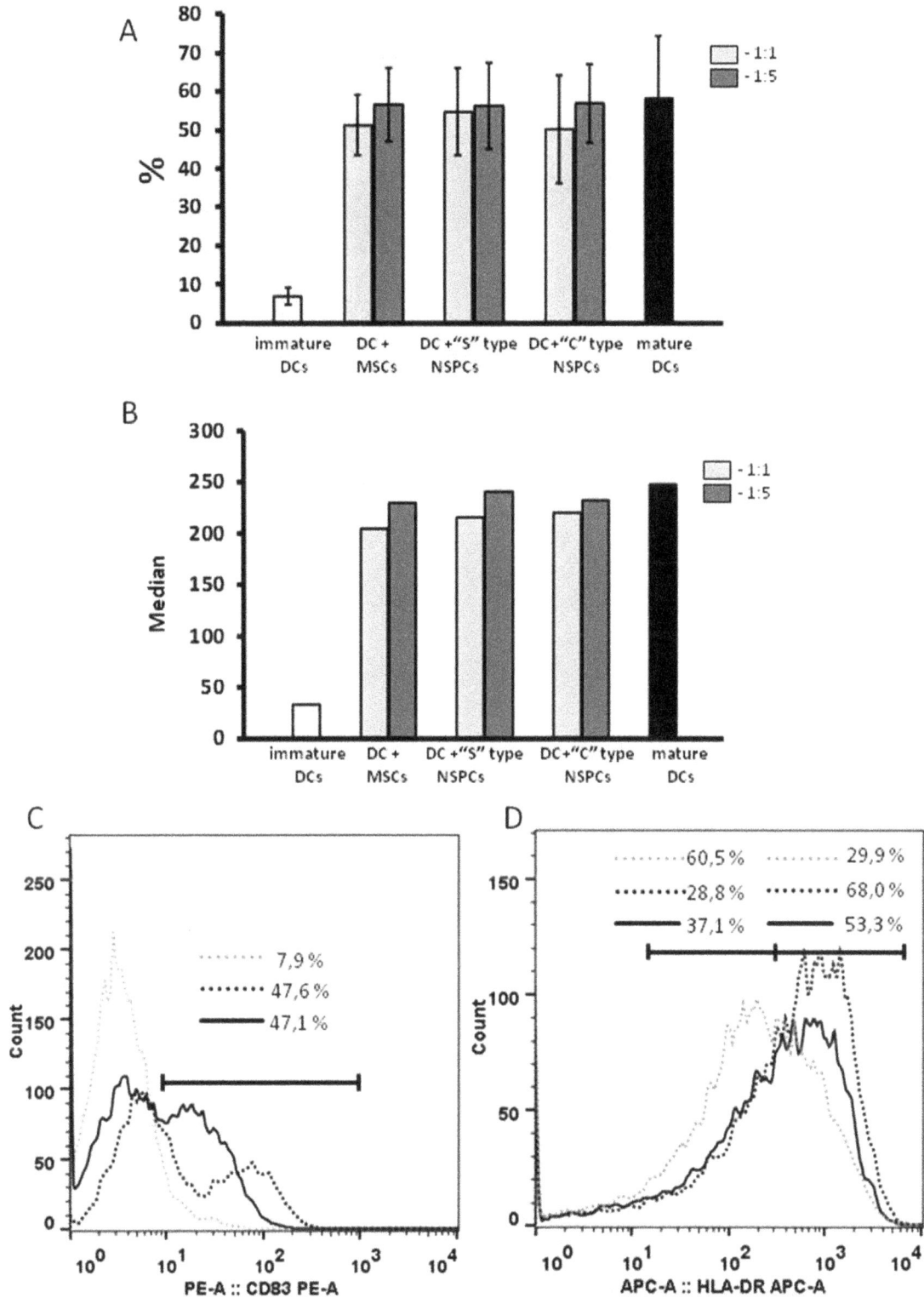

Figure 3.   Effects of neural stem/progenitor cells (NSPCs) grown with or without fetal calf serum (FCS) upon maturation of dendritic cells (DCs). NSPCs were co-cultivated with immature DCs at 1:1 and 1:5 NSPCs/DCs ratios in the presence of bacterial lipopolysaccharide (LPS). After 3 days in co-culture the cells were suspended, double stained with fluorescent monoclonal antibodies (MoAbs) against CD83 and HLA-DR and analyzed by flow cytometry. (A, B) Combined data for 3 "C" type (serum-free medium) and 4 "S" type (FCS-containing medium) NSPCs cultures. (A) Percentage of DCs expressing CD83. (B) Median of fluorescence intensity of MoAbs against HLA-DR. (C, D) Histograms showing CD 83 (C) and HLA-DR (D) expression level for DCs co-cultured with S163 (representative experiment). Black curves – C163 co-culture; black broken curves – MSCs co-culture; grey broken curves – DCs monoculture without LPS. The percentages of cells within the defined populations given on top.

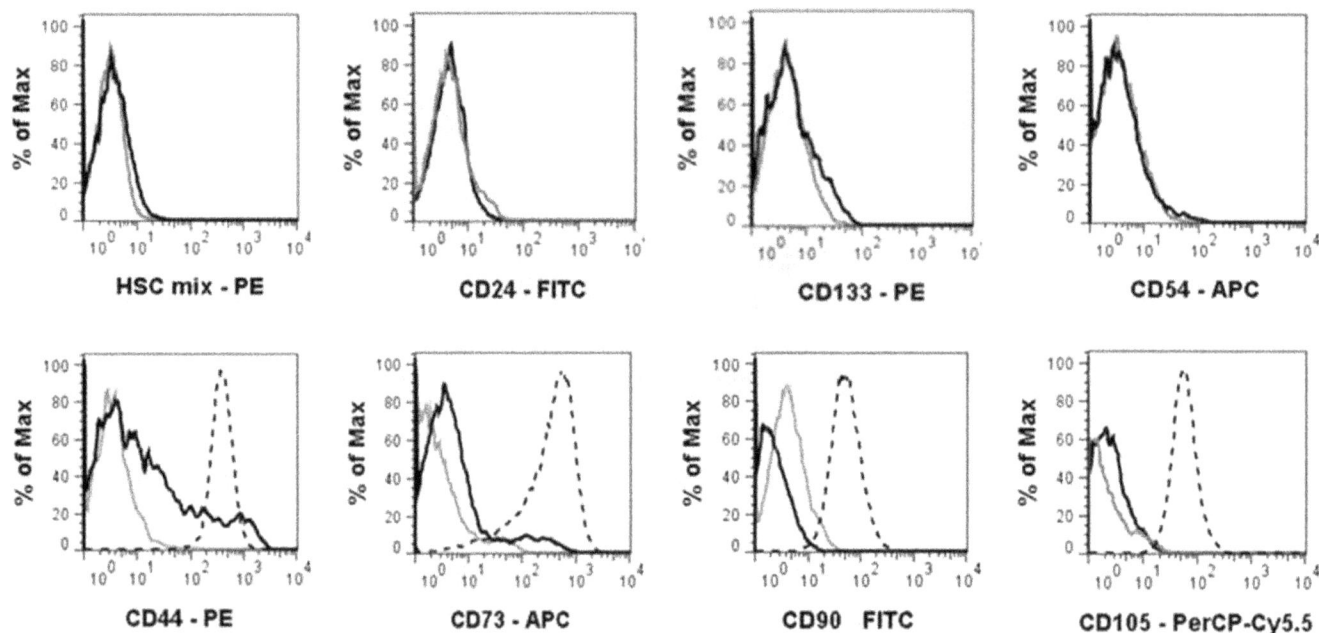

Figure 4. Expression of surface markers by neural stem/progenitor cells (NSPCs) from serum-containing and serum-free cultures derived from the same autopsy specimen.
Cell suspensions from S235 and C235 cultures were treated with fluorochrome-conjugated monoclonal antibodies (MoAbs) and analyzed by flow cytometry. Black curves - S235; grey curves – C235; broken curves – mesenchymal stem cells (MSCs). HSC mix – fluorochrome-conjugated MoAbs cocktail against hematopoietic markers: CD19, CD11b, CD34, CD45, HLA-DR.

Discussion

Our data suggest that the presence or absence of FCS in the culture medium is crucially important for the formation of two alternate NSPC phenotypes ("S" and "C" phenotypes, respectively) characterized by the ability to block DCs differentiation from monocytes. The short time exposure to FCS is probably not sufficient for the formation of "S" type cultures, because "S" phenotype is established only after passaging of NSPCs culture, as seen from our experiments with C235 and S235 cultures. It is not yet clear if DCs' differentiation block is induced by the majority of cells in NSPCs "S" cultures or by a minor subpopulation.

It was suggested that serum exposure promotes NSPCs differentiation into astroglia[16]. Subsequently, gene expression profiling of human NSPCs following their serum-induced astrocyte differentiation revealed elevated levels of the expression of 45 genes including GFAP[19]. Moreover, astrocytes can suppress *in vitro* monocyte/microglial activation and function[20]. Therefore, it seems likely that NSPCs' ability to control DCs differentiation may be associated with their serum-induced differentiation into astrocytes direction. However, this suggestion is opposed by certain results of our current studies. Here, as well as in our earlier publication we showed that NSPCs maintained in FSC-containing medium supposed to promote astrocytic diffentiation, still capable of expressing such "stemness" markers as nestin and Lex/SSEA1, as well as an early marker of neuronal differentiation βIII-tubulin. Their expression is mostly localized in neurosphere-like floating cell aggregates[21]. Probably, maintaining of NSPCs cultures in serum-containing media results in the accumulation of the least differentiated cells in neurospheres, while more differentiated cells adhere to cultural plastic and are eliminated at passaging.

Data concerning the interactions of NSPCs with DCs obtained by other researchers are scarce. On one hand, NSPCs derived by differentiation of human embryonic stem cells had almost no effect on monocytes differentiation *in vitro*[22]. On the other, human fetal NSPCs grown in serum-free conditions inhibited differentiation of monocytes into DCs[23]. This discrepancy may be caused by various reasons including the differences of cellular composition of the tested cultures and culture conditions. Data presented here show that NSPCs' impact on DCs differentiation from monocytes depends on the culture conditions of NSPCs.

The mechanism of FCS effect and difference between "C" and "S" phenotypes need further investigation including the possible role of BMP4 and other candidate factors on NSPCs and their co-cultures with monocytes. It is obvious, though, that culture conditions can result in differences in cell phenotypes. Importantly, dependence of essential cell properties from culture conditions can greatly complicate the process of development of cell-based therapies. Manufacture of clinical-grade cell products involves adaptation of laboratory culture methods, including drastic increase of cell production and exclusion of xenogeneic proteins achieved by substitution of FCS for human blood serum or utilizing serum-free media. That means that the results of basic and preclinical research carried out with cells grown using common laboratory methods, in some cases can be irrelevant to the effects of the controlled quality cell product obtained in a GMP facility and used for clinical studies. Our results show yet again that all preclinical studies with cultured cells have to be conducted using cells produced in exactly the same conditions and with the same equipment as the future clinical grade product. Dependence of clinically relevant properties of cell therapy products from the presence of certain factors, including serum components in the culture medium suggests that the effects of cell transplantation may depend upon the administration route. Really, after intravenous or intra-arterial administration transplanted cells find themselves in direct contact with all serum components, while after intracutaneous injection cells find themselves in a dramatically different environment.

Conclusion.

Addition of FCS instead of conventional combinations of growth factors to the NSPCs culture medium results in substantial modification of the immunological properties of the cultured cells manifested as the ability to suppress the *in vitro* differentiation of DCs from peripheral blood monocytes. At the same time, the patterns of cell types constituting the culture are similar in the presence or absence of FCS. In a broader prospective, it means that cells with almost identical phenotypes can display opposite immunomodulation properties. It should be taken into account when developing NSPCs-based cell products for regenerative medicine.

References

1. Andres RH, Horie N, Slikker W, Keren-Gill H, Zhan K, Sun G, Manley NC, Pereira MP, Sheikh LA, McMillan EL, Schaar BT, Svendsen CN, Bliss TM, Steinberg GK. Human neural stem cells enhance structural plasticity and axonal transport in the ischaemic brain. Brain. 2011; 134(Pt 6): 1777–89.

2. Lee ST, Chu K, Jung KH, Kim SJ, Kim DH, Kang KM, Hong NH, Kim JH, Ban JJ, Park HK, Kim SU, Park CG, Lee SK, Kim M, Roh JK. Anti-inflammatory mechanism of intravascular neural stem cell transplantation in haemorrhagic stroke. Brain. 2008; 131(Pt 3): 616–29.

3. Pluchino S, Furlan R, Martino G. Cell-based remyelinating therapies in multiple sclerosis: evidence from experimental studies. Curr. Opin.Neurol. 2004; 17(3): 247–55.

4. Ottoboni L, De Feo D, Merlini A, Martino G. Commonalities in immune modulation between mesemchymal stem cells (MSCs) and neural stem/precursor cells (NPCs). Immunol Lett. 2015; 168(2): 228-39.

5. Pluchino S, Zanotti L, Rossi B, Brambilla E, Ottoboni L, Salani G, Martinello M, Cattalini A, Bergami A, Furlan R, Comi G, Constantin G, Martino G. Neurosphere-derived multipotent precursors promote neuroprotection by an immunomodulatory mechanism. Nature. 2005; 436(7048): 266–71.

6. Ben-Hur T. Immunomodulation by neural stem cells. J Neurol Sci. 2008; 265(1-2): 1024.

7. Pluchino S, Zanotti L, Brambilla E, Rovere-Querini P, Capobianco A, Alfaro-Cervello C, Salani G, Cossetti C, Borsellino G, Battistini L, Ponzoni M, Doglioni C, Garcia-Verdugo JM, Comi G, Manfredi AA, Martino G. Immune Regulatory Neural Stem/Precursor Cells Protect from Central Nervous System Autoimmunity by Restraining Dendritic Cell Function. PLoS One. 2009; 4(6): e5959.

8. Fainstein N, Vaknin I, Einstein O, Zisman P, Ben Sasson SZ, Baniyash M, Ben-Hur T. Neural precursor cells inhibit multiple inflammatory signals. Mol Cell Neurosci. 2008; 39(3): 335–41.

9. Einstein O, Fainstein N, Vaknin I, Mizrachi-Kol R, Reihartz E, Grigoriadis N, Lavon I, Baniyash M, Lassmann H, Ben-Hur T. Neural precursors attenuate autoimmune encephalomyelitis by peripheral immunosuppression. Ann Neurol. 2007; 61(3): 209–18.

10. Steptoe RJ, Thomson AW. Dendritic cells and tolerance induction. Clin Exp Immunol. 1996; 105(3): 397-402.

11. Dauer M, Obermaier B, Herten J, Haerle C, Pohl K, Rothenfusser S, Schnurr M, Endres S, Eigler A. Mature dendritic cells derived from human monocytes within 48 hours: a novel strategy for dendritic cell differentiation from blood precursors. J. Immunol. 2003; 170(8): 4069-76.

12. Karalkin PA, Lupatov AY, Yarygin KN. Endocytosis of micro- and nanosized particles by human dendritic cells. Biochemistry (Moscow) Supplement Series A: Membrane and Cell Biology. 2009; 3(4): 410-16.

13. Christopherson K, Hromas R. Chemokine regulation of normal and pathologic immune responses. Stem Cells. 2001; 19(5): 388-96.

14. Jiang XX, Zhang Y, Liu B, Zhang SX, Wu Y, Yu XD, Mao N. Human mesenchymal stem cells inhibit differentiation and function of monocyte-derived dendritic cells. Blood. 2005; 105(10): 4120-26.

15. Nauta AJ, Kruisselbrink AB, Lurvink E, Willemze R, Fibbe WE. Mesenchymal stem cells inhibit generation and function of both CD34-derived and monocyte-derived dendritic cells. J. Immunol. 2006; 177(4): 2080-87.

16. Reynolds BA. Weiss S. Clonal and population analyses demonstrate that an EGF-responsive mammalian embryonic CNS precursor is a stem cell. Dev Biol. 1996; 175 (1): 1-13.

17. Poltavtseva RA, Revishchin AV, Aleksandrova MA, Korochkin LI, Viktorov IV, Sukhikh GT. Neural stem and progenitor cells of human embryos and fetuses as a basis of new biomedical technologies. Ontogenez 2003; 34 (3): 211-15

18. Lupatov AY, Karalkin PA, Suzdaltseva YG, Burunova VV, Yarygin VN, Yarygin KN. Cytofluorometric analysis of phenotypes of human bone marrow and umbilical fibroblast-like cells. Bull Exp Biol Med. 2006; 142 (4): 521-26.

19. Obayashi S, Tabunoki H, Kim SU, Satoh J. Gene expression profiling of human neural progenitor cells following the serum-induced astrocyte differentiation. Cell Mol Neurobiol. 2009; 29 (3): 423-38.

20. Kostianovsky AM, Maier LM, Anderson RC, Bruce JN, Anderson DE. Astrocytic regulation of human monocytic/microglial activation. J Immunol. 2008; 181(8): 5425-32.

21. Aleksandrova MA, Poltavtseva RA, Marei MV, Sukhikh GT. Analysis of Neural Stem Cells from Human Cortical Brain Structures In Vitro. Bull Exp Biol Med. 2016; 161(1): 197-208.

22. Shahbazi M, Kwang TW, Purwanti YI, Fan W, Wang S. Inhibitory effects of neural stem cells derived from human embryonic stem cells on differentiation and function of monocyte-derived dendritic cells. J Neurol Sci. 2013; 330: 85–93.

23. Pluchino S, Gritti A, Blezer E, Amadio S, Brambilla E, Borsellino G, Cossetti C, Del Carro U, Comi G, Hart B, Vescovi A, Martino G. Human neural stem cells ameliorate autoimmune encephalomyelitis in non-human primates. Ann Neurol. 2009; 66 (3): 343–54.

Abbreviations

NSPCs:	Neural stem/progenitor cells
DCs:	Dendritic cells
MSCs:	Mesenchymal stem cells
MHC:	Major histocompatibility complex
FCS:	Fetal calf serum
EGF:	Epidermal growth factor
FGF-2:	Basic fibroblast growth factor
GM-CSF:	Granulocyte macrophage colony-stimulating factor
IL-4:	Interleukine-4
LPS:	Lipopolysaccharide
TNF-α:	Tumor necrosis factor-α
MoAbs:	Monoclonal antibodies
GFAP:	Glial fibrillary acidic protein

Potential Conflicts of Interests

None

Acknowledgements

This research work was supported by grant No 14-25-00179 from Russian Science Foundation.

The date analysis and preparation of the manuscript was performed within the framework of the Program for Basic Research of State Academies of Sciences for 2013–2020. The authors are grateful to Alexander Samokhin for technical assistance.

Ethical standards

The work protocols were approved by the Research Center of Obstetrics, Gynecology and Perinatology ethical committee in full accordance with the national regulations.

Corresponding Author

Alexey Yu Lupatov, Institute of Biomedical Chemistry, Pogodinskaya str. 10, 119121 Moscow, Russia, alupatov@inbox.ru.

8

Safety and Feasibility of Autologous Mesenchymal Stem Cell Transplantation in Chronic Stroke in Indian patients

Bhasin A[1], Kumaran SS[2], Bhatia R[1], Mohanty S[3], Srivastava MVP[1]

Abstract

Introduction: Stem cell (SC) therapy has been envisioned as a therapeutic vehicle to promote recovery in resistant neurological diseases. Knowing the logistics and paradigms in recovery processes after Stroke, clinicians have pioneered the transplantation therapy. This study presents four-year follow up of our previous trial transplanting bone-marrow-derived animal-free culture expanded intravenous mesenchymal stem cells (MSCs) in chronic stroke which was published in 2010.

Methods: We performed an open-label, pilot trial on 12 patients with chronic stroke. Patients were allocated to two groups, those who received intravenous autologous *ex vivo* cultured mesenchymal stem cells (MSC group) or those who did not (control group), all followed for four years from the day of cell transplantation.

Results: The reports have been optimistic regarding safety as we did not find any cell related side effects / mortality till 208th week. We observed that modified Barthel Index showed statistical significant improvement at 156 and 208 weeks of transplantation (95 % CI : -10.27 to 0.07; p =0.041) follow up in the MSC group as compared to controls. The 2nd and 3rd quartile for mBI in MSC group was 89 & 90 respectively suggesting good performance of patients in the stem cell group. The impairment scales i.e., Fugl Meyer, Ashworth tone scale, strength of hand muscles (MRC) did not show any significant improvement at 208th week which is similar to our previous published report.

Conclusion: This follow up study primarily indicates safety, tolerance and applicability of autologous mesenchymal stem cells in Stroke. MSCs may act as "chaperones" or work through paracrine mechanisms leading to functional recovery post stroke.

Key Words: Stem cell transplantation, Stroke, Recovery

Introduction

The knowledge and use of stem cells in regenerative medicine and drug development has been a soulful interest in biomedical field[1]. Evidence of neurogenesis in the adult brain is well proven refuting the dilemma regarding CNS regeneration. With an enthralling research opportunities in medicine targeting treatment opportunities, cell transplantation and gene therapies act as panacea to improve the quality and expectancy of life in resistant neurological disorders. Stroke is associated with high mortality and severe morbidity and reports suggest that 50% stroke survivors suffer residual neurological deficits[2,3]. Because of the changed morbidity spectrum, the focus of interest is shifting towards behavioral recovery, although rehabilitation motor therapy is important for maximization of functional recovery after stroke[4,5]. Stem cell therapy recently has been divided under two groups; "replacement therapy" and "neurotrophic therapy". Clinical trials of differentiated tumor cell lines, neural progenitor cells from primordial porcine striatum, and autologous bone marrow-derived mesenchymal stem cells (MSCs) have been conducted[6].

Neurorestorative processes contributing to functional improvement after chronic stroke include neurogenesis, angiogenesis, and synaptic plasticity. Cell transplantation is a cellular approach that has the potential to induce all of the neurorestorative processes essential for facilitating recovery of neurological function. Bone marrow-derived mesenchymal stem cells (MSCs) have great potential as therapeutic agents in stroke management, since they are easily accessible and can be rapidly expanded *ex vivo* for autologous transplantation. Increasing evidence suggests that bone marrow cells migrate throughout the brain and differentiate into neurons and glial cells[7-9].

MSC as neurorestorative therapy: Cognizance from our last trial

The latest consensus reported improvement of stroke outcomes after systemic stem cell injection which relies on the paracrine / autocrine hypothesis of these cells i.e, non-cell-autonomous properties, release of relevant trophic factors, rather than on engraftment into the lesioned area. However, several variables related to the optimal patient, such as age, type of stroke, location size of the lesion, and timing of treatment, remain to be

Author Names in full: Ashu Bhasin[1], Senthil S. Kumaran[2], Rohit Bhatia[1], Sujata Mohanty[3], M V Padma Srivastava[1]

[1]Department of Neurology, [2]Department of NMR, [3]Stem Cell Facility, All India Institute of Medical Sciences (AIIMS), New Delhi, India.

addressed[10,11]. MSCs are excellent candidates for cell transplantation as they are easily accessible, and can be preserved with minimal loss of potency. Transplantation by these cells have been safe and has been widely used in clinical trials (NCT 01714167) of neurological, cardiovascular and immunological diseases with encouraging results[12]. Our last report on MSC infusion in six chronic stroke patients established the safety and tolerance of MSC derived using serum-free media for expansion unlike bovine serum[13]. There was no significant difference in baseline clinical and radiological scores between the MSC and control groups, suggesting that the two groups were comparable to study the effectiveness of therapy after 8 and 24 weeks. There was no significant difference in FM and mBI scores after therapy (8 weeks: p = 0.87, t = 0.161 and p = 0.95, t = 0.065, respectively; and at follow-up (p=0.65 and p=0.75, respectively). A meagre reduction in the Ashworth tone scale was observed between the two groups. The adult brain can regenerate neurons lost after brain ischemia. Repair mechanisms in stroke are related to acute injury (first epoch) and is said to occur in the initial few hours after acute event when changes in blood flow, metabolism and ischemic cascade are most active. A second epoch is related with upregulation of growth factors which continue for days to weeks and is referred to as endogenous repair related events. A third epoch occurs weeks to months after stroke when spontaneous recovery mechanisms plateau representing a stable but modifiable early and late chronic phase. The purpose of this study was to attain maximum restoration possible and eventual return to normalcy of function. We followed up those six patients till four years. This short article presents safety, feasibility and tolerance of bone marrow derived mesenchymal stem cells after four years of infusion. It also studies the efficacy end points in terms of clinical and laboratory parameters at the end of 208 weeks (4 years).

Methods

Twelve patients (n=12) diagnosed with stroke (index event) 3 months to 2 years, MRC (Medical Research Council) grade of muscle power for the wrist and hand extensor or flexor muscles of at least 2, NIHSS (National Institute of Health Stroke Scale) between 4 and 15 who were conscious and comprehendible were recruited. All the patients were assessed on muscle power (MRC), tone (modified Ashworth) and Fugl Meyer (FM) scale for upper limbs and modified Barthel index (mBI) at baseline, 8weeks, 24, 78, 156 and 208 weeks[14,15]. The study was approved by Institute Committee for Stem Cell Research and Therapy (ICSCRT) and written informed consent was obtained from all the subjects. The trial is registered with CTRI (Ref/2011/08/002677).

Procedure

Bone Marrow Aspiration, Expansion and Transplantation

Bone marrow was aspirated under aseptic conditions from the posterior superior iliac crest of 6 chronic stroke patients. The bone marrow was diluted with phosphate-buffered saline, layered over Ficoll density medium and centrifuged at 1,800 rpm. for 25 min. Using Stem Pro MSC SFM basal medium (A-10334, Invitrogen), the mononuclear cell were plated at a density of 10^6 cells/cm^2 in T-25 tissue culture flask and incubated at 37 ° C/5% CO^2 . The cells were harvested and seeded at 3,000 or 10,000 cells/cm^2 in triplicate wells of 6-well plates. Trypan blue dye was used to test viability. MSC cultures of all patients were harvested using TrypLE TM Express (Invitrogen) on reaching 70–90% confluency. Non-adherent cells were removed after 24 h and fresh media was again added for incubation[16, 17]. The whole procedure took around 21±7 days. All samples were tested for mycoplasma and endotoxins at every third passage using commercially available kits according to the manufacturer's instructions. Aseptic infusion technique was followed

and cells were directly dissolved in 250-ml saline bottle and infused intravenously over 2–3 h using a sterile 50-ml syringe. The control group was administered with neurophysiotherapy regime only for 8 weeks.

Statistics

Mean difference between groups was compared using t test. We used both parametric and non-parametric tests for the outcome measures. Mortality was defined as death of a subject enrolled in the study till the end point which includes all cause mortality (cardiac, non cardiac and vascular) and the survival time was the day the patient received stem cell transplantation till the follow up or the end of study. Individual changes in FM and mBI between baseline and 8, 78, 156 weeks and 208 weeks were analyzed by parametric t test. A p < 0.05 was taken to indicate statistical significance. All statistical analyses were conducted using SPSS 12.0 (Chicago, IL).

Result

Baseline Characteristics of Patients

A total of twelve (n=12) patients were included in this study allocated to both the groups. Their mean age was 42.8±16.4 years (mean ± SD). The laboratory tests after the stem cell transplantation were normal for all patients as described till the last follow up.. The mean cell viability at transplantation was 98%, the cells were sterile and endotoxin free during expansion and at the time of injection. There were no early and late adverse reactions observed in patients during and after transplantation. Flow-cytometric analysis showed phenotype markers such as CD90, CD73, CD105 and were negative for HLA class II. The mean CD90, CD73 and CD105 were 61, 57.1 and 40%, respectively.

Mortality and adverse events

The IRB approved only six patients for MSC transplantation as pilot study in the year 2010, none of the patients reported malignancies, tumor or any cystic malformations when examined at fours years. These patients were screened with regular clinical examination, laboratory and radiology (i.e., MRI scans) investigations. They were telephonically interviewed (if it was not possible for them for a hospital visit) for any delayed reactions of skin, untreated infections or any other alarming symptoms. One of the patient (id 6) reported skin allergy/ rash after 9 months of transplantation (table 2). He underwent hospitalization for the same but it was found that the infection was unrelated to cells. Recurrent stroke or TIAs were not reported in all the six subjects.

Clinical Results

In the MSC or experimental group (males: females = 2:4), all were right handed dominant with age = 42±16.4 years (mean ± SD); the mean FM score was 44±11.6 at baseline and 53±7.1 at 208th week (p=0.026, t = -2.26), at 78 weeks (45.5 ± 7.2) exhibiting statistically significant improvement between all time points (p<0.05) (table 1). The second quartile for the experimental group for mBI and FM at 208 weeks was 92 and 54 respectively whereas control group showed a median of 51.7 and 47.4 respectively. Repeated measures ANOVA was found to be statistically significant at all time measurements i.e., at baseline and at 8, 24 weeks 78, 156 and 208 weeks (p<0.05). The control group showed significant improvement also between baseline and four year assessment. The mean FM scores at baseline was 16.8±6.1 and at 208 weeks was 48 ± 5.2 (p=0.002) respectively. These patients also showed statistically significant improvement between baseline and 24, 24 and 78, 156 to 208 weeks (p≤0.05) for both FM and mBI scores.

Table 1. Clinical outcomes and demographics in experimental / (MSC) and control group

No	Group	Age/sex	Months after stroke	Area of lesion All MCA territory	Baseline		24 weeks		78 weeks		156 Weeks		208 weeks	
					FM (/66)	mBI (/100)	FM (/66)	mBI (/100)	FM (/66)	mBI (/100)	FM ((/66)	mBI (/100)	FM (/66)	m BI (/100)
1	E	28/F	11	Rt fronto-parietal (I)	22	52	44	80	52	88	56	90	59	92
2	E	20/F	12	Rt fronto-parietal (H)	11	30	30	60	38	74	42	82	42	82
3	E	59/F	7	Rt frontal (I)	11	40	32	70	41	82	46	86	50	88
4	E	35/F	8	Lt int capsule (H)	14	32	28	65	38	78	45	88	49	92
5	E	55/M	9	Right frontal (I)	22	52	44	78	52	86	58	90	58	92
6	E	55/M	8	Right frontal (I)	20	58	42	82	52	90	56	90	60	94
Mean		**42**	**9.3**		**16.6**	**44**	**36.6**	**72.5**	**45.1**	**83**	**50.5**	**87.6**	**53**	**90**
1	C	40/M	10	Lt frontal (I)	11	40	30	65	38	72	41	78	43	78
2	C	28/M	12	Rt parietal (I)	20	52	38	78	48	84	52	88	55	90
3	C	42/M	8	Rt int capsule (I)	12	35	36	65	42	72	47	77	47	77
4	C	30/M	12	Lt tempor parietal(I)	11	42	30	68	38	78	42	82	42	86
5	C	60/M	7	Left caudate (I)	24	55	33	73	42	80	46	84	48	84
6	C	50/M	8	Right frontoparietal (H)	23	50	38	72	47	82	51	86	53	88
Mean	C	**46.5**	**9.3**		**16.8**	**45.6**	**34.1**	**70.1**	**42.5**	**78**	**46.5**	**82.5**	**48**	**83.8**

Table 2. Onsetof morbidities and reactions in both the groups. None were related to cell transplantation

Morbidities and reactions	MSC group	Control group
Early reactions		
Fever	1	0
Infection (pneumonia,UTI etc)	0	0
Pain	2	0
drowziness	0	1
Long term effects		
Tumor formation	0	0
Systemic cancer	0	0
Brain tumor	0	0
Seizures	1	2
Psychological illnes	1	2

Comparison between MSC and Control Group

The baseline characteristics between the two groups were matched (p>0.05) suggesting that the two groups were comparable to study the effectiveness of therapy after 8, 24, 78, 156 and 208 weeks. Only mBI was statistically significant at 208 weeks (95 % CI: -12.9 to 0.49; p=0.05) and at 156 weeks (95 % CI: -1.26 to 1.76; p=0.04) (figures 1& 2) whereas there was no significant difference in FM scores at four yearly examination (95% CI:-3.01 to 2.01, p=0.19). The estimated difference between the two proportions for Fugl Meyer scale was 5 at 4 years. We did not report any significant improvement in power and tone measured on MRC and Ashworth tone scale for upper and lower limbs.

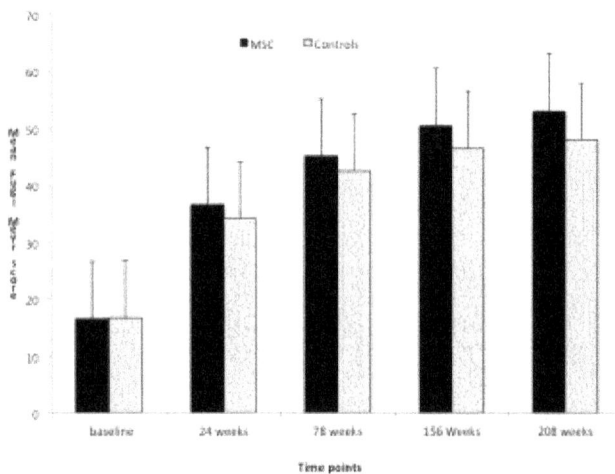

Figure 1. Graph showing mean Fugl Meyer scores between experimental and control groups at all time points.

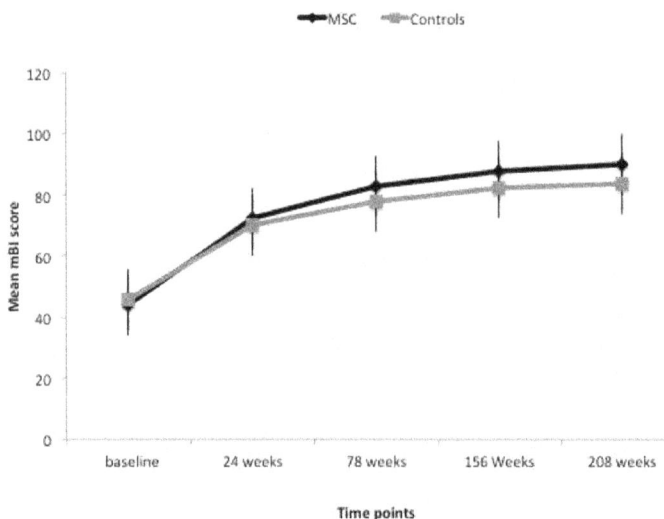

Figure 2. Graph showing mean modified Barthel Index in experimental and control groups at all time points.

Discussion

We had studied safety and feasibility of *ex vivo* culture expanded mesenchymal stem cells with animal serum free media in our published trials[13, 18, 19]. Owing to ethical concerns of using these cells, it was necessary to monitor these patients for more safety concerns and potential late complications i.e., tumorogenesis and genetic mutations. Our first study was morally based on the safety,

feasibility, practicality and procurement of mesenchymal cells in which we did not report any significant improvement in the functional outcomes till 24 weeks. In this report, we present safety and efficacy of mesenchymal stem cells at 208 weeks (4years) in six chronic stroke patients. In this mid- to long-term follow up, we present only the clinical data and not the functional imaging results, as two of the patients could not undergo MRI due to claustrophobia and hence BOLD and DTI results are not explained in this.

Bang *et al* in their 5 year follow up[21] reported the risk of zoonoses raising the possibility that administration of MSCs contaminated by xenogeneic proteins lead to a risk of immunologic rejection of the injected cells and serious complications such as autoimmune reactions against one's own stem cells[22,23]. As we used no animal medium for the culture expansion so the risk of occurence of GVHD was not expected and hence not reported in our patients.

The results of the present study showed that intravenous transplantation of *ex vivo* culture expanded MSCs is safe based on results of four-years of follow up. There was no mortality or any comorbidities during this period. Supraventricular tachyarrhythmia was reported in patients who received hematopoietic stem cell transplantation. Similarly, it is hypothesized that seizures may be caused by aberrant innervation from newly formed neural circuits after cell transplantation. We did not report any such incidence in our patients. In addition, it is also reported that, vascular occlusion can be caused by MSCs at the time of infusion via occlusion of the arteries of the brain or other organs or by restenosis[24]. Fortunately, our six patients tolerated the transplantation well and are still under long-term follow-up for any such event occurence. In our study no immune suppressants were required following transplantation, eliminating the risks associated with MSC therapy[25-27]. This is the first known study with a relatively long term follow up establishing the safety and tolerance of MSC derived using serum-free media for expansion unlike bovine serum used in the earlier study[21].

A score of 92 i.e., 75th percentile of mBI in experimental group as compared to 85 in control reflects a 7 point difference suggesting that control group also recovered well. In our published study, we presented that intravenous delivery of cells as safe, well tolerated by patients till 6 months but we failed to prove any remarkable difference between the two groups. A four-year long follow up can be considered a good reference to scale stroke recovery, very likely the patients must have opted for alternative systems of medicine i.e., acupuncture, acupressure, naturopathy and other uncontrolled physiotherapy regimes. Till 24 weeks as last reported, there was no improvement in the activities of daily living scale whereas when examined at 208 weeks, patients performed functionally better in the MSC group than in the control group with modified Barthel index being statistically significant (p<0.05). Enhancing neurogenesis can be a candidate explanation of the therapeutic mechanism of MSCs. Preclinical studies showed the importance of neurogenesis in an animal model of stroke and transplanted MSCs might enhance this process[28,29]. It has been proven that stem cells home in the infarcted regions thus promoting functional recovery in chronic stroke rats[30,31]. As reported earlier, cell-enhanced recovery has been reported with chronic delivery of cells even 1 month after ischemia[32].

We did not observe any significant improvement in MRC, Ashworth tone scale, Fugl Meyer and volume of lesion at four years between the two groups. The recovery observed was in aspects of functional gains although it was reported from patients with stem cell therapy that their performance and task oriented activity had increased compared to the pre stem cell status. Owing to ethical concerns and rampant use of stem cells without regulation, the institute ethics committee gave approval for six patients initially. The control group also showed improvement with an increased clinical and ADL scores which would question the psychoimmunological or placebo effects of mesenchymal stem cells.

The interval between the onset of stroke and the time of cell therapy may be an important criteria for selecting patients for cell therapy. Stroke is classically divided into an acute, sub-acute and chronic phase. Each phase is defined by a complex array of events with overlapping and distinct kinetics that led to tissue regeneration and remodelling. Cell transplantation at a chronic phase is thought to augment the neurobehavioural responses after injury via neurotrophic approach. The homogeneity of the subject group i.e., the type of stroke, etiology, premorbid status are few questions which need to be answered and stated before planning a trial[33,34]. Recently, there have been various efforts to enhance the therapeutic beneficial effects of stem cells (including blood-brain barrier manipulation, chronic preconditioning and genetically modified MSCs) and to reduce possible adverse effects of MSCs. We hope the therapeutic effects and safety of MSCs will be improved with these efforts and further studies.

The Indian government has regularized stem cell research practices in the country with the premier research institutes like Indian council of Medical Research and the Department of Biotechnology having laid down stem cell research guidelines in 2013 according to which all clinical trials in India should be approved by IC-SCRT and national apex committee (NAC) along with CDSCO draft on compensation towards injury due to participation in clinical research[35,36]. Phase II of a randomized controlled transplantation of autologous stem cells in stroke by our group is currently undergoing which would help to delineate the efficacy of these cells in a more scientific manner and amend the pitfalls in the current study. A very recent study published by Prasad et al [37] investigated the safety and efficacy of intravenous mononuclear stem cell transplantation in sub-acute ischemic stroke in which fifty-eight patients received a mean of 280.75 million BMSCs at median of 18.5 days after stroke onset. There was no significant difference between BMSCs arm and control arm in the Barthel Index score (63.1 versus 63.6; p=0.92), modified Rankin scale shift analysis (p=0.53) or score >3 (47.5% versus 49.2%; p=0.85), NIHSS score (6.3 versus 7.0; p=0.53) which is similar to our study as there was no statistically significant improvement observed between study and control group.

Conclusion

As no study is flawless, we also faced several limitations which require mention. First, owing to the experimental nature of treatment, the sample size was very small to state the efficacy of the cells[32, 33]. Altogether all current human studies imply that stem cell therapy in brain is feasible, the limited data obtained from this research thus far provide little consistent evidence of any clinical benefit. Further trials are needed to determine the optimal cell population and method of administration is needed to improve the outcome of cell therapy for stroke[38, 39]. The results of the present study showed some potential of MSC in regard to the functional improvement in patients nevertheless the trial primarily explains the tolerance, forbearance and safety associated with MSCs transplantation widening their scope for translational medicine.

References

1.   Eriksson PS, Perfilieva E, Bjork-Eriksson T. Neurogenesis in the adult human hippocampus. Nat Med. 1998; 4(11): 1313-7.

2.   Stahnisch FW, Nitsch R. Cajal's concept of neuronal plasticity: the ambiguity lives on. Trends Neurosci. 2002; 25(11): 589-91.

3.   Lee JS, Hong JM, Moong GJ, Lee PH, Bang OY. Long-Term Effects of MSC Treatment in Stroke. Stem Cells. 2010; 28(6):1099-106.

4.   Bjorklund A, Lindvall O. Cell replacement therapies for central nervous system disorders. Nat Neurosci. 2000; 3(6):537-44.

5.   Weimann JM, Charlton CA, Brazelton TR, Hackman RC, Blau HM. Contribution of transplanted bone marrow cells to purkinje neurons in human adult brains. Proc Natl Acad Sci USA. 2003; 100(4):2088-93.

6.   Sigrid C, Schwarz J. Translation of stem cell therapy for neurological diseases. Translational Research. 2010; 156(3): 155-60.

7.   Gogel S, Gubernator M, Minger SL. Progress and prospects: stem cells and neurological diseases. Gene Ther. 2011;18(1):1-6

8.   Chen J, Chopp M. Neurorestorative treatment of stroke: cell and pharmacological approaches. NeuroRx. 2006;3(4):466-73.

9.   Prockop DJ. Marrow stromal cells as stem cells for non hematopoietic tissues. Science. 1997;276(5309):71-4.

10. Conget PA, JJ Minguell. Phenotypical and functional properties of human bone marrow mesenchymal progenitor cells. J Cell Physiol. 1999;181(1):67-73.

11. Caplan AI. Why are MSCs therapeutic? New data: new insight. J Pathol. 2009;217(2):318-24.

12. Castro Henrique P, Coehlo Pimentel P, Fonseca M, Freitas GR, Otero RM. The rise of Cell Therapy trials of Stroke. Review of Registered and published studies. Stem Cells Dev. 2013 ;22(15):2095-111.

13. Bhasin A, Srivastava M, Mohanty S, Kumaran S, Bhatia R, Garg A, Airan B. Autologouss mesenchymal stem, cells in chronic stroke. Cerebrovasc Dis Extra. 2011;1(1):93-104.

14. Loewen SC, Anderson BA: Reliability of modified motor assessment scale and the Barthel index. Phys Ther. 1988;68(7):1077-81.

15. Oldfield RC: The assessment and analysis of handedness: the Edinburgh inventory. Neuropsychologia. 1971;9(1):97-113.

16. Chase LG, Lakshmipathy U, Rao SM, Vemuri MC. A novel serum-free medium for the expansion of human mesenchymal stem cells. Stem Cell Res Ther. 2010;1(1):8.

17. Lindroos B, Boucher S, Chase L, Kuokkanen H, Huhtala H, Haataja R. Serum-free, xeno-free culture media maintain the proliferation rate and multipotentiality of adipose stem cells in vitro. Cytotherapy. 2009;11(7):958-72.

18. Bhasin A, Srivastava MVP, Bhatia R, S Mohanty S, Kumaran S, Bose S. Stem cell therapy. A clinical trial in Stroke. Clin Neurol Neurosurg. 2013;115(7):1003-8.

19. Bhasin A, Srivastava MVP, Bhatia R, Mohanty S, Senthil S. Autologous Intravenous mononuclear stem cell therapy in chronic ischemic stroke. J Stem Cells Regen Med. 2012;8(3):181-9.

20. Wei X, Yang X, Han ZP, Qu F, Shao L, Shi Y. Mesenchymal stem cells: a new trend for cell therapy. Acta Pharmacol Sin. 2013;34(6):747-54.

21. Bang OY, Lee JS, Lee PH, Lee G. Autologous mesenchymal stem cell transplantation in stroke patients. Ann Neurol. 2005;57(6):874-82.

22. Spees JL, Gregory CA, Singh H, Tucker HA, Peister J, Lynch PJ, Hsu SC, Smith J, Prockop DJ. Internalized antigens must be removed to prepare hypoimmunogenic mesenchymal stem cells for cell and gene therapy. Mol Ther. 2004;9(5):747-56.

23. Cobo F, Talavera P, Concha A. Diagnostic approaches for viruses and prions in stem cell banks. Virology. 2006;347(1):1-10.

24. Hidalgo JD, Krone R, Rich MW, Blum K, Adkins D, Fan MY, Brown R, Devine S, Grawbert T, Blum W, Tomasson M, Goodnough LT, Vij R, Dipersio J, Khoury H. Supraventricular tachyarrhythmias after hematopoietic stem cell transplantation: Incidence, risk factors and outcomes. Bone Marrow Transplant. 2004;34(7):615-9.

25. Aggarwal S, Pittenger MF. Human mesenchymal stem cells modulate allogeneic immune cell responses. Blood. 2005;105(4):1815-22.

26. Zhang R, Zhang Z, Wang L, Wang Y, Gousev A, Zhang L, Ho KL, Morshead C, Chopp M. Activated neural stem cells contribute to stroke-induced neurogenesis and neuroblast migration toward the infarct boundary in adult rats. J Cereb Blood Flow Metab. 2004;24(4):441-8.

27. Kokaia Z, Thored P, Arvidsson A, Lindvall L. Regulation of stroke-induced neurogenesis in adult brain–recent scientific progress. Cereb Cortex. 2006;16 Suppl 162-7.

28. Jin K, Wang X, Xie L, Mao XO, Zhu W, Wang Y, Shen J, Mao Y, Banwait S, Greenberg DA. Evidence for stroke-induced neurogenesis in the human brain. Proc Natl Acad Sci U S A. 2006 ;103(35):13198-202.

29. Willing A, Lixian J, Milliken M, Poulus S, Zigova T, Song S, Hart C, Sanchoz- Ramos J, Sanberg PR. Intravenous versus intrastriatal cord blood administration in a rodent model of stroke. J Neurosci Res. 2003;73(3):296-307.

30. Shen LH, Li Y, Chen J, Zacharek A, Gao Q, Kapke A, Lu M, Raginski K, Vangpuri P, Smith A, Chopp M. Therapeutic benefit of bone marrow stromal cells administered 1 month after stroke J Cereb Blood Flow Metab. 2007;27(1):6-13.

31. Chen J, Zhang ZG, Li Y, Wang L, Xu YX, Gautam SC, Lu M, Zhu Z, Chopp M. Intravenous administration of human bone marrow stromal cells induces angiogenesis in the ischemic boundary zone after stroke in rats. Circ Res. 2003;92(6):692-9.

32. Shen LH, Li Y, Chen J, Cui Y, Zhang C, Kapke A, Lu M, Savant-Bhonsale M, Chopp M. One-year follow-up after bone marrow stromal cell treatment in middle-aged female rats with stroke. Stroke. 2007;38(7):2150-6.

33. Freeman TB, Vawter DE, Leaverton PE, Godbold JH, Hauser RA, Goetz CG, Olanow CW. Use of placebo surgery in controlled trials of a cellular-based therapy for parkinson's disease. N Engl J Med. 1999;341(13):988-92.

34. Lindvall O, Kokaia Z, Martinez-Serrano A. Stem cell therapy for human neurodegenerative disorders-how to make it work. Nat Med. 2004;10 Suppl:S42-50.

35. Mannello F, Tonti GA. Concise review: No breakthroughs for human mesenchymal and embryonic stem cell culture: Conditioned medium feeder layer, or feeder-free; medium with fetal calf serum, human serum, or enriched plasma; serum-free, serum replacement nonconditioned medium, or ad hoc formula? Stem Cells. 2007;25(7):1603-9.

36. Savitz SI, Rosenbaum DM, Dinsmore JH,Wechsler LR, Caplan LR. Cell transplantation for stroke. Ann Neurol. 2002;52(3):266-75.

37. Prasad K, Sharma A, Garg A, Mohanty S, Bhatnagar S, Johri S, Singh KK, Nair V, Sarkar RS, Gorthi SP, Hassan KM, Prabhakar S, Marwaha N, Khandelwal N, Misra UK, Kalita J, Nityanand S; INVEST study group. Intravenous autologous mononuclear stem cell therapy for ischemic stroke: a multicentric randomized trial. Stroke. 2014;45(12):3618-24.

38. Mittal S. Stem cell research. India Perspective. Perspect Clin Res. 2013;4(1):105-7.

39. Bhasin A, Sriavstava MV, Bhatia R, Kumaran S, Mohanty S. Stem cells in neurological diseases. Indian Perspective. J Of Stem Cell Res and Therapy. 2014; 4: 3-10.

Abbreviations

MSC:	Mesenchymal Stem cells
mBI :	modified Barthel Index
FM :	Fugl Meyer scale
DTI :	Diffusion tensor imaging
MRC :	Medical Research Council scale for power assessment

Potential Conflicts of Interests

None

Acknowledgments

We acknowledge the Department of Science and Technology, India for the grant in aid support.

Corresponding Author

M V Padma Srivastava, Department of Neurology, All India Institute of Medical Sciences, New Delhi, India, 110029
vasanthapadma123@gmail.com

9

Increased motility of mesenchymal stem cells is correlated with inhibition of stimulated peripheral blood mononuclear cells *in vitro*

Bertolo A[1#], Pavlicek D[1#], Gemperli A[1,2], Baur M[3,4], Pötzel T[3], Stoyanov J[1,5,6]

Abstract

Immunomodulatory properties of mesenchymal stem cells (MSC) are key components of their successful applications in clinical setting. However, treatments based on MSC immunomodulation need understanding of cell characteristics before cell transplantation. We used live-imaging to test the suitability of the MSC motility as a parameter for quick prediction of the immunomodulatory potential of human MSC in regulating the activity of stimulated peripheral blood mononuclear cells (PBMC) *in vitro*. Bone marrow MSC, from various donors and *in vitro* passages, were cultured with or without stimulated PBMC. After seven days, immunomodulation was assessed by measuring PBMC proliferation, IgG production and cytokine secretion in MSC and PBMC monocultures and co-cultures, and results were correlated to MSC motility. In co-culture, we observed that MSC successfully inhibited PBMC activity, reducing PBMC proliferation and IgG production compared to PBMC monoculture. MSC modulated PBMC to reduce the secretion of TNFα and IL-10, increase IL-6, G-CSF and MCP-1, while GM-CSF was not affected. By live-imaging tracking of cell trajectories, we observed that fast moving MSC were inhibiting more efficiently stimulated PBMC compared to slow ones. In co-culture, fast MSC were more effective in inhibiting IgG production (~30% less IgG), and secreted higher levels of IL-10 (~10% increase) and GM-CSF (~20% increase) compared to slower cells. Furthermore, fast MSC in monocultures produced 2.3-fold more IL-6, 1.5-fold MCP-1 and 1.2-fold G-CSF in comparison to slower cells. In conclusion, live-imaging cell tracking allowed us to develop an indicative assay of the immune-regulatory potential of MSC prior to *in vivo* administration.

Key Words: Human mesenchymal stem cells, Immunomodulatory potential, In vitro cell motility, Stem cell transplantation

Introduction

Human mesenchymal stem cells (MSC) are multipotent stromal cells with the ability to undergo extensive proliferation[1,2], produce a large number of cytokines[3], and the potential to differentiate into several cell lineages, such as adipocytes, chondrocytes, myocytes and osteoblasts[4]. Because of these defining characteristics, MSC emerged as one of the favorite candidates for cell-based therapies and tissue engineering approaches. Clinical trials have shown the beneficial effects of MSC application in critical health conditions like myocardial infarction[5], spinal cord injuries[6] and liver cirrhosis[7]. Additionally to their tissue restorative capacity, MSC also showed extensive immunomodulatory effects[8] making them potentially applicable in the treatment of immune-related diseases, such as graft versus host disease[9], systemic lupus erythematosus and multiple sclerosis[10].

The exact mechanism by which MSC regulate the immune system is still a matter of debate, but it is likely to be a co-effect of direct contact between cells and secretion of soluble factors. The complexity of the immunomodulatory mechanism is represented by the involvement of more than a dozen soluble factors which were shown to act on both innate and adaptive immune cells[11,12]. Among the most discussed secreted immunosuppressive factors are indoleamine-pyrrole 2,3-dioxygenase[13], prostaglandin E2[14], transforming growth factor-β[15] and nitric oxide[16]. Secretion of those soluble factors is dependent on the microenvironment

of the MSC, for example tumor necrosis factor α (TNF-α), interleukin 1-β (IL1-β) or interferon-γ (IFN-γ) are required for the activation of MSC induced immunomodulation[17,18]. MSC were reported to mediate a shift from a T_h1 driven response to rather an anti-inflammatory T_h2 response[19] which is characterized by lower levels of interleukin-2 (IL-2), IFN-γ and TNF-α and higher concentrations of interleukin-4 (IL-4), IL-5, IL-10 and IL-13. MSC can also secrete interleukin-6 (IL-6) which was shown to inhibit the differentiation of monocytes into antigen presenting dendritic cells[20]. Furthermore, IL-6 produced by MSC promotes neutrophil survival and expansion when combined with granulocyte macrophage colony-stimulating factor (GM-CSF)[21]. Additionally, it was found that by producing monocyte chemoattractant protein-1 (MCP-1 or CCL2), MSC are able to inhibit IgG production of plasma cells[22,23] and induce T-cells apoptosis via the FAS ligand-dependent FAS pathway[24].

Despite all promising researches, clinical trials with autologous MSC transplantations can have uncertain outcomes, partially caused by the wide intra- and inter-donor variability of MSC populations[25]. Such variations include diverse differentiation potential, cell morphology[26] or cell motility. Nowadays, there is a consensus that MSC therapies would be better predictable and more reproducible if we could evaluate and then use only cells with standardized characteristics.

We have demonstrated previously that *in vitro* MSC motility can be

Author Names in full: Alessandro Bertolo[1#], David Pavlicek[1#], Armin Gemperli[1,2], Martin Baur[3,4], Tobias Pötzel[3], Jivko Stoyanov[1,5,6]

[1]Swiss Paraplegic Research, Nottwil, Switzerland, [2]Department of Health Sciences and Health Policy, University of Lucerne, Lucerne, Switzerland, [3]Cantonal Hospital of Lucerne, Lucerne, Switzerland, [4]Swiss Paraplegic Centre, Nottwil, Switzerland, [5]Institute for Surgical Technology and Biomechanics, University of Bern, Bern, Switzerland, [6]Center for Applied Biotechnology and Molecular Medicine, University of Zurich, Zurich, Switzerland.

# These authors contributed equally

a useful parameter to quickly characterize and distinguish the differentiation potential of MSC populations[27]. Despite the observation that MSC were moving randomly and without directionality, we could determine that slow moving MSC were more likely to be senescent when compared with fast moving ones. However, average moving cells outperformed the rest with their ability to differentiate showing that MSC motility is a good predictor for the differentiation potential. We then wanted to investigate if a correlation with the immunomodulatory capacity of MSC also exists.

In this study, we tested the suitability of the MSC motility as a parameter for quick prediction of the immunomodulatory potential of the cells. We investigated by live-imaging microscopy the *in vitro* motility of human MSC isolated from different donors at various culture passages and correlated the velocity to their immunomodulatory capacities in co-culture with allogeneic peripheral blood mononuclear cells (PBMC). Immunomodulation was assessed by measuring the PBMC proliferation, IgG production and cytokine secretion (listed in Table 1) in the MSC and PBMC co-cultures and results were compared to PBMC and MSC monocultures.

Table 1. List of analysed cytokines and their expression by MSC

Cell type	Immunomodulation	Cytokines [Ref]
MSC	Pro-Inflammatory	IL-6[3, 33]
	Anti-Inflammatory	IL-6[3, 33], MCP-1[20]
PBMC	Pro-Inflammatory	TNF-α[38], IL-10[32]
	Anti-Inflammatory	IL-6[33], IL-10[39], MCP-1[20], G-CSF[34, 40]

Materials and Methods

Mesenchymal stem cells (MSC) isolation and expansion

Bone marrow (BM) samples were harvested from the iliac crest of donors undergoing spine surgery. The study was ethically approved by the ethics committee of Canton of Lucerne (Study number: 730). Written informed consent was obtained from all the participants and this procedure was also approved by the approving body. MSC were isolated from BM of ten donors (4 females and 6 males; average age: 43 years; range: 17-59 years). The BM aspirates were immediately resuspended in 3.8% sodium citrate and phosphate buffered saline (PBS, Applichem - Axonlab, Baden, Switzerland) and then filtered through a 100 µm cell strainer to remove clots (Falcon - Faust, Schaffhausen, Switzerland). Mononuclear cells were separated by H-Lympholyte Cell Separation Media gradient centrifugation (density 1.077 g/mL; Cedarlane - Bio Concept, Allschwil, Switzerland) in Leucosep tubes (Huberlab, Reinach, Switzerland) at 800 g for 15 minutes, washed with PBS, centrifuged again at 210 g for 10 minutes and plated at a density of 1×10^5 cells/cm^2 in tissue culture flasks (TPP – Faust) in α-MEM, supplemented with 10% fetal bovine serum (FBS) (both Amimed – Bio Concept), (100 units/mL) penicillin / (100 mg/mL) streptomycin, 2.5 µg/ml amphotericin B (both Gibco – LuBioScience GmbH, Lucerne, Switzerland) at 37°C in a humid atmosphere containing 5% CO$_2$. After two days, non-adherent cells were discarded, whereas adherent cells were cultured in growing medium consisting of DMEM/Ham's F12, supplemented with 10% foetal bovine serum (FBS) (both Amimed), (100 units/mL) penicillin / (100 mg/mL) streptomycin (Pen-Strep), 2.5 µg/ml Amphotericin B (all Gibco) and 5 ng/ml recombinant basic fibroblast growth factor

(bFGF, Peprotech – LuBioScience), followed by media change three times per week. At 80% confluency, MSC were frozen and stored at - 150°C.

Phenotypic characterization of MSC

Bone marrow-derived mononuclear cells (1×10^6 cells) were plated in 10 cm-Primaria cell-culture dishes (Falcon) and cultured with growing medium. After 14 days, cell colonies were washed with PBS, fixed with 100% methanol, and stained with Giemsa solution (all these reagents were from Applichem).

Following cell culture expansion, CD44, CD90 and CD105 positive and CD14 negative MSC markers were analyzed by flow cytometry. Briefly, cells were incubated with CD14-FITC (NB100-77759, Novus Biological - LuBioScience), CD44-FITC (NBP1-41278, Novus Biological), CD90-FITC (NBP1-96125, Novus Biological) and CD105-FITC (MCA1557A488T, AbD Serotec - LuBioScience) antibodies in PBS for one hour at 4°C, washed and resuspended in PBS. Cell fluorescence was evaluated with FACScalibur flow cytometer (Becton Dickinson) and data were analyzed using FlowJo v.10.0 software (Treestar, Ashland, OR, USA).

Peripheral blood mononuclear cells (PBMC) isolation and characterization

Venous blood (45 ml) was collected from a healthy male donor (27 years old) in S-Monovettes containing EDTA (S-Monovettes, 9 ml K3E; Sarstedt, Nümbrecht, Germany). Peripheral blood mononuclear cells (PBMC) were isolated by H-Lympholyte Cell Separation Media gradient centrifugation in a Leucosep tube at 800 g and room temperature, for 20 minutes. The PBMC-containing buffy coat was carefully retrieved and washed with PBS, followed by a centrifugation at 210 g and room temperature for 10 minutes. The obtained PBMC pellet was resuspended in RPMI-1640 medium (Amimed; Bio Concept) supplemented with 10% FBS, Pen-Strep and amphotericin B.

Flow cytometric analysis of PBMC with CD4 (APC Mouse Anti-Human CD4 Clone RPA-T4, BD Bioscience, Allschwil, Switzerland) and CD8 (PE Mouse Anti-Human CD8 Clone RPA-T8, BD Bioscience, Allschwil, Switzerland) surface markers was performed after seven days in co-culture with MSC and in PBMC monoculture. Cells were incubated with antibodies in PBS for 15 minutes at room temperature, washed and resuspended in PBS. Cell fluorescence was evaluated with FACScalibur flow cytometer and data were analyzed using FlowJo v.10.0 software.

PBMC stimulation before co-culture

PBMC were stimulated in a cocktail adapted from a previous work[28], consisting of 60 ng/ml human recombinant interleukin-2 (IL-2), 25 ng/ml Interleukin-10 (IL-10), 100 ng/ml Interleukin-21 (IL-21) (all from BioBasic Inc.; Stephan Klee Trading and Consulting, Sissach, Switzerland), the synthetic unmethylated oligodeoxynucleotide deoxycytosine-deoxyguanosine (CpG2429: tcgtcgttttcggcggccgccg, 360 nM[29] Microsynth AG, Balgach, Switzerland) and 2.5 µg/ml pokeweed mitogen (Sigma-Aldrich Chemie GmbH, Buchs, Switzerland) in RPMI-1640 medium (Amimed; Bio Concept) + 10% FBS. After addition of the stimulating cocktail, PBMC were incubated overnight at 37°C in the incubator (5% CO$_2$), then washed with PBS, centrifuged at 210 g at room temperature for 10 minutes, and re-suspended in media for co-culture with MSC, or as a control.

MSC and PBMC co-cultures

MSC were split in three groups for co-culture with PBMC, *in vitro* cell tracking and cell metabolic activity (day 0). To prepare co-culture with PBMC, *in vitro* cell tracking and cell metabolic activity (day 0). To prepare co-culture with PBMC, MSC (2×10^4 cells/well) were seeded in 96-well plates (each donor in quadruplicate; flat bottom culture test plates; TPP) in growing medium, and left for plastic attachment for 4 hours. After the incubation time, growing medium was removed and stimulated and unstimulated (negative control) PBMC (1.5×10^5 cells/well) were co-cultured with MSC in a final volume of 300 µl/well of RPMI-1640 medium (Amimed; Bio Concept) supplemented with 10% FBS, (100 units/mL), Pen-Strep and amphotericin B. This co-culture was maintained for 7 days at 37°C and 5% CO_2.

The ratio MSC:PBMC used (2:15) lies in range of previous work on immunosuppression[30]. To study the correlation between MSC immunomodulatory capacity and cell motility, our preliminary test showed that MSC inhibited more efficiently IgG production at the ratio of 2:15 than 1:15.

Cell metabolic activity

MSC (2×10^4 cells/well) were seeded in 96-well plates (each donor in triplicate; flat bottom culture test plates) in growing medium, left overnight to adhere to the plate and then the cell activity was assessed by resazurin reduction assay. MSC were incubated (day 1) in resazurin solution - 15 ng/mL resazurin, 2.5 ng/mL methylene blue, 0.1 mM potassium ferricyanide, 0.1 mM potassium ferrocyanide (all Applichem) in growing medium without bFGF - for 6 hours and bottom well fluoresce absorbance was measured (λex= 535 nm and λem= 595 nm) using a Multimode Detector (DTX 880; Beckman Coulter, Nyon, Switzerland).

In vitro cell tracking of MSC

MSC (day 0) at *in vitro* passage 2-3 (n=7) and passage 6 (n=3) were plated at a density of 5.6×10^3 cells/cm². After 3 hours, the movements of the adherent cells started to be recorded using an inverted phase-contrast microscope equipped with a high-sensitive camera (Olympus, Tokyo, Japan, http://www.olympus-global.com) at 40X magnification. The interval between image acquisitions was 10 minutes, using the Xcellence software program (Olympus) over a 24-hour period. Video sequences were analyzed using ImageJ (NIH, Bethesda, MD, http://www.nih.gov/ij) and the plugin MTrackJ, which allows manual tracking of individual cell trails. Analyses were only made for cells moving within the plane of focus. The full length of the track was determined as the distance from the first point to the last point of the track, and the cell speed was measured as mm/day. We defined three representative groups for cell motility: slow moving MSC (0.1-0.2 mm/day), medium moving MSC (0.4-0.5 mm/day) and fast moving MSC (0.9-1.0 mm/day).

PBMC proliferation assay

Before stimulation, the isolated PBMC were stained with the fluorescent cell proliferation indicator CytoTell green (AAT Bioquest; LuBioScience) according to the manufactures protocol (20 minutes incubation at room temperature in 1:600 diluted dye). The proliferative response is the percentage of cells that underwent at least 1 cell division. The proliferative response of stimulated PBMC in co-cultures (n=10) and PBMC controls (n=1) was measured after 7 days of incubation by flow cytometry (total of 30'000 events gated) using the intracellular CytoTell dilution method and the viability staining solution 7-AAD (eBioscience, Vienna, Austria). Data was analyzed using FlowJo software.

IgG production assay

After 7 days of incubation, the amount of secreted IgG antibody in the supernatant t of stimulated co-cultures (n=10), PBMC controls

(n=1) and reference donors (n=42; age range: 23-58 years (mean: 42.8 years), and interquartile range IQR: 19) was quantified using a standard indirect ELISA, as follow: a 96-well plate (Nunc MaxiSorp, Fluka Chemie GmbH, Buchs, Switzerland) was coated with 1 ng/µL Protein A (LuBioScience) in PBS and incubated overnight at 4 °C, then washed with PBS with a plate washer (Beckman-Coulter, Nyon, Switzerland), and non-specific binding sites were blocked for 2 hours at room temperature with blocking solution containing 5% TopBlock (LuBioScience) in PBS. After washing wells with PBS, cell culture supernatants (in triplicate for each donor) – cleared of cell debris by centrifugation and diluted threefold in PBS – were incubated for 2 hours at room temperature. Supernatants were then removed and the wells washed with PBS. Anti-human-IgG HRP-conjugated secondary antibody (A80-119P Bethyl) diluted 1:5000 in blocking buffer was incubated for 1 hour at room temperature. IgG were determined by colorimetric measurement of the product of the enzymatic reaction mediated by HRP and o-phenylenediamine solution (15.3 mg/mL in citrate buffer, pH 5.0, Applichem – Axonlab). The reaction was stopped with 10% sulphuric acid. Absorbance was measured at 450 nm by DTX 880 Multimode Detector and IgG concentration (ng/mL) was determined from dilutions of purified human IgG (Bethyl – LuBioScience).

Cytokine measurements

The concentrations of cytokines and chemokines were analyzed in the supernatants of monoculture of MSC, and co-cultures of PBMC and MSC after 7 days incubation, by Bio-Plex Pro Cytokine, Chemokine and Growth Factor Assay (Bio-Rad Laboratories AG – Cressier, Switzerland). Data were collected and analyzed using a Bio-Rad Bio-Plex 200 instrument equipped with Bio-Plex Manager software (Bio-Rad). We measured the concentrations of interleukin-2 (IL-2), interleukin-4 (IL-4), interleukin-6 (IL-6), interleukin-10 (IL-10), granulocyte-colony stimulating factor (G-CSF), granulocyte-macrophage colony-stimulating factor (GM-CSF), monocyte chemoattractant protein 1 (MCP1) and tumor necrosis factor-alpha (TNF-α).

Statistical analysis

Cytokine and IgG concentrations, and proliferative responses were presented in bar charts as mean ± standard deviation (SD). Non-parametric Mann-Whitney-Wilcoxon U-test for related variables was used to determine significant differences between samples, as a normal distribution of the data could not be guaranteed in this data set. For all tests, *p < 0.05* was considered significant. Data analysis was performed with SPSS 24.0 for Windows (SPSS Inc.).

Scatterplot were produced for culture concentration versus cell motility and smoothed via semiparametric regression models using the mixed model representation of penalized splines[31] as implemented in the SemiPar package in R (R Foundation for Statistical Computing, Vienna, Austria, http://www.r-project.org). Scatterplots and scatterplot smoothers were computed using R, version 2.14.2, for Windows (R Foundation for Statistical Computing). The confidence bands represent the certainty about the average trend. They capture the high variation in the data points. A single future prediction may not be well accordant to the suggested trend as interpolated; however, on average (of many predictions) it will be.

Results

Mesenchymal stem cells (MSC) characterization

The bone marrow-isolated MSC were initially characterized by their elongated fibroblastic cellular phenotype (Figure 1A) and by their ability to generate colony forming units (Figure 1B). Furthermore,

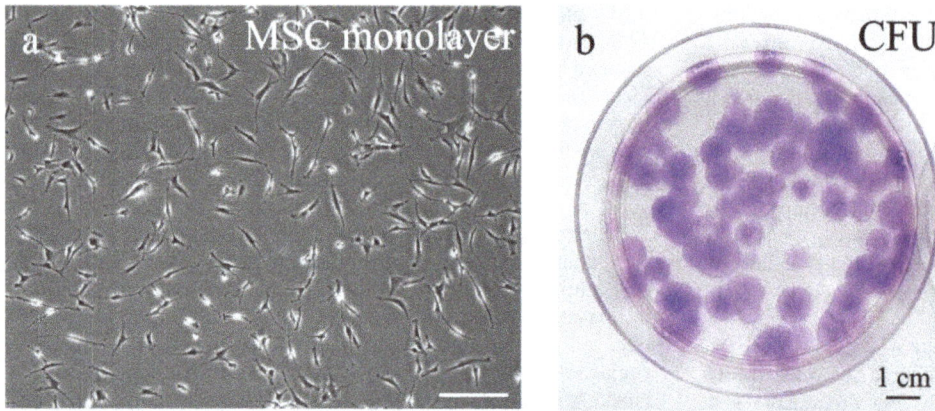

Figure 1 MSC characterization was based on their peculiar fibroblast-like morphology (a, entire scale bar is 200 μm), ability to form colonies (stained with Giemsa; b) and expression of the positive markers CD44 (blue line), CD90 (green line), CD105 (orange line) and the negative marker CD14 (red line), tested by flow cytometry analysis (grey line = unstained control; c).

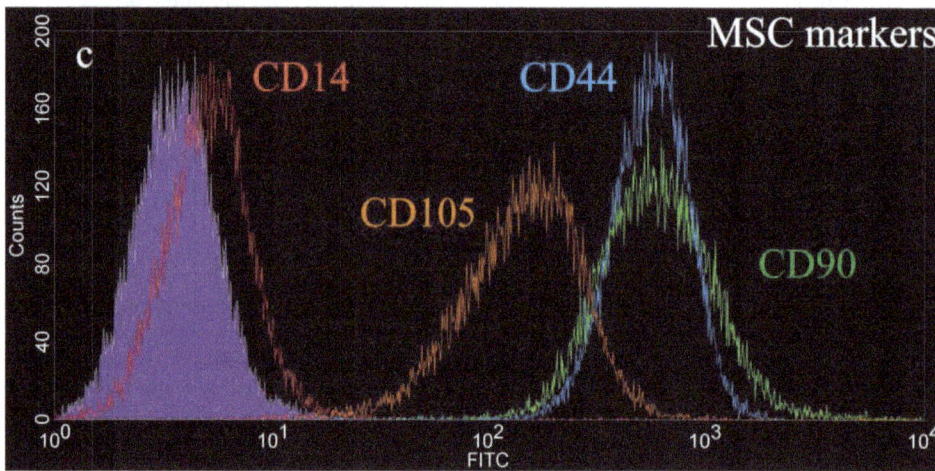

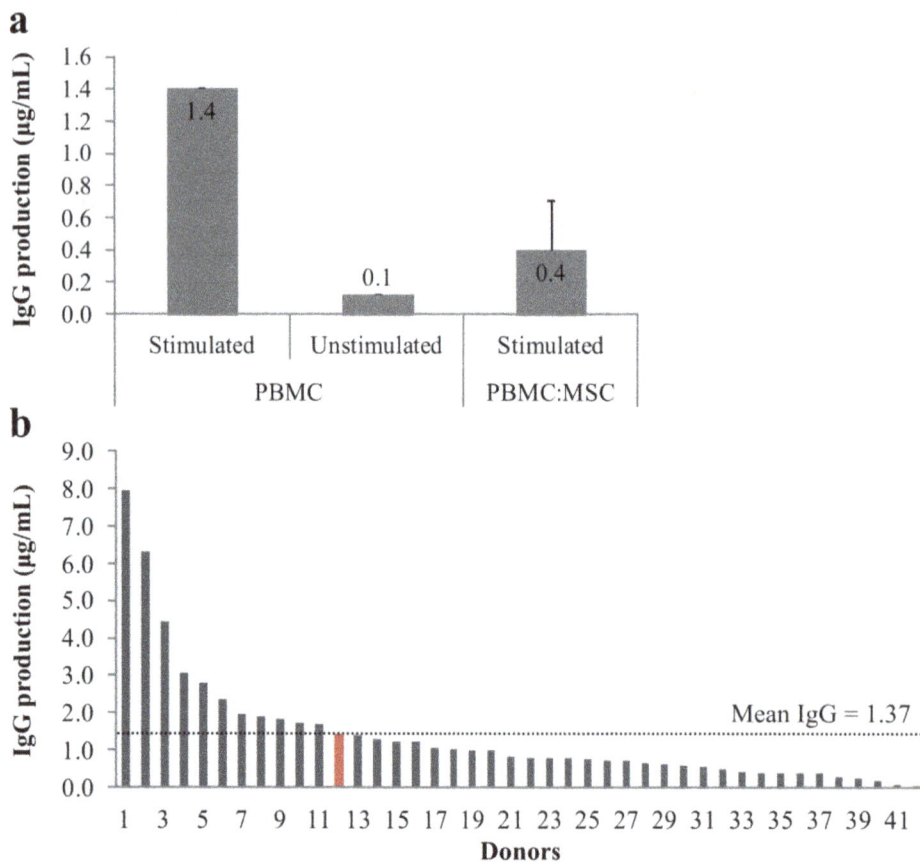

Figure 2 Effects of stimulation cocktail on IgG production by PBMC. After seven days culture, the immuno-suppressive action of MSC on PBMC (a) was determined by measuring IgG production in stimulated (n=1) and unstimulated (n=1) PBMC monocultures, as well as in stimulated PBMC and MSC co-cultures (n=10; data represented as mean ± SD). On the bottom (b), comparison of IgG production between 42 donors (red bar = sample used to test the immuno-suppressive action of MSC).

MSC were characterized by flow cytometry analysis with the positive mesenchymal stem cell markers CD44, CD90, and CD105 and the negative monocyte-related marker CD14 (Figure 1C).

IgG production by peripheral blood mononuclear cells (PBMC) in co-culture

IgG production inhibition by MSC was tested on stimulated allogeneic PBMC in co-culture for 1 week (Figure 2A). Monocultures of MSC and PBMC (unstimulated or stimulated) served as a control. When co-cultured with MSC, stimulated PBMC decreased IgG production by 71%, while unstimulated PBMC IgG production was only a tenth of the stimulated control. Overall, PBMC production of IgG by the donor used in this project was very close (1.41 µg/ml) to the mean IgG production calculated out of 42 donors (1.37 µg/ml, Figure 2B).

MSC modulated peripheral blood mononuclear cells (PBMC) activity in co-culture

After seven days culture, stimulated (column A) and unstimulated (column B) PBMC, and stimulated PBMC isolated from co-culture with MSC (column C) characterization was based on gating light scattered by cells (Figure 3: top row), CD4/CD8 ratio of T-cells (Figure 3: middle row) and cell morphology (Figure 3D). The viability (7-AAD assay) of the stimulated PBMC in monocultures was 95% and in co-cultures 96%. Forward (FSC) and side scattering profiles of stimulated PBMC showed a large spreading and activation of cells compared to unstimulated PBMC, and the results in monoculture were similar to co-culture with MSC. Analysis of mean FSC intensity showed that stimulated PBMC increased cell size of 26% in comparison to unstimulated PBMC, and in co-culture with MSC only of 13%. CD4/CD8 ratios of unstimulated PBMC in monocultures and in co-cultures with MSC were identical (ratio = 1.55), while stimulated PBMC in monoculture (ratio = 0.70) had a lower ratio compared to PBMC in co-culture (ratio = 1.09). Immunosuppression by MSC significantly prevented blastogenesis of stimulated PBMC already after three days of co-culture.

The immunosuppressive effects of MSC on PBMC were determined by cell proliferative response of $CD4^+$ T-cells and $CD8^+$ T-cells (Figure 4: top rows). MSC inhibited the proliferation of both $CD4^+$ (Figure 4D) and $CD8^+$ T-cells (Figure. 4E), especially $CD4^+$ T-cells (2.6-fold) in comparison to $CD8^+$ T-cells (1.6-fold), while unstimulated PBMC were not dividing at all.

We analyzed the concentration of eight inflammation-related cytokines in supernatants of controls (monocultures) and co-cultures (Figure 5), namely interleukin-6 (IL-6), granulocyte-colony stimulating factor (G-CSF), monocyte chemoattractant protein-1 (MCP-1), interleukin-10 (IL-10), tumor necrosis factor (TNF-α) and granulocyte-macrophage colony-stimulating factor (GM-CSF). The concentrations of interleukin-2 and -4 (IL-2 and IL-4) were at or below the detection limit (data not shown). Co-culture of MSC with stimulated PBMC led to substantially increased IL-6 (Figure 5A), G-CSF (Figure 5B) and MCP-1 (Figure 5C) concentrations. In comparison to stimulated PBMC monoculture, the average cytokine increase corresponded to 340-fold for IL-6, 600-fold for G-CSF and 30-fold for MCP-1. Furthermore, the increase in G-CSF significantly correlated with *in vitro* culture passage of MSC. In stimulated PBMC:MSC co-culture, late passage MSC (P6) produced ~20% more G-CSF *(p < 0.01)* and ~10% more IL-6 *(p < 0.05)* in comparison to early passage MSC (P2-P3) (data not shown). On the other hand, the presence of MSC inhibited the production of TNF-α (Figure 5D) and IL-10 (Figure 5E), 3.5- and 2.5-fold respectively. GM-CSF concentrations were not influenced by MSC (Figure 5F).

MSC modulated the secretion of cytokines also in unstimulated PBMC co-culture, resulting in a 400-fold increase of IL-6, 3-fold increase of G-CSF and 5-fold increase of MCP-1 productions, compared to PBMC monoculture. Although IL-10 and TNF-α levels were unaffected by the MSC, GM-CSF was inhibited 1.8-fold in comparison to PBMC monoculture.

Monoculture of MSC produced mostly IL-6 (2.7 ng/ml) followed by MCP-1 (2.3 ng/ml), and in lower amount GM-CSF (140 pg/ml), G-CSF (50 pg/ml), TNF-α (23 pg/ml) and IL-10 (8.4 pg/ml). Beside, compared to unstimulated cells, stimulation of PBMC in monoculture increased the production of TNF-α, IL-10 and GM-CSF, and reduced MCP-1 (no changes in IL-6 and G-CSF levels).

MSC in vitro motility and immunosuppressive potential

We measured cell motility of MSC by time-lapse microscopy recording. For each donor, 70 MSC were tracked for 24 hours and their motility was plotted against proliferative response of $CD4^+$ T-cells (Figure 6A) and $CD8^+$ T-cells (Figure 6B), and IgG production (Figure 6C) by stimulated PBMC in co-culture. We observed that mostly slow and fast moving MSC suppressed PBMC proliferation and IgG production, even though changes in proliferation were small in both cases. Slow moving MSC (0.1-0.2 mm/day) corresponded to $CD4^+$ T-cells proliferative response of 11.6%, medium moving MSC (0.4-0.5 mm/day) of 12.2% and fast moving MSC (0.9-1.0 mm/day) of 11.9%. Furthermore, slow moving MSC corresponded to $CD8^+$ T-cells proliferative response of 38.4%, medium moving MSC of 40.3% and fast moving MSC of 39.3%.

PBMC produced in correspondence of slow MSC 80% IgG (356 µg/ml), medium speed MSCs 100% (447 µg/ml) and fast moving MSCs 77% (345 µg/ml). The metabolic activity of MSC was plotted against cell motility (Figure 6D) and as expected fast moving MSC were also the most metabolically active. Compared to slow moving MSC, fast moving MSC were ~20% more active and medium moving ~10%.

MSC in vitro motility in monoculture and cytokine concentrations

The motility of MSC was plotted against cytokine concentrations in monocultures after one week of incubation (Figure 7). Fast moving stem cells produced 2.3-fold more IL-6 (Figure 7A), 1.2-fold more G-CSF (Figure 7B) and 1.5 fold-more MCP-1 (Figure 7C) than slower speed cells. On the other hand, GM-CSF (Figure 7E) was moderately reduced (6% difference between slow and fast) with increasing MSC speed. Secretion of IL-10 (Figure 7D) and TNF-α (Figure 7F) by MSC was low and independent of MSC motility.

MSC in vitro motility influence on cytokine production in co-culture with stimulated PBMC

In co-culture with stimulated PBMC, cell motility of MSC was plotted against cytokine productions after one week of incubation (Figure 8). Although IL-6 concentration was strongly increased compared to MSC monoculture, the difference between slow and fast MSC was only 1.6% (Figure 8A). Also, the concentrations of G-CSF (Figure 8B) and TNF-α (Figure 8F) were independent of MSC motility with a maximum difference of 3% respectively 4% between speeds. The production of MCP-1 (Figure 8C) was negatively correlated with MSC motility. In correspondence of slow MSC, MCP-1 production was 14% higher compared to fast MSC. On the other hand, increased IL-10 (Figure 8D) and GM-CSF (Figure 8E) were produced in correspondence of fast MSC. IL-10 and GM-CSF differences between slow and fast cells were 12% and 18% respectively.

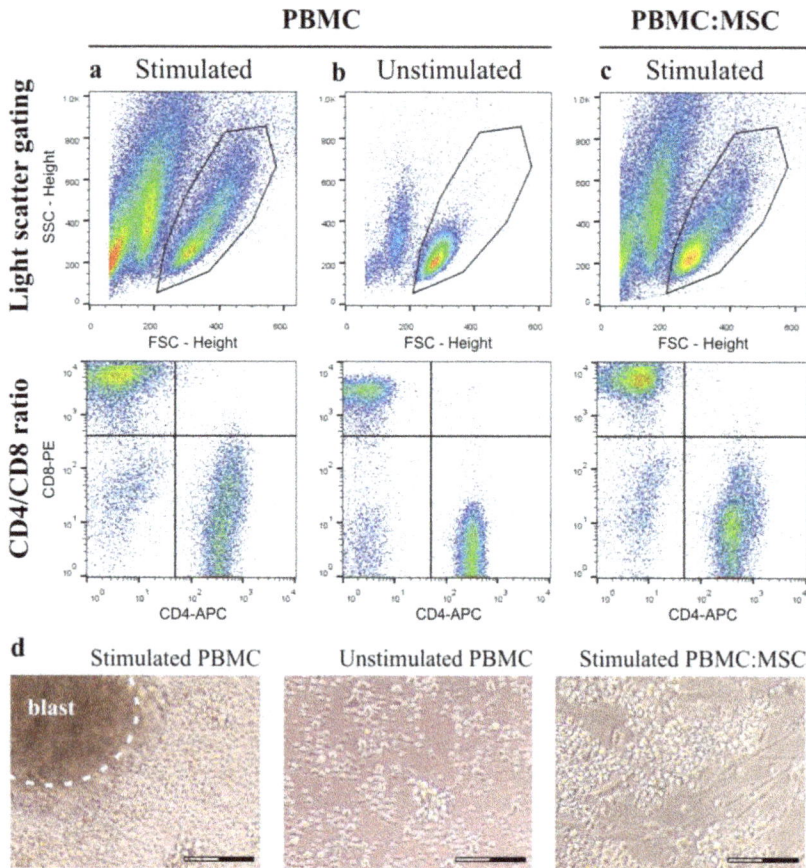

Figure 3 After seven days culture, stimulated (column a) and unstimulated (column b) PBMC, and stimulated PBMC (column c), isolated from co-culture with MSC, were morphologically characterized. Images from a representative sample show light scattered gating of cells (side scatter, SSC, and forward scatter, FSC; top row) and CD4/CD8 ratio of T-cells (middle row). On the bottom (d), microphotographs taken after three days show the presence or lack of lymphocyte blast formation in the same samples (entire scale bar is 100 μm).

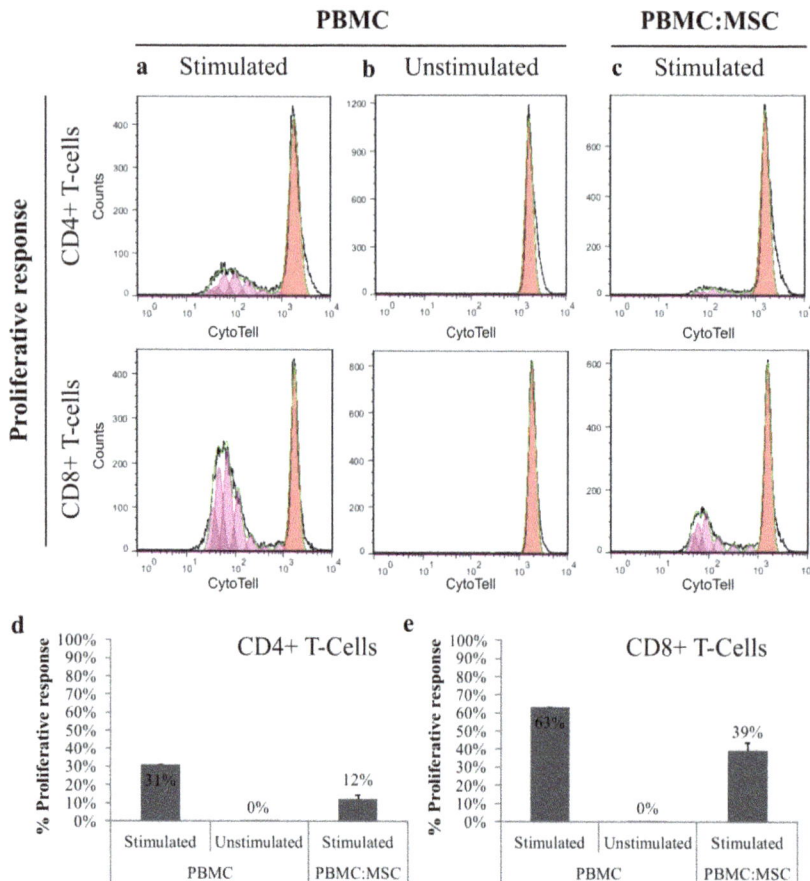

Figure 4 After seven days culture, effectiveness of immuno-suppressive action of MSC on PBMC was determined by measuring cell proliferative response of stimulated (column a) and unstimulated (column b) PBMC, and stimulated PBMC (column c), isolated from co-culture with MSC. Top rows represent the proliferative response of CD4[+] T-cells and CD8[+] T-cells, in a representative sample (CytoTell staining). Results of the proliferative response of CD4[+] T-cells (d) and CD8[+] T-cells (e) were summarized (stimulated (n=1) and unstimulated (n=1) PBMC monocultures, stimulated PBMC and MSC co-cultures (n=10); data represented as mean ± SD).

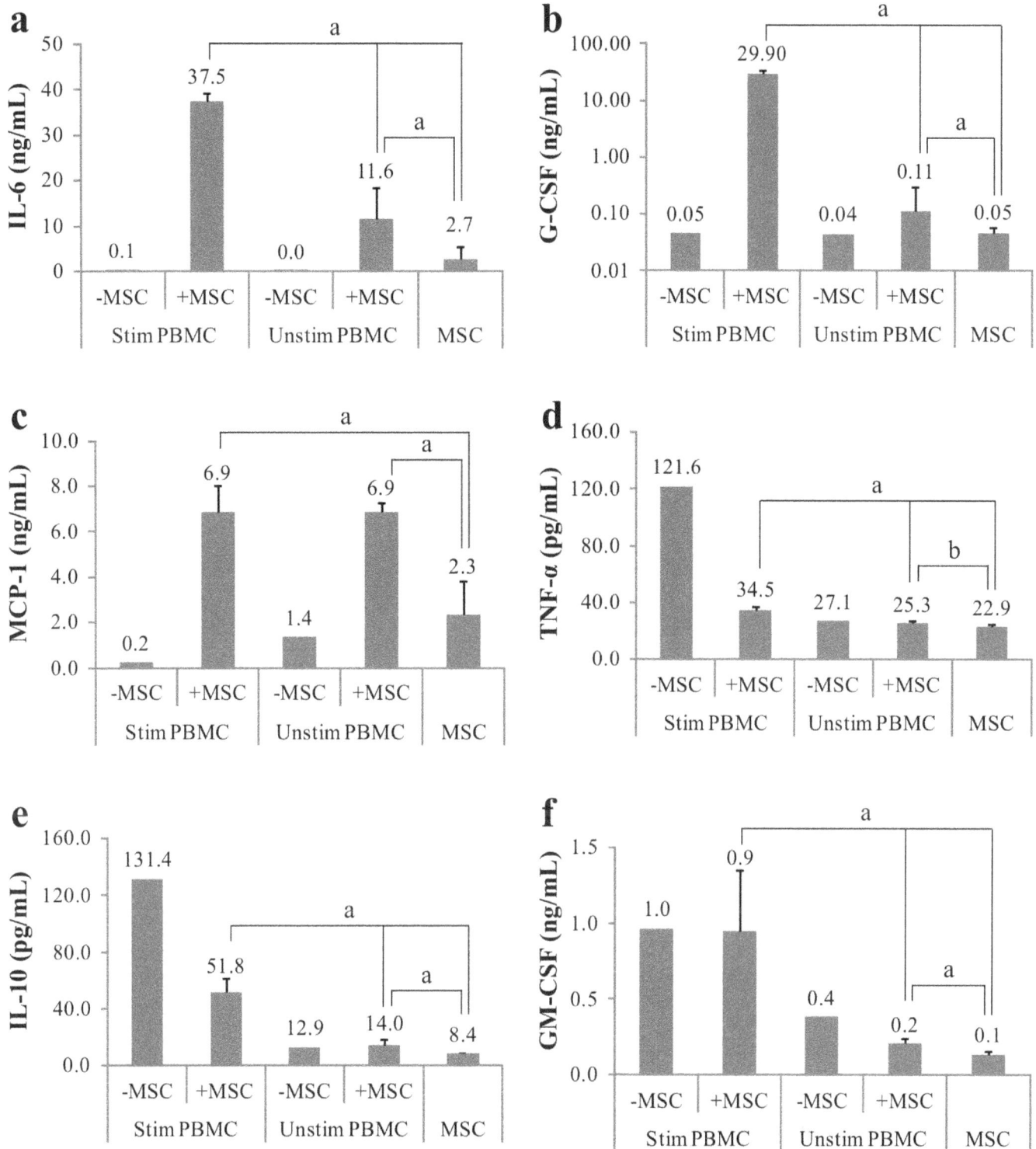

Figure 5 *MSC and PBMC had a reciprocal influence in the production of cytokines. After seven days, supernatant concentration of IL-6 (a), G-CSF (b), MCP-1 (c), TNF-α (d), IL-10 (e) and GM-CSF (f) was measured in MSC monoculture (n=10), stimulated (n=1) and unstimulated (n=1) PBMC monocultures, and co-culture with or without MSC (n=10). Data was acquired by Bio-Plex analysis and represented as mean ± SD (a = p<0.01; b = p<0.05).*

a   CD4+ T-cells proliferation

b   CD8+ T-cells proliferation

c   IgG production

d   Cell metabolic activity

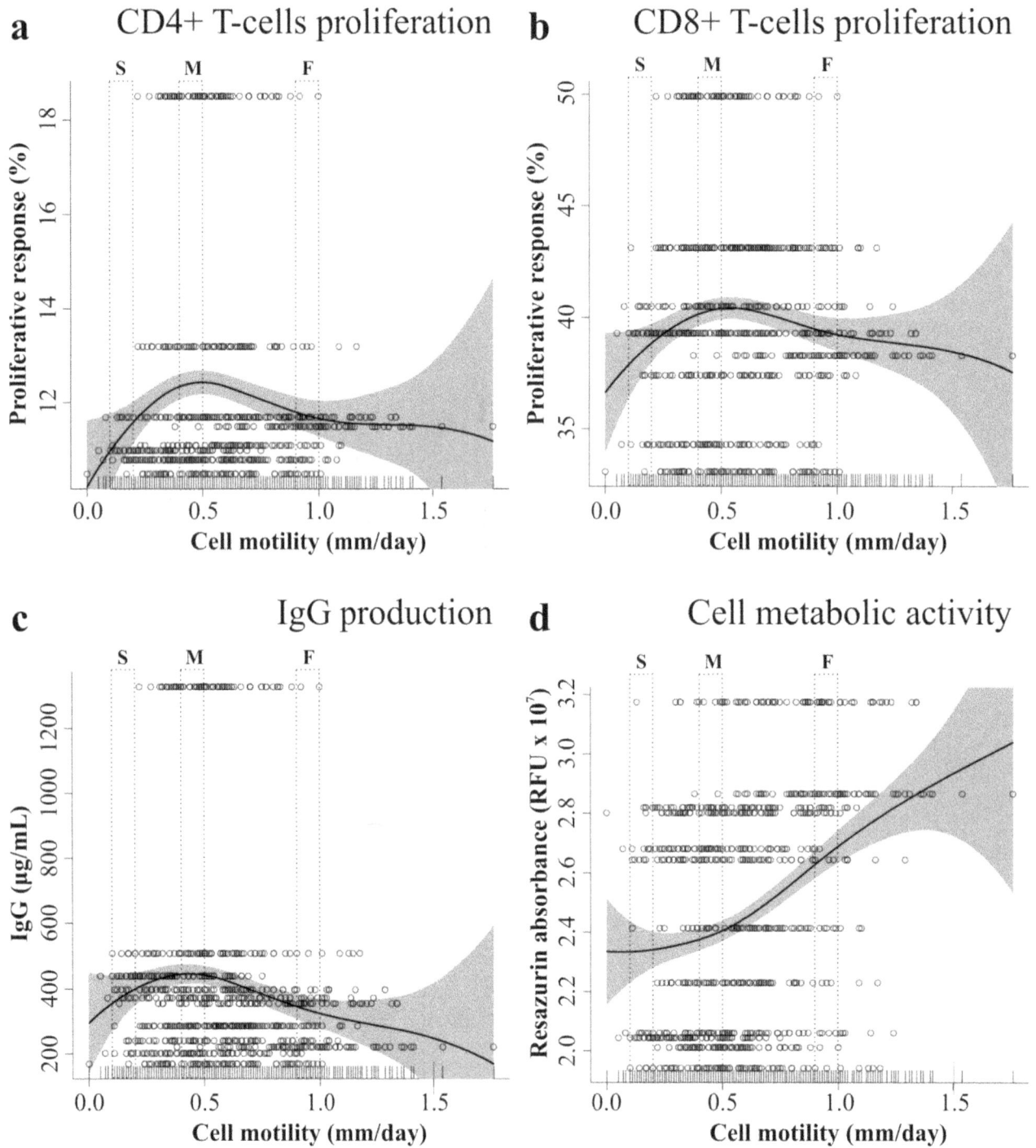

Figure 6 *Proliferative response of CD4⁺ T-cells (a) and CD8⁺ T-cells (b), and IgG production (c) of stimulated PBMC in co-culture with MSC plotted against cell motility. The metabolic activity (d) of MSC in monoculture was also plotted against cell motility. Each row (70 cells) represents a MSC population. Abbreviations: O = single cells; — = penalized spline smoother; grey area = confidence band. (S = slow, M = middle, F = fast moving cells)*

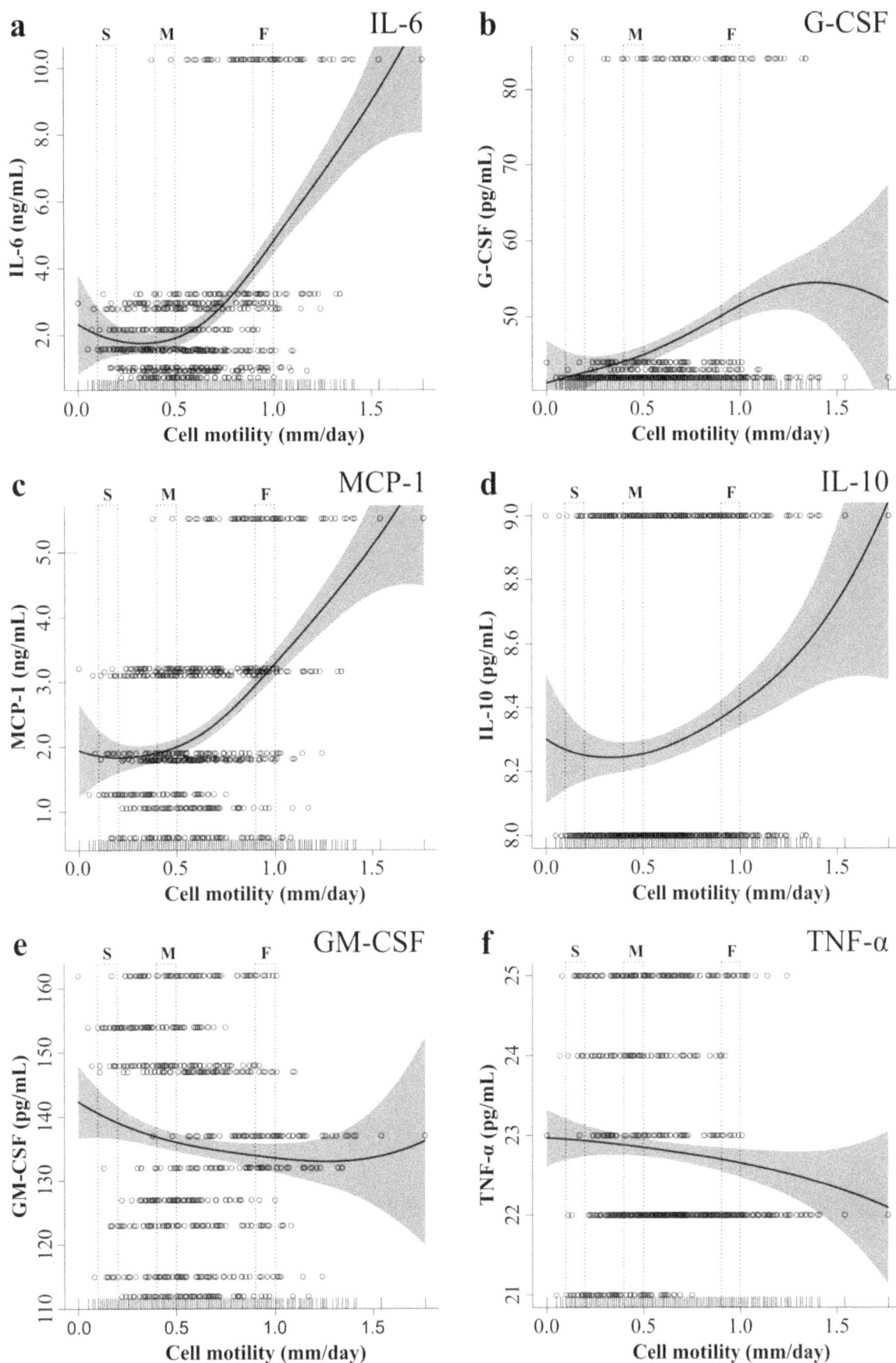

Figure 7 MSC monoculture concentration of IL-6 (a), G-CSF (b), MCP-1 (c), IL-10 (d), GM-CSF (e)) and TNF-α (f) plotted against cell motility. Each row (70 cells) represents a MSC population. Abbreviations: O = single cells; — = penalized spline smoother; grey area = confidence band. (S = slow, M = middle, F = fast moving cells)

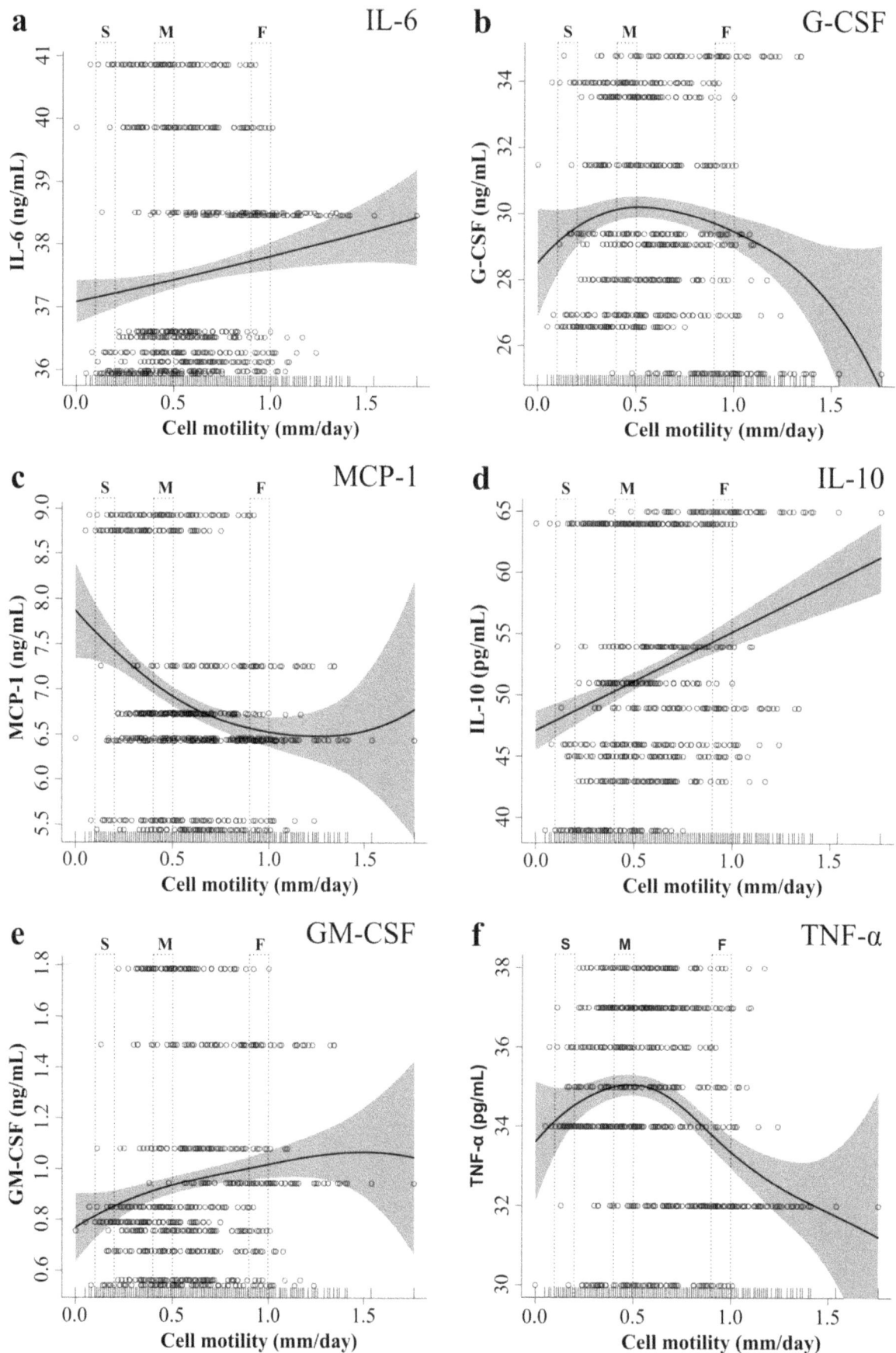

Figure 8 Stimulated PBMC + MSC co-culture concentration of IL-6 (a), G-CSF (b), MCP-1 (c), IL-10 (d), GM-CSF (e) and TNF-α (f) plotted against cell motility. Each row (70 cells) represents a MSC population. Abbreviations: O = single cells; — = penalized spline smoother; grey area = confidence band. (S = slow, M = middle, F = fast moving cells)

Discussion

In this study, we found that *in vitro* mesenchymal stem cells (MSC) motility correlates to some aspects of their immunosuppressive potential and production capacity of some cytokines. MSC immunomodulation effects were determined in mixed lymphocyte reaction assay, a broadly used method which provides direct contact and allows most fundamental interactions between cells. In co-cultures with peripheral blood mononuclear cells (PBMC), PBMC blastogenesis was prevented in all MSC co-cultured samples and MSC successfully inhibited CD4+ T-cells and CD8+ T-cells proliferation but also the production of IgG. We stratified the MSC populations according to our empirical observations in three representative cell motility groups: slow moving (0.1-0.2 mm/day), medium moving (0.4-0.5 mm/day) and fast moving (0.9-1.0 mm/day). In co-culture with PBMC, fast moving MSC inhibited more effectively IgG production and proliferation of PBMC in comparison to slower cells, and were the most metabolically active. Interestingly, in the case of PBMC co-cultured with fast MSC, reduced secretion of G-CSF and TNF-α were observed, along with increased IL-10 secretion. This particular combination of cytokine secretion is peculiar of M2 phenotype of macrophages (involved in parasite control, tissue remodelling, immune regulation and phagocytic activity), which are characterized by higher anti-inflammatory potential compared to M1 macrophages (producing pro-inflammatory cytokines, mediating resistance to pathogens and promoting T_h1 responses)[32]. The ability of MSCs to shift macrophages toward an M2 phenotype *in vitro* has been already described[33], and our data on secretion of cytokines suggest that fast moving MSC correlate better to M2 phenotype shift. Cytokine expression analysis of MSC in monoculture showed that IL-6 and MCP-1 were secreted in large amount by faster cells compared to slower ones. As a limitation, we cannot discuss properly the secretion origins of MCP-1 in co-cultures because in our experimental setting we cannot discriminate which type of cell – MSC or PBMC – produced this cytokine.

Our results suggest that within the same MSC population, sub-groups of cells have different roles in modulating the action of PBMC. There might be a possibility that the observed intra-donor variability of MSC motility extrapolates even to the stem cell variability between people. This speculation is supported by the observation that MSC isolated from patients with multiple sclerosis had functional differences compared to healthy controls, such as reduced anti-proliferative capacity and lower secretion of anti-inflammatory cytokines[34]. The dynamics occurring between sub-populations of MSC with different cell motility may play an important role for their overall immune-regulatory capacity. To better understand these dynamics, we also investigated the release of cytokines and chemokines by MSC, which are known to play a key role in the suppressive signalling.

Despite the complex nature of cytokine signalling, in co-cultures we could discriminate distinct responses related to MSC regulatory abilities. The correlation between MSC motility and immunomodulation was based on the measurement in culture medium of the cytokines IL-2, IL-4, IL-6, IL-10, TNF-α, G-CSF, GM-CSF and MCP-1, shown previously to be relevant because of their anti- and pro-inflammatory properties and expression by both MSC and PBMC (Table 1). Stimulated PBMC secreted large amount of IL-10, TNF-α and GM-CSF, while unstimulated PBMC produced mostly MCP-1 and GM-CSF. On the other hand, MSC in monocultures produced only relevant amount of MCP-1 and IL-6, and negligible quantity of the other cytokines, as previously described in the literature[35]. No cross-talk from the cytokines used in the stimulation cocktail was expected since the pre-stimulated PBMC were thoroughly washed ahead of their culturing.

The immuno-suppressive action of MSC in co-culture with stimulated PBMC was demonstrated by the reduced PBMC secretion of pro-inflammatory cytokines (TNF-α) and increased MSC secretion of anti-inflammatory cytokines (IL-6, MCP-1 and G-CSF). Unexpectedly, the anti-inflammatory cytokine IL-10 was reduced by MSC, but a growing body of evidence shows that IL-10 action is multifactorial and in some settings may not be the previously thought inhibitor of immune functions[36,37]. Furthermore, IL-10 was described to stimulate IgG isotype switch in B-lymphocytes[38] and ultimately has been used as a main component of PBMC stimulation cocktail. The secretion by stimulated PBMC of another important cytokine, IL-6, was observed in co-culture with MSC, indicating an anti-inflammatory action by IL-6 in this particular setting[39,40]. Also MCP-1 had an anti-inflammatory pattern, where its expression was higher in both co-cultures compared to monocultures. Not surprisingly, the other immuno-modulatory molecule G-CSF – which has also been proven to have an anti-inflammatory role[41] – was massively upregulated when MSC were co-culture with stimulated PBMC. *In vivo*, G-CSF is a hematopoietic cytokine produced by monocytes, macrophages, fibroblasts, and endothelial cells which regulates neutrophil mobilization during infections and inflammations[42]. We speculate that such a large production of G-CSF was triggered from MSC, what might mimic the innate immune-activation – namely instant blood-mediated inflammatory and anti-inflammatory reactions – observed *in vivo* after systemic injection of MSC[43]. As a matter of evidence[44], *in vitro* long-term expansion of MSC has been related to impaired inflammatory modulation and we observed the same pattern: co-cultures with high passage MSC (P6) were significantly producing more IL-6 and G-CSF than early passage MSC (P2 and P3). Similar results were reflected in a phase II clinical trial for the treatment of acute graft versus host disease (GvHD) where MSC transplantation failed to prevent the development of grade II acute GvHD in one patient because increased gene expression of IL-6 and CSF which possibly may have promoted T- and B-cell proliferation and macrophages activation[45]. Among all cytokines analysed, GM-CSF concentration was not affected by the presence of MSC and we concluded that it might not be involved in the immunomodulation process.

The limitation of our study is the experimental application of a single PBMC donor. However, the aim of this study was to compare MSC behaviours without introducing further confounders. Indeed, the results presented in this work focus on MSC cell motility and immunomodulatory potential rather than the effects of multiple sources of PBMC. To avoid misleading results, the choice of the PBMC donor was based on IgG production and selecting the closest donor to the mean value of the investigated population. Further limitation, is that we did not examine neither the functional outcomes that cell motility might have on specific immune cell subsets, nor the correlation of MSC hypoimmunogenicity to *in vitro* cell tracking.

Conclusion

We showed that MSC motility is a prospective indicator for MSC immunomodulatory potential. Although the heterogeneity of cell motility in MSC populations reduce the accuracy of the proposed method, it can be fruitfully used to indicate the overall potential of cell populations, especially in those with lower variability. In monoculture, fast MSC were more metabolically active and produced larger amounts of G-CSF, IL-6 and MCP-1. In co-culture with stimulated PBMC, fast MSC inhibited more efficiently IgG production, and correlated with higher IL-10 concentrations. The process of standardization of cell production – *i.e.* MSC extraction, expansion and administration – is fundamental in the application of MSC as a treatment. We believe that *in vitro* cell tracking can contribute to a better understanding of the immunomodulatory properties of MSC, beyond the standard MSC molecular markers. In combination with the previously demonstrated predictive value of live-imaging for differentiation potential[27], we think that the measurement of cell motility is a fast assay which can be used alone or complementary to other tests in order to improve the prediction of clinical outcomes.

References

1. Schallmoser K, Rohde E, Reinisch A, Bartmann C, Thaler D, Drexler C, Obenauf AC, Lanzer G, Linkesch W, Strunk D. Rapid large-scale expansion of functional mesenchymal stem cells from unmanipulated bone marrow without animal serum. Tissue engineering Part C, Methods. 2008;14(3):185-96.

2. Colter DC, Class R, DiGirolamo CM, Prockop DJ. Rapid expansion of recycling stem cells in cultures of plastic-adherent cells from human bone marrow. Proceedings of the National Academy of Sciences of the United States of America. 2000;97(7):3213-8.

3. Kyurkchiev D, Bochev I, Ivanova-Todorova E, Mourdjeva M, Oreshkova T, Belemezova K, Kyurkchiev S. Secretion of immunoregulatory cytokines by mesenchymal stem cells. World journal of stem cells. 2014;6(5):552-70.

4. Pittenger MF, Mackay AM, Beck SC, Jaiswal RK, Douglas R, Mosca JD, Moorman MA, Simonetti DW, Craig S, Marshak DR. Multilineage potential of adult human mesenchymal stem cells. Science. 1999;284(5411):143-7.

5. Miyahara Y, Nagaya N, Kataoka M, Yanagawa B, Tanaka K, Hao H, Ishino K, Ishida H, Shimizu T, Kangawa K, Sano S, Okano T, Kitamura S, Mori H. Monolayered mesenchymal stem cells repair scarred myocardium after myocardial infarction. Nat Med. 2006;12(4):459-65.

6. Uccelli A, Benvenuto F, Laroni A, Giunti D. Neuroprotective features of mesenchymal stem cells. Best practice & research Clinical haematology. 2011;24(1):59-64.

7. Eom YW, Kim G, Baik SK. Mesenchymal stem cell therapy for cirrhosis: Present and future perspectives. World journal of gastroenterology. 2015;21(36):10253-61.

8. Nauta AJ, Fibbe WE. Immunomodulatory properties of mesenchymal stromal cells. Blood. 2007;110(10):3499-506.

9. Le Blanc K, Frassoni F, Ball L, Locatelli F, Roelofs H, Lewis I, Lanino E, Sundberg B, Bernardo ME, Remberger M, Dini G, Egeler RM, Bacigalupo A, Fibbe W, Ringdén O; Developmental Committee of the European Group for Blood and Marrow Transplantation. Mesenchymal stem cells for treatment of steroid-resistant, severe, acute graft-versus-host disease: a phase II study. Lancet. 2008;371(9624):1579-86.

10. Wei X, Yang X, Han ZP, Qu FF, Shao L, Shi YF. Mesenchymal stem cells: a new trend for cell therapy. Acta pharmacologica Sinica. 2013;34(6):747-54.

11. Gao F, Chiu SM, Motan DA, Zhang Z, Chen L, Ji HL, Tse HF, Fu QL, Lian Q. Mesenchymal stem cells and immunomodulation: current status and future prospects. Cell death & disease. 2016;7:e2062.

12. Francois M, Galipeau J. New insights on translational development of mesenchymal stromal cells for suppressor therapy. J Cell Physiol. 2012;227(11):3535-8.

13. Meisel R, Zibert A, Laryea M, Gobel U, Daubener W, Dilloo D. Human bone marrow stromal cells inhibit allogeneic T-cell responses by indoleamine 2,3-dioxygenase-mediated tryptophan degradation. Blood. 2004;103(12):4619-21.

14. Aggarwal S, Pittenger MF. Human mesenchymal stem cells modulate allogeneic immune cell responses. Blood. 2005;105(4):1815-22.

15. Sotiropoulou PA, Perez SA, Gritzapis AD, Baxevanis CN, Papamichail M. Interactions between human mesenchymal stem cells and natural killer cells. Stem Cells. 2006;24(1):74-85.

16. Ren G, Zhang L, Zhao X, Xu G, Zhang Y, Roberts AI, Zhao RC, Shi Y. Mesenchymal stem cell-mediated immunosuppression occurs via concerted action of chemokines and nitric oxide. Cell stem cell. 2008;2(2):141-50.

17. English K. Mechanisms of mesenchymal stromal cell immunomodulation. Immunology and cell biology. 2013;91(1):19-26.

18. DelaRosa O, Lombardo E, Beraza A, Mancheño-Corvo P, Ramirez C, Menta R, Rico L, Camarillo E, García L, Abad JL, Trigueros C, Delgado M, Büscher D. Requirement of IFN-gamma-mediated indoleamine 2,3-dioxygenase expression in the modulation of lymphocyte proliferation by human adipose-derived stem cells. Tissue Eng Part A. 2009;15(10):2795-806.

19. Batten P, Sarathchandra P, Antoniw JW, Tay SS, Lowdell MW, Taylor PM, Yacoub MH. Human mesenchymal stem cells induce T cell anergy and downregulate T cell allo-responses via the TH2 pathway: relevance to tissue engineering human heart valves. Tissue engineering. 2006;12(8):2263-73.

20. Melief SM, Geutskens SB, Fibbe WE, Roelofs H. Multipotent stromal cells skew monocytes towards an anti-inflammatory interleukin-10-producing phenotype by production of interleukin-6. Haematologica. 2013;98(6):888-95.

21. Cassatella MA, Mosna F, Micheletti A, Lisi V, Tamassia N, Cont C, Calzetti F, Pelletier M, Pizzolo G, Krampera M. Toll-like receptor-3-activated human mesenchymal stromal cells significantly prolong the survival and function of neutrophils. Stem Cells. 2011;29(6):1001-11.

22. Rafei M, Hsieh J, Fortier S, Li M, Yuan S, Birman E, Forner K, Boivin MN, Doody K, Tremblay M, Annabi B, Galipeau J. Mesenchymal stromal cell-derived CCL2 suppresses plasma cell immunoglobulin production via STAT3 inactivation and PAX5 induction. Blood. 2008;112(13):4991-8.

23. Deshmane SL, Kremlev S, Amini S, Sawaya BE. Monocyte chemoattractant protein-1 (MCP-1): an overview. Journal of interferon & cytokine research : the official journal of the International Society for Interferon and Cytokine Research. 2009;29(6):313-26.

24. Akiyama K, Chen C, Wang D, Xu X, Qu C, Yamaza T, Cai T, Chen W, Sun L, Shi S. Mesenchymal-stem-cell-induced immunoregulation involves FAS-ligand-/FAS-mediated T cell apoptosis. Cell stem cell. 2012;10(5):544-55.

25. Kim N, Cho SG. Clinical applications of mesenchymal stem cells. The Korean journal of internal medicine. 2013;28(4):387-402.

26. Prockop DJ, Sekiya I, Colter DC. Isolation and characterization of rapidly self-renewing stem cells from cultures of human marrow stromal cells. Cytotherapy. 2001;3(5):393-6.

27. Bertolo A, Gemperli A, Gruber M, Gantenbein B, Baur M, Pötzel T, Stoyanov J. In vitro cell motility as a potential mesenchymal stem cell marker for multipotency. Stem cells translational medicine. 2015;4(1):84-90.

28. Heidt S, Hester J, Shankar S, Friend PJ, Wood KJ. B cell repopulation after alemtuzumab induction-transient increase in transitional B cells and long-term dominance of naive B cells. American journal of transplantation : official journal of the American Society of Transplantation and the American Society of Transplant Surgeons. 2012;12(7):1784-92.

29. Jurk M, Schulte B, Kritzler A, Noll B, Uhlmann E, Wader T, Schetter C, Krieg AM, Vollmer J. C-Class CpG ODN: sequence requirements and characterization of immunostimulatory activities on mRNA level. Immunobiology. 2004;209(1-2):141-54.

30. Melief SM, Zwaginga JJ, Fibbe WE, Roelofs H. Adipose tissue-derived multipotent stromal cells have a higher immunomodulatory capacity than their bone marrow-derived counterparts. Stem cells translational medicine. 2013;2(6):455-63.

31. Ruppert D, Wand MP, Carroll RJ. Semiparametric regression during 2003-2007. Electronic journal of statistics. 2009;3:1193-256.

32. Kim J, Hematti P. Mesenchymal stem cell-educated macrophages: a novel type of alternatively activated macrophages. Exp Hematol. 2009;37(12):1445-53.

33. Mosser DM. The many faces of macrophage activation. J Leukoc Biol. 2003;73(2):209-12.

34. de Oliveira GL, de Lima KW, Colombini AM, Pinheiro DG, Panepucci RA, Palma PV, Brum DG, Covas DT, Simões BP, de

Oliveira MC, Donadi EA, Malmegrim KC. Bone marrow mesenchymal stromal cells isolated from multiple sclerosis patients have distinct gene expression profile and decreased suppressive function compared with healthy counterparts. Cell Transplant. 2015;24(2):151-65.

35. Park CW, Kim KS, Bae S, Son HK, Myung PK, Hong HJ, Kim H. Cytokine secretion profiling of human mesenchymal stem cells by antibody array. International journal of stem cells. 2009;2(1):59-68.

36. Rasmusson I, Ringden O, Sundberg B, Le Blanc K. Mesenchymal stem cells inhibit lymphocyte proliferation by mitogens and alloantigens by different mechanisms. Experimental cell research. 2005;305(1):33-41.

37. Xu G, Zhang L, Ren G, Yuan Z, Zhang Y, Zhao RC, Shi Y. Immunosuppressive properties of cloned bone marrow mesenchymal stem cells. Cell research. 2007;17(3):240-8.

38. Malisan F, Brière F, Bridon JM, Harindranath N, Mills FC, Max EE, Banchereau J, Martinez-Valdez H. Interleukin-10 induces immunoglobulin G isotype switch recombination in human CD40-activated naive B lymphocytes. The Journal of experimental medicine. 1996;183(3):937-47.

39. Scheller J, Chalaris A, Schmidt-Arras D, Rose-John S. The pro- and anti-inflammatory properties of the cytokine interleukin-6. Biochimica et biophysica acta. 2011;1813(5):878-88.

40. Schindler R, Mancilla J, Endres S, Ghorbani R, Clark SC, Dinarello CA. Correlations and interactions in the production of interleukin-6 (IL-6), IL-1, and tumor necrosis factor (TNF) in human blood mononuclear cells: IL-6 suppresses IL-1 and TNF. Blood. 1990;75(1):40-7.

41. Hartung T. Anti-inflammatory effects of granulocyte colony-stimulating factor. Current opinion in hematology. 1998;5(3):221-5.

42. Bajrami B, Zhu H, Kwak HJ, Mondal S, Hou Q, Geng G, Karatepe K, Zhang YC, Nombela-Arrieta C, Park SY, Loison F, Sakai J, Xu Y, Silberstein LE, Luo HR. G-CSF maintains controlled neutrophil mobilization during acute inflammation by negatively regulating CXCR2 signaling. The Journal of experimental medicine. 2016;213(10):1999-2018.

43. Moll G, Rasmusson-Duprez I, von Bahr L, Connolly-Andersen AM, Elgue G, Funke L, Hamad OA, Lönnies H, Magnusson PU, Sanchez J, Teramura Y, Nilsson-Ekdahl K, Ringdén O, Korsgren O, Nilsson B, Le Blanc K. Are therapeutic human mesenchymal stromal cells compatible with human blood? Stem Cells. 2012;30(7):1565-74.

44. von Bahr L, Sundberg B, Lönnies L, Sander B, Karbach H, Hägglund H, Ljungman P, Gustafsson B, Karlsson H, Le Blanc K, Ringdén O. Long-term complications, immunologic effects, and role of passage for outcome in mesenchymal stromal cell therapy. Biology of blood and marrow transplantation : journal of the American Society for Blood and Marrow Transplantation. 2012;18(4):557-64.

45. Kuzmina LA, Petinati NA, Parovichnikova EN, Lubimova LS, Gribanova EO, Gaponova TV, Shipounova IN, Zhironkina OA, Bigildeev AE, Svinareva DA, Drize NJ, Savchenko VG. Multipotent Mesenchymal Stromal Cells for the Prophylaxis of Acute Graft-versus-Host Disease-A Phase II Study. Stem cells international. 2012;2012:968213.

Abbreviations

MCS:	Mesenchymal stem cells
FBS:	Fetal bovine serum
PBMC:	Peripheral blood mononuclear cells
IL-2:	Interleukin-2
IL-4:	Interleukin-4
IL-6:	Interleukin-6
IL-10:	Interleukin-10
G-CSF:	Granulocyte-colony stimulating factor
GM-CSF:	Granulocyte-macrophage colony-stimulating factor
MCP1:	Monocyte chemoattractant protein 1
TNF-α:	Tumor necrosis factor-alpha
GvHD:	Graft versus host disease

Potential Conflicts of Interests

None

Acknowledgements

The authors thank Dr W. Wei-Lynn Wong and her team at the University of Zurich for her technical support.

Financial support

This work was supported by the Swiss Paraplegic Foundation, the Center for Applied Biotechnology and Molecular Medicine (Grant CABMM to J. Stoyanov from 3 march 2015) and the Swiss National Foundation (Grant CR2313_159744).

Corresponding author

Alessandro Bertolo, Biomedical Laboratories, Swiss Paraplegic Research, Guido A. Zäch Strasse 4, 6207 Nottwil, Switzerland. e-mail: alessandro.bertolo@paraplegie.ch

Randomized controlled trial comparing hyaluronic acid, platelet-rich plasma and the combination of both in the treatment of mild and moderate osteoarthritis of the knee

Lana JFSD[1,4], Weglein A[3], Sampson S[2], Vicente EF[1], Huber SC[1,7], Souza CV[4], Ambach MA[5], Vincent H[6], Urban-Paffaro A[7], Onodera CMK[7], Annichino-Bizzacchi JM[7], Santana MHA[8], Belangero WD[8]

Objective: This study aims at evaluating the clinical effects of Platelet Rich Plasma (PRP) and Hyaluronic Acid (HA) as individual treatments for mild to moderate Osteoarthritis (OA) and it also examines the potential synergistic effects of PRP in combination with HA. Research continues to emerge examining the potential therapeutic efficacy of HA and PRP as autologous injectable treatments for joint arthritis. However, there is a paucity of research investigating the effects of combining HA and PRP on pain and functional status in patients with OA.

Design: In this multi-center, randomized, controlled, double blind, prospective trial, 105 patients with mild to moderate knee osteoarthritis, who met the study criteria, were randomly allocated to one of three interventions: HA (n=36), PRP (n=36), or HA+PRP (n=33). Each patient received 3 intra-articular knee injections of their assigned substance, with 2 week intervals between each injection. Clinical outcomes were evaluated using the Western Ontario and McMaster Universities Arthritis Index (WOMAC) and Visual Analogue Scale (VAS) questionnaire at baseline and after 1,3,6 and 12 months.

Results: The study showed that the PRP group have significant reduction in VAS scores at 1 (p= 0.003), 3 (p= 0.0001), 6 (p= 0.0001) and 12 (p= 0.000) months when compared to HA. In addition, the PRP group illustrated greater improvement in WOMAC physical activity scale at 12 months (p= 0.008) when compared to the HA group. Combining HA and PRP resulted in a significant decreases in pain (p=0.0001) and functional limitation (p=0.0001) when compared to HA alone at 1 year post treatment; and significantly increased physical function at 1 (p=0.0004) and 3 (p=.011) months when compared to PRP alone.

Conclusion: The findings of the study support the use of autologous PRP as an effective treatment of mild to moderate knee osteoarthritis. It also shows that the combination of HA and PRP resulted to better outcomes than HA alone up to 1 year and PRP alone up to 3 months. Furthermore, the results suggest that combination of PRP and HA could potentially provide better functional outcomes in the first 30 days after treatment with both PRP and HA alone.

Key Words: Hyaluronic acid, Joint pathology, Knee, Osteoarthritis, Platelet-rich plasma

Introduction

Osteoarthritis of the knee joint has a great impact on physical performance and is considered one of the ten major causes of disability in the world. Standard conservative treatments for knee osteoarthritis include: weight loss, physical exercises, use of non-steroid anti-inflammatory agents, analgesics, injection of hyaluronic acid (HA) and injection of glucocorticoids[1,2]. Although, standard conservative measures can provide symptomatic improvements, they are not without their limitations. Steroid injections are common practice among practitioners, including orthopedic surgeons, however, prolonged use of such pharmacological treatments may have adverse effects on existing cartilage[3]. Also, chronic use of anti- inflammatory medications may cause nephrotoxicity and gastrointestinal side effects[3]. However, recently, Orthobiologic injections have emerged as a potentially safe and efficacious option for joint Osteoarthritis.

Hyaluronic Acid (HA) is currently a widely used injectable treatment for degenerative joint pathology. It is a glycosaminoglycan that acts as a backbone for proteoglycans of the extracellular matrix[4], providing increased joint lubrication. Studies have demonstrated that HA has positive therapeutic efficacy for knee osteoarthritis with initial efficacy at 4 weeks, and peak effectiveness at 8 weeks which lasts for up to 6 months[5]. When compared to continuous oral NSAIDS or other anti-inflammatory medications, HA has illustrated comparable, if not greater, therapeutic effects on knee OA with a better safety profile[5,6].

Autologous platelet rich plasma (PRP) has also emerged as an alternative in the context of injectable treatment for OA. PRP is comprised of a potent cellular milieu containing platelet concentrations above baseline, as well as an undifferentiated mixture of anti-inflammatory, pro-inflammatory, anabolic and catabolic mediators in an attempt to stimulate a supra-physiologic response and elicit the body's natural healing potential. Currently, most studies on PRP are anecdotal or case reports with small sample sizes. However, larger randomized controlled trials have demonstrated superior efficacy in areas such as tendinopathies[7] and knee osteoarthritis[8].

Author Names in full: José F. S. D. Lana[1,4], Adam Weglein[3], Steve E. Sampson[2], Eduardo F. Vicente[1], Stephany Cares Huber[1,7], Clarissa V. Souza[4], Mary A. Ambach[5], Hunter Vincent[6], Aline Urban-Paffaro[7], Carolina M. K. Onodera[7], Joyce M. Annichino-Bizzacchi[7], Maria Helena A. Santana[8], William D. Belangero[4]

[1]Bone and Cartilage Institute – (IOC) Indaiatuba – Brazil, [2]David Geffen School of Medicine at UCLA – USA, [3]Regenerative Ortho Med Clinic – USA [4]Institute of Orthopedics and Traumatology of University of Campinas (UNICAMP) - Brazil , [5] Orthohealing Center – USA,[6]Department of Physical Medicine and Rehabilitation: UC Davis,[7] Hemocentro of Campinas, University of Campinas (UNICAMP)- Brazil, [8] School of Chemical Engineering University of Campinas (UNICAMP) – Brazil

Although many studies have suggested both HA and PRP have potential to enhance the cartilage healing process and slow down the progression of OA[9, 10, 11], comparative trials have shown that PRP can be superior to HA in treating knee OA[12, 13]. Furthermore, PRP with its potent mixture of growth factors and cytokines has also been shown to increase the production of HA from native synoviocytes[14]. These findings suggest a potential additive effect of combining PRP with HA in treating OA. However, there is not much research examining such synergistic effects.

The main objective of our study was to evaluate the effectiveness of HA and PRP as monotherapies for mild to moderate OA and compare the results to the combination of PRP+HA.

Materials and Methods

Research design

The study is a double-blind, randomized and controlled prospective with three groups receiving three different lines of treatment. After the selection, the patients were randomized 1: 1: 1 by lot, in the three different treatment groups.   The selection and randomization was performed by a biomedical team responsible for research. After review and approval by the institutional ethics committee, volunteer participants were blinded and subjected to a standardized injection protocol performed by one interventionist. The participants then completed the WOMAC and VAS questionnaires at baseline and at 30, 90, 180 and 360 days after treatment.

Patients and sampling

The study was conducted in two orthopedic clinics as well as one ambulatory regenerative medicine clinic in Brazil from January 2011 to April 2014. One hundred and twenty patients were enrolled in our study, but 105 (87.5%) were ultimately included, as fifteen patients were lost for follow up after randomization. The local ethics committee of University of Uberaba approved the study (authorization number 0042.0.227.000-11) and all volunteer participants signed informed consent and were randomly allocated to one of the three groups of intervention, namely, HA, PRP, or PRP+HA groups, as evidenced in the figure 1. The following inclusion criteria for patient selection were used: age between 40 to 70 years, history of chronic pain for at least four months and/or joint edema and radiographic evidence of mild to moderate OA according to Kellgren-Lawrence classification (grade I, II and III)[15]. The exclusion criteria were considered to be: coagulopathies, axial deviation of lower limb larger than 5° for valgus and varus knee, severe cardiovascular diseases, diabetes mellitus and, immunosuppressive status, patients on anticoagulants, antithrombotic and anti-platelet drugs and non-steroid anti-inflammatory medication, patients with less than 11mg/dL of hemoglobin and less than 150.000 mm³ platelets, auto-immune diseases, history of previous surgery in the affected joint and OA grade IV according to Kellgren-Lawrence classification. In addition, C reactive protein (CRP) and Uric acid levels were also assessed in all patients and abnormal levels were used as exclusion criteria.

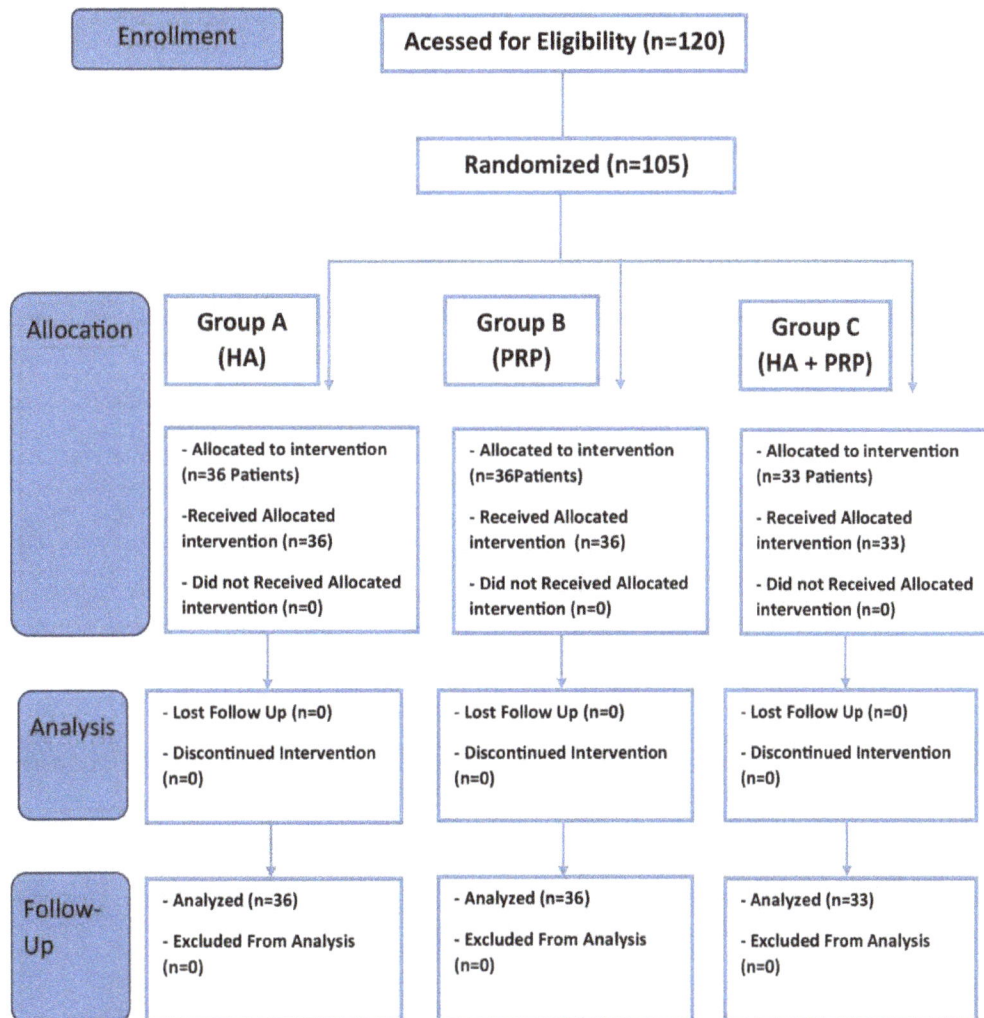

Figure 1: *Flow-chart and details for all phases of research.*

In order to evaluate the systemic inflammation, the levels of CPR were measured in 30, 90, 180 and 360 days after the first application of PRP.

Assessment and Outcomes

Patients were assessed at screening for clinical and demographic characteristics and baseline assessment. Patients were followed for over one year and were submitted to four more follow-up evaluations: +30 (one month), +90 (3 months), +180 (6 months) and 360 days (1 year), where they completed VAS and WOMAC questionnaires. The version of the Western Ontario and McMaster Universities Arthritis Index (WOMAC)[16] used in the study was translated and validated to Brazilian Portuguese[17]. The WOMAC scores are presented by Likert scale in which each question has a score ranging from 0 to 100, distributed as follows: 0 = none; 25 = little; 50 = Moderate; 75 = severe; 100 = very intense. Each of the five scores is calculated as the sum of the items included[18].

The primary analysis is the **median change** in VAS and WOMAC scores from pre-treatment baseline to 360 days across the three groups. Since VAS and WOMAC outcomes did not follow normal distribution, median values were used. To control for baseline differences, we subtracted the baseline and compared changes from baseline. This makes for a more fair comparison where differences are not due to differences at baseline. The secondary analysis is the median change in VAS and WOMAC scores from pre-treatment baseline to 30, 90 and 180 days.

Intervention

Patients were asked to discontinue the use of any anti-inflammatory drugs two weeks before initiation of treatment until trial completion. The procedure was performed in a procedure room at a clinic setting. Ultrasound guidance at knee medial compartment in 30° degree of flexion was used in the procedure.

Injections were performed under ultrasound guidance three times in the affected knee(s), with interval of two weeks between them. The injections were administered using the lateral mid-patellar approach using strict sterile technique. Lidocaine 2% with epinephrine was used for local anesthesia (without intra articular anesthesia), buffering with 0,2 ml of sodium bicarbonate (8.4%). The PRP group received 5 ml of platelet rich plasma (white blood cells (WBC) rich, red blood cells (RBC) poor, activated with serum), while the HA group received 2.0 ml (20 mg of HA) of high molecular weight (2.4 - 3.6 million daltons) non cross-linked hyaluronic acid extracted from bacteria cells (Eufflexa-Ferring 10mg/ml HA). The PRP+HA group received both treatments, with the 2.0 ml injection of HA first, followed by the 5 ml of PRP. All the patients treated with PRP alone or in combination of HA used the same volume of PRP which is 5 ml. After the injections, patients were instructed to apply local icepack, three times a day for 30 minutes each in the first 2 days after injection and switch to hot packs in the third and fourth days after injection. Patients took Dipirone 1.0 g twice a day for the first two days after procedure.

PRP Preparation

Blood was collected from the patients after a fasting period of four hours. About 60 ml of total blood was drawn under aseptic conditions, primarily from the median or antecubital vein. Basal platelet count was performed and the PRP was collected. 8.5 ml of the anticoagulant ACD (citric acid, sodium citrate, dextrose) was used to preserve the blood cells and to maintain physiologic pH [19, 20].

The first centrifugation was carried out at (300G for 5 minutes), with the purpose of separating the blood components into three main layers: red blood cells (RBC) or erythrocytes, white blood cells (WBC) or buffy coat and plasma. Studies under way at UNICAMP – University of Campinas, Brazil, suggest that at this speed there is a better recuperation of the platelets contained in the sample[21]. The whole top part of the content of the tubes (plasma and buffy coat) is collected, avoiding the collection of erythrocytes[22]. This content continues on to the second centrifugation at a higher speed rotation (700G for 17 minutes), which will promote a higher sedimentation of platelets and leukocytes. In this manner, it is possible to obtain a higher concentration of platelets in the final product, with no alteration to its integrity and causing no harm in the liberation of the platelet growth factors[23,24]. Platelet count was performed pre and post centrifugation in a hematological counter (ABX Micro 60-OT, Horiba ABX) to ensure the highest level of quality control.

Activation is carried out with only autologous thrombin, in the proportion of 0.8 ml of thrombin for 5 ml of PRP.

Statistical Analyses

Descriptive analyses are provided for demographic and clinical characteristics. The Kolmogorov-Smirnov and Shapiro-Wilk tests were applied to check distributions for normality. Chi-square tests were used to compare binary outcomes and the, Kruskall-Wallis and Wilcoxon tests were applied to compare distributions of continuous data The primary analysis is the median change in VAS and WOMAC scores from pre-treatment baseline to 360 days across the three groups. A two-sided p value less than 0.05 was considered statistically significant. Computation were carried out using IBM SPSS v 21 and SAS versión 9.4.

Results

The mean age was 60.9 years (45-70), 90 patients (84.8%) were female. In all of the 105 patients, a mild adverse reaction in the form of a knee swelling was reported 3-5 days after the application. It was not a reported as a major complication by any patient. It was verified that the majority of patients in all the groups have grade II of OA by Kellgren-Lawrence in the right knee. Also, it was observed that the patients were overweight through BMI in all the groups of treatment. The majority of the population was brown and has as comorbidities hypothyroidism, dyslipidemia and hypertension. Half of the patients in all the groups were physically active, practicing walking or aquatic activities, without axial impact. These data were presented in Table 1. It was found that statistical differences in the groups related to race (p=0.0076) and comorbidities (p=0.0266). This difference in race was observed in the group treated with association of PRP+HA in comparison to HA (p=0.0201) and PRP (p=0.0246). In regard to the comorbidities, a significant difference was observed between the groups that were treated with HA+PRP and PRP (p=0.0031).

In the baseline only WOMAC pain were significant (HA-PRP p=0.0073; HA+PRP – PRP p=0.0165), evidenced that the group of HA present more pain than the other two groups, as verified in Table 2. Three days after the treatment, it was verified thru VAS that the HA groups continued with significant more pain than the other groups (HA-PRP p=0.0034; HA+PRP-PRP p=0.0113). It was also observed that there was a significant improvement on the WOMAC physical in the group treated with HA+PRP when compared to the other groups (HA+PRP-HA p=0.0001; HA+PRP-PRP p=0.0004), as described in Table 3. According to the VAS, in 90 days, it was verified that the groups treated with PRP alone (p=0.0001) or in combination (p=0.0000) showed significant less pain than HA. Also an improvement in WOMAC physical was observed in the group HA+PRP when compared with the other groups (HA- HA+PRP p=0.0052; PRP-HA+PRP P=0.0110) as reported in Table 4. At the 180 day mark, significantly less pain was observed in the groups treated with PRP alone or in the combination and an improvement in the WOMAC physical was observed only for the group HA+PRP in comparison with HA (p=0.0262), as observed in the Table 5. This tendency was verified at 360 days, as demonstrated in Table 6. It was verified that the groups treated with PRP alone (p=0.0000) or in combination (p=0.0000) showed significant less pain in comparison to HA according to VAS. Also, these groups showed a significant improvement in WOMAC physical in comparison to HA (HA+PRP-HA p=0.0001; PRP-HA p=0.0089).

In summary, the PRP group had significantly greater median VAS improvement at 30, 90, 180, 360 days and significantly greater WOMAC PA improvement at 360 days when compared to the HA group. The HA + PRP group had statistically significant decrease from baseline of the median VAS and WOMAC PA when compared to the HA group. Thus, combining HA and PRP resulted to less pain and less functional limitation compared to HA alone at 30, 90, 180 and 360 days. When comparing HA + PRP group to PRP alone, the combination resulted in a statistically significant improvement in median WOMAC PA values at 30 and 90 days only. Figures 3 and 4 summarizes the median VAS and WOMAC PA change from baseline, respectively. The median changes from day 0 baseline in WOMAC

pain and WOMAC stiffness were not statistically different among the three groups at any time.

Relative to PRP, our final PRP product consisted of platelets, leukocytes and circulating fibrinogen, with a small residue of red cells (Figure 2). The PRP platelet concentration varied between 800,000 and 1,600,000 per mm^3 of plasma, which corresponds to 5 to 8 times the basal concentration in all patients. The basal concentration of platelets was 155.000 to 315.000 mm^3 and white blood cells (WBC) were 9.7 ± 3.4 per mm^3.

In relation to the inflammation, the level of CPR showed evidence that the group treated with PRP alone or in association had an increase in the CPR levels after 90 days and a decrease at the end of the follow-up. On the other hand, the group treated with HA showed an increase in 30 days with a posterior decrease in 90 days, but at the end of follow-up the levels of CPR were higher than baseline, as verified in the Table 7. In baseline, PRP group had the highest CPR value, being significant in comparison of HA+PRP and HA (p=0.0013). 30 days after the first application, HA group showed the highest value of CPR in comparison to other groups (p=0.0152). In 90 days, it was observed that the HA group had the lowest value when compared with other groups of PRP alone or in association (p<0.0001). In 180 and 360 days after treatment it was verified the same pattern. Patients treated with HA presented highest values of CPR in comparison to the groups treated with PRP (p<0.001).

Table 1: Patients Casuistic (n= 105)*

	HA group (n= 36)	**PRP group (n= 36)**	**HA+PRP group (n= 33)**
Sex, F:M, (%)	33 (91.7): 3 (8.3)	29(80.6): 7(19.4)	27 (81.8): 6 (18.2)
Age, mean ± SD (range)	60 ± 6.6 (45-70)	60.9 ± 7(48-70)	62 ± 6.1(48-70)
Kellgren-Laurence grade, 1:2:3 (%)	9(25):16(44):11 (31)	9(25):14(39):13(36)	5(15.2):14(42.4):14(42.4)
Limb, R:L:both (%)	17(47.2):13(6.1):6(16.7)	14(39):16(44):5(15)	21(64):7(21):5(15)
BMI	28.24 ± 8.77	27.42 ± 6.89	29.15 ± 7.31
Caucasian	14 (38.9%)	8 (22.2%)	4 (12.1%)
Brown	19 (52.8%)	27 (75%)	21 (63.6%)
Black	3 (8.3%)	1 (2.8%)	8 (24.2%)
Hypothyroidism	4 (11.1%)	3 (8.3%)	6 (18.2%)
Dyslipidemia	12 (33.3%)	12 (33.3%)	8 (24.2%)
HT	15 (41.7%)	11 (30.6%)	19 (57.6%)
Physical Activity (walk or aquatic activity without axial impact, up until 3x per week)	16 (44.4%)	23 (63.8%)	17 (51.5%)

* P statistically significant in race (p=0.0076) and comorbidities (p=0.0266).

HA= hyaluronic acid; PRP= platelet-rich plasma; WBC= white blood cells; F= female; M= male; SD= standard deviation; R= right; L= left; BMI = body mass index; HT = hypertension

Table 2: Baseline comparisons of VAS, WOMAC Pain, WOMAC stiffness and WOMAC physical activity (PA). Median (range) reported.

Outcome	HA (n=36)	PRP (n=36)	HA+PRP (n=33)	HA vs PRP	P values HA vs HA+PRP	PRP vs HA+PRP
VAS	7.0 (5-10)	7.5 (3-10)	7.0 (5-10)	0.2100	0.1447	0.7680
WOMAC Pain	388 (125-500)	288 (100-500)	275 (100-500)	**0.0173**	**0.0165**	0.5662
WOMAC Stiffness	75 (25-200)	125 (25-200)	125 (25-200)	0.0972	0.0582	0.5278
WOMAC PA	988 (425-1425)	913 (425-1425)	950 (450-1425)	0.1993	0.5954	0.3282

Table 3: Median change from base (pre) to 30 days. Median (range) reported.

Outcome	HA	PRP	HA+PRP	HA vs PRP	P values HA vs HA+PRP	PRP vs HA+PRP
VAS	-3.0 (-7, 0)	-4.5 (-8, 0)	-4.0 (-8,-1)	**0.0034**	**0.0113**	0.9417
n	35	36	33			
WOMAC Pain	-200 (-450, 25)	-175 (-350, 75)	-175 (-375, 25)	0.1420	0.1191	0.8355
n	36	34	33			
WOMAC Stiffness	- 50.0 (-175, 0)	-50.0 (-150, 25)	-75 (-100, -25)	0.7900	0.1028	0.2334
n	23	22	19			
WOMAC PA	-362.5 (-1075, 200)	-375.0 (-1050, 275)	-650 (-1125, -75)	0.1909	**0.0001**	**0.0004**
n	36	36	33			

Table 4: Median change from base (pre) to 90 days. Median (range) reported.

Outcome	HA	PRP	HA+PRP	HA vs PRP	P values HA vs HA+PRP	PRP vs HA+PRP
VAS	-3.0 (-6, 0)	-6.0 (-8, 1)	-6.0 (-9, -1)	**0.0001**	**0.0000**	0.1795
n	36	35	33			
WOMAC Pain	-187.5 (-450, 75)	-225.0 (-375, 0)	-200 (-375, -25)	0.5113	0.2652	0.6617
n	36	33	33			
WOMAC Stiffness	-50.0 (-125, 25)	-100.0 (-175, 0)	-75.0 (-125, -25)	0.1282	0.1382	0.7284
n	22	22	19			
WOMAC PA	-512.5 (-1225, 500)	-550.0 (-1150, 25)	-725.0 (-1225, -25)	0.4368	**0.0052**	**0.0110**
n	36	36	33			

Table 5: Median change from base (pre) to 180 days. Median (range) reported.

Outcome	HA	PRP	HA+PRP	HA vs PRP	P values HA vs HA+PRP	PRP vs HA+PRP
VAS	-3.0 (-7, 4)	-5.0 (-9, -1)	-5.0 (-9, -1)	**0.0001**	**0.0000**	0.2235
n	36	35	33			
WOMAC Pain	-162.5 (-450, 250)	-225.0 (-450, 0)	-200 (-450, -25)	0.1555	0.3029	0.5579
n	36	34	33			
WOMAC Stiffness n	-62.5 (-125, 0) 14	-62.5 (-125, 0) 18	-100 (-150, 25) 14	0.9226	0.0953	0.0698
WOMAC PA	-462.5 (-1350, 600)	-625.0 (-1400, 0)	-675.0 (-1300, -250)	0.0909	**0.0262**	0.1629
n	36	36	33			

Table 6: Comparison of median VAS, WOMAC pain, WOMAC stiffness and WOMAC physical activity (PA) change from baseline to 360 days. Median (range) reported

Outcome	HA	PRP	HA+PRP	HA vs PRP	P values HA vs HA+PRP	PRP vs HA+PRP
VAS	-2 (-7, 2)	-5 (-9, 1)	-5 (-9, -1)	**0.0000**	**0.0000**	0.6783
n	33	32	25			
WOMAC Pain	-188 (-450, 50)	-238 (-425, 0)	-200 (-450, 50)	0.2273	0.6546	0.3057
n	34	30	33			
WOMAC Stiffness n	-75 (-125, 50) 15	-100 (-175, 0) 14	-88 (-175, 0) 12	0.3192	0.4674	0.7537
WOMAC PA	-450 (-1350, 375)	-775 (-1300, 0)	-825 (-1325, -300)	**0.0089**	**0.0001**	0.1982
n	36	34	33			

Table 7: Results of mean and standard deviation of CPR levels of different groups in the follow-up

CPR levels	HA	PRP	HA+PRP	P values
Baseline	2.6 ± 1.7	3.3 ± 2.3	2.6 ± 1.6	0.0013
+30	4.7 ± 1.7	3.6 ± 1.3	3.8 ± 1.4	0.0152
+90	2.6 ± 1.4	4.4 ± 1.4	4.2 ± 1.6	<0.0001
+180	6.0 ± 2.3	3.1 ± 1.6	3.4 ± 1.6	<0.0001
+360	6.3 ± 2.3	2.8 ± 1.4	3.0 ± 1.4	<0.0001

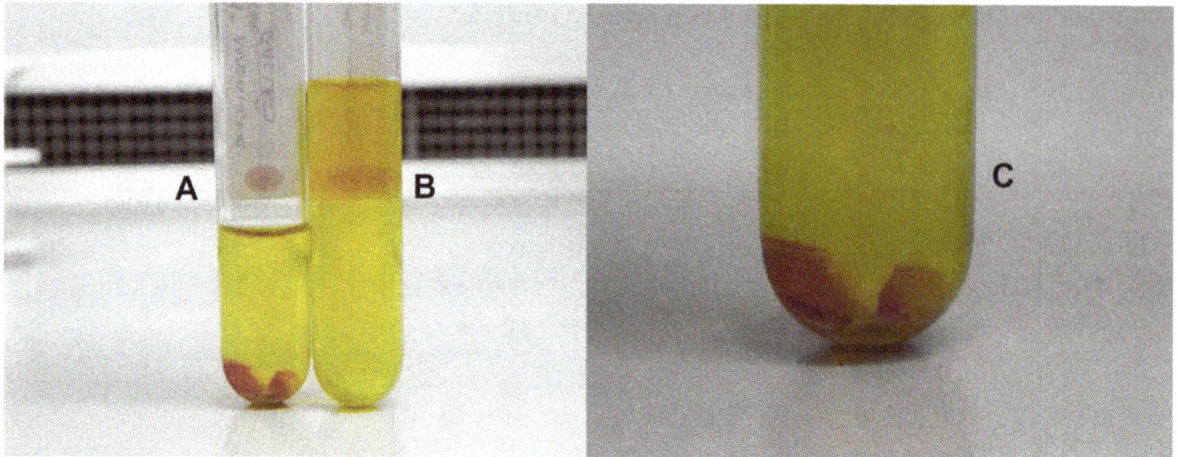

Figure 2: *(A) Platelet-Rich Plasma and leukocytes (L-PRP) containing the white series (buffy coat) and residual red cells; (B) top part of the collected plasma after the second centrifugation, which corresponds to the platelet poor plasma (PPP), approximately 80% of the total centrifuged volume; C) Cellular fraction in evidence before PRP suspension.*

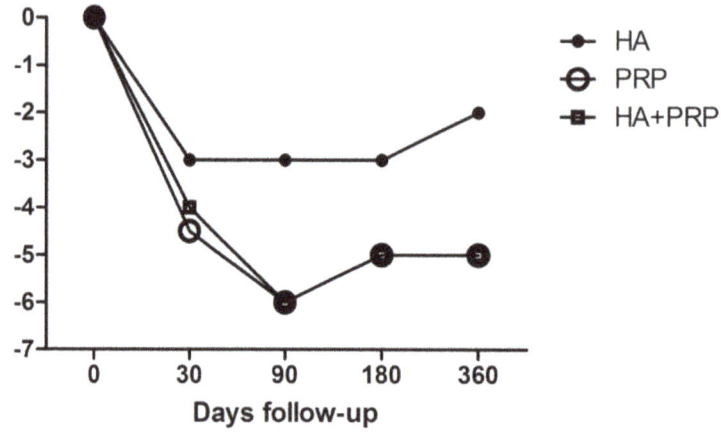

Figure 3: Median VAS change from Baseline

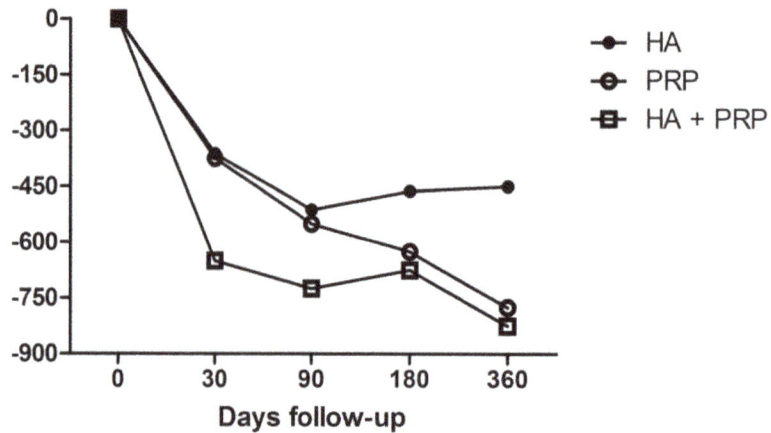

Figure 4: Median WOMAC PA change from baseline

Discussion

The use of buffy-coat or leukocyte layer together with PRP was incentivized by studies that highlighted the antimicrobial[25, 26] and immune-regulatory[27, 28] actions of the leukocytes, as well as proving that the majority of the platelets are found in this layer, together with the leukocytes after the centrifugation[29]. There are controversies as to the use of the leukocytes as studies suggests that with the presence of leukocytes, the neutrophils are enabled to liberate metalloproteins that cause degradation to the extracellular matrix and even release free radicals [30]. However, the macrophages are responsible for the removal of the debris, phagocytic function and also have an important role in the balance of the pro-inflammatory and anti-inflammatory aspects of healing. As it is not possible to fractionate the different types of white blood cells, it may be that the absence of macrophages could be more harmful to the cure than any secondary harm inflicted by the presence of the neutrophils. We believe that this increase in CPR levels in the first 90 days of the treatment in groups treated with PRP can be explained due to the increase of inflammatory activity in the joint because of the WBC.

It was furthermore demonstrated that the polymerization and final architecture of the fibrin network considerably influences the intensity and speed of the liberation of growth factors, mainly TGFβ1 and the presence of the leukocytes maintains a fundamental role in the development of this network[31].

Relative to activation of PRP, the use of chemical activators cause instability in the fibrin network and rapid growth factor release. On the other hand, if the PRP is activated in a more physiological manner, a stable tetramolecular network is formed and it has direct influence in the speed and amount of liberation of the growth factors[31].

Recently, there has been a lot of interest in new treatments aimed at stimulating repair or replacing damaged cartilage in joints. There are currently limited high-level studies in the literature to demonstrate the real efficacy of PRP injections. Sampson et al[32] presented a pilot study involving 14 patients with primary and secondary knee OA where treatment with PRP resulted to significant improvement in function and relief of pain and symptoms. Most of the patients expressed favorable outcome at 12 months after treatment. Kon et al[33] published a study involving 100 patients with chronic degenerative condition of the knees treated with intraarticular knee injections and followed at 6 and 12 months. They showed statistically significant improvement in all clinical scores and concluded that their preliminary results indicate that treatment with PRP injections is safe and has the potential to reduce pain and improve knee function and quality of life in younger patients with low degree of articular degeneration. Sanchez et al[34] performed an observational cohort study of 30 patients with knee OA and showed significant reduction of the WOMAC pain subscale at 5 weeks for the autologous preparation rich in growth factors (PRGF) group. They also demonstrated percent reductions in the physical function and overall WOMAC at 5 weeks associated in favor of the PRGF group.

In our study, the patients enrolled have some significant differences between the groups when evaluated the race and comorbidities. In relation to race, it was verified that in the group that used association of PRP and HA, we had more black and less Caucasian people than the other groups. However, in Brazil we have extreme population miscegenation and arthritis does not have relevance in context with race. In relation to comorbidities, it was verified that the group that used PRP + HA had more patients with hypothyroidism and hypertension.

When PRP was compared to HA, the PRP group had significantly greater median VAS improvement at 30, 90, 180, 360 days and significantly greater WOMAC PA improvement at 360 days compared to the HA group. This supports the findings of other studies that showed PRP having superior results versus HA in the treatment of knee OA. Sanchez et al[34] showed that PRP is better in pain, physical activity and overall WOMAC scores in 5 weeks compared to HA. Spakova et al[10] showed statistically significant better results in the PRP group compared to HA at 3 and 6 month follow up periods in both WOMAC and numeric rating scale (NRS) scores. Kon et al[35] showed that the PRP group showed better results than the HA group at 6 months follow up in the International Knee Documentation Committee and VAS scores and concluded that autologous PRP injections showed more and longer efficacy than HA injections in reducing pain and symptoms and recovering articular function. Patel et al[36] evaluated PRP and placebo in treatment of OA using the same methodology as our study with WOMAC and VAS. It was verified that the groups treated with a single or double injection of PRP had an improvement in relation of placebo, however, in 6 months occurred the deterioration of the results. Our study showed an improvement even after 1 year and this can be explained due to one more application and the use of PRP rich in leukocytes.

Many studies have suggested that the application of hyaluronic acid and PRP may have potentially positive effects on cartilage repair and slow down the progression of OA[9-11]. However, to our knowledge, there is lack of studies in literature that examined the combination use of HA and PRP. Studies show that HA provides appropriate matrix and supportive scaffold material for cartilage repair and enhances the mechanical properties of the cartilage[37-39]. Thus, it is hypothesized that their combination may be synergistic. According to literature, combining PRP and HA may benefit from their dissimilar biological mechanisms and helping with the signaling molecules as inflammatory molecules, catabolic enzymes, cytokines and growth factors. Also, it was demonstrated that the association of HA+PRP showed synergic effects in the potentials regenerative and anti-inflammatory in comparison to HA or PRP alone. This association can alter the inflammatory cytokines in the degeneration process of the chondrocytes through specific mediators (CD44, TGF-βRII) and also promote the regeneration of cartilage and inhibit inflammation in OA. The time to all these modifications happen is between 30-90 days after application, which explains the 30-90 days of improvement in WOMAC PA[40,41].

The results of our study showed that the HA + PRP group had statistically significant decrease from baseline of the median VAS and WOMAC PA when compared to the HA group. Thus, combining HA and PRP resulted to less pain and less functional limitation compared to HA alone at 30, 90, 180 and 360 days.

When comparing HA + PRP group to PRP alone, the combination resulted to a statistically significant improvement in median WOMAC PA values at 30 and 90 days only. The lubrication and support to the extracellular matrix that the HA provided seemed to enable earlier functional benefit to the PRP injection. This combination may result to better rehabilitation and earlier return to activities of daily activities.

The median changes from day 0 baseline in WOMAC pain and WOMAC stiffness were not statistically different among the three groups (HA, PRP and HA+PRP) at any time. No overall WOMAC score comparisons were made.

When the inflammation was evaluated, it was verified that the groups that treated with PRP alone or in combination presented lower levels of CPR at the end of follow-up in comparison to HA. Interestingly, in these groups an increase in CPR levels was observed at 90 days. This increase could be explained due to the inflammatory process of cells in the regenerative phase of treatment and also peak of improvement in treatments based in cell therapy.

Study Limitations

The study utilized self-reported questionnaires such as WOMAC and VAS to assess pain and functional outcomes, which could potentially limit the objectivity of results. In addition, advanced imaging such as MRI was not performed because of high costs, but could have provided more objective data as to the benefit of treatments. Although functional tests can provide more objective responses to treatment, they were not included in the study and should be considered for future studies. Another limitation was the absence of a gold standard or true control group using saline.

Conclusion

Our results suggest that the use of autologous PRP and its combination with HA are safe and effective methods for treatment of mild to moderate osteoarthritis of the knee. The PRP group had significantly greater reduction in VAS scores at 30, 90, 180 and 360 days and significantly greater WOMAC physical activity improvement at 360 days compared to the HA group. Combining HA and PRP resulted to significantly less pain and less functional limitation compared to HA alone up to 1 year after treatment. HA+ PRP combination also resulted to significantly more physical function early in the treatment (1 month and 3 months) as compared to PRP alone. More randomized controlled studies with larger numbers of patients are needed to confirm these findings and to investigate the persistence of the beneficial effects observed.

References

1. Conaghan PG, Dickson J, Grant RL, Care and management of osteoarthritis in adults: summary of NICE guidance. BMJ. 2008; 336 (7642): 502–3.
2. Hinton R, Moody RL, Davis AW, Thomas SF. Osteoarthritis: diagnosis and therapeutic considerations. Am. Fam. Physician. 2002; 65 (5): 841–8.
3. Michael JWP, Schlüter-Brust KU, Eysel P.The epidemiology, etiology, diagnosis, and treatment of osteoarthritis of the knee. Dtsch. Arztebl. Int. 2010; 107 (9): 152–62.
4. Gigante A, Callegari L. The role of intra-articular hyaluronan (Sinovial) in the treatment of osteoarthritis. Rheumatol. Int. 2011; 31 (4): 427–44.
5. Bannuru RR, Natov NS, Dasi UR, Schmid CH, McAlindon TE. Therapeutic trajectory following intra- articular hyaluronic acid injection in knee osteoarthritis--meta-analysis. Osteoarthritis Cartilage. 2011; 19 (6):611–9.
6. Bannuru RR, Vaysbrot EE, Sullivan MC, McAlindon TE. Relative efficacy of hyaluronic acid in comparison with NSAIDs for knee osteoarthritis: a systematic review and meta-analysis. Semin. Arthritis Rheum. 2014; 43 (5): 593–9.
7. Mishra AK, Skrepnik NV, Edwards SG, Jones GL, Sampson S, Vermillion DA, Ramsey ML, Karli DC, Rettig AC. Efficacy of platelet-rich plasma for chronic tennis elbow: a double-blind, prospective, multicenter, randomized controlled trial of 230 patients. Am J Sport. Med. 2014; 42 (2): 463–71.
8. Patel S, Dhillon MS, Aggarwal S, Marwaha N, Jain A. Treatment with platelet-rich plasma is more effective than placebo for knee osteoarthritis: a prospective, double-blind, randomized tria. Am J Sport. Med. 2013; 41 (2): 356–64.
9. Filardo G, Kon E, Martino AD, Matteo BD, Merli ML, Cenacchi A, Fornasari PM, Marcacci M. Platelet- rich plasma vs hyaluronic acid to treat knee degenerative pathology: study design and preliminary results of a randomized controlled trial. BMC Musculoskelet. Disord.2012; 13 (1):229.
10. Spaková T, Rosocha J, Lacko M, Harvanová D, Gharaibeh A. Treatment of Knee Joint Osteoarthritis with Autologous Platelet-Rich Plasma in Comparison with Hyaluronic Acid. Am. J. Phys. Med. Rehabil. 2012; 91(5): 411-7
11. Lubowitz JH, Provencher MT, Poehling GG. Cartilage treatment and biologics current research. Arthroscopy. 2013; 29 (10): 1597–8.
12. Kon E, Mandelbaum B, Buda R, Filardo G, Delcogliano M, Timoncini A, Fornasari PM, Giannini S, Marcacci M. Platelet-rich plasma intra-articular injection versus hyaluronic acid viscosupplementation as treatments for cartilage pathology: from early degeneration to osteoarthritis. Arthroscopy. 2011; 27 (11):1490–501.
13. Spaková T, Rosocha J, Lacko M, Harvanová D, Gharaibeh A. Treatment of knee joint osteoarthritis with autologous platelet-rich plasma in comparison with hyaluronic acid. Am. J. Phys. Med. Rehabil. 2012;91 (5): 411– 17.
14. Anitua E, Sánchez M, Nurden AT, Zalduendo MM, Fuente M de la, Azofra J, Andía I. Platelet - released growth factors enhance the secretion of hyaluronic acid and induce hepatocyte growth factor production by synovial fibroblasts from arthritic patients. Rheumatology (Oxford). 2007; 46 (12): 1769–72.
15. KELLGREN JH, LAWRENCE JS. Radiological assessment of osteo-arthrosis. Ann. Rheum. Dis.1957; 16 (4): 494–502.
16. Bellamy N, Buchanan WW, Goldsmith CH, Campbell J, Stitt LW. Validation study of WOMAC: a health status instrument for measuring clinically important patient relevant outcomes to antirheumatic drug therapy in patients with osteoarthritis of the hip or knee. 1988; 15(12):1833-40.
17. I. MF, Translation and validation of specific quality of life questionnaire for osteoarthritis WOMAC (Western Ontario and McMaster Universities Osteoarthritis Index) for the Portuguese language. 2002.
18. Bellamy N. WOMAC: a 20-year experiential review of a patient-centered self-reported health status questionnaire. J. Rheumatol. 2002; 29 (12): 2473–6.
19. Lei H, Gui L, Xiao R. The effect of anticoagulants on the quality and biological efficacy of platelet- rich plasma. Clin. Biochem. 2009; 42 (13–14): 1452–60.
20. Andrade MGS, de Freitas Brandão CJ, Sá CN, de Bittencourt TCBDSC, Sadigursky M. Evaluation of factors that can modify platelet-rich plasma properties. Oral Surg. Oral Med. Oral Pathol. Oral Radiol. Endod. 2008; 105(1): e5–e12.
21. Perez AGM, Lichy R, Lana JFSD, Rodrigues AA, Luzo ACM, Belangero WD, Santana MHA. Prediction and modulation of platelet recovery by discontinuous centrifugation of whole blood for the preparation of pure platelet-rich plasma. Biores. 2013; 2(4): 307–14.
22. Jacobson M, Fufa D, Abreu EL, Kevy S, Murray MM. Platelets, but not erythrocytes, significantly affect cytokine release and scaffold contraction in a provisional scaffold model. Wound Repair Regen.2008; 16(3): 370–8.
23. Weibrich G, Kleis WKG, Hafner G, Hitzler WE, Wagner W. Comparison of platelet, leukocyte, and growth factor levels in point-of-care platelet-enriched plasma, prepared using a modified Curasan kit, with preparations received from a local blood bank. Clin. Oral Implants Res. 2003; 14 (3): 357–62.
24. Weibrich G, Kleis WKG, Buch R, Hitzler WE, Hafner G. The Harvest Smart PRePTM system versus the Friadent-Schutze platelet-rich plasma kit. Comparison of a semiautomatic method with a more complex method for the preparation of platelet concentrates. Clin. Oral Implants Res. 2003;14 (2): 233–39.
25. Cieslik-Bielecka A, Gazdzik TS, Bielecki TM, Cieslik T. Why the platelet-rich gel has antimicrobial activity?. Oral Surg. Oral Med. Oral Pathol. Oral Radiol. Endod. 2007; 103 (3): 303–5; author reply 305–6.
26. Moojen DJ, Everts PA, Schure RM, Overdevest EP, van Zundert A, Knape JT, Castelein RM, Creemers LB, Dhert WJ. Antimicrobial activity of platelet-leukocyte gel against Staphylococcus aureus. J Orthop Res. 2008;26(3):404-10.
27. Dohan DM, Choukroun J, Diss A, Dohan SL, Dohan AJJ, Mouhyi J, Gogly B. Platelet-rich fibrin (PRF): a second-generation platelet concentrate. Part III: leucocyte activation: a new feature for platelet concentrates?. Oral Surg. Oral Med. Oral Pathol. Oral Radiol. Endod. 2006; 101 (3): e51–5.

28. El-Sharkawy H, Kantarci A, Deady J, Hasturk H, Liu H, Alshahat M, Van Dyke TE. Platelet-rich plasma: growth factors and pro- and anti-inflammatory properties. J. Periodontol. 2007; 78(4): 661–9.

29. Weibrich G, Kleis WKG, Hitzler WE, Hafner G. Comparison of the platelet concentrate collection system with the plasma-rich-in-growth-factors kit to produce platelet-rich plasma: a technical report. Int. J. Oral Maxillofac. Implants. 2005;20(1): 118–23.

30. Toumi H, Best TM. The inflammatory response: friend or enemy for muscle injury? Br. J. Sports Med. 2003;37(4): 284–6.

31. Dohan EDM, Bielecki T, Jimbo R, Barbé G, Del Corso M, Inchingolo F, Sammartino G. Do the fibrin architecture and leukocyte content influence the growth factor release of platelet concentrates? An evidence-based answer comparing a pure platelet-rich plasma (P-PRP) gel and a leukocyte- and platelet- rich fibrin (L-PRF). Curr. Pharm. Biotechnol. 2012; 13(7): 1145–52.

32. Sampson S, Reed M, Silvers H, Meng M, Mandelbaum B. Injection of platelet-rich plasma in patients with primary and secondary knee osteoarthritis: a pilot study. Am. J. Phys. Med. Rehabil. 2010; 89(12):961–9.

33. Kon E, Buda R, Filardo G, Di Martino A, Timoncini A, Cenacchi A, Fornasari PM, Giannini S, Marcacci M. Platelet-rich plasma: intra-articular knee injections produced favorable results on degenerative cartilage lesions. Knee Surg. Sports Traumatol. Arthrosc. 2010; 18 (4): 472–9.

34. Sánchez M, Anitua E, Azofra J, Aguirre JJ, Andia I. Intra-articular injection of an autologous preparation rich in growth factors for the treatment of knee OA: a retrospective cohort study. Clin Exp Rheumatol. 2008;26(5):910-3.

35. Kon E, Mandelbaum B, Buda R, Filardo G, Delcogliano M, Timoncini A, Fornasari PM, Giannini S, Marcacci M. Platelet-rich plasma intra-articular injection versus hyaluronic acid viscosupplementation as treatments for cartilage pathology: from early degeneration to osteoarthritis. Arthrosc. J. Arthrosc. Relat. Surg. 2011; 27 (11):1490–1501.

36. Patel S, Dhillon MS, Aggarwal S, Marwaha N, Jain A. Treatment with platelet-rich plasma is more effective than placebo for knee osteoarthritis: a prospective, double-blind, randomized trial. Am. J. Sports Med. 2013: 41(2): 355-64.

37. Levett PA, Hutmacher DW, Malda J, Klein TJ. Hyaluronic acid enhances the mechanical properties of tissue-engineered cartilage constructs. PLoS One. 2014; 9(12): e113216.

38. Ge Z, Li C, Heng BC, Cao G, Yang Z. Functional biomaterials for cartilage regeneration. J. Biomed. Mater. Res. A. 2012; 100 (9): 2526–36.

39. Matsiko A, Levingstone TJ, O'Brien FJ, Gleeson JP. Addition of hyaluronic acid improves cellular infiltration and promotes early-stage chondrogenesis in a collagen-based scaffold for cartilage tissue engineering. J Mech Behav Biomed Mater. 2012;11:41-52.

40. Andia I, Abate M. Knee osteoarthritis: hyaluronic acid, platelet-rich plasma or both in association? Expert Opin Biol Ther. 2014;14(5):635-49.

41. Chen W, Lo W, Hsu W, Wei H, Liu H, Lee C, Chen ST, Shieh Y, Williams DF, Deng W. Synergistic anabolic actions of hyaluronic acid and platelet-rich plasma on cartilage regeneration in osteoarthritis therapy. Biomaterials. 2014;35(36):9599-607.

Abbreviations

PRP: Platelet Rich Plasma
HA: Hyaluronic Acid
BMC: Bone Marrow Concentrate
RBC: Red Blood Cells
WBC: White Blood Cells
WOMAC: Western Ontario and McMaster Universities Arthritis Index
VAS: Visual Analogue Scale
BMI: Bone Mass Index

Potential Conflicts of Interests

The authors have no conflicts of interest and received no sponsorship for any of the products used in the trial.

Corresponding Author

Jose F.S.D. Lana, Bone and Cartilage Institute, Instituto do Osso e da Cartilagem (IOC), Avenida Presidente Kennedy, número 1386, Salas 26, 28 e 29, Indaiatuba, São Paulo, Brazil, Zip Code: 13334-170; Email: josefabiolana@gmail.com

11

Oct4B, CD90, and CD73 are upregulated in bladder tissue following electro-resection of the bladder

Takeuchi T[1], Tonooka A[2], Okuno Y[1], Hattori-Kato M[1], Mikami K[1]

Aim: We tested the hypothesis that stimulation by electro-resection of bladder tissue induces stem cells in the tissue repair process. **Materials & Methods**: After primary transurethral resection of a bladder tumor and surrounding tissue (TUR-Bt), second TUR-Bt was performed. Tissues excised by second TUR-Bt were immunohistochemically stained for Oct4, a marker of pluripotency, and for CD90 and CD73, markers of mesenchymal stromal cells, when no bladder tumor cells remained. **Results and Conclusions**: Oct4B protein was sporadically stained in the cytoplasm of interstitial cells in four out of eight cases. CD90 and CD73 are upregulated in interstitial and vascular endothelial cells without CD45 expression. Mesenchymal stromal cells, but not pluripotent stem cells, may be mainly involved in bladder tissue repair.

Key Words: Oct4B, CD90, CD73, Electric, Stimulation, Bladder

Introduction

In 2014, Obokata *et al.*, reported a cellular reprogramming phenomenon with acid treatment called stimulus-triggered acquisition of pluripotency (STAP). Unfortunately, their article was retracted because of misconduct, and the trial to replicate of the STAP cell phenomenon by other groups failed[1]. Nevertheless, the idea that strong environmental stimuli may reprogram differentiated somatic cells into less-differentiated ones is still worth pursuing.

The POU family transcription factor Oct4 (octamer-binding transcription factor 4) is an essential regulator of pluripotency and is of central significance in nuclear reprogramming[2]. It is one of the four reprogramming Yamanaka factors generating induced pluripotent stem cells[3]. Mesenchymal stromal cells (MSCs) are a rare population of non-hematopoietic stromal cells that reside in the bone marrow and connective tissues. They have the potential to differentiate into mesenchymal tissues such as bone, cartilage, muscle, and adipose tissues and, therefore, can be significant in tissue repair[4]. CD90 (thymus cell antigen 1) and CD73 (ecto-5'-nucleotidase) are surrogate positive markers of MSCs, while MSCs lack CD45 (leukocyte common antigen) expression[5, 6].

Transurethral electro-resection of intravesical tumors (TUR-Bt) is the first step in the treatment of bladder cancer. To confirm the completeness of endoscopic resection of bladder tumors, secondary resection of bladder tissue at the site of the preceding resection is performed within a few months. When no tumors remain in the resected specimens, the bladder is often preserved *in situ*. In the patients, the bladder tissue after primary electro-resection undergoes tissue repair. We hypothesized that the STAP phenomenon can be introduced by the stimulus of electro-resection in the bladder tissue during regeneration and that various levels of stem cell markers such as Oct4, CD90, and CD73 would appear in the bladder tissue resected by the secondary electro-resection.

Materials and Methods

Following endoscopic primary bipolar electro-resection of bladder tumors in saline (the TURis system, Olympus, Tokyo, Japan), secondary resection of bladder tissue at the primary resection site was performed. Those electro-resections were done at 280 watts.

Eight bladder paraffin-embedded specimens of secondary resections without remaining bladder tumors on examination with hematoxylin-eosin staining were immunohistochemically stained using anti-human Oct4 rabbit monoclonal antibody raised against amino acids 250-350 of human origin (EPR2054, Abcam, Cambridge, UK), anti-human Oct4 mouse monoclonal antibody raised against amino acids 1-134 of human origin (sc-5279, Santa Cruz Biothcnology, Inc., Dallas, Texas, USA), anti-human CD90/Thy1 rabbit monoclonal antibody (EPR3132, Abcam, Cambridge, UK), anti-human CD73 mouse monoclonal antibody (sc-32299, Santa Cruz Biotchnology, Inc., Dallas, Texas, USA), and anti-human CD45 mouse monoclonal antibody (IR751, Dako Japan, Tokyo, Japan). The mean interval between the primary and secondary electro-resection for the eight patients was 58 days. EPR2054 antibody detects both Oct4A and Oct4B proteins, while sc-5279 identifies Oct4A protein only.

The pathological diagnoses of corresponding primary tumors were all urothelial cancer and those specimens were also stained for Oct4 and CD90 as above. Two paraffin-embedded specimens of bladders excised at autopsy (died of cardiac infarction and pancreatic cancer), two paraffin-embedded specimens of testicular embryonal cancers, and paraffin-embedded specimens of primary TUR-Bts were similarly stained.

Author Names in full: Takumi Takeuchi[1], Akiko Tonooka[1], Yumiko Okuno[1], Mami Hattori-Kato[1], Koji Mikami[1]

[1] *Department of Urology, Kanto Rosai Hospital, Kizukisumiyoshi-cho, Nakahara-ku, Kawasaki, Japan,* [2] *Department of Pathology, Kanto Rosai Hospital, Kizukisumiyoshi-cho, Nakahara-ku, Kawasaki, Japan.*

Results

As summarized in Table 1, the pT stages of primary electro-resection were pT1 or possibly more than pT1, and tumor grades were G2 to G3 in the eight cases with no tumors in the secondary electro-resected specimens. Both EPR2054 and sc-5279 detected Oct4-expressing cells in the nucleus of embryonal cell cancer cells (Figure 1). DAPI staining for nuclear co-localization of Oct4A was not performed. Control autopsy bladder tissues did not show Oct4-expressing cells at all (Figure 2) by either EPR2054 or sc-5279. In four out of the eight cases, Oct4 protein was sporadically stained with EPR2054 in the cytoplasm of interstitial cells located in the specimens of second TUR-Bt (Figure 3 and Figure 4), but sc-5279 did not detect Oct4A protein in the specimens, revealing that Oct4 detected by EPR2054 is Oct4B. In bladder tumors resected by the primary TUR-Bt, Oct4A was not detected by sc-5279. Oct4 was sporadically demonstrated in five out of the eight bladder tumors in the cytoplasm of interstitial cells, but not in tumor cells by EPR2054, showing that the detected Oct4 was Oct4B *(Data not shown)*.

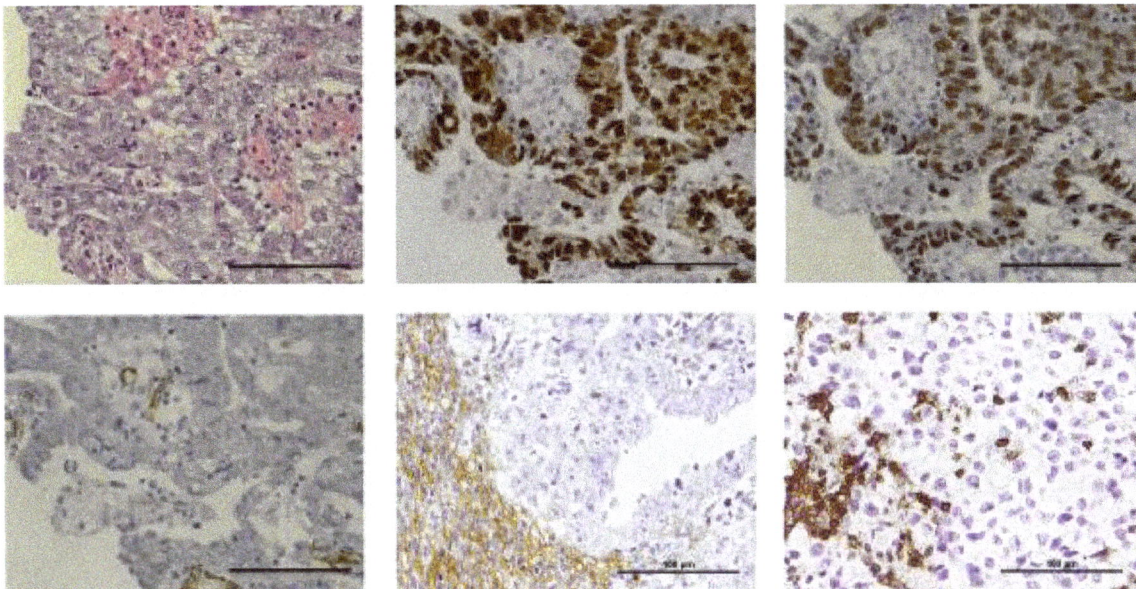

Figure 1: *Immunohistochemistry of embryonal cell cancer. Upper left: hematoxylin and eosin staining. Upper middle: Oct4 staining with EPR2054. Upper right: Oct4A staining with sc-5279. Lower left: CD90 staining. Lower middle: CD73 staining. Lower right: CD45 staining. 400x in the original picture, and Bar=100 μm. Oct4A was expressed in the nucleus of embryonal cell cancer cells. CD90 was weakly positive in the vascular endothelial cells. CD73 was negative in embryonal cell cancer, while CD45 was expressed in lymphocytes infiltrating cancer. In the stroma surrounding embryonal cell carcinomas, CD73 was strongly positive.*

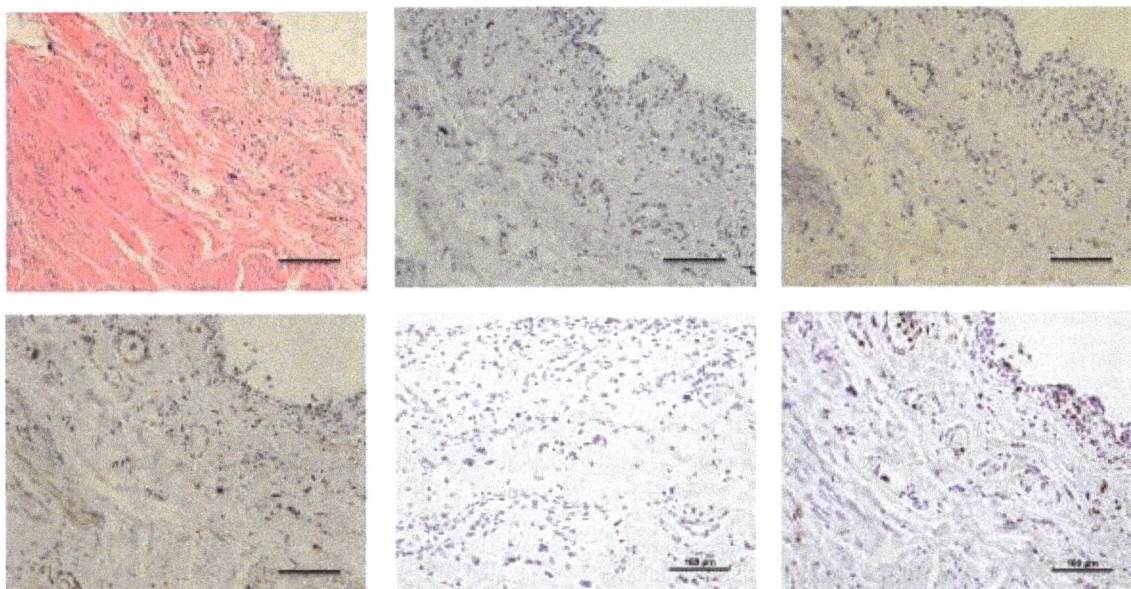

Figure 2: *Immunohistochemistry of representative (died of cardiac infarction) control autopsy bladder tissue. Upper left: hematoxylin and eosin staining. Upper middle: Oct4 staining with EPR2054. Upper right: Oct4A staining with sc-5279. Lower left: CD90 staining. Lower middle: CD73 staining. Lower right: CD45 staining. 200x in the original picture, and Bar=100 μm. Oct4A, Oct4B, and CD73 were negative. CD90 was weakly positive in the vascular endothelial cells. CD45 was expressed in lymphocytes.*

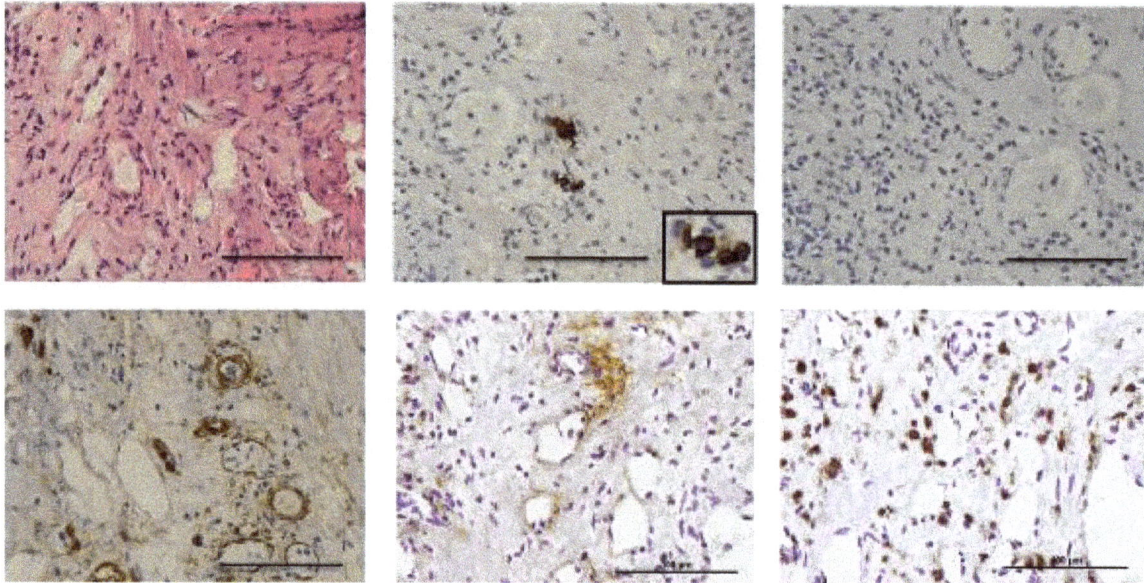

Figure 3: *Immunohistochemistry of a representative specimen of second TUR-Bt. Upper left: hematoxylin and eosin staining. Upper middle: Oct4 (Oct4B) staining with EPR2054 (a portion of positive cells is magnified at the corner). Upper right: Oct4A staining with sc-5279. Lower left: CD90 staining. Lower middle: CD73 staining. Lower right: CD45 staining. 400x in the original picture, and Bar=100 μm. Oct4B was expressed in the cytoplasm of interstitial cells. Oct4A was negative. CD90 and CD73 were expressed in the interstitial and vascular endothelial cells. CD45 was expressed in lymphocytes infiltrating tissue.*

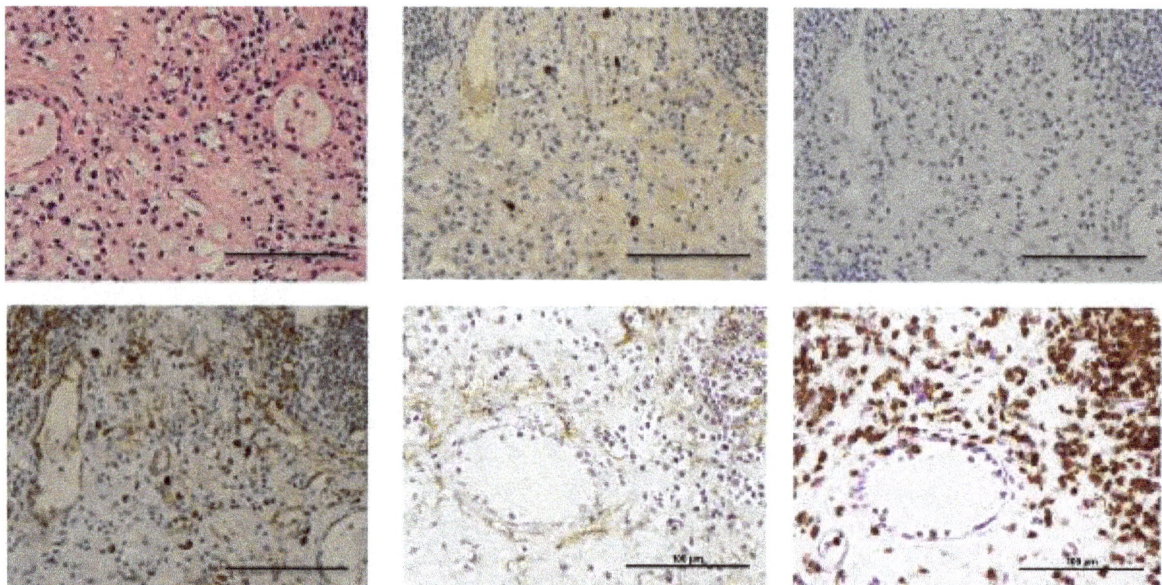

Figure 4: *Immunohistochemistry of a representative specimen of second TUR-Bt. Upper left: hematoxylin and eosin staining. Upper middle: Oct4 (Oct4B) staining with EPR2054. Upper right: Oct4A staining with sc-5279. Lower left: CD90 staining. Lower middle: CD73 staining. Lower right: CD45 staining. 400x in the original picture, and Bar=100 μm. Oct4B was expressed in the cytoplasm of interstitial cells. Oct4A was negative. CD90 and CD73 were expressed in the interstitial and vascular endothelial cells. CD45 was expressed in lymphocytes infiltrating tissue.*

CD90 expression was weakly positive in the vascular endothelial cells and CD73 was basically negative in control autopsy bladders and embryonal cell carcinomas, while CD45 was detected in lymphocytes there. In the stroma surrounding embryonal cell carcinomas, CD73 was strongly positive. CD90 and CD73 were markedly up-regulated in the interstitial cells in addition to showing enhanced expression in vascular endothelial cells in all electro-resected specimens by the second TUR-Bt (p=0.0016 by the chi-square test, compared with autopsy controls). CD45 was not detected in either interstitial or endothelial cells, being expressed only in lymphocytes infiltrating the electro-resected specimens. In bladder tumors resected by the primary TUR-Bt, CD90 was stained in vascular endothelial and interstitial cells, and possibly smooth muscle cells *(Data not shown)*.

The clinical courses after second TUR-Bt are listed in Table 1. Six patients underwent BCG bladder instillation as an adjuvant therapy. Intravesical tumor recurrence occurred in one case. One case has shown no tumor recurrence without additional therapy since second TUR-Bt and another has undergone total cystectomy without any remaining tumor in the cystectomy specimen.

Table 1

Patient	Age	Pathology of 1st TUR-BT	Intervals	Oct4B	Oct4A	CD90	CD73	CD45	Clinical course after 2nd TUR-BT
1	72	UC, pT1≦, G2>G3	35	+	-	+	+	-	No remaining tumor in Cx specimen,
2	77	UC, pT1, G3	80	+	-	+	+	-	No bladder recurrence for 1,103 days
3	65	UC, pT1≦, G3>G2	59	-	-	+	+	-	BCG+, no bladder recurrence for 1,069 days
4	69	UC, pT1, G2>G3	73	-	-	+	+	-	BCG+, no bladder recurrence for 939 days
5	63	UC, pT1≦, G2>G3	63	-	-	+	+	-	BCG+, no bladder recurrence for 838 days
6	54	UC, pT1, G2	56	+	-	+	+	-	BCG+, no bladder recurrence for 659 days
7	76	UC, pT1, G2>G3	56	-	-	+	+	-	BCG+, no bladder recurrence for 544 days
8	81	UC, pT1, G2>G3	42	+	-	+	+	-	BCG+, CIS after 600 days

Patients were all males except # 2. UC: urothelial cancer. Intervals: intervals (days) between 1st and 2nd TUR-BTs. Oct4B: Oct4B protein expression in the 2nd TUR-BT specimens stained with EPR2054 antibody, but not with sc-5279 antibody; Oct4A: Oct4A protein expression in the 2nd TUR-BT specimens stained with sc-5279 antibody; CD90, CD73: CD90 and CD73 protein expressions in the 2nd TUR-BT specimens, CD45: CD45 protein expression except in infiltrating lymphocytes in the 2nd TUR-BT specimens, Cx: cystectomy; BCG: intravesical BCG (Bacille de Calmette et Guérin) instillation, CIS: carcinoma in situ.

Discussion

In the present study, Oct4-positive cells were observed in electro-stimulated bladder tissue. However, it is important to identify which isoform of Oct4 is expressed and to take the function of expressed Oct4 into consideration. There are three splice variants of Oct4: Oct4A, Oct4B, and Oct4B1, caused by alternative splicing of Pou5f1 mRNA. Oct4B mRNA produces three isoforms: Oct4B-164, Oct4B-190, and Oct4B-265, by alternative translation[7]. Only Oct4A has been shown to be a definite marker of pluripotency and self-renewal of cells.

In applying immunohistochemistry to specimens, an antibody against exon 1a of the Oct4 gene uniquely stains Oct4A protein, but not Oct4B and Oct4B1 isoforms because Oct4B and Oct4B1 mRNAs are missing exon 1a[8]. Additionally, Oct4A is generally located in the nucleus, while Oct4B and Oct4B1 are in the cytoplasm[9-11]. In our study, Oct4 protein expression was detected in the cytoplasm with EPR3132 antibody against exons 4-5, but not with that against exon 1a (sc-5279). This indicates that Oct4B-positive cells appeared in the tissue following electro-resection of the bladder. EPR3112 will not detect Oct4B1, as the Oct4B1 protein is truncated due to the stop codon TGA located in exon 2b harbored as a cryptic exon[12].

The functions of Oct4B and Oct4B1 are basically unknown. Oct4B has been reported to be expressed in the cytoplasm of various tumor cells[13-15]. It increases with tumor proliferation and angiogenesis, and

protects tumors from apoptosis[16-18]. Oct4B1 was originally regarded as a putative marker of stemness[12, 19] and is expressed in human colorectal cancer[20]. Additionally, two isoforms of OCT4B, OCT4B-190 and OCT4B-265, as well as Oct4B1 have been reported to be upregulated in response to various kinds of stress[7, 11, 21]. Electro-resection of bladder tissue and the subsequent reactions in the present study may have caused the stress-triggered appearance/infiltration of Oct4B protein-expressing cells.

CD90 and CD73, markers of MSCs, were enhanced in the tissue resected by the second TUR-Bt, while CD45 expression was limited to infiltrating lymphocytes. Then, electric stimulation administered to the bladder tissue in the primary TUR-Bt may have induced the recruitment and activation of MSCs that participate in the repair of bladder tissues. CD90 has been reported to be overexpressed in activated tumor endothelial cells compared with normal endothelial cells[22, 23]. Vascular endothelial cells in the regenerating tissue may be similar to tumor endothelial cells.

Conclusion

Electro-resection of bladder tissue induced the appearance of Oct4B protein-expressing interstitial cells as well as enhanced CD90 and CD73 expression in the vascular endothelial and interstitial cells. Not pluripotent stem cells, but the more downstream MSCs may be mainly involved in tissue repair of the bladder.

References

1. De Los Angeles A, Ferrari F, Fujiwara Y, Mathieu R, Lee S, Lee S, Tu HC, Ross S, Chou S, Nguyen M, Wu Z, Theunissen TW, Powell BE, Imsoonthornruksa S, Chen J, Borkent M, Krupalnik V, Lujan E, Wernig M, Hanna JH, Hochedlinger K, Pei D, Jaenisch R, Deng H, Orkin SH, Park PJ, Daley GQ. Failure to replicate the STAP cell phenomenon. Nature. 2015; 525(7570): E6-9.

2. Radzisheuskaya A, Silva JC. Do all roads lead to Oct4? The emerging concepts of induced pluripotency. Trends Cell Biol. 2014; 24(5): 275-284.

3. Takahashi K, Yamanaka S. Induction of pluripotent stem cells from mouse embryonic and adult fibroblast cultures by defined factors. Cell. 2006; 126(4): 663-676.

4. Augello A, Kurth TB, De Bari C. Mesenchymal stem cells: a perspective from in vitro cultures to in vivo migration and niches. Eur Cell Mater. 2010; 20: 121-133.

5. Barda-Saad M, Rozenszajn LA, Ashush H, Shav-Tal Y, Ben Nun A, Zipori D. Adhesion molecules involved in the interactions between early T cells and mesenchymal bone marrow stromal cells. Exp Hematol. 1999; 27(5): 834-844.

6. Barry F, Boynton R, Murphy M, Haynesworth S, Zaia J. The SH-3 and SH-4 antibodies recognize distinct epitopes on CD73 from human mesenchymal stem cells. Biochem Biophys Res Commun. 2001; 289(2): 519-524.

7. Gao Y, Wei J, Han J, Wang X, Su G, Zhao Y, Chen B, Xiao Z, Cao J, Dai J. The novel function of OCT4B isoform-265 in genotoxic stress. Stem Cells. 2012; 30(4): 665-672.

8. Liedtke S, Stephan M, Kögler G. Oct4 expression revisited: potential pitfalls for data misinterpretation in stem cell research. Biol Chem. 2008; 389(7): 845-850.

9. Cauffman G, Van de Velde H, Liebaers I, Van Steirteghem A. Oct-4 mRNA and protein expression during human preimplantation development. Mol Hum Reprod. 2005; 11(3): 173-181.

10. Lee J, Kim HK, Rho JY, Han YM, Kim J. The human OCT-4 isoforms differ in their ability to confer self renewal. J Biol Chem. 2006; 281(44): 33554-33565.

11. Farashahi-Yazd E, Rafiee MR, Soleimani M, Tavallaei M, Salmani MK, Mowla SJ. OCT4B1, a novel spliced variant of OCT4, generates a stable truncated protein with a potential role in stress response. Cancer Lett. 2011; 309(2): 170-175.

12. Gao Y, Wang X, Han J, Xiao Z, Chen B, Su G, Dai J. The novel OCT4 spliced variant OCT4B1 can generate three protein isoforms by alternative splicing into OCT4B. J Genet Genomics. 2010; 37(7): 461-465.

13. Alexander RE, Cheng L, Grignon DJ, Idrees MT. Cytoplasmic OCT4 staining is a sensitive marker of neuroendocrine differentiation. Hum Pathol. 2014; 45(1): 27-32.

14. Di J, Duiveman-de Boer T, Zusterzeel PL, Figdor CG, Massuger LF, Torensma R. The stem cell markers Oct4A, Nanog and c-Myc are expressed in ascites cells and tumor tissue of ovarian cancer patients. Cell Oncol. (Dordr). 2013; 36(5): 363-374.

15. Alexander RE, Cheng L, Grignon DJ, Idrees M. Cytoplasmic staining of OCT4 is a highly sensitive marker of adrenal medullary-derived tissue. Am. J Surg Pathol. 2-13; 37(5): 727-733.

16. Cortes-Dericks L, Yazd EF, Mowla SJ, Schmid RA, Karoubi G. Suppression of OCT4B enhances sensitivity of lung adenocarcinoma A549 cells to cisplatin via increased apoptosis. Anticancer Res. 2013; 33(12): 5365-5373.

17. Li SW, Wu XL, Dong CL, Xie XY, Wu JF, Zhang X. The differential expression of OCT4 isoforms in cervical carcinoma. PLoS One. 2015; 10(3): e0118033.

18. Asadi MH, Mowla SJ, Fathi F, Aleyasin A, Asadzadeh J, Atlasi Y. OCT4B1, a novel spliced variant of OCT4, is highly expressed in gastric cancer and acts as an antiapoptotic factor. Int J Cancer. 2011; 128(11): 2645-2652.

19. Papamichos SI, Kotoula V, Tarlatzis BC, Agorastos T, Papazisis K, Lambropoulos AF. OCT4B1 isoform: the novel OCT4 alternative spliced variant as a putative marker of stemness. Mol Hum Reprod. 2009; 15(5): 269-270.

20. Gazouli M, Roubelakis MG, Theodoropoulos GE, Papailiou J, Vaiopoulou A, Pappa KI, Nikiteas N, Anagnou NP. OCT4 spliced variant OCT4B1 is expressed in human colorectal cancer. Mol Carcinog. 2012; 51(2): 165-173.

21. Wang X, Zhao Y, Xiao Z, Chen B, Wei Z, Wang B, Zhang J, Han J, Gao Y, Li L, Zhao H, Zhao W, Lin H, Dai J. Alternative translation of OCT4 by an internal ribosome entry site and its novel function in stress response. Stem Cells. 2009; 27(6): 1265-1275.

22. Ohmura-Kakutani H, Akiyama K, Maishi N, Ohga N, Hida Y, Kawamoto T, Iida J, Shindoh M, Tsuchiya K, Shinohara N, Hida K. Identification of tumor endothelial cells with high aldehyde dehydrogenase activity and a highly angiogenic phenotype. PLoS One. 2014; 9(12): e113910.

23. Schubert K, Gutknecht D, Köberle M, Anderegg U, Saalbach A. Melanoma cells use Thy-1 (CD90) on endothelial cells for metastasis formation. Am J Pathol. 2013; 182(1): 266-76.

Abbreviations

STAP   : Stimulus-triggered Acquisition of Pluripotency
MSC   : Mesenchymal Stromal Cells
TUR-Bt : Transurethral electro-resection of intravesical tumors
BCG   : Bacille de Calmette et Guérin

Potential Conflicts of Interests

None

Ethical standards

The experiment was conducted with the human subjects' understanding and consent. The Ethical Committee of Kanto Rosai Hospital approved the experiments.

Acknowledgements

This study was supported by a grant-in-aid for scientific research proposed by Kanto Rosai Hospital.

Corresponding Author

Takumi Takeuchi, Department of Urology, Kanto Rosai Hospital, 1-1 Kizukisumiyoshi-cho, Nakahara-ku, Kawasaki, Japan. 211-8510; E-mail address: takeuchit@abelia.ocn.ne.jp

12

StemRegenin 1 selectively promotes expansion of Multipotent Hematopoietic Progenitors derived from Human Embryonic Stem Cells

Tao L[1], Togarrati PP[2], Choi KD[3], Suknuntha K[4]

Abstract

Human embryonic stem cell (hESC)-derived hematopoietic stem/progenitor cells hold tremendous potential as alternative cell sources for the treatment of various hematological diseases, drug discovery and toxicological screening. However, limited number of hematopoietic stem/progenitor cells generated from the differentiation of hESCs hinders their downstream applications. Here, we show that aryl hydrocarbon receptor antagonist StemRegenin 1 (SR1) selectively promotes expansion of hESC-derived lin⁻CD34⁺ hematopoietic progenitors in a concentration-dependent manner. The colony-forming cell (CFC) activity was found to be enriched in the CD34⁺ cells that were expanded with SR1; however, these cells have less colony-forming activity as compared to unexpanded cells (1,338 vs. 7 of CD34⁺ cells to form 1 colony, respectively). Interestingly, SR1 showed a bipotential effect on the proliferation of CD34 negative population, that is low dose of SR1 (1 μM) enhanced cell proliferation, whereas it was repressed at higher doses (>5 μM). In summary, our results suggest that SR1 has the potential to facilitate expansion of hESC-derived lin⁻CD34⁺ hematopoietic progenitors, which further retain the potential to form multilineage hematopoietic colonies.

Key Words: SR1, Hematopoietic progenitor, Human embryonic stem cell, CD43

Introduction

A member of the family of basic helix-loop-helix transcription factors, aryl hydrocarbon receptor (AHR) is well known for regulating the function of xenobiotic-metabolizing enzymes, and the toxicity and carcinogenic properties of several compounds[1]. AHR has also been proven to play an important role in the regulation of pluripotency and stemness of hematopoietic stem cells (HSCs). Inhibition of AHR by StemRegenin 1 (SR1) has been shown to lead to a 50-fold increase in cells expressing CD34 and a 17-fold increase in cells that retain the ability to engraft immunodeficient mice[2].

Conventional sources such as umbilical cord blood, bone marrow, and peripheral blood contain very limited number of HSCs. Additionally, cumbersome tissue extraction procedures, risk of blood-borne pathogen contamination and MHC mismatch issues are the major problems associated with the shortage of available HSCs required to meet the therapeutic demand at the blood banks and clinics. Alternatively, human embryonic stem cells (hESCs) have the potential to form massive numbers of HSCs when cultured under hematopoietic differentiation inducing conditions.

Hematopoietic development from hESCs using mouse bone marrow stromal cell line, OP9, as feeder starts with the formation of primitive hematovascular mesodermal precursors (HVMPs), defined phenotypically as KDR^bright APLNR⁺PDGFRα^low/-. A transient population of VE - cadherin⁺CD73⁻CD235a/CD43⁻

hemogenic endothelial progenitors (HEPs) gradually emerge from HVMP (day 4) which subsequently undergoes endothelial-to-hematopoietic transition[3]. A more committed CD43⁺CD235a/41a⁻ multipotent hematopoietic progenitors (MPs) with hematopoietic colony-forming ability can be obtained from hESC/OP9 cocultures after 8 days of differentiation[4]. Although MPs can be expanded for additional 8 days in culture when supplemented with hematopoietic cytokines, they gradually lose CD34 expression and colony forming ability[5].

Multipotent hematopoietic progenitors are developmental intermediate between hematopoietic stem cells (HSCs) and mature hematopoietic cells of all lineages (i.e., erythro-megakaryocytic, myeloid, and lymphoid). They have immunophenotypic profile similar to HSCs such as CD34 expression and lacking of lineage markers (CD11b, CD14, CD2, CD3, CD7, CD19, CD38, CD41a, CD45RA, HLA-DR, and CD235a)[4]. Currently, therapeutic potential of blood cell products obtained from hESC-derived HSCs/MPs have been intensely investigated. Specifically, hESC-derived natural killer (NK) cells demonstrated cellular cytotoxic activity and effectively eradicated human tumor cells *in vivo*[6]. The Food and Drug Administration (USFDA) recently approved a chimeric antigen receptor (CAR) T lymphocytes for the treatment of acute lymphoblastic leukemia and a model of CAR T lymphocyte generated from induced pluripotent stem cells for cancer therapy has been reported[7]. Hence, *in vitro* expansion of hESC-derived MPs to achieve sufficient number of cells for cancer immunotherapy and other medical applications is a prerequisite.

Author Names in full: Tao Lihong[1],Togarrati Padma Priya[2],Choi Kyung-Dal[3],Suknuntha Kran[4]

[1]Wisconsin National Primate Research Center, University of Wisconsin, Madison, WI, USA [2]Cell Therapy Core, Blood Systems Research Institute, San Francisco, CA, U.S.A,
[3]Lillehei Heart Institute, Department of Medicine, University of Minnesota, Minneapolis, MN, USA, [4]Department of Pharmacology, Faculty of Science, Mahidol University, Bangkok, Thailand

Aim of the present study was to evaluate effects of SR1 in the expansion of MPs derived from hESC/OP9 co-culture. Our data would highlight an effective strategy for the *in-vitro* expansion of hematopoietic progenitors derived from hESCs that would provide an unlimited source of cells for devising cellular therapies for various hematological disorders and malignancies.

Materials and Methods

Maintenance of WA01 and their differentiation into hematopoietic lineage on OP9 feeders

The human embryonic stem cell (hESC) line WA01 was obtained from WiCell and maintained in an undifferentiated state on irradiated mouse embryonic fibroblasts (MEFs). OP9 stromal cells were procured from ATCC and were maintained on gelatin-coated 10 cm dishes (BD Biosciences) in the OP9 growth medium consisting of 20% FBS (Gibco) in α-MEM medium (Invitrogen). Hematopoietic differentiation of WA01 cells on OP9 feeders was performed as previously described[4,8] in differentiation medium containing α-MEM basal medium supplemented with 10% FBS (HyClone), 100 μM monothioglycerol (MTG; Sigma Aldrich) and ascorbic acid (50 μg/ml) (Sigma Aldrich). MPs were derived on day 8 of WA01/OP9 co-culture.

Isolation of WA01-derived lin⁻CD43⁺CD235a/41a⁻ MPs

Cells were obtained by digesting the differentiated WA01/OP9 co-cultures with collagenase IV (1 mg/ml) (Invitrogen) followed by treatment with 0.05% trypsin-EDTA (Invitrogen) for 15 minutes at 37°C. Single cells were obtained by passing the digested cells through a 100-μM cell strainer (BD Biosciences) and counted. Cells were labeled with CD43 monoclonal antibody (clone 1G10) for CD43⁺ hematopoietic cell enrichment using magnetic-activated cell separation columns according to manufacturer's intruction (Miltenyi Biotec). Subsequently, CD43-enriched cells were stained with CD34, CD235a, and CD41a monoclonal antibodies, and lin⁻CD34⁺CD43⁺CD235a/CD41a⁻ MP cells were isolated by fluorescence-activated cell sorting (FACSAria, BD Biosciences). All monoclonal antibodies were from BD Biosciences.

Flow cytometric analysis of expanded MPs

Expanded MPs were stained with CD34 and CD43 monoclonal antibodies for flow cytometric analysis. Isotype-matched controls were used to set threshold for background. Data was acquired on a FACS Canto flow cytometer (BD Biosciences). 7-aminoactinomycin D (7AAD) was used to discriminate live cells from dead cells, and the stained live single cells were analyzed on FlowJo (Tree Star, Inc.).

Hematopoietic colony-forming unit (CFU) assay

Single cells were plated at a density of 200 cells/35-mm dish in MethoCult GF H4435 (StemCell Technologies). Colonies were scored after 14 days according to their morphology as granulocyte (G), macrophage (M), granulocyte/macrophage (GM), and multilineage colonies containing erythroid and non-erythroid cells (GEMM) as previously described[4,9].

Cell proliferation assay

lin⁻CD34⁺CD43⁺CD235a/CD41a⁻ MPs were plated in duplicate in 96-well plates containing 4x10³ cells/well. Cells were cultured in serum-free medium containing 10%BIT (StemCell Technologies), 100 μM 2-mercaptoethanol, and ExCyte (Millipore) in IMDM supplemented with 10 ng/ml IL3, and 50 ng/ml IL6 and SCF. SR1 was added to the

cultures at concentrations ranging from 1, 5 and 10 μM (Cayman Chemical). Viable cell count was determined using trypan blue (Gibco).

RNA-Seq analysis

To visualize the comparative gene expression levels of genes expressed in WA01, HVMPs, HEs, and MPs, a heat map was constructed using MultiExperiment Viewer v4.2 (http://www.tm4.org). RNA-seq data was obtained from NCBI GEO DataSets (acession number: GSE39661). The gene expression levels were estimated in transcripts per million (tpm) as described earlier[3]. TPM for MP was averaged from D8 CD43⁺CD235a⁻ and D8 CD43⁺CD235a⁺ subset.

Statistical analysis

Data obtained from three experiments were reported as mean ± SEM. Significance of the data was determined by ANOVA followed by Bonferroni *post hoc* test. Pearson correlation between CD34 expression and colony-forming cell (CFC) was determined. p value < 0.05 was considered statistically significant. All the graphs and statistics were done on Prism software (GraphPad).

Results

Expression profile of aryl hydrocarbon receptor and its associated genes are upregulated in hematopoietic progenitors derived from differentiated pluripotent stem cells

In this study, we have examined the gene expression profile of WA01 and its differentiated hematopoietic derivatives such as HVMPs, Hemogenic endothelia (HEs), and MPs, which was previously generated by our group[3]. It was revealed that several AHR-associated genes (Figure 1A) namely *CYP1A1*, *CYP1A2*, *CYP1B1*, *AHRR*, *ARNT*, *AHR*, *EP300*, *TIPARP*, and *AIP* were upregulated as cells acquired CD43 expression, suggesting that AHR signaling is activated in committed hematopoietic cells (Figure 1B). This information prompted us to further evaluate whether inhibition of AHR activity will lead to the sustained maintenance of naive multipotent phenotype and functionality of MPs.

SR1 promotes expansion of MPs without deteriorating cell viability

To generate MPs, OP9 stromal cells were used to induce hematopoietic differentiation in WA01. The experimental outline for the generation of MPs and examination of their colony-forming activities are shown in Figure 1C. On day 8 of WA01/OP9 co-culture, MPs are found to be enriched within CD43⁺glycophorin A⁻ (CD235a) CD41a⁻ population[5]. Approximately 2-5x10⁴ of MPs can be obtained from a single 10 cm dish containing hESC/OP9 co-cultures. Effects of SR1 at concentrations >1 μM (high dose) has been shown anti-proliferative in cynomolgus, rhesus, and dog[2], however, such effects of SR1 on human CD34⁺ cells remains poorly understood. Hereby, we have evaluated the effects of high doses SR1 on MPs grown under serum free conditions through viable cell count analysis, flow cytometry and CFU assays. We limited our experiments to a short 7-day assay because WA01-derived MPs slowly lose CD34 expressions and almost completely disappear within the first week[5]. Our data showed that after 7 days of expansion cultures, SR1 at 1 μM slightly increased total cell expansion of MPs (p>0.5), whereas at 10 μM doses it markedly inhibited expansion (Figure 1D). Interestingly, flow cytometric analyses using live/dead staining marker (7AAD) showed that a reduction in expansion resulted from anti-proliferative effects of SR1 at high dose, not the cell death (Figure 1E).

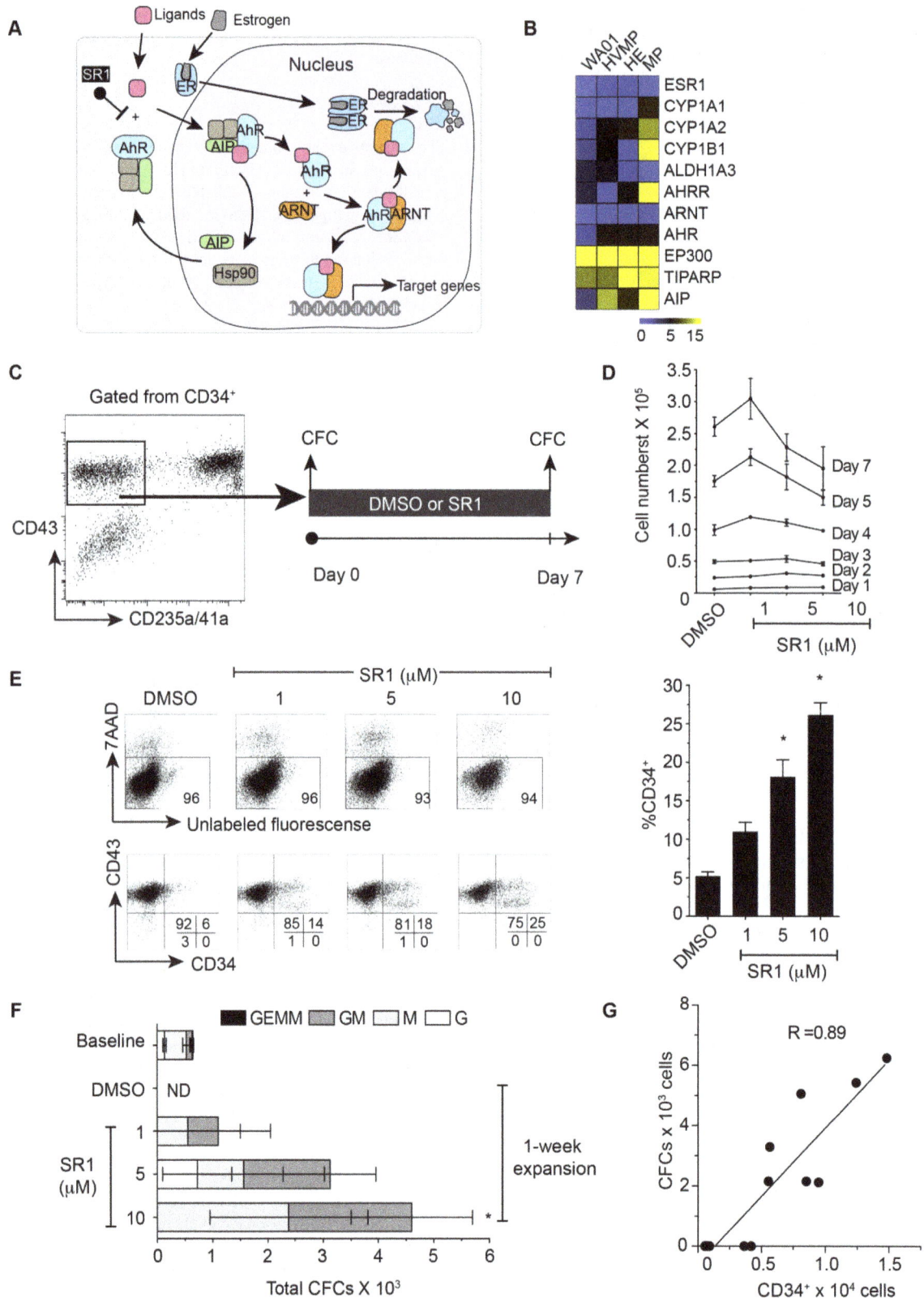

Figure 1. *Aryl hydrocarbon signaling and its effects on multipotent hematopoietic progenitor cells. (A) Schematic diagram showing current mechanisms of AHR regulation. (B) Heat map showing the expression of genes associated with AHR signaling and estrogen receptor in WA01, HVMP, HE, and MP. (C) Schematic diagram showing the experimental outline. FACS-sorted live CD235a/41a⁻CD34⁺CD43⁺ cells from day 8 WA01/OP9 coculture shown in the gate were cultured in the presence or absence of SR1 for 7 days. The sorted cells (day 0) and expanded cells (day 7) were plated in methylcellulose for the colony-forming cell (CFC) assay. (D) Cross-sectional presentation of total viable cell numbers on a day-to-day basis. * indicates significant difference compared with DMSO. (E) Representative flow cytometric dot plots showing the effect of SR1 on cell viability after 7-day expansion using 7AAD (upper panel) and CD43 vs CD34 expression on the expanded cells (lower panel). Right bar graph summarizes a percentage of CD34 expression shown in the dot plots. (F) Absolute number of colony-forming cells in WA01-derived MPs (baseline, day 0), expanded cells with DMSO only, and expanded cells with 1, 5 and 10 μM SR1 (G) Correlation between colony-forming cells and CD34 expression. Error bars represent SEM from 3 experiments. * indicates p < 0.05 compared to DMSO. HVMP = hematovascular mesodermal precursor, HE = hemogenic endothelium, MP = multipotent hematopoietic progenitor, ER = estrogen receptor, AHR = aryl hydrocarbon receptor, AIP = AHR interacting protein, ARNT = AHR nuclear translocator, Hsp90 = heat shock protein 90, SR1 = StemRegenin 1, ND = not detectable*

SR1 enhances CD34 expression and its hematopoietic progenitor activity in a dose-dependent manner

At the late stage of MP maturation, mature cells retain CD43, but lose CFU activity[5]. Therefore, we examined the expression of another hematopoietic progenitor cell marker CD34 and its colony-forming activity through culturing MPs for 7-days in the absence or presence of SR1 (Figure 1E). We found that SR1 maintained CD34 expression on MPs in a dose-dependent fashion, but had no effect on the CD43 expression (Figure 1E). To evaluate the colony-forming ability of CD34$^+$ at different stages of culture, 200 cells of sorted CD34$^+$ (unexpanded) were plated in methylcellulose medium containing hematopoietic cytokines as a baseline control (baseline). After 7-day expansion, 200 cells from each condition (DMSO, 1, 5, 10 µM of SR1) were plated in the same medium as baseline control. We could not detect any hematopoietic colonies from the expanded cultures grown without SR1 (Figure 1F). We noticed that colonies obtained from MPs after expansion were slightly smaller than those colonies obtained from unexpanded MPs indicating a gradual decrease in their proliferative potential. We hypothesized that CFCs might be enriched within the expansion cultures of CD34$^+$ population. Thus, we performed correlation analysis on CD34 and CD43 vs. CFCs. We found a strong positive correlation between CD34 vs. CFCs (R=0.89, p=0.0001) (Figure 1G), but not CD43. Estimated frequency of colony forming cell in CD34$^+$ population from expanded cultures was 1,338 cells to form 1 colony.

Discussion

The abilities of HSCs to self-renew and differentiate into mature cells highlight their potential as a valuable source for cell replacement therapy for various hematological diseases and high-throughput platform for drug discovery and toxicological screening. Limited availability of HSCs in the conventional donor cell sources, and the difficulty of *ex vivo* expansion of HSCs that retain all their functional attributes, pose as the major hurdles in the clinical applications of HSCs in treating various blood disorders and malignancies. With the discovery of hESC[10], cells with HSC-like phenotype can be generated unlimitedly in a dish[11]. hESC-derived cells as an attractive complementary cell source for therapeutic interventions, disease modeling and drug-screening. Although several groups describe efficient methods to generate *de novo* HSC-like cells from hESCs (reviewed earlier[12]), yield of cells remains one of the major hindrances in its downstream applications. Ectopic expression of *HOXB4* and *BMI1* transcription factors has been demonstrated to promote *ex vivo* expansion of HSCs[13,14]; however, use of virus-mediated gene transfer is the major drawback in the clinical translation of these findings. Therefore, optimization of *in vitro* expansion conditions to generate sufficient quantities of hESC-derived HSC-like cells is the need of the hour.

SR1 has been widely used in several protocols to promote HSC and hematopoietic cell expansión[2,15,16] and is currently under phase I/II clinical trial in patients with hematologic malignancies[17]. We found that several AHR target genes are upregulated when cells commit to hematopoietic lineage (lin$^-$CD34$^+$CD43$^+$). We demonstrated that SR1 favored expansion of progenitor cells regardless of the concentration used, but its effect on mature cells was found to be bipotential. Consistent to the report by Boitano, *et al*[2], SR1 at low dose (1 µM) facilitated mature cell proliferation, whereas high doses (>1 µM) suppressed total cell numbers. Flow cytometric analyses using 7AAD showed that SR1 did not cause cell death when used at high doses confirming the anti-proliferative effect is most likely. Although the effect of SR1 is mediated through direct binding and inhibition of the AHR[2], the precise mechanism of its bipotential effect on mature cells remains undescribed.

It is possible that SR1 at high dose has off target effects that initiate secondary signaling pathway. Functional study on the expanded cells showed that the effect on hematopoietic progenitor activity is concentration-dependent suggesting the benefit of high concentration of SR1 on MP expansion. Additionally, a strong positive correlation between CD34 *vs.* CFCs (R=0.89, *p*=0.0001) suggested an advantage of CD34 over CD43 as a marker for colony forming activity in the expanded cells. Notably, the numbers of colony-forming cells within the expanded CD34$^+$ population is much lower than unexpanded cells indicating that even though SR1 favors expansion of CD34$^+$ progenitor cells, some cells might undergo further differentiation.

Conclusion

In conclusion, our data demonstrates that high doses SR1 (>1 µM) selectively expand MP derived from WA01 (5-fold increase when used at 10 µM) without having deteriorating effects on cell viability. Mechanistic study of the bipotential effect of SR1 on MPs would provide insight to devise a novel approach for expansion of embryonic stem cell-derived blood products.

References

1. Mulero-Navarro S, Fernandez-Salguero PM. New Trends in Aryl Hydrocarbon Receptor Biology. Front Cell Dev Biol. 2016;4:45.
2. Boitano AE, Wang J, Romeo R, Bouchez LC, Parker AE, Sutton SE, Walker JR, Flaveny CA, Perdew GH, Denison MS, Schultz PG, Cooke MP. Aryl hydrocarbon receptor antagonists promote the expansion of human hematopoietic stem cells. Science. 2010;329(5997):1345-8.
3. Choi KD, Vodyanik MA, Togarrati PP, Suknuntha K, Kumar A, Samarjeet F, Probasco MD, Tian S, Stewart R, Thomson JA, Slukvin, II. Identification of the hemogenic endothelial progenitor and its direct precursor in human pluripotent stem cell differentiation cultures. Cell Rep. 2012;2(3):553-67.
4. Vodyanik MA, Thomson JA, Slukvin, II. Leukosialin (CD43) defines hematopoietic progenitors in human embryonic stem cell differentiation cultures. Blood. 2006;108(6):2095-105.
5. Choi KD, Vodyanik MA, Slukvin, II. Generation of mature human myelomonocytic cells through expansion and differentiation of pluripotent stem cell-derived lin-CD34+CD43+CD45+ progenitors. J Clin Invest. 2009;119(9):2818-29.
6. Woll PS, Grzywacz B, Tian X, Marcus RK, Knorr DA, Verneris MR, Kaufman DS. Human embryonic stem cells differentiate into a homogeneous population of natural killer cells with potent in vivo antitumor activity. Blood. 2009;113(24):6094-101.
7. Themeli M, Kloss CC, Ciriello G, Fedorov VD, Perna F, Gonen M, Sadelain M. Generation of tumor-targeted human T lymphocytes from induced pluripotent stem cells for cancer therapy. Nat Biotechnol. 2013;31(10):928-33.
8. Vodyanik MA, Slukvin, II. Hematoendothelial differentiation of human embryonic stem cells. Curr Protoc Cell Biol. 2007;Chapter 23:Unit 23.6.
9. Choi KD, Yu J, Smuga-Otto K, Salvagiotto G, Rehrauer W, Vodyanik M, Thomson J, Slukvin I. Hematopoietic and endothelial differentiation of human induced pluripotent stem cells. Stem Cells. 2009;27(3):559-67.
10. Thomson JA, Itskovitz-Eldor J, Shapiro SS, Waknitz MA, Swiergiel JJ, Marshall VS, Jones JM. Embryonic stem cell lines derived from human blastocysts. Science. 1998;282(5391):1145-7.
11. Vodyanik MA, Bork JA, Thomson JA, Slukvin, II. Human embryonic stem cell-derived CD34+ cells: efficient production in the coculture with OP9 stromal cells and analysis of lymphohematopoietic potential. Blood. 2005;105(2):617-26.
12. Togarrati PP, Suknuntha K. Generation of mature hematopoietic cells from human pluripotent stem cells. Int J Hematol. 2012;95(6):617-23.
13. Faubert A, Chagraoui J, Mayotte N, Frechette M, Iscove NN, Humphries RK, Sauvageau G. Complementary and independent function for Hoxb4 and Bmi1 in HSC activity. Cold Spring Harb Symp Quant Biol. 2008;73:555-64.

14. Antonchuk J, Sauvageau G, Humphries RK. HOXB4-induced expansion of adult hematopoietic stem cells ex vivo. Cell. 2002;109(1):39-45.

15. Gori JL, Chandrasekaran D, Kowalski JP, Adair JE, Beard BC, D'Souza SL, Kiem HP. Efficient generation, purification, and expansion of CD34(+) hematopoietic progenitor cells from nonhuman primate-induced pluripotent stem cells. Blood. 2012;120(13):e35-44.

16. Thordardottir S, Hangalapura BN, Hutten T, Cossu M, Spanholtz hydrocarbon receptor antagonist StemRegenin 1 promotes human plasmacytoid and myeloid dendritic cell development from CD34+ hematopoietic progenitor cells. Stem Cells Dev. 2014;23(9):955-67.

17. Wagner JE, Jr., Brunstein CG, Boitano AE, DeFor TE, McKenna D, Sumstad D, Blazar BR, Tolar J, Le C, Jones J, Cooke MP, Bleul CC. Phase I/II Trial of StemRegenin-1 Expanded Umbilical Cord Blood Hematopoietic Stem Cells Supports Testing as a Stand-Alone Graft. Cell Stem Cell. 2016;18(1):144-55.

Abbreviations

AHR:	Aryl hydrocarbon receptor
hESC:	human embryonic stem cell
SR1:	StemRegenin 1
CFC:	Colony-forming cell
HE:	Hemogenic endothelium
HEP:	Hemogenic endothelial progenitor
HVMP:	Hematovascular mesodermal precursor
MP:	Multipotent hematopoietic progenitors
FBS:	Fetal bovine serum
MTG:	Monothioglycerol
G:	Granulocyte
M:	Macrophage
GM:	Granulocyte/Macrophage
GEMM:	Granulocyte/Erythrocyte/Macrophage

Potential Conflicts of Interests

None

Funding

This work was supported by funds from the Department of Pharmacology, Faculty of Science, Mahidol University (A34/2557, grant to KS) and The Central Instrument Facility (CIF), Mahidol University (58/023, grant to KS)

Corresponding Authors

Suknuntha Kran, Department of Pharmacology, Faculty of Science, Mahidol University, 272 Rama VI rd, Ratchathewi, Bangkok, Thailand, 10400; E-mail: suknuntha@uwalumni.com

13

Mesenchymal stem cells-seeded bio-ceramic construct for bone regeneration in large critical-size bone defect in rabbit

Maiti SK[1], Ninu AR[2], Sangeetha P[2], Mathew DD[2], Tamilmahan P[2], Kritaniya D[3], Kumar N[1], Hescheler J[4]

Bone marrow derived mesenchymal stem cells (BMSC) represent an attractive cell population for tissue engineering purpose. The objective of this study was to determine whether the addition of recombinant human bone morphogenetic protein (rhBMP-2) and insulin-like growth factor (IGF-1) to a silica-coated calcium hydroxyapatite (HASi) - rabbit bone marrow derived mesenchymal stem cell (rBMSC) construct promoted bone healing in a large segmental bone defect beyond standard critical -size radial defects (15mm) in rabbits. An extensively large 30mm long radial ostectomy was performed unilaterally in thirty rabbits divided equally in five groups. Defects were filled with a HASi scaffold only (group B); HASi scaffold seeded with rBMSC (group C); HASi scaffold seeded with rBMSC along with rhBMP-2 and IGF-1 in groups D and E respectively. The same number of rBMSC (five million cells) and concentration of growth factors rhBMP-2 (50μg) and IGF-1 (50μg) was again injected at the site of bone defect after 15 days of surgery in their respective groups. An empty defect served as the control group (group A). Radiographically, bone healing was evaluated at 7, 15, 30, 45, 60 and 90 days post implantation. Histological qualitative analysis with microCT (μ-CT), haematoxylin and eosin (H & E) and Masson's trichrome staining were performed 90 days after implantation. All rhBMP-2-added constructs induced the formation of well-differentiated mineralized woven bone surrounding the HASi scaffolds and bridging bone/implant interfaces as early as eight weeks after surgery. Bone regeneration appeared to develop earlier with the rhBMP-2 constructs than with the IGF-1 added construct. Constructs without any rhBMP-2 or IGF-1 showed osteoconductive properties limited to the bone junctions without bone ingrowths within the implantation site. In conclusion, the addition of rhBMP-2 to a HASi scaffold could promote bone generation in a large critical-size-defect.

Key Words: Mesenchymal stem cells, Recombinant human bone morphogenetic protein, Insulin like growth factor, Silica-coated calcium

Introduction

Despite the benefits that minimally invasive surgery and osteosynthesis have brought to fracture management and bone healing, there are still many circumstances where bone healing remains challenging[1]. Large bone defects are serious complications that are most commonly caused by extensive trauma, tumour, infection, or congenital musculoskeletal disorders. In nonunion cases repairing of bone defects with composite biomaterials as defect filler can promote bone regeneration[2]. Currently, the gold standard for bone regeneration is the use of autogenous bone graft. In order to avoid morbidity at the donor site or if large amount of autogenous bone is needed, bone substitution materials can be used[3].

Bone substitution materials can be combined with cells such as mesenchymal stem cells (MSCs) to increase bone formation[4]. Bone-marrow-derived mesenchymal stem cells (BMSCs) represent an attractive cell population for tissue regeneration[5]. Bone marrow stem cells are pluripotent cells that have been used to facilitate bone repair because of their capability of differentiating into osteoblasts[6]. Several studies on the regeneration of bone have shown that cultured BMSCs, seeded on different bioabsorbable implants are able to induce bone formation *in vivo* and lead to improved healing of critical-size defects[4, 5].

Calcium phosphate bone substitutes such as hydroxyapatite (HA) and tricalcium phosphate (TCP) are currently used for bone substitution in many different clinical applications such as repair of bone defects after trauma or tumour and bone augmentation in spinal arthrodesis[7,8]. Although, these bone substitutes are osteoconductive, they often lack the osteogenecity needed to support bone healing in large defects and are slowly degraded in the body[1]. Studies had shown that coating of hydroxyapatite with a calcium silicate layer could encourage cell proliferation and osteogenic differentiation of human bone marrow-derived stromal cells[9]. Silica-calcium phosphate composite in comparison to calcium phosphate-rich biomaterials has a faster resorption rate owing to greater dissolution of Si ions[10].

The use of several growth factors have been studied in bone repair and these factors are known to play a role in differentiation of mesenchymal progenitor cells specific lineages like endothelial cells or osteoblasts[11,12]. Bone morphogenetic protein-2 (BMP-2) has been shown to accelerate bone healing in humans and animal models[13, 14]. BMP-2 acts by osteoinduction and is involved in the differentiation of mesenchymal progenitor cells into osteoblasts[1, 14]. The addition of recombinant human BMP (rhBMP-2) to a self-cross linkable cellulose hydrogels/biphasic calcium phosphate granules construct promotes bone regeneration in a critical-size segmental defect model of non-union in dogs[1]. It is also reported that protein, insulin-like growth factor (IGF-1) stimulates direct migration of human mesenchymal

Author Names in full: Swapan Kumar Maiti[1], Ajantha Ravindran Ninu[2], Palakkara Sangeetha[2], Dayamon D Mathew[2], Paramasivam Tamilmahan[2], Deepika Kritaniya[3], Naveen Kumar[1], Jurgen Hescheler[4]

[1]Principal Scientist, Surgery Division, Indian Veterinary Research Institute, Izatnagar, 243122, Uttar-Pradesh, India, [2]Ph.D Scholars, Surgery Division, Indian Veterinary Research Institute, Izatnagar, 243122, Uttar-Pradesh, India, [3]Senior Research Fellow, Surgery Division, Indian Veterinary Research Institute, Izatnagar, 243122, Uttar-Pradesh, India,[4]Director, Institute of Neurophysiology, Universität zu Köln, Robert-Koch-Strasse 39, D-50931, Köln, Germany

progenitor cells (MPC) and contributes to the recruitment of MPC in bone formation and bone healing[15].

Transplantation of human mesenchymal stem cells in a non-autogenous setting for bone regeneration in a rabbit critical-size defect (15mm) has been reported[5], but the regeneration potential of autogenous MSC with or without growth factors beyond standard critical-size defect was not reported. So, in the current study, we investigate the potential of cultured autogenic rabbit bone marrow-derived mesenchymal stem cells (rBMSC) seeded in a triphasic composite bio-scaffold (namely HASi) to generate new bone formation in an extensively large (30mm) segmental diaphyseal bone defect in rabbit model with or without growth factors rhBMP-2 and IGF-1.

Materials and Methods

Experimental design

The study was conducted on 30 female adult New Zealand White rabbits (2.86± 0.38 kg, 6-9 months old) divided into five equal groups (each n=6). They were kept in individual cages, fed a standard diet and allowed free mobilization during the study. The groups were compared as follows: The radial 30-mm segmental diaphyseal defect was filled with a HASi scaffold only (group B); HASi scaffold seeded with autogenous rBMSC (group C); HASi scaffold-seeded with autogenous rBMSC along with rhBMP-2 (group D) and HASi scaffold-seeded with autogenous rBMSC along with IGF-1 (group E). An empty defect served as the control group (group A).

The same number of rBMSC (five millions cells) and concentration of growth factors rhBMP-2 (50µg) and IGF-1 (50µg) were again injected around the bone defect on day 15 postsurgery in their respective groups.

Animals were treated in compliance with the guiding principles in the "Care and Use of Animals" policy of the authors' institutions. The institute Animal Ethical Committee for animal experiments has approved the design of the experiment.

Preoperatively, hematology was performed to ensure the absence of systemic diseases. The rabbits had no signs of bone or joint disease on the relevant limbs, as assessed by clinical examination and preoperative radiographs.

Bioceramic scaffold

A triphasic composite bio-scaffold (calcium silicate, hydroxyapatite and tricalcium phosphate) namely HASi with elements in the following percentage: calcium-66.36%, Phosphorus- 25.35%, Silicon-8.29% and porosity of 50 – 500 µm was used as ceramic bloc. Each HASi block was of 30 mm long and 5 mm in diameter were produced in an emulsion process as described earlier[16].

Isolation and culture of rBMSC

Isolation and culture of rBMSC was performed as described earlier[17]. The rBMSCs at passage-3 were used for this experiment.

Seeding of rBMSC into HASi ceramic blocks

The HASi bioscaffold were incubated at 4^0C in 50µM ml⁻1 fibronectin solution diluted in PBS for 24 h. Five million passage-3 rBMSC were resuspended in 4 ml of culture medium (DMEM) and transferred into a 5 ml tube. The HASi blocks were placed into the medium containing the cells. After 1.5 h of continuous spinning at 37^0C (35rpm), the ceramic blocks were placed into a 6-well plate.

The medium containing the cells was centrifuged twice at 800g for 5 min, and the resulting cell pellet was re-suspended in 70µl of culture medium and applied to the ceramic blocks. This MSC-seeded ceramic scaffold was used in group C. Tissue engineered bone construct for group D consisted of seeded HASi scaffold along with 50µg of rhBMP-2 suspended in 250 µl of DMEM, injected at the implant site, whereas, in group E, seeded HASi scaffold along with 50µg of IGF-1 suspended in 250 µl of DMEM injected at the implant site. In group B, only HASi block/scaffold was used at the implant site.

Surgical procedure

All the animals were acclimatized for two weeks to approaching and handling prior to surgery. Under general anesthesia with xylazine hydrochloride (5mg/kg, IM) and ketamine hydrochloride (50mg/kg, IM) and strict surgical asepsis, a unilaterally   critical-size bone defects were created in the radial diaphysis. A 4 cm super medial incision over the radius was given, soft tissue was dissected and the bone exposed by gentle retraction of the muscles. A Hohmann retractor was placed between ulna and radius to protect the ulna. A 30 mm segmental osteo-periosteal diaphyseal defect was created with an oscillating bone saw that was continuously cooled by irrigation with 0.9% sterile cold saline solution. The periosteum was removed with the bone and 5mm of periosteum was stripped from each side of the remaining radius. The bone gap was irrigated with sterile physiological saline solution and ceramic block (or nothing) fitted into the gap as per treatment protocol for different groups. Muscles, fascia and skin were separately closed over the defect with 4-0 resorpable sutures. A wooden splint with bandage was applied on the test bone for one week.

Postoperative care

Postoperatively, ceftriaxone sodium (22mg/kg, IM) administered intramuscularly for five days. Analgesic meloxicam (0.2 mg/kg, IM) was given for the first 3 postoperative days. There were no differences in quantity of meloxicam administered between the groups. Water and food were supplied ad libitum. After 90 days of experiment, the animals were sacrificed.

Radiological assessment

Craniocaudal and mediolateral radiographic view of each ostectomy site was assessed immediately after surgery to monitor the position of the implants, and at 7, 15, 30, 45, 60 and 90 days postoperatively to assess bone formation and bone union with the host bone at both proximal and distal junctions. The radiographs were graded with slight modification of the scoring system reported by Yang et al[18] (Table 1). For each category mean scores were calculated. These mean scores of each time interval were added separately for obtaining the total radiographic scores. Overall radiographic scores for each group were calculated by adding mean scores for each group at different intervals. Resorption of the implant was assessed qualitatively.

Microcomputed tomography assessment

Microcomputed tomography (µCT) technique was used for evaluation of three dimensional (3-D) trabecular new bone formation in different treatment groups. At day 90 after implantation, the constructs were explanted after euthanizing the animals, preserving both proximal and distal interfaces. Images were acquired under 70keV voltage with a constant 114 µA current. Spatial resolution was limited to 100-200 µm. A high- resolution protocol (slice thickness 120 µm, feed 60 µm, and pixel size 60 µm) was applied. An X-ray tomographic microscope, Micro-CT 40 was used in this study.

Table 1. Radiographic grading scale for analyzing the bone healing

Grading category	Score
Periosteal reaction	
None	0
Minimal (localized to the gaps)	1
Medium (extends over the gaps or towards ulna)	2
Moderate (1/4 to 1/2 of the defect area)	3
Full (1/2 to full length of defect)	4
Osteotomy line	
Both the osteotomy lines completely radiolucent	0
One of the osteotomy lines partially radiolucent	1
Both the osteotomy lines partially radiolucent	2
One of the osteotomy lines invisible	3
Both the osteotomy lines invisible	4
Construct appearance	
Unchanged/intact	0
Mild resorption (one localized area)	1
Moderate resorption (more than one localized area)	2
Mostly replaced	3
Fully replaced	4

Histopathological assessment

At day 90 post-implantation, the animals were sacrificed. The test bone sections throughout the length of the defect were collected from the site of surgical implant and washed thoroughly with sterile normal saline solution. Fixation was done in 10% formalin. The bone sections (longitudinal as well as transverse) were subjected to decalcification in Goodling and Stewart solution (15ml formic acid, 5ml formalin and 80ml distilled water). The decalcified bone sections were stained by H & E and Masson's trichrome stain. The sections were examined using a light microscope under different magnification. Bone healing was assessed in each group according to modified Lane and Sandhu[19] and Heiple et al[20]. Histopathological scoring system was presented in Table 2.

Both the radiographic and histological assessments were blindly performed.

Statistical analysis

All values were expressed as the mean plus or minus standard deviation (± SD). All the data were analyzed by analysis of variance (ANOVA) as per standard statistical methods, using SPSS software package (version 16). The various scores were compared with Kruskal-Wallis test. Significance was set for a p-value <0.05.

Results

Clinical assessment

The food and water intake was returned normal on day 3 in all experimental groups (B, C, D, E) whereas, it was on 6-8 days in control group. Weight bearing on the operated limb was mild to moderate from day 3 after surgery in all groups except group A. Complete weight bearing was seen after removal of wooden splint in all animals of groups B, C, D and E on day 7 after surgery. In the control group the animal did not bear weight normally throughout the experiment period. In three animals of group A, (empty control), a fracture of the treated leg was observed, so these three animals were sacrificed prior to the study endpoint. No animal of this group A was alive at day 90. The implanted biomaterials did not cause any apparent signs of irritation or infection and cutaneous wound healing was uneventful.

Radiographic assessment

The radiographic scoring was done based on mediolateral view as there was overlapping of the radius by ulna in craniocaudal view. Radiographic scores (mean ± SD) of construct appearance, osteotomy line, periosteal reaction, total and overall radiographic scores in all five groups at various time intervals are presented in Tables 3. Mediolateral views of radiograph of animals of five groups are presented in Figure 1. Overall radiographic scores of five groups are presented in Figure 2.

Table 2: Histopathological scoring system

Sl. No	Feature	Score
1.	**Osteogenesis**	
	No osteogenesis	0
	Weak osteogenesis	1
	Medium osteogenesis	2
	Good osteogenesis	3
	Perfect osteogenesis	4
2.	**Union**	
	No evidence of union	0
	Fibrous union	1
	Osteochondral union	2
	Bony union	3
	Complete organization of graft	4
3.	**Marrow**	
	None in the resected area	0
	Beginning to appear	1
	Present in greater than 1/2 defect	2
	Complete colonization by red marrow	3
	Mature fatty marrow	4
4.	**Cancellous bone/medullary bone**	
	No osseous cellular activity	0
	Early apposition of new bone	1
	Active apposition of new bone	2
	Reorganizing cancellous bone	3
	Complete re-organization of cancellous bone	4
5.	**Cortical/compact bone**	
	None	0
	Early appearance	1
	Formation underway	2
	Mostly re-organized	3
	Completely formed	4

Table 3. Radiographic scores (mean ±SD) of construct appearance, osteotomy line, periosteal reaction and total radiographic score at various time interval; overall radiographic scores (Mean ±SD), [a-e] Values in the same column with different superscript letter are significantly different (P<0.05)

Group and day (Interaction)	Construct appearance	Osteotomy line	Periosteal reaction	Total score
A×7	No construct	0.00±0.00	0.00±0.00	0.00±0.00[a]
B×7	0.00±0.00	0.00±0.00	0.00±0.00	0.00±0.00[a]
C×7	0.00±0.00	0.00±0.00	0.00±0.00	0.00±0.00[a]
D×7	0.00±0.00	0.00±0.00	0.00±0.00	0.00±0.00[a]
E×7	0.00±0.00	0.00±0.00	0.00±0.00	0.00±0.00[a]
A×15	No construct	0.00±0.00	0.00±0.00	0.00±0.00[a]
B×15	0.00±0.00	0.00±0.00	0.00±0.00	0.00±0.00[a]
C×15	0.00±0.00	0.50±0.55	0.33±0.52	0.83±0.02[c]
D×15	1.67±0.52	1.67±0.52	0.50±0.55	3.84±0.02[d]
E×15	0.00±0.00	0.67±0.52	0.17±0.41	0.84±0.02[c]
A×30	No construct	1.17±0.41	0.00±0.00	1.17±0.41[a]
B×30	0.65±0.55	0.85±0.52	0.00±0.00	1.50±0.02[a]
C×30	1.00±0.63	1.50±0.55	0.67±1.03	3.17±0.26[c]
D×30	2.50±0.55	3.17±1.33	1.50±0.55	7.17±0.45[d]
E×30	1.50±0.55	1.50±0.55	1.67±1.37	4.67±0.47[c]
A×60	No construct	1.67±0.52	0.00±0.00	1.67±0.52[a]
B×60	1.50±0.55	1.33±0.52	0.55±0.55	3.38±0.02[a]
C×60	1.67±0.52	2.67±0.52	2.33±0.82	6.67±0.17[c]
D×60	2.67±0.52	3.50±0.84	3.33±1.03	9.50±0.26[d]
E×60	2.67±0.52	3.00±0.89	2.00±1.26	7.67±0.17[e]
A×90	No construct	2.00±0.00	0.67±0.82	2.67±0.82[a]
B×90	1.83±0.41	2.33±0.52	1.67±0.52	5.83±0.06[b]
C×90	2.00±0.63	3.50±0.55	3.33±0.82	8.83±0.14[c]
D×90	3.50±0.84	3.83±0.41	3.33±0.03	10.66±0.23[d]
E×90	2.83±0.00	3.17±0.75	3.83±0.41	9.83±0.03[e]

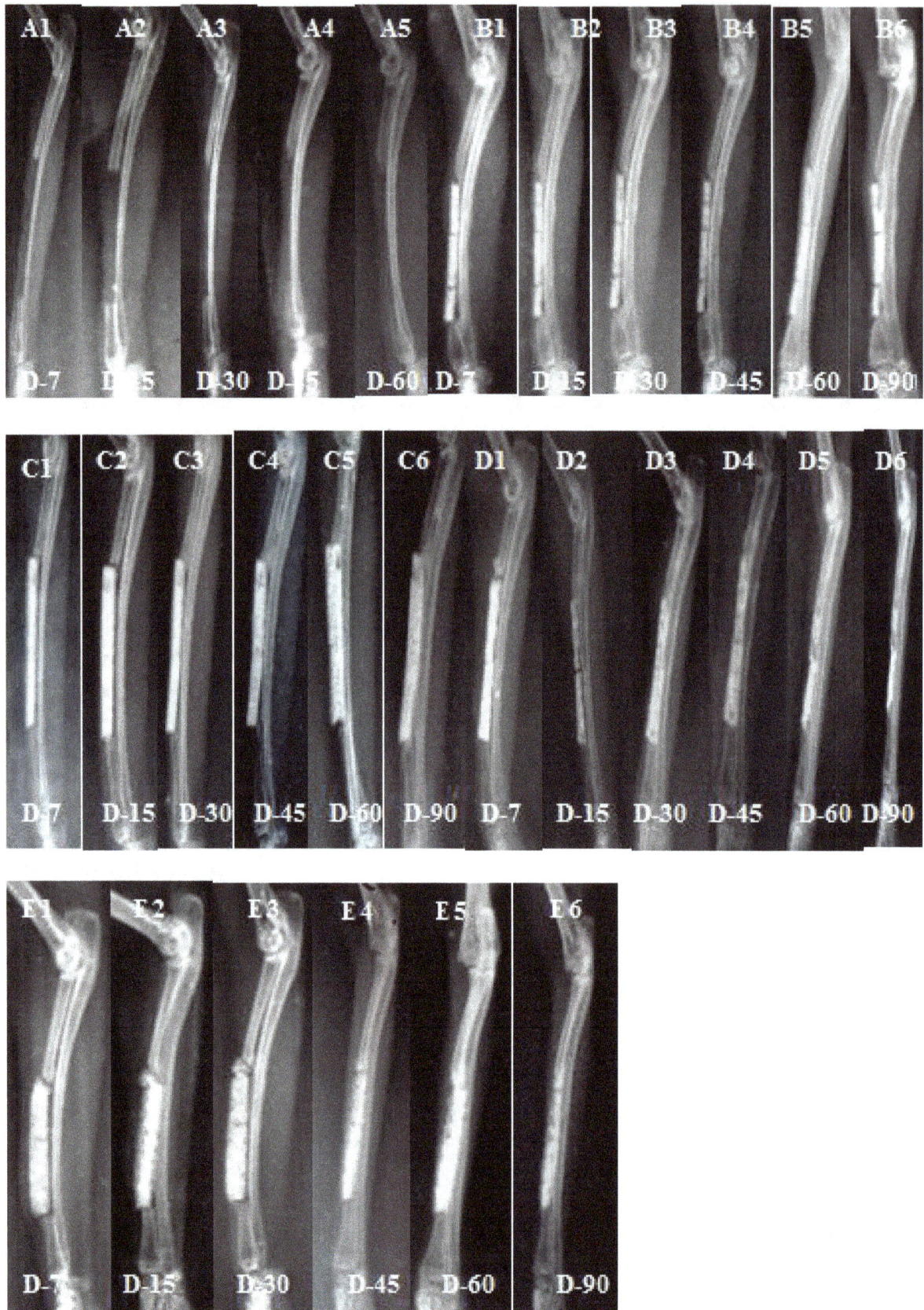

Figure 1: *Mediolateral radiographs of groups A, B, C, D and E at different intervals.   A1: gr A at day 7, A2: gr A at day 15, A3: gr A at day 30, A4: gr A at day 45, A5: gr A at day 60; B1: gr B at day 7, B2: gr B at day 15, B3: gr B at day 30, B4: gr B at day 45, B5: gr B at day 60, B6: gr B at day 90; C1: gr C at day 7, C2: gr C at day 15, C3: gr C at day 30, C4: gr C at day 45, C5: gr C at day 60, C6: gr C at day 90; D1: gr D at day 7, D2: gr D at day 15, D3: gr D at day 30, D4: gr D at day 45, D5: gr D at day 60, D6: gr D at day 90; E1: gr E at day 7, E2: gr E at day 15, E3: gr E at day 30, E4: gr E at day 45, E5: gr E at day 60, E6: gr E at day 90.*

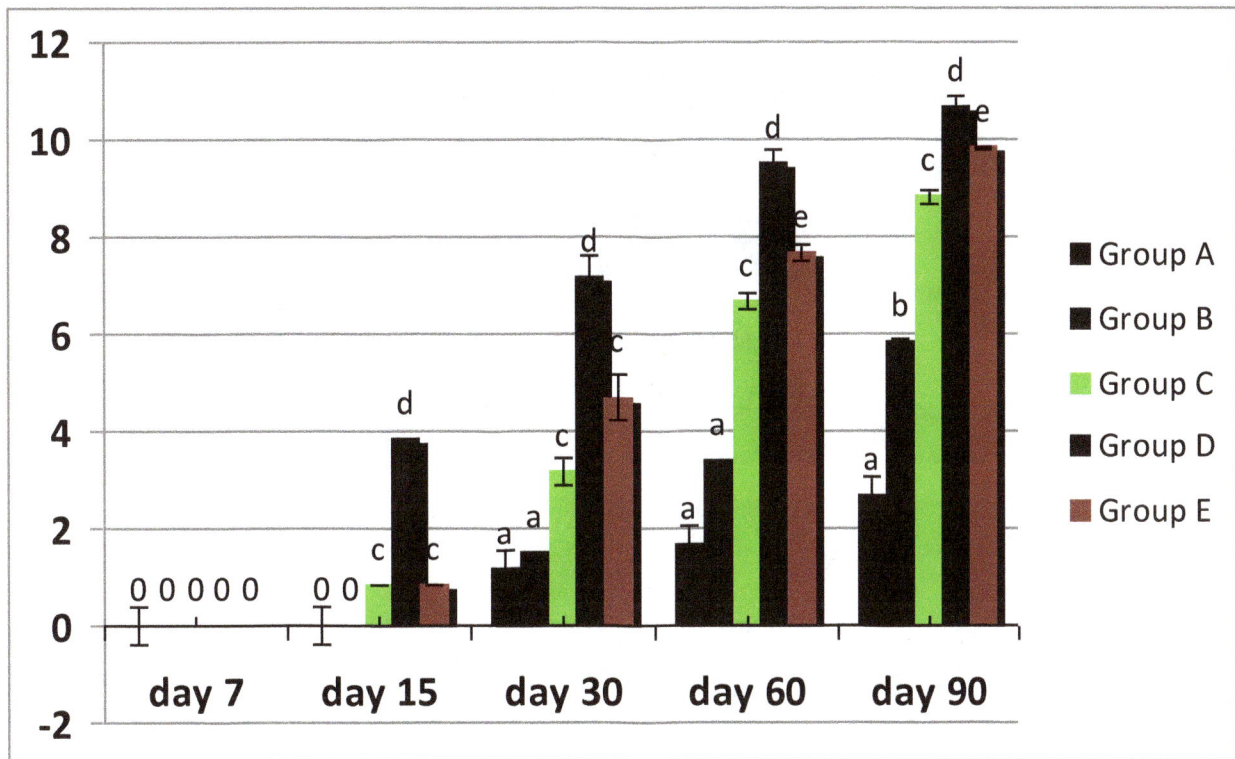

Figure 2: *Histogram showing of total radiographic score (mean +SD) in different groups at different time intervals*

In control group (A), at day 30, the osteotomy line at defect site became invisible marking the progress of bone repair near this cut end. At day 45, a slight increase in radio-opacity was seen near this defect, marking the beginning of callus formation. On day 60, the area of radio-opacity was seen to be spread a little more and the defect remaining unbridged. No animal of control group survived at day 90 as there was complete fracture of remaining ulna caused complete lameness and unable to stand or walk. In group B, mild resorption of the construct started at day 45 and at day 60, the resorption was moderate. There was gap between the construct and the cut ends of host bone till day 60, but there was increased bone density at the junction of construct with the ulna at day 90. There was no evidence of bridging at either proximal or distal end of ceramic block with the host bone. Osteogenic process was very negligible. In group C, bridging of the bone and construct at proximal end was seen from day 30 onwards. At day 60, there was close attachment of the construct with the adjacent ulna and bridging between composite construct and cut end of the host bone. At day 90, good amount of new bone formation was noticed and the construct also underwent moderate resorption by this time. In group D, bridging between host bone and implant in both proximal and distal interfaces was evident at day 30. At day 45, there was close union between composite scaffold and the adjacent ulna. At day 60, a major portion of the construct underwent resorption and the boundary between implant and normal bone disappeared, which indicated that the implant had been replaced by early new bone. This was more pronounced at day 90 (AP view). In group E, there was bony union between scaffold and ulna on day 45, whereas, bridging of both the proximal and distal defect ends with the host bone was seen at day 60. Moderate resorption of construct and bridging with adjacent ulna was more evident at day 90.

Statistical analysis of total radiographic score at day 15 showed that group D was significantly ($P<0.05$) different from other groups. On day 60, there was significant difference ($P<0.05$) between group C and group E. On day 90, all groups showed significant ($P<0.05$)

variation from each other. Overall radiographic score showed that group D had the highest score, followed by groups E, C, B and A.

Micro Computed Tomography assessment

Micro computed tomography assessment was able to distinguish between the three phases present inside the defects: newly formed bone, remaining triphasic bioceramic block and non-mineralized tissues. The μCT scanned slices of bone biopsy from different groups are presented in Figure 3. The transverse and longitudinal sections revealed the unbridged cut ends of the host radius and there was no osteogenic reaction in-between radius and adjacent ulna in any of the animal group A. In other groups, newly formed trabecular bone at the defect site in radius bone was seen. The HASi component in defect site was almost intact in group B, whereas it was in the process of resorption in groups C, D and E. In group C, signs of osteogenesis and process of remodeling were observed. In group D, transverse and longitudinal bone sections showed the establishment of periosteal continuity in between the cut ends of old host bone (radius) and continuation of medullary cavity at the defect site. Newly formed trabecular bone was under remodeling process in groups D and E.

Histopathological assessment

Histopathological sections at bone defect site of different groups at day 90 are presented in Figure 4. In control group (A) majority of the defect area was occupied by fibrous tissue (Figure 4A). In group B, very little new woven bone formation, which was discontinuous in nature, was seen at the junction of scaffold and cut ends of the host bone (Figure 4B). The scaffold was in the process of resorption and localized regions of new bone formation were seen as dispersed islands. In group C, new woven bone formation at the junction of scaffold and cut ends of host bone and osteochondral union between the ulna and scaffold was seen (Figure 4C). There was invasion of periosteum from the adjacent ulna into the defect area.

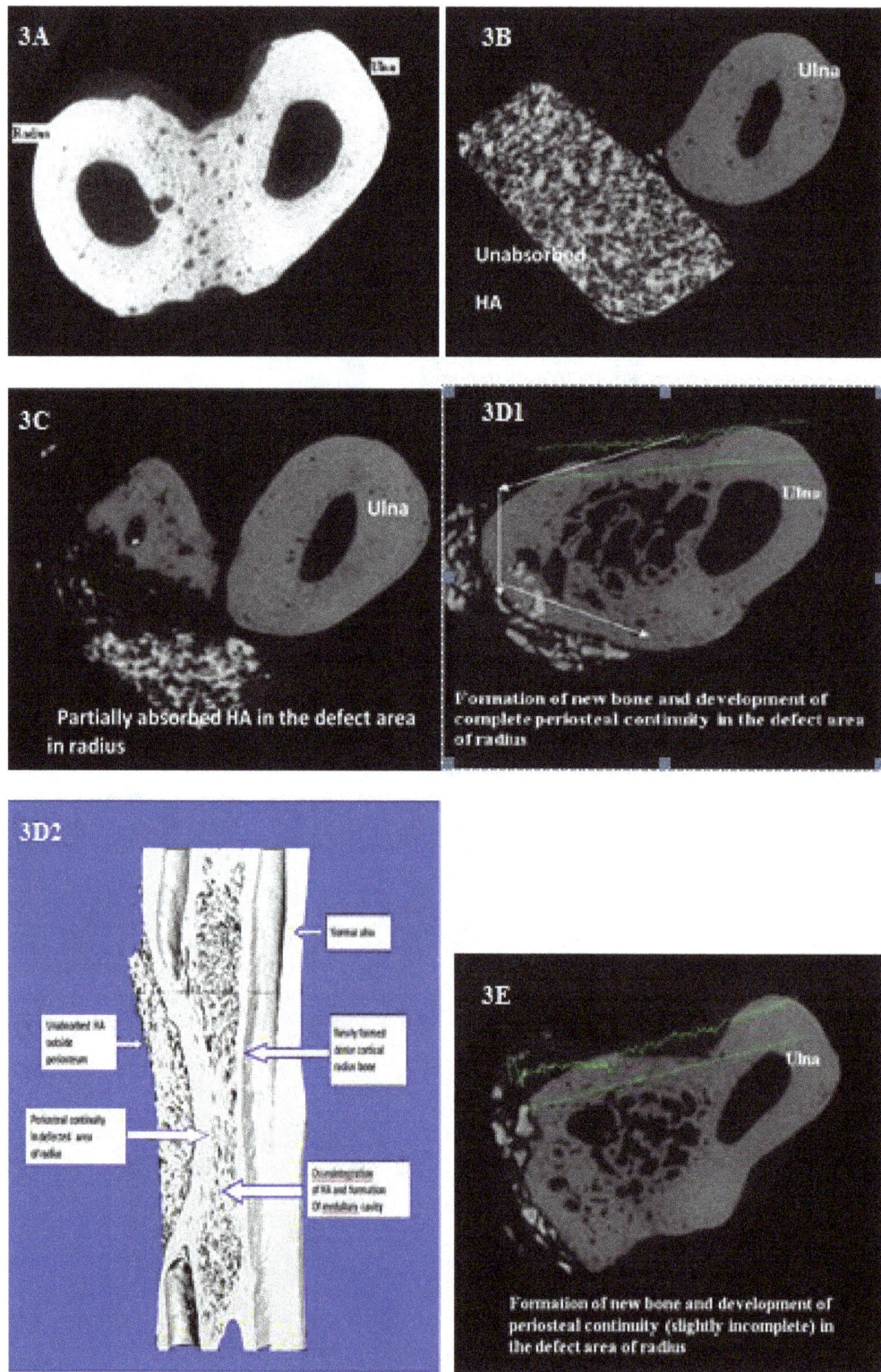

Figure 3: 3D transverse bone biopsy slice of groups A, B, C, D and E at day 90.   3A: normal bone biopsy of gr A, 3B: bone biopsy slice of gr B, 3C: bone biopsy slice of gr C, 3D1& 3D2: bone biopsy slice of gr D, 3E bone biopsy slice of gr E

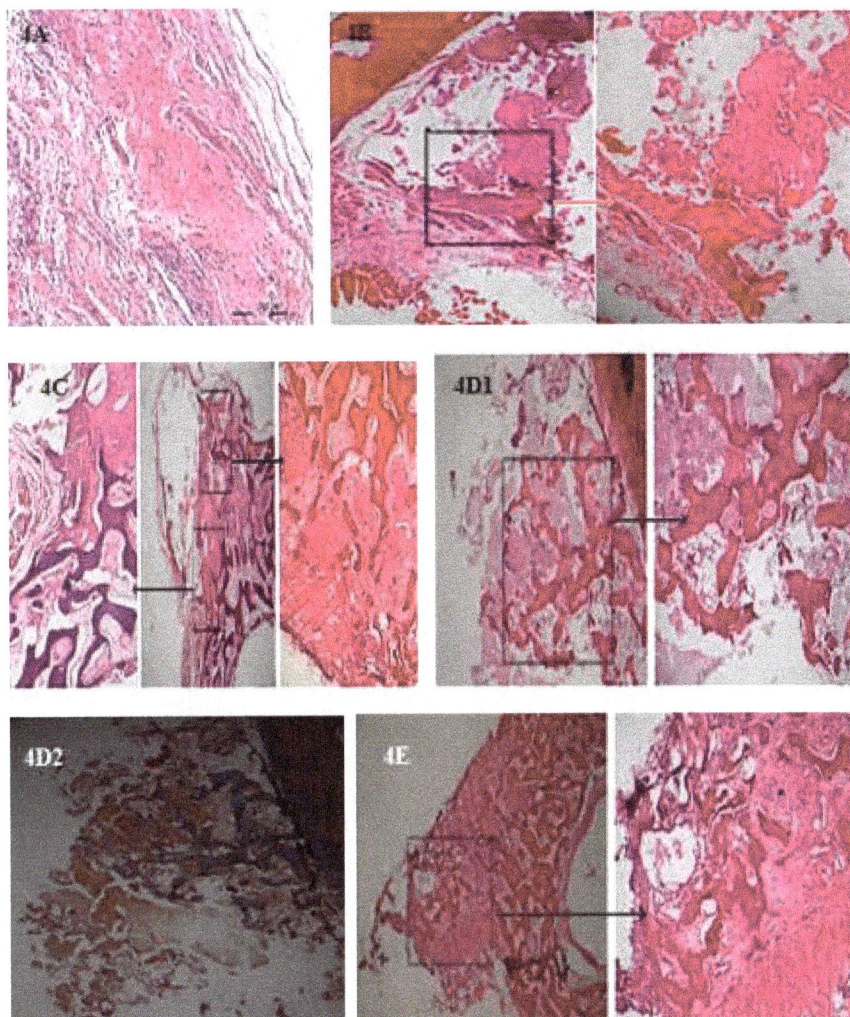

Figure 4: *Histopathological section at bone defect site of different groups at day 90;   4A: Longitudinal section gr A showed fibrous tissue proliferation at the cut ends, H&E, 100X;   4B: Transverse section of gr B showed few areas of new bone formation at the junction of scaffold and host bone, H&E, 40X, 100X;   4C: Transverse section of gr C showed osteochondral union between the ulna and scaffold, H&E, 40X, 100X;   4D1: Transverse section of gr D showed extensively bony union of scaffold with adjacent ulna, H&E, 40X, 100X;   4D2: Transverse section of gr D showed newly formed bone in the defect area repreasented by areas of mineralization (blue staining) and new osteoid (deep red staining) Masson's Trichome, 40x;   4E: Transverse section of gr E showed osteochondral union between the ulna and scaffold, H&E, 40X, 100X.*

Table 4. The total histological scores (mean ± SD) of bone healing in different groups. [a-e] values with different superscript letters vary significantly in the last column.

Group	Osteogenesis	Union	Marrow	Cancellous/ medullary bone	Cortical/compact bone	Total score
A	1.00±0.00	1.33±0.00	0.00±0.00	0.00±0.00	0.00±0.00	2.33±0[a]
B	2.00±0.00	1.33±1.15	0.67±0.58	0.67±0.58	0.00±0.00	4.67±0.33[b]
C	1.67±0.58	2.66±0.58	0.33±0.58	1.33±0.58	0.00±0.00	5.99±0.21[c]
D	3.00±0.00	3.00±0.00	2.00±0.00	3.00±0.00	1.66±0.58	12.66±0.58[d]
E	2.33±0.58	2.33±0.58	1.00±0.00	2.00±0.00	0.00±0.00	7.66±0.33[e]

The scaffold was under active resorption and replaced by newly formed woven bone at some places. In group D, abundant new dense bone tissue formation and close bony union of scaffold with the host bone at both cut ends as well as with the adjacent ulna was seen (Figure 4D1). Scaffold was under active resorption and many places it was replaced by newly formed woven bone. Increased vascularisation near the junction between scaffold and the adjacent ulna was seen. Marrow formation was also evident in more than half of the implant area indicative of remodeling. Osteogenesis process was of intramembraneous type without any intermediate cartilage formation. Masson's trichrome staining revealed close association of newly formed bone in the defect area with the host bone represented by more areas of mineralization (blue staining) and new osteoid (deep red staining) tissue (Figure 4D2). In group E, osteochondral union was seen between the scaffold and cut ends of host bone as well as with the ulna (Figure 4E). Three-fourth of the scaffold had undergone cartilaginous transition and areas of new bone formation were evident. The total histological scores of bone healing for different groups are presented in Table 4. Group D had the highest score, followed by groups E, C, B and A.

Discussion

The aim of the present work was to study the effect of BMSC with growth factors   (rhBMP-2 and IGF-1) seeded on a resorbable bio-ceramic scaffold (HASi) in the regeneration of bone at very large critical-sized defect, using an autogenous approach.

The rabbit radial critical-sized defect creates a weight bearing model in which the implanted scaffold will sensitize the surrounding mechanical load and act as a mechanical and structural rapport to the defect. In addition, since the ulna can also serve as an internal splint for the radius, no external fixation is needed. Even then, in this study since the defect size was too large, we used a custom-designed external splint which was maintained for 7 days. Transplantation of mesenchymal stem cells for bone regeneration in a rabbit critical-size defect (15mm) has been already reported[5], but the regeneration potential of autogenous MSC with or without growth factors beyond critical-size defect was not reported so far. So, in this study, we created large (30mm) segmental radial diaphyseal bone defect in rabbit model and we found that this model was very much suitable for this experiment. The only limitation of this model was without any scaffold or external fixation animal was unable to walk properly.

No significant bone formation and consolidation of the defect was achieved in any animal in which the defect was left untreated (control group). Since the purpose of the present study was to investigate the influence of MSC with or without growth proteins; empty scaffolds were used as an additional control group. The scaffold used in the present study was HASi-a triphasic bio-ceramic adding silicon in hydroxyapatite and tricalcium phosphate. In the bio-ceramic group (B) there was no evidence of bridging at either proximal or distal end of ceramic block with the host bone at day 90 post implantation. Osteogenic process was very negligible. Silica coated hydroxyapatite has osteoinductive properties[21], in addition to faster resorption rate resulting from the greater dissolution of Si ions[10]. Nevertheless, with regard to the results of the present study, HASi alone is not able to lead to healing of large critical-size-defects. Although, more new bone formation could be seen in animal treated with HASi alone compared with the empty controls, but it failed to bridge the defect even at day 90 post implantation. Similarly, reconstruction of 1.5cm segmental bone defects in the rabbit ulna using porous polylactic-co-glycolic acid (PLGA) scaffold failed to bridge completely even at 12 weeks post implantation[22]. In our view, even if this bio-ceramic implant (HASi) or other bio-implants include hydroxyapatite (HA) or its combination of tri-calcium phosphate (HA-TCP) or PLGA kept for

further longer duration, it might be failed to bridge the large bone defect completely. For this, further study wad suggested using different bio-materials for implantation in very large (3cm) radial bone defect in rabbit model.

In an additional control group, a combination of autogenous MSC and HASi was transplanted into the defect area. In these animals, increased bone formation was found compared with HASi alone. Radiological, μCT and histological analysis showed bony union between the scaffold and cut ends of the host bone as well as with the adjacent ulna. This observation confirms previous *in vivo* and *in vitro* experiments which demonstrated the benefit of the addition of mesenchymal stem cells on bio-scaffold for improved bone regeneration[3,5]. Mesenchymal stem cells (MSCs) are non-hematopoietic stromal stem cells, capable of self-replication and of differentiating into, and contributing to the regeneration of mesenchymal tissues such as bone, cartilage, ligament, tendon, muscle and adipose tissue. MSCs promote infiltration of osteoprogenitor cells, and thus enhance their subsequent mineralization and bone formation[22, 23]. MSC-derived osteoblast cells are anchorage dependent and require a supportive matrix in order to survive and flourish. So the selection of a suitable scaffold is another important criterion to be considered to fabricate a tissue-engineered construct. Silica coated hydroxyapatite scaffold (HASi) has significantly increased cell viability, proliferations and differentiation of osteoblast from different source in an *in vitro* culture[9]. The enhanced viability and proliferation of cells on HASi can be attributed to the multiphase composition (HA, tricalcium phosphate and calcium silicate) as well as silica content of HASi[21]. Silica-coated hydroxyapatite (HASi) could induce the osteogenic differentiation of rabbit BMSC by day 17 post-seeding in absence of any osteogenic induction media[24]. Since HASi has been provided a favorable 3D microenvironment for the osteogenic response, our aim was to use this tissue-engineered construct for bone regeneration and repair in a very large radial segmental defects in rabbits. Generally, cell proliferation and differentiation are two interdependent processes having a counteracting relationship. However, HASi was capable of inducing osteogenesis and cell proliferation in a parallel relationship, when it seeded with human BMSC[9]. This is in confirmation of our study where rabbit BMSC-seeded HASi scaffold promotes proliferation and osteogenic differentiation of mesenchymal stem cells in segmental bone defects.

In vivo bone formation can be influenced by the type and form of biomaterial, the pore size and pore distribution, interconnectivity and the resorption of the bi-omaterial[25]. The bio-material used (HASi) in our study was manufactured in blocks, consequently this cannot be compared to other studies where granules or powders were used [5]. For example Krebsbach *et al*[26] found more bone formation with HA/TCP powder than in HA/TCP blocks. In our study, blocks were used as scaffolds because of the better bio-mechanics and the easier future clinical use in segmental bone defects[3]. The bio-material used in the present study comprised open pores in the range of 50- 500μm, and geometry wise; it is fully interconnected with a large surface area to volume ratio. The latter quality to have seems to have improved the migration and distribution of osteoprogenitor cells throughout the scaffold material.   Secretion of osteoclasts is stimulated by Si ions and this in turn confirms the osteointegrative, osteoconductive and degradation properties of triphasic HASi bio-ceramic scaffold[27]. In this study, HASi block seems inevitability causing close union between scaffold and adjacent ulna due to its osteoconductive properties, which is seems to be good as it not only unite the adjacent splint bone near the defect site, also it provided further mechanical stability to the injured bone.

Bone development, growth, and repair predominantly occur through the process of endrochondral ossification, characterized by remodeling of cartilaginous templates. The same route efficiently supports engineering of bone marrow as a niche for hematopoietic stem cells-mesenchymal stem cells (MSC)[28]. Mesenchymal stem cells are known to have the ability to undergo osteogenic differentiation under suitable conditions[29].Their proliferation and differentiation capacity may be enhanced by exposing them to growth factors. Growth factors are protein signaling agents that act locality to stimulate formation and proliferation of osteoblasts and thereby promote bone healing. The rhBMP-2-treated constructs in group D encouraged the formation of abundant bone tissue bridging both proximal and distal interfaces as well as with adjacent ulna as early as eight weeks after surgery. At day 90 after surgery, μCT and histopathological analysis showed newly formed bony tissue within the implantation site, well-differentiated mineralized lamellar bone surrounding the HASi granules, characterized by the number of osteocytic lacunae and Haversian systems and the presence of osteoid border at the surface of new bony trabeculae. Periosteal continuity was complete at the defect site with host bone. Direct ossification of the scaffold and dense woven bone along with marrow formation were also noticed in some animals of this group, suggest the possibility of direct formation of osteoblasts from the osteoprogenitor cells by the action of rhBMP-2. The results confirmed that rhBMP-2 accelerate osteogenesis at the defect site by the process of osteoinduction.

BMP-2 has the highest osteoinductive potential among all the bone morphogenetic proteins[1]. There are differences between species in their sensitivity to bone morphogenetic proteins, so the result can be difficult to extrapolate from one species to another[30]. A minimum threshold dose of BMP-2 is necessary for a beneficial effect to occur, but a higher dose does not necessarily result in a better outcome[13, 31]. Bone morphogenetic proteins (BMPs) are hydrophobic, non-species specific glycoprotein, belongs to the expanding transforming growth factor-beta super family and has pleiotropic function that range from extra skeletal and skeletal organogenesis to bone generation and regeneration. It induces de novo bone formation in post fetal life through the process of direct (intra membranous) and endrochondral ossification and their response is dose dependent[32]. It is reported that a 2-cm ostectomy corresponds to a critical-size defect that does not heal spontaneously without the addition of bone grafts or any bone substitute[1]. Such an experimental non-union model provides very limited osteoconduction as bone contact was only present at both proximal and distal cortical junctions. The rhBMP-2 appeared to have osteoinductive properties that were quite efficient in such surgical conditions, and combining with this material (HASi) might ensure early healing. Bone morphogenetic protein-2 accelerates the rate of development of the callus and cortical union after fracture of the rabbit tibia, but it does not affect the amounts of bone and cartilage produced. Bone morphogenetic protein-2 stimulates bone and cartilage formation so that the callus develops and matures more rapidly[33]. In agreement with this study, recombinant human bone morphogenetic protein-2 accelerates healing in a rabbit ulnar osteotomy model[34].

It appears difficult to decide on an ideal concentration, since these studies varied in term of the BMP-2 carrier and the size of the defect. In this study, the same number of rBMSC (five millions cells) and concentration of growth factors rhBMP-2 (50μg) and IGF-1 (50μg) were again injected around the bone defect on day 15 postsurgery in groups C, D and E respectively, as the defect size was almost double than standard radial critical-size bone defect (15mm) in rabbit model[5]. In our study, local injection of 100μg rhBMP-2 allowed bone regeneration in an extensively large (30mm) radial diaphyseal critical-size defect in rabbit model. It is reported that rhBMP-2 when injected (120 μg) at the site of bone defect accelerates the rate of development of callus and cortical union after fracture of the rabbit tibia and ulna[33, 34]. However, further experiment was needed for

examining the beneficial effect of rhBMP-2 injected locally. Further studies also needed to assess the kinetic release of rhBMP-2 from our HASi construct.

Histological and μCT analysis in group E revealed that there was osteochondral union and cartilaginous transition between implant and host bone at defect site as well as with the adjacent ulna. Completion of cancellous bone formation and regions of increased neo-vascularisation with moderate resorption of construct took place at day 90 post surgery. New bone formation was more than group C, but comparatively less than group D. This could be because of IGF-1 is known to induce stem cells to differentiate towards the endothelial precursor germ layer, with significantly more endothelial cells at later stages[35]. There was cartilaginous transition of scaffold and new bone formation in group E as IGF-1 increases collagen and non-collagenous protein synthesis in vitro[36, 37, 38]. Previous studies also showed the ability of IGF to promote in vivo bone healing[39, 40]. Insulin-like growth factor-1 plus MSCs can improve bone healing mostly through endrochondral ossification[41].

Among the five groups, in vivo study showed that a radial segmental defect of 30mm did not show any sign of osteogenesis or bone healing in control (left untreated) group. There was little sign of osteogenesis in scaffold group; however, it provided very good mechanical as well as structural support to the defect, but it also unable to bridge the bone defect at day 90 post implantation. In scaffold-MSC seeded group, osteogenesis was better than the group where only scaffold was applied, probably due to the addition of MSCs, which promote infiltration of osteoprogenitor cells, and thus enhance their subsequent mineralization and bone formation. Addition of growth factors in scaffold-MSC construct accelerated the healing of critical sized bone defect. Among the two growth proteins, rhBMP-2-treated constructs encouraged the formation of abundant bone tissue bridging both proximal and distal interfaces as well as with adjacent ulna as early as eight weeks after surgery. IGF-1 treated construct also encourage new bone formation and bridging the defect but osteogenesis was comparatively less than rh-BMP-2 treated group. The HASi was acted as suitable bioscaffold for development of MSC-seeded tissue engineering construct for bone regeneration because of their biocompatibility and osteoconductivity.

Conclusion

The findings of this study shows that in vitro seeding of autogenous rBMSC on bioscaffold HASi could hasten the osteoconductive properties of scaffold and can be alternative to autogenous bone graft in the treatment of large bone defects and non-union. Addition of growth proteins particularly rhBMP-2 to autogenous MSC seeded HASi bio-ceramic construct could accelerate bone regeneration in a large critical-size-bone defect model controlled study.

References

1. Minier K, Toure A, Fusellier M, Fellah B, Bouvy B, Weiss P, Gauthier O. BMP-2 delivered from a self-cross linkable Ca/P hydrogel construct promotes bone regeneration in a critical-size segmental defect model of non-union in dogs. Vet Comp Orthop Traumatol 2014; 27 (6): 411-21.
2. Li Ye, Chen SK, Li L, Qin L, Wang XL, Lai YX. Bone defect animal models for testing efficacy of bone substitute biomaterials. J Orthop Translatiom 2015; 3(3): 95-104
3. Kasten P, Vogel J, Luginbuhl R, Niemeyer P, Tonak M, Lorenz H. Ectopic bone formation associated with mesenchymal stem cells in a resorbable calcium deficient hydroxyapatite carrier. Biomaterials 2005; 26(29): 5879-89.
4. Bruder SP, Kraus KH, Goldberg VM, Kadiyala S. The effect of implants loaded with autologous mesenchymal stem cells on the healing of canine segmental bone defects. J Bone Joint Surg Am 1998; 80(7):985-96.

5. Niemeyer P, Szalay K, Luginbuhl R, Sudkamp NP, Kasten P. Transplantation of human mesenchymal stem cells in a non-autogenous setting for bone regeneration in a rabbit critical –size-defect model. Acta Biomaterialia 2010; 6 (3): 900-08.

6. Kim HJ, Park JB, Lee JK, Park EY, Park EA, Riew KD, Rhee SK. Transplanted xenoxenic bone marrow stem cells survive and generate new bone formation in the poterolateral lumber spine of non-immunosuppressed rabbits. Eur Spine 2008; 17 (11): 1515-21.

7. Daculsi G, Passuti N, Martin S, Deudon C, Legeros RZ, Raher S. Macroporous calcium phosphate ceramic for long bone surgery in humans and dogs. Clinical and histological study. J Biomed Mater Res 1990; 24 (3):379-96.

8. Baur TW, Smith ST. Bioactive materials in orthopedics surgery: overview and regulatory considerations. Clin Orthop Rev 2002; 395(2):11-22.

9. Nair MB, Bernhardt A, Lode A, Heinemann C, Thieme S, Hanke T, Varma H, Gelinsky M, John A. A bioactive triphasic ceramic-coated hydroxyapatite promotes proliferation and osteogenic differentiation of human stromal cells. J Biomed Mater Res A 2009a; 90 (2): 533-42.

10. El-Ghannam AR. Advanced bioceramic composite for bone tissue engineering: design principles and structure-bioactivity relationship. J Biomed Mater Res A 2004: 69 (3): 490-501.

11. Linkhart TA, Mohan S, Baylink DJ. Growth factors for bone growth and repair: IGF, TGF-beta and BMP. Bone 1996; 19 (1 Suppl): 1S-12S.

12. Devescovi V, Leonardi E, Ciapetti G, Cenni E. Growth factors in bone repair. Chir Organi Mov 2008; 92(3):161-68

13. Sciadini MF, Jojnson KD. Evaluation of recombinant human bone morphogenetic protein-2 as a bone-graft substitute in a canine segmental defect model. J Orthop Res 2000; 18 (2):289-302.

14. Pluhar GE, Manley PA, Heiner JP, Vanderby R Jr, Seeherman HJ, Markel MD. The effect of recombinant human bone morphogenetic protein -2 on femoral reconstruction with an intercalary allograft in a dog model. J Orthop Res 2001; 19 (2): 308-17

15. Fiedler J, Brill C, Blum WF, Brenner RE. IGF-1 and IGF-2 stimulate directed cell migration of bone marrow derived human mesenchymal progenitor cells. Biochem Biophys Res Comm 2006; 345 (3): 1177-83.

16. LeGeros RZ. Properties of osteoconductive biomaterials: calcium phosphates. Clin Orthop Relat Res 2002; 395 (2): 81-98.

17. Maiti SK, Shiva Kumar MU, Srivastava L, Kumar N, Ninu AR. Isolation, proliferation and morphological characteristics of bone marrow derived mesenchymal stem cells (BM-MSC) from different animal species. Trends Biomater Artif Org 2012; 27(1): 29-35.

18. Yang, C.Y., Simmons. D.J. and Lozano. R. The healing of grafts combining freeze-dried and demineralized allogeneic bone in rabbits. Clin Orthop Relat Res 1994; 298 (1):286-95.

19. Lane, J. M. and Sandhu, H. S. Current approach to experimental bone grafting. Orthop Clin North Am 1987; 18(2): 213–25.

20. Heiple, K. G., Goldberg, V. M., Powell, A. E., Bos, G. D. and Zika, J. M. Biology of cancellous bone grafts. Orthop Clin North Am 1987: 18(2): 179–85.

21. Nair MB, Varma HK, Menon KV, Shenoy SJ, John A. Reconstruction of goat femur segmental defects using triphasic ceramic-coated hydroxyapatite in combination with autologous cells and platelet-rich plasma. Acta Biomater 2009c; 5 (5): 1742-55.

22. Zhang X, Qi YY, Zhao TF, Li D, Dai X S, Niu L, He RX. Reconstruction of segmental bone defects in the rabbit ulna using periosteum encapsulated mesenchymal stem cells-loaded poly (lactic-co-glycolic acid) scaffolds. Chin Med J 2012; 125 (22): 4031-36.

23. Wang X, Wang Yu, Gou W, Lu Q, Peng J, Lu S. Role of mesenchymal stem cells in bone regeneration and fracture repair: a review. Int Orthop 2013; 37 (12): 2491-98.

24. Ninu AR, Maiti SK, Palakkara S, Kritaniya D, Mahan T, Kumar N. In vitro osteoinduction potential of a novel silica coated hydroxyapatite bioscaffold seeded with rabbit mesenchymal stem cell. J Stem Cell Res Ther 2016; 2(1): 00009.

25. Mankani MH, Kuznetsov SA, Fowler B, Kingman A, Robey PG. In vivo bone formation by human bone marrow stromal cells: effect of carrier particle size and shape. Biotechnol Bioeng 2001; 72 (1): 96-107.

26. Krebsbach PH, Kuznetsov SA, Satomura K, Emmons RV, Rowe DW, Robey PG. Bone formation in vivo: comparison of osteogenesis by transplanted mouse and human marrow stromal fibroblasts. Transplantation 1997; 63 (8):1059-69..

27. Nair MB, Varma HK, Menon KV, Shenoy SJ, John A. Tissue regeneration and repair of goat segmental femur defect with bioactive triphasic ceramic-coated hydroxyapatite scaffold. J Biomed Mater Res A 2009b; 91(3): 855-65.

28. Scotti C, Tonnarelli B, Papadimitropoulos A, Piccinini E, Todorov A, Centola M, Barbero A, Martin I. Engineering small-scale and scaffold-based bone organs via endochondral ossification using adult progenitor cells. Methods Mol Biol 2016; 1416: 413-14.

29. Birmingham E, Niebur GL, McHugh PE, Shaw G, Barry FP, McNamara LM. Osteogenic differentiation of mesenchymal stem cells in regulated by osteocyte and osteoblast cells in a simplified bone niche. Cell Mater 2012; 23 (1):13-27

30. Itoh T, Mochizuki M, Nishimura R, Matsunaga S, Kadsawa T, Kobuko S, Yokota S, Sasaki N. Repair of ulnar segmental defect by recombinant human bone morphogenetic protein -2 in dogs. J Vet Med Sci 1998; 60:451-58.

31. Boraish S, Paul O, Hawkes D, Wickham M, Lorich DG. Complications of recombinant human BMP-2 for treating complex tibial plateau fractures: a preliminary report. Clin Orthop Relat Res 2009; 467 (12):3257- 62.

32. Maiti S K, Singh G R. Bone morphogenetic proteins-novel regulators of bone formation. Indian J Exp Biol 1998; 36 (3): 237-44

33. Bax BE, Wozney JM, Ashhurst DE. Bonemorphogenetic protein-2increases the rate of callus formation after fracture of the rabbit tibia. Calcif Tissue Int 1999: 65 (1): 83-89.

34. Bouxsein ML, Turek TJ, Blake CA, D'Augusta D, Li X, Stevens M, Seeherman HJ, Wozney JM. Recombinant human bone morphogenetic protein-2 accelerates healing in a rabbit ulnar osteotomy model. J Bone Joint Surg Am 2001; 83(8): 1219-30.

35. Piecewicz SM, Pandey M, Roy B, Xiang SH, Zetter Br, Sengupta S. Insulin-like growth factors promote vasculogenesis in embryonic stem cells. PloS ONE 2012; 7 (2): e32191.

36. Canalis E, McCarthy T, Centrella M. Isolation and characterization of insulin like growth factor 1 (Somatomedin-C) from cultures of fetal rat calvariae. Endocrinology 1988; 122(1):22-27.

37. Hock JM, Centella M, Canalis E. Insulin-like growth factor-1 has independent effects on bone matrix formation and cell replication. Endocrinology 1988; 122 (1): 254-60.

38. McCarthy TL, Centella M, Canalis E. Insulin-like growth factor and bone. Connect Tissue Res 1989; 20(1): 277-82.

39. Schmidmaier G, Wildemann B, Bail H, Luke M, Fuchs T, Stemberger A, Flyvbjerg A, Hass NP, Raschke M. Local application of growth factors Insulin-like growth factor and transforming growth factor-beta-1 from a biodegradable poly (D, L-Lactide) coating of osteosynthetic implants accelerates fracture healing in rats. Bone 2001; 28(4):341-50.

40. Blumenfeld I, Srouji S. Lanir Y, Laufer D, Livne E. Enhancement of bone healing in old rats by TGF-beta and IGF-1. Expt Geronto 2002; 37(4):553-65.

41. Myers TJ, Yan Y, Granero-Molto F, Weis JA, Longobardi L, Li T, Li Y, Contaldo C, Ozkan H, Spagnoli A. Systemically delivered insulin-like growth factor-1 enhances mesenchymal stem cell-dependant fracture healing. Growth Factors 2012; 30 (4):230-41.

Abbreviations

BMSC: Bone marrow derived Mesenchymal Stem Cell
DMEM: Dulbecco's modified Eagle Medium
FBS: Fetal Bovine Serum
HASi: Silica-coated Calcium Hydroxyapatite
IGF: Insulin-like Growth Protein
MSC: Mesenchymal Stem Cell
PBS: Phosphate Buffered Saline
rhBMP: Recombinant human Bone Morphogenetic Protein
µCT: Micro Computed Tomography
gr: Group

Potential Conflicts of Interests

None

Acknowledgements

The authors wish to thank Dr K. P. Singh, Principal Scientist, CADRAD, IVRI, Izatnagar (UP), India for his technical assistance in evaluation of histological sections and Prof. H. Varma, Sree Chitra Tirunal Institute for Medical Sciences and Technology, Trivandrum, Kerala (India) for his technical assistance for designing and preparation of HASi bio-ceramic. Senior author, wish to acknowledge to Prof Dimitry Spitkovsky, Institute of Neurophysiology, Köln University, Germany for his whole-hearted stem cell research support during his stay at Germany as "Visiting Professor".

This research was supported by a research grant from Department of Biotechnology (DBT), Government of India.

Corresponding Author

Swapan Kumar Maiti, Principal Scientist, Surgery Division, Indian Veterinary Research Institute, Izatnagar-243 122, Uttar-Pradesh, India Email:swapanivri@gmail.com; maiti_62@rediffmail.com

The Effect of Pro-Neurogenic Gene Expression on Adult Subventricular Zone Precursor Cell Recruitment and Fate Determination After Excitotoxic Brain Injury

Jones KS[1], Connor BJ[1]

Despite the presence of on-going neurogenesis in the adult mammalian brain, neurons are generally not replaced after injury. Using a rodent model of excitotoxic cell loss and retroviral (RV) lineage tracing, we previously demonstrated transient recruitment of precursor cells from the subventricular zone (SVZ) into the lesioned striatum. In the current study we determined that these cells included migratory neuroblasts and oligodendrocyte precursor cells (OPC), with the predominant response from glial cells. We attempted to override this glial response by ectopic expression of the pro-neurogenic genes Pax6 or Dlx2 in the adult rat SVZ following quinolinic acid lesioning. RV-Dlx2 over-expression stimulated repair at a previously non-neurogenic time point by enhancing neuroblast recruitment and the percentage of cells that retained a neuronal fate within the lesioned area, compared to RV-GFP controls. RV-Pax6 expression was unsuccessful at inhibiting glial fate and intriguingly, increased OPC cell numbers with no change in neuronal recruitment. These findings suggest that gene choice is important when attempting to augment endogenous repair as the lesioned environment can overcome pro-neurogenic gene expression. Dlx2 over-expression however was able to partially overcome an anti-neuronal environment and therefore is a promising candidate for further study of striatal regeneration.

Key Words: Adult neurogenesis, Pax6, Dlx2, Regeneration, Oligodendrocyte progenitor cell, Neuroblast

Introduction

Compensatory adult neurogenesis has been demonstrated in many models of brain injury and neurodegeneration, including stroke, trauma, epilepsy, excitotoxic lesioning, Huntington's and Parkinson's disease[1-9]. However, complete neuronal repair is yet to be achieved. In the normal adult mammalian brain, neurogenesis is predominantly observed from the subventricular zone (SVZ) of the lateral ventricles and throughout the olfactory bulb system, as well as the dentate gyrus of the hippocampus. Specifically in the SVZ, slow dividing Type B stem cells generate rapidly proliferating Type C cells (transiently amplifying precursors or TAPs) that can generate both neuroblasts and oligodendrocytes[7, 10]. TAPs have been found to be heterogeneous and express combinations of the pro-neurogenic genes *Mash1, Pax6, Ngn2, Dlx2* and the oligodendrocyte lineage gene *Olig2*[2, 11-16]. Neural cell loss or injury in the adult brain can alter endogenous neurogenesis and elicit a compensatory repair process. Specifically, alterations in the expression of *Mash1, Pax6, Ngn2, Dlx2* and/or *Olig2* have been observed in the adult SVZ and parenchyma in various models of neural cell loss, consistent with their potential roles in the endogenous repair process[2, 8, 9, 16-19].

If endogenous repair is to be restorative, attraction of the appropriate cellular phenotype to repopulate and repair damaged areas of the brain is essential. After injury, SVZ neural progenitor cells (NPCs) have been found to be redirected to areas of neural cell loss and either, 1) stay in their original neuronal lineage program[20, 21]; 2) change their lineage program to a different neuronal subtype[22, 23]; or 3) have their lineage altered to a different cell type altogether[24]. However, the plasticity of these cell lineages differ between injury and disease models in the appropriate recruitment and differentiation of sub-type specific cells. Why this happens is not well understood. We previously showed that quinolinic acid (QA) -induced striatal cell loss stimulates a transient neurogenic response from SVZ-derived precursor cells, with increased proliferation and redirected migration of cells away from the SVZ and rostral migratory stream to the injury site[6]. Retrovirus (RV) GFP lineage tracing found the phenotype of redirected cells appeared to change over time from a neuronal to glial morphology[25]. Classically, endogenous repair studies have focused on the proliferation of SVZ progenitors labelled with Bromodeoxyuridine or with RV-GFP, to track the migration of DCX+ precursor cells to areas of neural damage and determine the neural phenotypes generated, while ignoring non-DCX+ migratory cells[6, 22, 23, 25, 26]. To address this, the current study examined the phenotypic profiles of all RV-GFP labelled cells migrating from the SVZ into the QA lesioned striatum over time. Interestingly, GFP+ cells observed in the injured striatum included migratory neuroblasts as well as bipolar *Olig2+* cells, with the predominant response observed from glial cells.

We attempted to override this glial response by ectopic expression of the pro-neurogenic genes, *Pax6* or *Dlx2* in the adult rat SVZ following QA acid lesioning. Pro-neurogenic transcription factor delivery has been examined as a way to enhance a neurogenic response following neural injury[2, 17-19, 27, 28]. Based on the presence

---

Author Names in full: Kathryn S. Jones[1], Bronwen J. Connor[1]

[1] Centre for Brain Research, Department of Pharmacology and Clinical Pharmacology, School of Medical Science, Faculty of Medical and Health Sciences, University of Auckland..

of oligodendrocyte precursor cells (OPCs) in response to QA-induced striatal cell loss, we investigated the effect of over-expressing the pro-neurogenic factors *Pax6* and *Dlx2*. Studies have demonstrated the requirement of *Pax6* as a 'master regulator' of neurogenesis in the adult brain. *Pax6* acts to suppress the glial transcription factor *Olig2* in the adult SVZ and to reprogram postnatal glia and reactive astrocytes into neurons[12, 13, 15, 29, 30]. Repression of *Olig2* or overexpression of *Pax6* was able to promote neuroblast generation in a cortical stab wound injury and post striatal ischemia[18, 19]. *Olig2* has also been shown to interfere with *Dlx2* expression and neuroblast fate in the normal SVZ[31]. Therefore, in order to determine if the observed gliogenic fate post QA lesioning could be overcome, we delivered retrovirus expressing either *Pax6* or *Dlx2* with *GFP* directly to SVZ precursor cells at time points where significant progenitor cell recruitment had been observed. Interestingly, only RV-Dlx2 over-expression enhanced both neuroblast recruitment and the percentage of recruited cells that retained a neuronal fate when compared to RV-GFP control animals. Surprisingly, RV-Pax6 expression resulted in increased OPC numbers with no change in neurogenesis when compared to controls. These findings suggest that signals released from damaged tissue can selectively override pro-neurogenic gene expression. Therefore, a better understanding of interactions between neural precursor cells and inflammatory signals is required in order to successfully regenerate cells endogenously for injury or disease.

Materials and Methods

All experimental protocol were approved by the University of Auckland. Animal work was carried out with strict accordance to guidelines set by the University of Auckland Animal Ethics Committee in accordance with the New Zealand Animal Welfare Act 1999 and conformed to international guidelines for the ethical use of animals. Retroviral generation was approved by the University of Auckland and conformed to the Environmental Protection Authority of New Zealand.

Retroviral generation

pMXIG-GFP, pMXIG-Dlx2-GFP and pMXIG-Pax6-GFP plasmids were kindly donated by Professor Magdalena Gotz (Department of Physiological Genomics, Ludwig-Maximilians University, Munich, Germany)[12, 13, 29]. RV-GFP, RV-Pax6-GFP and RV-Dlx2-GFP retroviral particles were generated and concentrated as per previously described methods[25].

Surgical procedures

Adult male Wistar rats weighing 250-300g (three months of age; University of Auckland Vernon Jansen Unit) were used in this study. The animals were housed in a temperature and humidity controlled room that was kept on a 12 hour light and dark cycle. Food and water were available *ad libitum*. Animal welfare was monitored daily. Every effort was made to minimize the number of animals used and their suffering. For excitotoxic lesions, 400nl of fresh 50nM quinolinic acid (QA) pH 7.4 was injected unilaterally into the striatum at the following coordinates: AP +0.7mm, ML -2.5mm relative to bregma, and DV -5.0mm relative to dura. Control animals did not receive a sham injection as our previous findings have demonstrated that sham surgery resulted in no significant difference to SVZ proliferation or neural precursor cell migration[25]. For RV injections, 2µl of concentrated retrovirus (RV-GFP, RV-Pax6-GFP or RV-Dlx2-GFP, titre 1x10^8 colony forming units (cfu)/ml) containing 80µg/ml polybrene) was injected unilaterally at the following co-ordinates: AP +0.2mm, ML -1.7mm, relative to bregma and DV -3.4mm relative to

dura. RV-GFP was injected two days prior to lesioning, on the day of lesioning and two, three, five and seven days post lesion (n=3-5 per time point)[25]. RV-Pax6-GFP and RV- Dlx2-GFP were injected on the day of lesioning or two days post lesion (n=5-6 per virus per time point). RV control animals received an injection of either RV-Pax6-GFP or RV-Dlx2-GFP into the SVZ but received no QA or sham lesion (n =3-4). All animals, including controls, were transcardially perfused five days post RV injection to allow the same amount of time for cells to respond to lesion-induced signals and migrate. Perfusion was with ice cold 0.9% saline, followed by 400ml 4% paraformaldehyde in 0.1M phosphate buffer pH 7.4. Brains were removed and post fixed overnight at 4°C in 4% paraformaldehyde, then cryoprotected in 30% sucrose in 0.1M phosphate buffer pH 7.2. Sectioning was carried out in sagittal orientation with 40µm between each section.

Immunohistochemistry

Sections were washed 3 x 5 minutes in 1X PBS and 3 x 5 minutes in 1X PBS + 0.2% Triton X-100. Primary antibodies were incubated at room temperature overnight in immunobuffer containing 3% donkey or goat serum in 1X PBS + 0.2% Triton. Primary antibodies used were: GFP (chicken polyclonal, 1:500, Abcam), GFP (rabbit polyclonal, 1:1000, Abcam), Doublecortin C-terminus (goat polyclonal, 1:300, Santa Cruz), NG2 (rabbit polyclonal, 1:300, Chemicon), GFAP (mouse monoclonal, 1:2000, Sigma), Pax6 (rabbit polyclonal, 1:1000, Covance), Dlx2 (rabbit polyclonal, 1:500, Abcam), Olig2 (rabbit polyclonal, 1:500, Chemicon), Brg1 (mouse monoclonal, Santa Cruz 1:100). Sections were then incubated at room temperature for 4 hours in secondary antibodies in immunobuffer. Secondary conjugated antibodies used were goat anti-chicken Alexa Fluor 488, donkey anti-rabbit Alexa Fluor 488, donkey anti-goat Alexa Fluor 594, donkey anti-rabbit Alexa Fluor 594, donkey anti-mouse Alexa Fluor 647 and donkey anti-rabbit Alexa Fluor 647 (all 1:500, Invitrogen).

Quantitative PCR

SVZ tissue was isolated from the brains of QA lesioned animals at 1, 2, 3 and 7 days post lesion (n=3-4). RNA was extracted using the Qiagen Lipid Tissue RNeasy Mini Kit and cDNA synthesized using the SA Bioscience RT^2 First Strand Kit with 400ng purified RNA. Quantitative SYBRgreen PCR was performed on an ABI 7900HT machine and the RT^2 Profiler PCR Array System using a customised SA Biosciences Rat Neurogenesis and Neural Stem Cell PCR Array (PARN 404). SA Bioscience software calculated fold regulatory changes using the ΔΔ Ct method[32] between gene expression in the QA lesioned SVZ compared to control SVZ, normalised to the arthritic mean Ct of the three most stable housekeeping genes of five run (*Rplp1* – Ribosomal protein, large P1, *Rpl13a* – Ribosomal protein L13A and *Ldha* – Lactate dehydrogenase A. Also run were *Hprt1* – Hypoxanthine phosphoribosyltransferase 1 and *Actb* – Beta actin).

Microscopy

GFP-labelled cell counts and morphological analysis was performed under a 40x oil lens on a Zeiss Axioplan fluorescent microscope. DCX, NG2, GFAP, Dlx2, Pax6 and Olig2 immunostaining was imaged at 40x on a Zeiss inverted LSM fluorescent confocal microscope in z series with 3.4µm between each slice, with a tile scan to cover the entire striatum.

Statistical Analysis

The number of GFP-labelled cells observed in the lesioned striatum was totalled from 12 sections per animal, per time point, per virus. Cell numbers were totalled per animal and an average GFP-labelled cells per section calculated. For RV-GFP morphology analysis over time a two way ANOVA was performed. For comparisons of RV-GFP-labelled cells per timepoint a one way ANOVA followed by an all-pair wise Dunnet's multiple comparison post hoc test was performed to compare between groups. GFP-labelled cell co-expression with DCX, Olig2, NG2 or GFAP was quantified from three sections per animal, per time point, per virus. Group values were averaged and reported as the mean +/- standard error of the mean. For comparisons between RV-GFP, RV-Dlx2-GFP and RV-Pax6-GFP labelled cells, a one way ANOVA followed by an all-pair wise Dunnet's multiple comparison post hoc test to compare between groups was used. Control GFP (no QA lesion), day 0 and day 2 RV injection groups were analyzed separately. For qPCR, the normalized fold changes for each group of animals was compared to the normalized fold change of the control group using the student's t test, provided by the SA Biosciences software. Results were considered significant if p<0.05.

Results

Excitotoxin-induced striatal cell loss stimulates recruitment of neuroblasts and oligodendrocyte precursor cells from the subventricular zone into the lesioned striatum

Replication incompetent, pseudotyped GFP retrovirus was injected into the SVZ of QA lesioned animals or non-lesioned controls at a range of time points prior to or following QA injection (Figure 1a-b). Retrovirus has previously been shown to only infect fast dividing cells, including *in vivo* in the adult rodent SVZ[33-36], allowing birth dating and tracking of migration of newborn SVZ-derived precursor cells. Sham-injected (0.9% saline) controls were carried out previously[25] and no striatal migration from SVZ-labelled progenitors was found, with GFP labelled cells remaining within the RMS and migrating normally to the olfactory bulb. Therefore, no chemotaxic property due to injury or inflammation was caused by the surgery alone. To minimize the number of animals used in this study sham controls were not repeated. GFP+ cells recruited into the QA lesioned striatum were quantified 5 days post RV-GFP injection to allow time for migration. In unlesioned control animals GFP cells were found in the SVZ, throughout the RMS (Figure 1c) and olfactory bulb but not in the striatum. In lesioned animals, in agreement with our previous observations[25], GFP-labelled cell recruitment was observed by cells born either two days prior to QA lesioning through to 7 days following QA lesioning, with both bipolar and multipolar phenotypes observed (Figure 1d-i). Significantly more GFP-labelled cells were recruited into the QA lesioned striatum from SVZ progenitors that were born on the day of QA lesioning or two days post QA lesion when compared to controls (Figure 1j; one way ANOVA=0.0032; Dunnett's post hoc test between time points and control p<0.05). At 3, 5 and 7 dpl (days post lesion) small numbers of GFP+ cells labelled were found in the striatum, SVZ and RMS, but the number of GFP cells in the striatum was not significantly different compared to non-lesioned controls.

GFP-labelled cells exhibited either bipolar or multipolar phenotypes[37] and the ratio of these cell types was altered in a temporal manner[25] (Figure 1d-i, k), with a significant change in morphology observed over time (two way ANOVA F6,51=2.941 p=0.019). GFP+ cells labelled on the day of QA lesioning exhibited similar numbers of bipolar and multipolar morphologies, with significantly more bipolar cells in the striatum compared to controls (Figure 1k; one way ANOVA p=0.0016, Dunnett's post hoc test p<0.01). In contrast, there were significantly more multipolar cells labelled 2 days following QA lesioning when compared to controls (Figure 1k; one way ANOVA p=0.013; Dunnett's post hoc test p<0.05). These results suggest that a switch in cell fate may be occurring within the QA lesioned striatum over time.

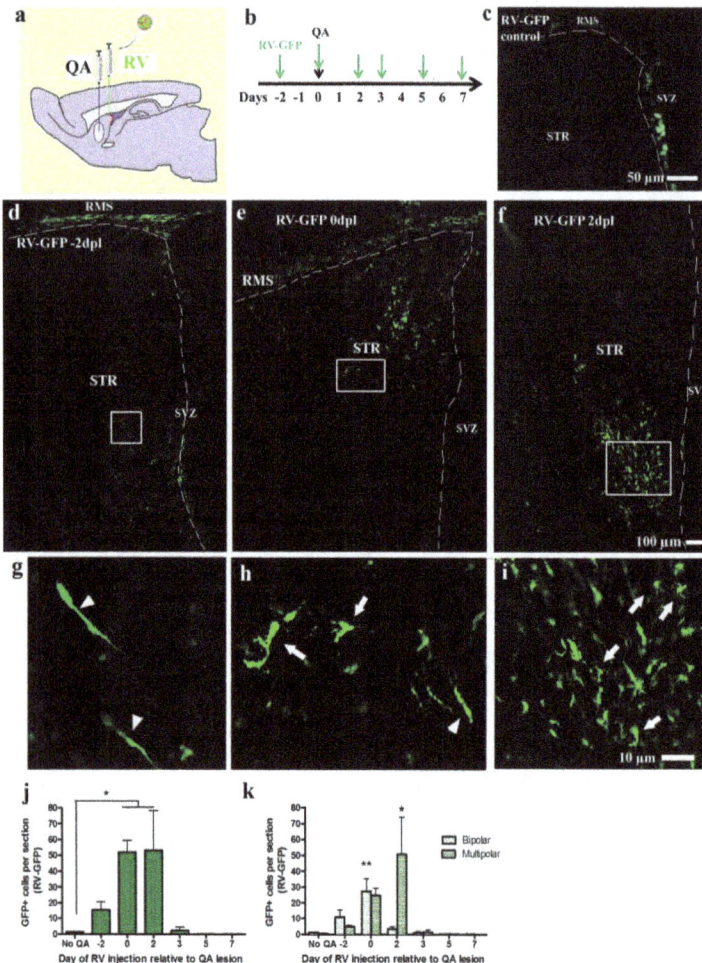

*Figure 1: GFP-labelled cells from the SVZ are recruited into the QA-lesioned striatum and are both bipolar and multipolar. (a-b) Diagram and timeline of QA and RV-GFP injections. GFP-positive cells (green) are found in the SVZ and RMS of non-lesioned controls (c) and in the SVZ, RMS and striatum of lesioned animals (d-f). Confocal images showing GFP cells recruited into the striatum (STR, outlined) labelled in the SVZ two days prior (d), on the day (e), or two days post QA lesioning (f). (g-i) Magnified images of boxes from d-f showing cell morphology. (j-k) Graphs demonstrating (j) the number of GFP-labelled cells per striatal section (12 sections per animal, 3-5 animals per group, one way ANOVA. * P<0.05) and (k) the subdivision of total GFP-labelled cells per section into bipolar and multipolar phenotypes (one way ANOVA, * p<0.05, ** p<0.01) over time (two way ANOVA p<0.05). Scale bar c = 50 μm, d-f = 100 μm and g-I = 10 μm.*

Bipolar cells recruited from the SVZ are routinely described as neuroblasts. Interestingly, while we observed a significant increase in the number of DCX/GFP labelled cells migrating into the striatum from cells labelled on the day of QA lesioning compared to unlesioned controls (Figure 2a, c and g; one way ANOVA p<0.0001; Dunnett's post hoc test p<0.001), characterization also indicated the recruitment of bipolar OLIG2/GFP labelled OPCs from the SVZ (Figure 2b and d). GFP-labelled multipolar cells were found to almost exclusively co-label with the oligodendrocyte markers, OLIG2 and/or NG2 (Figure 2b, e and f). However, both bipolar and multipolar GFP-labelled cell populations contained lineage negative cells that could not be characterized with any of the markers examined including DCX, NG2, GFAP, OLIG2, MASH1, DLX2, or PAX6 (Figure 2h-i). Striatal lineage negative cells were generated from GFP-positive cells at all time points following QA lesioning and were especially prominent in the bipolar cell population. While positive staining was observed with MASH1/GFP, DLX2/GFP and OLIG2/GFP in cells within the SVZ (Supplementary Figure 1) and for DLX2/GFP and DCX/GFP throughout the RMS (Supplementary Figure 2), RV-GFP-labelled cells in the striatum were never found to express either MASH1 or PAX6 indicating either specific recruitment of subtypes of neural precursor cells in the different regions of the brain or down-regulation of specific pro-neurogenic genes in recruited cells. Further, GFAP expression was never observed in any GFP-labelled cells in either the striatum or the SVZ indicating that RV-GFP was not transducing slow dividing Type B stem cells in the SVZ or proliferating GFAP+ glia and that there was no recruitment of GFAP+ glia or stem cells from the SVZ into the lesioned striatum (Supplementary Figure 7). DCX has previously been observed to co-label with NG2 in the cortex, however confocal imaging confirmed that DCX+ neuroblasts in the SVZ and migrating DCX+ cells in the lesioned striatum did not label with NG2 (Supplementary Figure 3), confirming their neuronal fate.

RV-Pax6 over-expression alters the number of striatal GFP cells with multipolar-glial cell phenotypes

Previous studies have shown *Pax6* and *Dlx2* to have a potent neurogenic effect in the adult brain, and *Pax6* coupled with *Olig2* repression able to promote neurogenesis in injury models[13, 18, 19, 29-31]. Based on these previous studies and our lineage tracing results, we investigated whether RV delivery of the pro-neurogenic genes *Pax6* or *Dlx2* directly to precursor cells in the SVZ could overcome the predominantly gliogenic fate of recruited cells migrating into the QA lesioned striatum. We also examined whether *Pax6* or *Dlx2* over-expression would reprogram lineage negative cells towards a neuronal fate. RV-Dlx2-GFP or RV-Pax6-GFP was injected into the SVZ of non-lesioned control animals and reliable co-expression of transgenes with GFP was observed (Supplementary Figure 4a-c and 5a-c). GFP+ cells remained in the SVZ and RMS of unlesioned animals and did not migrate into the striatum (Supplementary Figure 6[25]). RV-Dlx2-GFP or RV-Pax6-GFP was injected into the SVZ either on the day of QA lesioning or 2 days following QA lesioning (Figure 3a), the time points when significant recruitment of GFP-labelled cells was previously observed (Figure 1j). To determine the effect of *Pax6* or *Dlx2* on the recruitment of GFP-labelled cells from the SVZ, total GFP+ cell number was quantified in the striatum for both RV-Pax6 and RV-Dlx2 treated animals. Percentages of GFP-labelled cells in the striatum expressing DCX, OLIG2, NG2 and GFAP were also calculated to examine the effect of *Pax6* or *Dlx2* over-expression on precursor cell lineage following recruitment to the striatum.

Surprisingly, over-expression of *Dlx2* and *Pax6* gave very different results in relation to the number of GFP-labelled cells recruited to the QA lesioned striatum, even though the viruses had identical titres and therefore infected a similar number of cells upon injection into the SVZ. Percentages of cells exhibiting a neuronal fate once recruited into the damaged area were also different between groups. We observed that injection of RV-Pax6 in the SVZ on the day of QA lesioning (day 0) led to a significant reduction in the total number of GFP labelled cells recruited to the lesioned striatum (Figure 3b, red bars), including a decrease in the number of bipolar cells (Figure 3c) and DCX+ neuroblasts (Figure 3d) when compared to RV-GFP controls (green bars). However, when RV-Pax6 was injected two days post lesion, an increase in the recruitment of GFP-labelled cells to the striatum was observed (Figure 3b).

Interestingly, the morphology of these cells was predominantly not bipolar (Figure 3c) and the number of DCX+ cells was unchanged when compared to RV-GFP control animals (Figure 3d). Instead, we observed a significant increase in a multipolar phenotype of GFP-labelled cells in the lesioned striatum in animals injected with RV-Pax6 two days post lesion (Figure 3f) and an increase in NG2 cell number when compared to RV-GFP controls (Figure 3g). However, when the percentage of striatal GFP cells co-expressing subtype specific markers was examined following RV-Pax6 over-expression, we observed that Pax6-GFP+ cells redirected into the QA lesioned striatum retained the same fate profile as RV- GFP controls with no

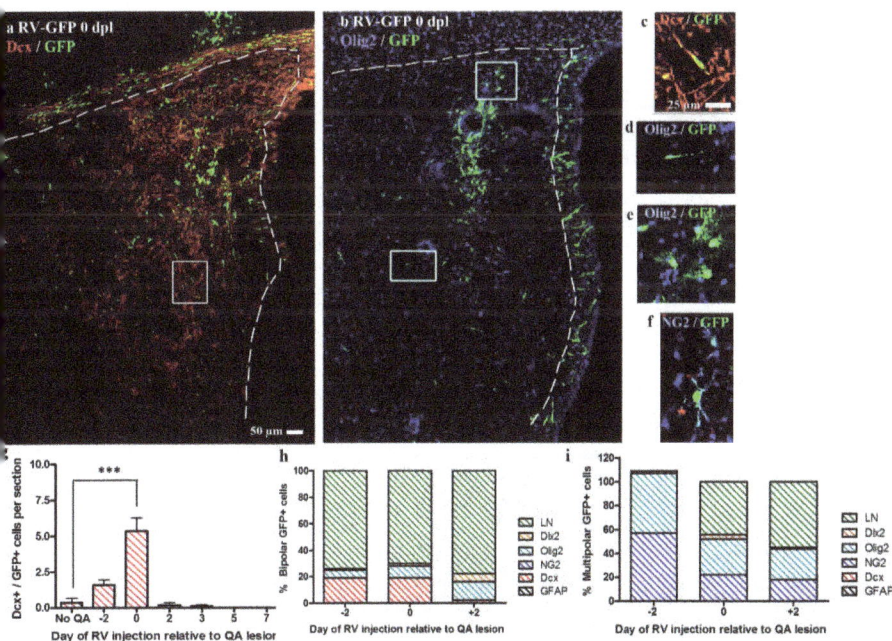

Figure 2: GFP-labelled cells recruited into the QA-lesioned striatum are neuroblasts and oligodendrocyte precursor cells. *Striatal GFP cells (green, outlined area) express (a) DCX (red) and (b) OLIG2 (blue). Bipolar GFP cells can be either neuronal or oligodendrocyte lineage. (c) A bipolar DCX/GFP neuroblast (from box in a), (d) a bipolar OLIG2/GFP oligodendrocyte precursor cell (from the lower boxed region in b). Many multipolar GFP cells are OLIG2/GFP oligodendrocyte precursor cells. (e) OLIG2+ multipolar GFP cells (from the upper boxed region in b) and (f) NG2+ (blue) / GFP+ (green) cells. (g) Graph demonstrating the number of DCX/GFP cells per striatal section (one way ANOVA p<0.0001). (h and i) Graphs demonstrating the percentage of bipolar (h) and multipolar (i) GFP-labelled cells expressing DLX2, OLIG2, NG2, DCX, GFAP or lineage negative (LN). Scale bars a-b = 50 µm, c-f = 25 µm.*

significant alteration observed in the percentage of bipolar cells that expressed either OLIG2 or DCX (Figure 3j-k) or percentage of multipolar cells expressing NG2 when compared to RV-GFP control animals (Figure 3l). These results indicate that Pax6 over-expression was unable to promote SVZ-derived precursor cells to a neuronal fate following recruitment into the QA lesioned striatum.

Dlx2 enhances neuroblast recruitment and retention of a neuronal fate in the QA-lesioned striatum

In contrast to *Pax6*, injection of RV-Dlx2 in the SVZ had no effect on the total number of GFP-labelled cells recruited into the striatum at either time point examined (Figure 3b, blue bars). Further, RV-Dlx2 had no effect on the morphology of GFP+ cells or on DCX+, OLIG2+ or NG2+ cell numbers when injected on the day of QA

lesioning (Day 0, Figure 3c-g). However, we observed that injection of RV-Dlx2 2 days following lesioning significantly increased both the number of bipolar GFP-labelled cells (Figure 3c) and the number of DCX/GFP neuroblasts compared to controls (Figure 3d) while not changing the number of multipolar cells or affecting OLIG2 or NG2 cell number (Figure 3e-g). Notably, when labelled at 2 days post lesion, the percentage of bipolar cells was significantly increased in the striatum (Figure 3h) and the percentage of DCX/GFP neuroblasts was also significantly increased to ~ 25% of the bipolar GFP+ population when compared to controls (Figure 3j, m-o). This occurred in conjunction with a significant reduction in multipolar cell fate (Figure 3i), while percentages of OLIG2/GFP and NG2/GFP expressing cells remained unchanged (Figure 3k-l). This may indicate that ectopic *Dlx2* expression can induce lineage negative GFP cells to a neuronal fate.

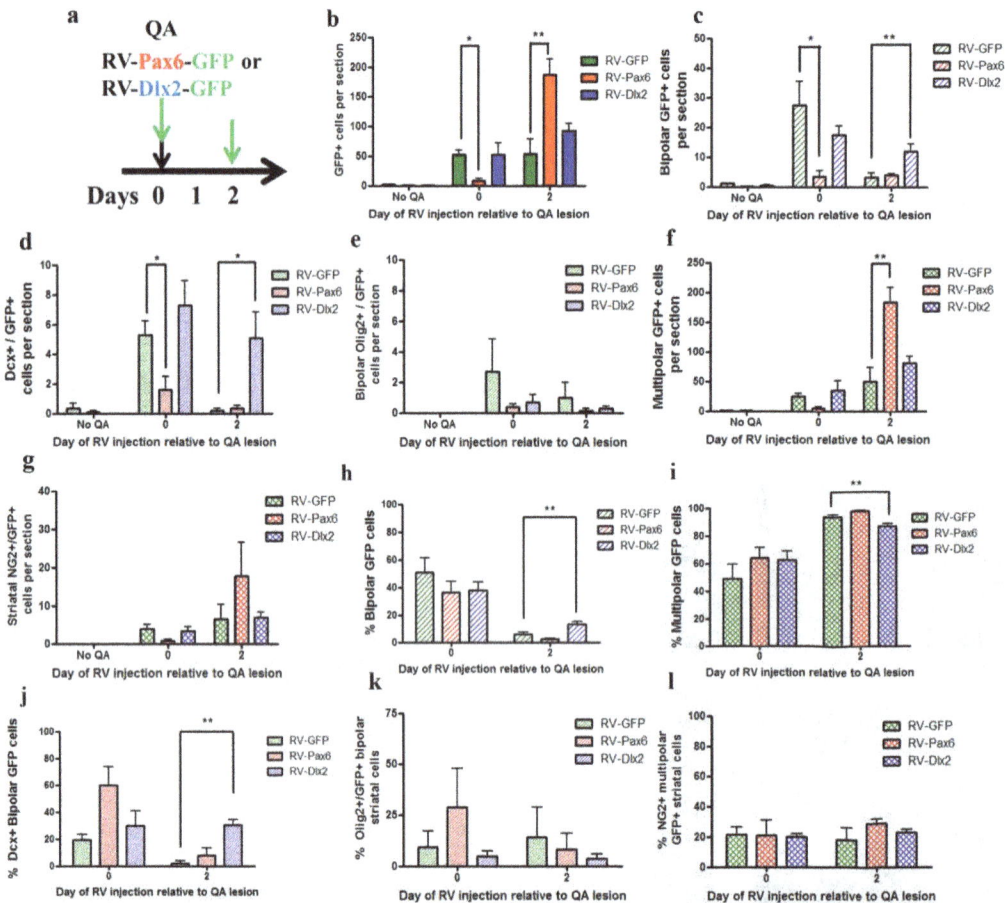

Figure 3: Ectopic expression of Pax6 or Dlx2 in SVZ-derived precursor cells following QA-induced striatal lesioning alters GFP-labelled cell number, morphology and fate in the striatum. (a) Time line of QA and RV-Pax6 or RV-Dlx2 injections. (b-l) Graphs demonstrating: (b) the number of GFP-labelled cells per striatal section; (c) the number of bipolar GFP-labelled cells per striatal section; (d) the number of DCX/GFP cells per striatal section; (e) the number of bipolar OLIG2/GFP cells per striatal section; (f) the number of multipolar cells per striatal section; (g) the number of NG2/GFP cells per striatal section; (h) the percentage of GFP-labelled cells exhibiting a bipolar morphology; (i) the percentage of GFP-labelled cells exhibiting a multipolar morphology; (j) the percentage of bipolar DCX/GFP cells; (k) the percentage of bipolar OLIG2/GFP cells; and (l) the percentage of multipolar NG2/GFP cells in the QA lesioned striatum (all one way ANOVAs * P<0.05; ** P<0.01). (m-o) Images of GFP (green)/DCX (red) labelling from (m) RV-Dlx2-GFP in no-lesion controls (n) RV-GFP day 2 controls and (o) RV-Dlx2-GFP day 2 animals. Scale m-o = 100 μm.

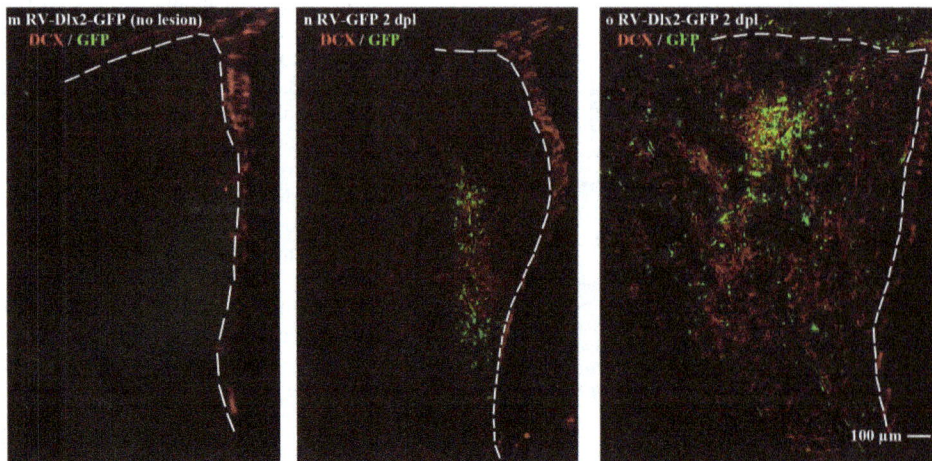

Interestingly, while both ectopic DLX2 and PAX6 could be detected in 83-92% of all RV-GFP labelled cells in SVZ of non-lesioned control animals (Supplementary Figure 4 a-c and 5 a-c), down-regulation of transgenes was observed in the majority of GFP-labelled cells recruited into the striatum from animals injected at 2 days post lesion (Figure 4 a-f). Only 2-3% of striatal GFP+ cells remained expressing PAX6 and DLX2. Similarly while *Brg1*, an essential gene for the pro-neurogenic function of bipolar SVZ PAX6 progenitor cells[38], was observed in the SVZ of bipolar RV-PAX6-GFP cells (Figure 4 g-j) and some GFP+ multipolar cells near to the RMS, it was absent in multipolar RV-PAX6-GFP+ cells in the striatum, of which some also stained for NG2 (Figure 4k, l-s). This further indicates the loss of neuronal function in RV-PAX6 recruited cells. These findings indicate that *Dlx2*, while downregulated in many GFP cells of the striatum, does retain a significant effect on both the recruitment and regulation of DCX+ neuroblasts within the damaged striatum at acute time points post QA lesion.

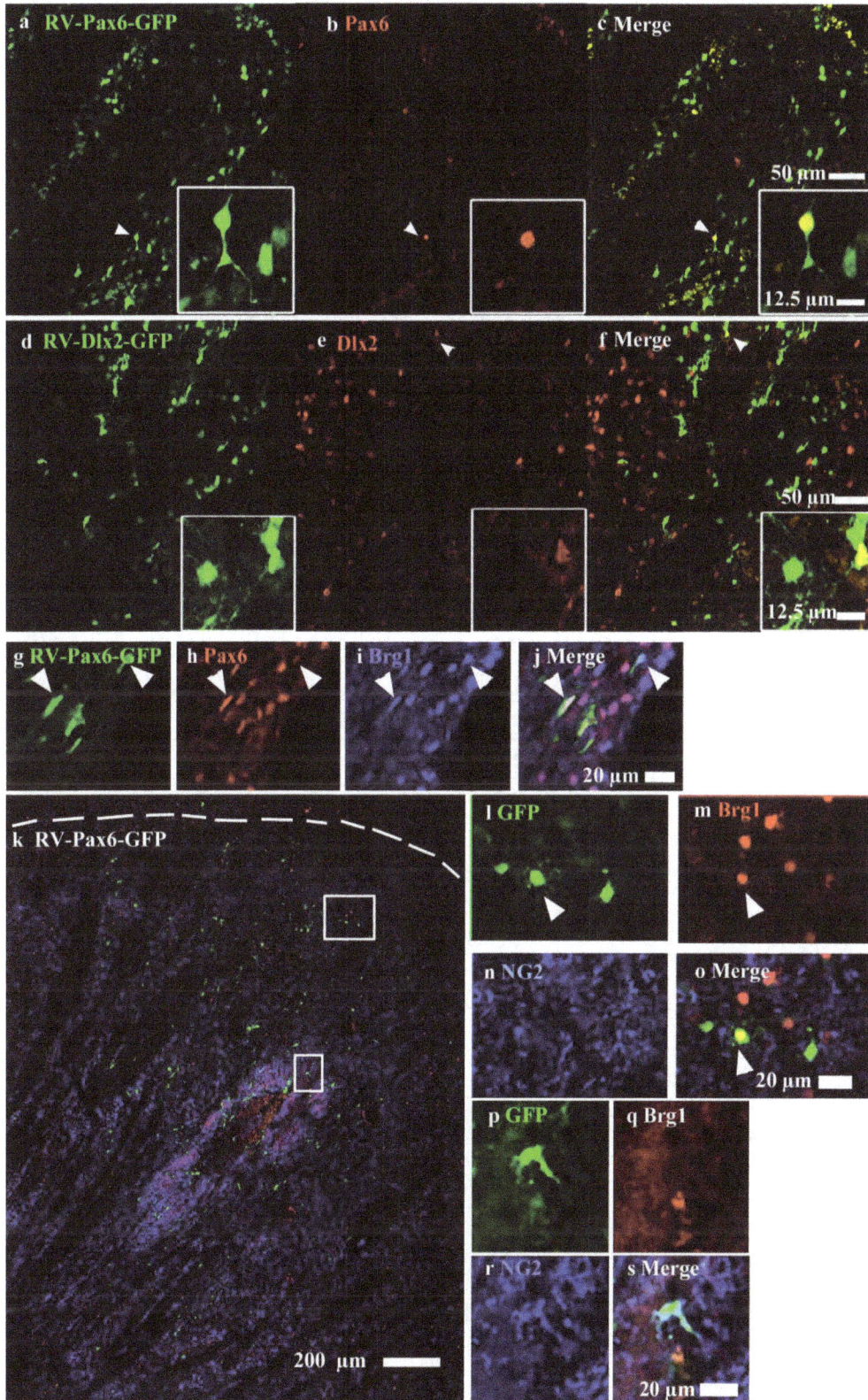

Figure 4: Down-regulation of transgene expression in the QA lesioned stratum and BRG1 expression.

PAX6 expression from RV-Pax6-GFP (a-c) and DLX2 expression from RV-Dlx2-GFP (d-f) is down-regulated in the lesioned striatum from cells labelled at 2dpl. Arrowheads show few remaining positive co-expressing cells. (g-j) Bipolar RV-Pax6-GFP cells (green) in the SVZ co-express PAX6 (red) and BRG1 (blue). Arrowheads indicate two triple labelled cells. (k-s) In RV-Pax6-GFP animals, a few BRG+ / multipolar GFP+ cells are observed close to the SVZ and RMS (l-o, upper boxed area), however all GFP+ multipolar cells further into the lesioned area and all NG2 / GFP+ cells are BRG negative (p-s, lower boxed area). Scales a-f = 50 μm, boxed area a-f 12.5 μm, g-j and l-s = 20 μm and k = 200 μm

The expression of signalling molecules in the SVZ following QA-induced striatal injury

Using quantitative PCR, we examined mRNA expression of a number of signalling molecules in the SVZ at 1, 2, 3 and 7 days post lesion in order to identify QA lesion-induced changes that may be implicated in the phenotypic switch of neural precursor cells in the lesioned environment. Changes in mRNA expression were observed in many of the main signalling families, including the BMP and Notch pathways and in molecules that are known to regulate the proliferation and migration of neural precursor cells (Table 1).

Bmp4, *Hey1*, *Heyl*, *Tnr* and *pleiotropin* mRNA expression was reduced in the first 1-2 days post QA lesion, then *Bmp4*, *Tnr* and *pleiotropin* significantly increased at 3 days post lesion, and *Hes1* at 7dpl when compared to unlesioned controls. *Stat3* was increased throughout the time course, while *Noggin* was significantly increased at day 3. Further, a range of genes including *Robo1*, *Smad4* and *BMP2* were significantly reduced from day 1 up to days 3 to 7 post QA lesion. In addition, we observed a significant increase in the expression of *Fgf2* and *Bdnf* mRNA from 1 to 3 days post QA lesion while expression of *Fgf13* and *Vegf* mRNA was reduced when compared to unlesioned controls.

Gene	1 dpl Fold Δ	Sig.	2 dpl Fold Δ	Sig.	3 dpl Fold Δ	Sig.	7 dpl Fold Δ	Sig.
Bdnf	11.4	*	18.4	*	4.0	*	11.2	ns
Fgf2	4.1	***	1.7	*	1.8	**	1.6	ns
Fgf13	-2.8	**	-1.7	*	-3.2	**	1.3	ns
Vegf	-2.6	***	-1.9	***	-2.0	***	-1.7	***
Bai1	-3.3	**	-1.4	**	-1.5	*	1.1	ns
Artn	-1.8	**	1.0	ns	-2.2	**	1.0	ns
Fez1	-2.9	***	-1.6	***	-1.4	**	-1.2	ns
Ptn	-1.6	***	1.1	ns	1.7	***	1.0	ns
Mdk	-1.3	**	-1.5	**	1.1	ns	1.4	ns
Nrg1	-2.1	***	1.4	ns	-2.9	**	1.1	ns
Bmp2	-3.0	**	-3.6	**	-2.2	*	-2.1	*
Bmp4	-2.4	**	-1.4	ns	2.4	**	1.7	*
Smad4	-1.3	**	-1.4	***	-1.2	ns	1.0	ns
Noggin	-1.6	ns	1.1	ns	1.8	**	1.3	ns
Stat3	4.2	***	2.2	**	2.6	***	2.0	**
Nrp2	2.3	***	1.7	**	2.1	**	3.7	ns
Nrp1	1.1	ns	1.6	ns	2.0	**	2.1	*
Robo1	-2.7	***	-1.4	**	-1.6	*	-1.1	ns
Ntn1	-2.2	***	-1.5	**	-1.2	ns	-1.3	ns
Hes1	1.1	ns	1.1	ns	1.5	ns	1.8	**
Heyl	-3.1	***	-1.7	**	1.1	ns	-1.2	ns
Hey1	-3.0	***	-1.8	**	-1.1	ns	-1.3	ns
Notch2	1.0	ns	-1.1	ns	1.5	ns	1.3	ns
Tnr	-2.2	***	-2.1	ns	2.0	***	1.2	ns

*Table 1: mRNA expression levels of signalling molecules in the SVZ following QA striatal lesioning. Fold changes shown in blue represent significant (sig.) down-regulation greater than 1.5 fold compared to unlesioned control; fold changes shown in red represent significant up-regulation greater than 1.5 fold compared to unlesioned control. Sign. = Significance; dpl = days post lesion; * P<0.05, ** P<0.01, *** P <0.001, ns=not significant.*

Discussion

While compensatory adult neurogenesis has been demonstrated in many models of brain injury, the correct cell types are not always generated for successful endogenous repair. We previously described transient SVZ precursor cell recruitment into the striatum following an excitotoxic injury, which exhibited a predominantly glial response[6, 25]. We have now confirmed that recruited cells of a bipolar morphology represent both neuroblasts and oligodendrocyte progenitor cells and that a proportion of multipolar cells are oligodendrocyte progenitors, but not astrocytes. Results observed in a Nestin-CreER[T2]:R26R-YFP mouse stroke model reported similar percentages of recruited Dcx and NG2 progenitors as reported in our RV-GFP study, at 6 weeks post injury, but also identified a large percentage of GFAP+ astrocytes recruited into the striatum[39]. Astrocyte recruitment is not observed in our QA lesion model at the time points we examined, indicating endogenous repair mechanisms do vary between disease models and perhaps between species[39].

Pro-neurogenic transcription factor delivery has been trialled as a mechanism to enhance the regenerative response to neural damage, with studies demonstrating moderate success when injecting pro-neurogenic transcription factors directly into damaged brain parenchyma[12, 17-19, 27, 28]. The current study therefore aimed to convert the observed gliogenic response to a neurogenic one by individually over-expressing the pro-neurogenic genes *Pax6* or *Dlx2* in SVZ-derived neural precursors. Interestingly we found that only ectopic *Dlx2* expression was able to overcome signals released from damaged tissue and enhance both neuroblast recruitment and the percentage of recruited cells that retained a neuronal fate in the QA lesioned striatum. We propose this may reflect the importance the microenvironment plays in regulating neural cell fate following injury or disease.

While it is believed that *Dlx2* and *Pax6* may have similar roles in promoting adult SVZ neurogenesis[12, 40], very different results were observed in the current study following *Dlx2* over-expression when compared to *Pax6*. This may be explained by different complements of chemokine receptors on PAX6+ and DLX2+ precursor cells, as inflammatory-induced chemoattractants play an essential role in neuroblast and OPC recruitment[3, 41-44] and have been shown to be expressed in the QA lesioned striatum[41, 42]. While DLX2+ precursor cells have been observed to migrate towards chemoattractants during forebrain development[45], expression of chemokine receptors specifically on adult SVZ-derived PAX6+ or DLX2+ precursor cells has never has been examined. We thus propose the pan-cell type decrease in Pax6-GFP cells observed in the striatum of animals labelled at the time of QA lesioning may indicate that RV-Pax6 over-expression has generated PAX6+ precursor cells (possibly TAPs) which either do not express the complement of chemokine receptors required to respond to migratory cues released from the QA lesioned striatum at the time of lesioning or chemokines that attract PAX6+ precursor cells may not be secreted from the QA lesioned striatum at this immediate time point. Lack of appropriate chemokine signalling is likely because PAX6+ cells labelled two days post lesioning were recruited in large numbers to lesioned striatum. It is also possible that the RV-Pax6 cells are recruited into the striatum to a similar extent as the GFP and RV-Dlx2 cells, but do not survive at the early time point, while increasing proliferation at the latter time point. Further analysis is required however to identify the chemokine/signalling molecule(s) responsible for this *Pax6*-dependant effect.

In contrast, *Dlx2* over-expression at both time points examined did not lead to a change in the number of recruited GFP+ cells to the striatum, suggesting these cells may be responding to a different chemokine or complement of chemokines. Over-expression of *Dlx2* has been shown to promote reprogramming of adult cortical astroglia into functional GABAergic neurons *in vitro*, under both normal conditions and in cortical astrocytes responding to injury[46, 47]. *Dlx2* is also believed to repress oligodendrogenesis by suppressing *Olig2* in the adult SVZ through a BMP mediated mechanism[31]. Consistent with this, RV-DLX2 expression did increase total bipolar GFP+ cell recruitment and DCX+ cell number, in conjunction with a reduction in multipolar GFP+ cell number when compared to RV-GFP control animals. However, as OLIG2+ and NG2+ cell numbers remained unchanged this suggests that instead of suppressing *Olig2* expression, *Dlx2* may be altering the fate of the lineage negative GFP+ cells identified in controls. While DCX has been observed to co-label with NG2 in the cortex[48], confocal imaging confirmed that DCX+ neuroblasts in the SVZ and migrating into the lesioned striatum do not express NG2, establishing their neuronal fate in the striatum. Unfortunately, staining for mature neuronal markers was not able to be performed due to the immature fate of the cells. Therefore, in contrast to *Pax6*, *Dlx2* over-expression in SVZ precursor cells has a significant neurogenic effect within the QA lesioned striatum.

In contrast to previous work[18, 19], we observed that over-expression of *Pax6* in SVZ-derived precursor cells was unable to promote an increase in DCX+ cell recruitment in the QA lesioned striatum. Instead, ectopic PAX6 expression appeared to promote an oligo-glial cell fate. Ninkovic and colleagues[38] have reported that adult SVZ neurogenesis regulated by *Pax6* is co-dependant on a Brg-containing BAF chromatin remodelling complex. Loss of either *Pax6* or *Brg1* alters the fate of adult SVZ-derived precursor cells. Specifically, in the parenchyma surrounding the SVZ and RMS, loss of *Pax6* or *Brg1* altered neuroblast lineage to OLIG2+ and/or NG2+ OPCs, starting in the RMS and this effect was specific to PAX6 progenitors. While we saw positive staining of RV-PAX6-GFP cells with PAX6 and BRG1 in the SVZ, we also observed an absence of PAX6 and BRG1 in RV-PAX6-GFP cells in the striatum that acquired a multipolar fate and some of which were positive for NG2. This suggests signals released after QA lesioning may be promoting the alteration of SVZ-derived *Pax6*-expressing cells to an oligodendroglial fate, resulting in the reduction in DCX+ neuroblasts observed. We also observed some BRG1+ immunostaining for RV-DLX2-GFP cells in both bipolar and multipolar cells of the striatum (data not shown), indicating a different regulatory role for *Brg1* to the one it plays for *Pax6*. This is unsurprising as *Brg1* control of neurogenesis was found to be specific for *Pax6*[38]. Jablonska and colleagues (2010) also found alterations in BMP signals in the SVZ which led PAX6+ neuronal precursor cells to switch their molecular, cellular and migratory paths towards an oligodendrocyte lineage following white matter injury[24]. In the current study we also observed alterations in SVZ BMP signalling following QA lesion that could have impacted the increase in glial cell fate found with RV-Pax6. In addition to dynamic changes in *Bmp2* and *Bmp4* expression, we found significant up-regulation of *Stat3*, *Fgf2*, *Bdnf*, *Hes1*, and *Noggin*. These changes were coupled with significant decreases in many other molecules and growth factors indicating the complex environmental regulation within the SVZ precursor pool after injury.

It is interesting to observe such dynamic changes in signalling molecules in the SVZ after a striatal lesion, but it is difficult to fully understand how or in fact which of these molecules are acting specifically on the Dlx2 and Pax6 TAPS or neuroblasts of the SVZ, as to date very few studies have been performed to examine the range of receptors on these cells. Further, when tissue is collected for gene expression analysis the entire SVZ is pooled, resulting in a heterogeneous mix of all cell types. This means only the 'big picture' and not effects on specific cell types can be observed. Further studies are needed to tease out the specific effects of each signalling factor on the individual cells of the SVZ.

Interestingly, two recent papers have identified parenchymal astrocytes in the mouse striatum that can respond to QA lesion or stroke induced signals, up-regulate *Mash1* and generate DCX+ neuroblasts contributing to striatal regeneration[8, 9]. A role for decreased *Notch* signalling within these cells in the striatum was implicated for this endogenous repair mechanism. We also observed down-regulation in some components of the Notch signalling pathway in the SVZ immediately following lesioning, further supporting that lesion-induced cues can alter Notch regulation of SVZ neurogenesis. It is exciting to note that the rodent brain appears to retain the capacity for both acute recruitment of cells from the SVZ immediately following injury (within the first 2 days following QA lesion) and a longer term ability to regenerate neuroblasts from striatal astrocytes activating a neurogenic programme (from 2 weeks post injury)[8, 9, 25, 39]. Our study only examined acute time points following striatal lesioning which may be why we did not observe parenchymal astrocyte neurogenesis. Long term survival and differentiation studies on RV-Pax6 and RV-Dlx2 cells will offer more information on fate-switching and the endogenous repair potential from both recruited SVZ cells and neurogenic striatal astrocytes.

Conclusion

The current study demonstrates that RV-Dlx2 over-expression in SVZ-derived progenitors can stimulate acute neuroblast recruitment and retention of a neuronal fate in an excitotoxic lesion model at a previously non-neurogenic time point. In contrast, over-expression of *Pax6* in SVZ-derived progenitor cells was not successful at inhibiting an oligodendrocyte fate and resulted in increased multipolar cell numbers with no change in neuronal recruitment. This indicates a complex interaction between signals released from the lesioned environment and gene expression in recruited cells. To promote successful endogenous repair after injury, we first need to better understand which lesion-induced signals are recruiting the subsets of SVZ progenitors into the striatum, and also how they are altering cell fate determination during this endogenous repair process.

References

1. Curtis MA, Penney EB, Pearson AG, van Roon-Mom WM, Butterworth NJ, Dragunow M, Connor B, Faull RL. Increased cell proliferation and neurogenesis in the adult human Huntington's disease brain. Proc Natl Acad Sci U S A. 2003; 100(15): 9023-27.

2. Jones KS, Connor B. Proneural transcription factors Dlx2 and Pax6 are altered in adult SVZ neural precursor cells following striatal cell loss. Mol Cell Neurosci. 2011; 47(1): 53-60.

3. Cayre M, Canoll P, Goldman JE. Cell migration in the normal and pathological postnatal mammalian brain. Prog Neurobiol. 2009; 88(1): 41-63.

4. Kernie SG, Parent JM. Forebrain neurogenesis after focal Ischemic and traumatic brain injury. Neurobiol Dis. 2010; 37(2): 267-74.

5. Zhang RL, Zhang ZG, Chopp M. Ischemic stroke and neurogenesis in the subventricular zone. Neuropharmacology. 2008; 55(3): 345-52.

6. Tattersfield AS, Croon RJ, Liu YW, Kells AP, Faull RL, Connor B. Neurogenesis in the striatum of the quinolinic acid lesion model of Huntington's disease. Neuroscience. 2004; 127(2): 319-32.

7. Ninkovic J, Gotz M. Fate specification in the adult brain--lessons for eliciting neurogenesis from glial cells. Bioessays. 2013; 35(3): 242-52.

8. Nato G, Caramello A, Trova S, Avataneo V, Rolando C, Taylor V, Buffo A, Peretto P, Luzzati F. Striatal astrocytes produce neuroblasts in an excitotoxic model of Huntington's disease. Development. 2015; 142(5): 840-45.

9. Magnusson JP, Goritz C, Tatarishvili J, Dias DO, Smith EM, Lindvall O, Kokaia Z, Frisen J. A latent neurogenic program in astrocytes regulated by Notch signaling in the mouse. Science. 2014; 346(6206): 237-41.

10. Alvarez-Buylla A, Garcia-Verdugo JM. Neurogenesis in adult subventricular zone. J Neurosci. 2002; 22(3): 629-34.

11. Parras CM, Galli R, Britz O, Soares S, Galichet C, Battiste J, Johnson JE, Nakafuku M, Vescovi A, Guillemot F. Mash1 specifies neurons and oligodendrocytes in the postnatal brain. Embo J. 2004; 23(22): 4495-4505.

12. Brill MS, Snapyan M, Wohlfrom H, Ninkovic J, Jawerka M, Mastick GS, Ashery-Padan R, Saghatelyan A, Berninger B, Gotz M. A dlx2- and pax6-dependent transcriptional code for periglomerular neuron specification in the adult olfactory bulb. J Neurosci. 2008; 28(25): 6439-52.

13. Hack MA, Saghatelyan A, de Chevigny A, Pfeifer A, Ashery-Padan R, Lledo PM, Gotz M. Neuronal fate determinants of adult olfactory bulb neurogenesis. Nat Neurosci. 2005; 8(7): 865-72.

14. Roybon L, Deierborg T, Brundin P, Li JY. Involvement of Ngn2, Tbr and NeuroD proteins during postnatal olfactory bulb neurogenesis. Eur J Neurosci. 2009; 29(2): 232-43.

15. Kohwi M, Osumi N, Rubenstein JL, Alvarez-Buylla A. Pax6 is required for making specific subpopulations of granule and periglomerular neurons in the olfactory bulb. J Neurosci. 2005; 25(30): 6997-7003.

16. Brill MS, Ninkovic J, Winpenny E, Hodge RD, Ozen I, Yang R, Lepier A, Gascon S, Erdelyi F, Szabo G, Parras C, Guillemot F, Frotscher M, Berninger B, Hevner RF, Raineteau O, Gotz M. Adult generation of glutamatergic olfactory bulb interneurons. Nat Neurosci. 2009; 12(12): 1524-33.

17. Zhang RL, Chopp M, Roberts C, Jia L, Wei M, Lu M, Wang X, Pourabdollah S, Zhang ZG. Ascl1 lineage cells contribute to ischemia-induced neurogenesis and oligodendrogenesis. J Cereb Blood Flow Metab. 2011; 31(2): 614-25.

18. Kronenberg G, Gertz K, Cheung G, Buffo A, Kettenmann H, Gotz M, Endres M. Modulation of fate determinants Olig2 and Pax6 in resident glia evokes spiking neuroblasts in a model of mild brain ischemia. Stroke. 2010; 41(12): 2944-49.

19. Buffo A, Vosko MR, Erturk D, Hamann GF, Jucker M, Rowitch D, Gotz M. Expression pattern of the transcription factor Olig2 in response to brain injuries: implications for neuronal repair. Proc Natl Acad Sci U S A. 2005; 102(50): 18183-188.

20. Wei B, Nie Y, Li X, Wang C, Ma T, Huang Z, Tian M, Sun C, Cai Y, You Y, Liu F, Yang Z. Emx1-expressing neural stem cells in the subventricular zone give rise to new interneurons in the ischemic injured striatum. Eur J Neurosci. 2011; 33(5): 819-30.

21. Yang Z, You Y, Levison SW. Neonatal hypoxic/ischemic brain injury induces production of calretinin-expressing interneurons in the striatum. J Comp Neurol. 2008; 511(1): 19-33.

22. Arvidsson A, Collin T, Kirik D, Kokaia Z, Lindvall O. Neuronal replacement from endogenous precursors in the adult brain after stroke. Nat Med. 2002; 8(9): 963-70.

23. Parent JM, Vexler ZS, Gong C, Derugin N, Ferriero DM. Rat forebrain neurogenesis and striatal neuron replacement after focal stroke. Ann Neurol. 2002; 52(6): 802-13.

24. Jablonska B, Aguirre A, Raymond M, Szabo G, Kitabatake Y, Sailor KA, Ming GL, Song H, Gallo V. Chordin-induced lineage plasticity of adult SVZ neuroblasts after demyelination. Nat Neurosci. 2010; 13(5): 541-50.

25. Gordon RJ, Tattersfield AS, Vazey EM, Kells AP, McGregor AL, Hughes SM, Connor B. Temporal profile of subventricular zone progenitor cell migration following quinolinic acid-induced striatal cell loss. Neuroscience. 2007; 146(4): 1704-18.

26. Thored P, Arvidsson A, Cacci E, Ahlenius H, Kallur T, Darsalia V, Ekdahl CT, Kokaia Z, Lindvall O. Persistent production of neurons from adult brain stem cells during recovery after stroke. Stem Cells. 2006; 24(3): 739-47.

27. Tepavcevic V, Lazarini F, Alfaro-Cervello C, Kerninon C, Yoshikawa K, Garcia-Verdugo JM, Lledo PM, Nait-Oumesmar B, Baron-Van Evercooren A. Inflammation-induced subventricular zone dysfunction leads to olfactory deficits in a targeted mouse model of multiple sclerosis. J Clin Invest. 2011; 121(12): 4722-34.

28. Grande A, Sumiyoshi K, Lopez-Juarez A, Howard J, Sakthivel B, Aronow B, Campbell K, Nakafuku M. Environmental impact on direct neuronal reprogramming in vivo in the adult brain. Nat Commun. 2013; 4: 2373.

29. Hack MA, Sugimori M, Lundberg C, Nakafuku M, Gotz M. Regionalization and fate specification in neurospheres: the role of Olig2 and Pax6. Mol Cell Neurosci. 2004; 25(4): 664-78.

30. Heins N, Malatesta P, Cecconi F, Nakafuku M, Tucker KL, Hack MA, Chapouton P, Barde YA, Gotz M. Glial cells generate neurons: the role of the transcription factor Pax6. Nat Neurosci. 2002; 5(4): 308-15.

31. Colak D, Mori T, Brill MS, Pfeifer A, Falk S, Deng C, Monteiro R, Mummery C, Sommer L, Gotz M. Adult neurogenesis requires Smad4-mediated bone morphogenic protein signaling in stem cells. J Neurosci. 2008; 28(2): 434-46.

32. Livak KJ, Schmittgen TD. Analysis of relative gene expression data using real-time quantitative PCR and the 2(-Delta Delta C(T)) Method. Methods. 2001; 25(4): 402-08.

33. Miller DG, Adam MA, Miller AD. Gene transfer by retrovirus vectors occurs only in cells that are actively replicating at the time of infection. Mol Cell Biol. 1990; 10(8): 4239-42.

34. Aguirre A, Gallo V. Reduced EGFR signaling in progenitor cells of the adult subventricular zone attenuates oligodendrogenesis after demyelination. Neuron Glia Biol. 2007; 3(3): 209-20.

35. Ming GL, Song H. Adult neurogenesis in the mammalian central nervous system. Annu Rev Neurosci. 2005; 28: 223-50.

36. Lewis PF, Emerman M. Passage through mitosis is required for oncoretroviruses but not for the human immunodeficiency virus J Virol. 1994;68(1):510-6.

37. Nishiyama A. Polydendrocytes: NG2 cells with many roles in development and repair of the CNS. Neuroscientist. 2007; 13(1): 62-76.

38. Ninkovic J, Steiner-Mezzadri A, Jawerka M, Akinci U, Masserdotti G, Petricca S, Fischer J, von Holst A, Beckers J, Lie CD, Petrik D, Miller E, Tang J, Wu J, Lefebvre V, Demmers J, Eisch A, Metzger D, Crabtree G, Irmler M, Poot R, Gotz M. The BAF Complex Interacts with Pax6 in Adult Neural Progenitors to Establish a Neurogenic Cross-Regulatory Transcriptional Network. Cell Stem Cell. 2013; 13(4): 403-18.

39. Li L, Harms KM, Ventura PB, Lagace DC, Eisch AJ, Cunningham LA. Focal cerebral ischemia induces a multilineage cytogenic response from adult subventricular zone that is predominantly gliogenic. Glia. 2010; 58(13): 1610-19.

40. de Chevigny A, Core N, Follert P, Wild S, Bosio A, Yoshikawa K, Cremer H, Beclin C. Dynamic expression of the pro-dopaminergic transcription factors Pax6 and Dlx2 during postnatal olfactory bulb neurogenesis. Front Cell Neurosci. 2012; 6: 6.

41. Connor B, Gordon RJ, Jones KS, Maucksch C. Deviating from the well travelled path: Precursor cell migration in the pathological adult mammalian brain. J Cell Biochem. 2011; 112(6): 1467-74.

42. Gordon RJ, McGregor AL, Connor B. Chemokines direct neural progenitor cell migration following striatal cell loss. Mol Cell Neurosci. 2009; 41(2): 219-32.

43. Tsai HH, Frost E, To V, Robinson S, Ffrench-Constant C, Geertman R, Ransohoff RM, Miller RH. The chemokine receptor CXCR2 controls positioning of oligodendrocyte precursors in developing spinal cord by arresting their migration. Cell. 2002; 110(3): 373-83.

44. Banisadr G, Frederick TJ, Freitag C, Ren D, Jung H, Miller SD, Miller RJ. The role of CXCR4 signaling in the migration of transplanted oligodendrocyte progenitors into the cerebral white matter. Neurobiol Dis. 2011; 44(1): 19-27.

45. Tiveron MC, Rossel M, Moepps B, Zhang YL, Seidenfaden R, Favor J, Konig N, Cremer H. Molecular interaction between projection neuron precursors and invading interneurons via stromal-derived factor 1 (CXCL12)/CXCR4 signaling in the cortical subventricular zone/intermediate zone. J Neurosci. 2006; 26(51): 13273-78.

46. Blum R, Heinrich C, Sanchez R, Lepier A, Gundelfinger ED, Berninger B, Gotz M. Neuronal network formation from reprogrammed early postnatal rat cortical glial cells. Cereb Cortex. 2010; 21(2): 413-24.

47. Heinrich C, Blum R, Gascon S, Masserdotti G, Tripathi P, Sanchez R, Tiedt S, Schroeder T, Gotz M, Berninger B. Directing astroglia from the cerebral cortex into subtype specific functional neurons. PLoS Biol. 2010; 8(5): e10000373.

48. Tamura Y, Kataoka Y, Cui Y, Takamori Y, Watanabe Y, Yamada H. Multi-directional differentiation of doublecortin- and NG2-immunopositive progenitor cells in the adult rat neocortex in vivo. Eur J Neurosci. 2007; 25(12): 3489-98.

Abbreviations

RV:	Retroviral
SVZ:	Subventricular zone
OPC :	Oligodendrocyte precursor cells
TAPs :	Transiently Amplifying Precursors
NPCs :	Neural Progenitor Cells
RV :	Retrovirus
QA :	Quinolinic Acid
DPL:	Days post lesion
DPI:	Days post injection

Potential Conflicts of Interests

None

Acknowledgments

The authors would like to thank Professor Magdalena Gotz for kindly donating the plasmids for use in this study.

Sponsors / Grants

Funding was provided by the Neurological Foundation of New Zealand (66 Grafton Rd, Grafton, Auckland, New Zealand), and the Health Research Council of New Zealand (Level 3, 110 Stanley St, Grafton, Auckland 1010). Jones KS was supported by a Neurological Foundation of NZ Postgraduate Scholarship.

Additional Information

Supplementary Information accompanies this article. Supplementary figures are linked to the online version of the article.

Corresponding Author

Bronwen J Connor, Centre for Brain Research, Department of Pharmacology and Clinical Pharmacology, School of Medical Science, Faculty of Medical and Health Sciences, University of Auckland, 85 Park Road, Grafton, Auckland, New Zealand 1023. Email: b.connor@auckland.ac.nz

Comparing the *in vivo* and *in vitro* effects of hypoxia (3% O$_2$) on directly derived cells from murine cardiac explants versus murine cardiosphere derived cells

Amirrasouli MM[1,2,3], Shamsara M[2]

Abstract

Coronary heart disease (CHD) is still one of the main causes of death in the world, despite significant advances in clinical treatments. Stem cell transplantation methods have the potential to improve cardiac function and patients' outcome following heart attack, but optimal cell types, cell preparation methods and cell delivery routes are yet to be developed. Mammalian hearts contain a small fraction of progenitor cells which, in culture, migrate out of the cardiac explants, known as explant-derived cell (EDCs) and contribute to spheroids known as cardiospheres (Csphs). Following further culture and cell passaging, Csphs give rise to cardiosphere-derived cells (CDCs). EDCs, Csphs and CDCs show *in vitro* and *in vivo* angiogenesis and tissue regeneration in myocardial ischemia. However, CDC and Csph formation is time consuming, expensive and not always successful. Therefore, this study aims to compare EDCs with CDCs and assess the effect of hypoxic preconditioning on their pro-angiogenic potential. The data showed that preconditioning EDCs in hypoxic cell culture enhances cell growth, viability and expression of stem cell and pro-angiogenic markers more than CDCs. *In vivo* experiments using a sub-dermal matrigel plug assay showed that EDCs and CDCs alone have limited pro-angiogenic potential; however, hypoxic preconditioning of EDCs and CDCs significantly enhances this process. Further research will increase our understanding of cardiac stem cell mediated angiogenesis and improve clinical therapies for myocardial infarction (MI) patients.

Key Words: Coronary heart disease (CHD); Stem cell transplantation, Cardiac progenitors; Explant-derived cell (EDCs); Cardiospheres (Csphs), Cardiosphere-derived cells (CDCs); Hypoxia; Angiogenesis.

Introduction

Stem cell transplantation studies following heart attack aim to establish a way to supply adequate blood and reduce the infarct size. Transplantation of cardiac progenitor cells (cardiosphere-derived cells (CDCs) and cardiospheres (Csphs)) has been shown to be effective either by paracrine or endocrine neovascularisation[1-4]. However, a major dilemma in stem cell transplantation studies is their low survival rate after transplantation. Therefore, improving cell retention after transplantation such as hypoxia preconditioning of the candidate cells could improve the efficiency of stem cell therapy. Hypoxia preconditioning has been shown to stimulate numerous endogenous mechanisms such as reducing apoptosis and enhancing myocyte protection[5]. Studies have shown that hypoxia preconditioning of EDCs and CDCs markedly improves cell migration (*in vitro*) and cell recruitment into the ischemic myocardium[6-10]. Here, we showed that the expression of stem cell (Sca-1, Abcg2), endothelial and angiogenic markers (Eng, Flk1, Vegf) increased significantly in EDCs and CDCs preconditioned with hypoxia and interestingly, this response was more significant in EDCs. In order to assess the ability of CDCs and EDCs to promote neovascularization *in vivo*, we used a mouse model of angiogenesis with subcutaneous injection of matrigel combined with CDCs or EDCs. The results showed that EDCs and CDCs have limited angiogenic capacity alone. However, this characteristic was significantly enhanced in both cell types upon preconditioning with hypoxia (3% O$_2$).

Material and methods

Mice

Mice (C57BL/6) were obtained from Jackson laboratory and CAG-farnesylated-eGFP mice were obtained from Prof. A. Medvinski (Edinburgh University). All animal experiments were performed under a UK Home Office Licence and the Iranian National Institute of Genetic Engineering and Biotechnology (NIGEB) guidelines for laboratory animal care.

Cell culture

Adult murine cardiac stem cells were expanded using a similar method as described by Amirrasouli[11]. Briefly, following dissection of adult murine hearts, they were minced into small fragments and digested with 0.05% trypsin for 10 minutes. The partially digested tissue fragments were then moved to 35 mm cell culture plates pre-coated with 1 mg/ml fibronectin (BD Biosciences)

Author Names in full: Muhammad Mehdi Amirrasouli[1,2,3], Mehdi Shamsara[2]

[1]Department of Cardiovascular Medicine, Institute of Genetic Medicine, International centre for life, School of Medicine, Newcastle University, UK, [2]National Institute of Genetic Engineering and Biotechnology (NIGEB), Shahrak-e- Pajoohesh, 15th Km, Tehran -Karaj Highway, Tehran, Iran, [3]Molecular Genetics Department, Ghanoon Medial Laboratory, West Hakim highway, Tehran, Iran

and cultured in IMDM (Gibco Invitrogen) supplemented with 20% foetal calf or bovine serum (heat inactivated), 1% L-Glutamine (Gibco Invitrogen), 0.1mM 2-mercaptoethanol (Gibco Invitrogen), 100 unit/ml penicillin and 100μg/ml streptomycin. After 4 weeks, the explant cultures were randomly selected to culture in a typical CO_2 incubator normoxia (20% O_2, 48 hours) or hypoxia (3% O_2/48 hours).

Csphs and CDC culture

To culture Csphs, EDCs were seeded at a density of 10^5 cells per well of a 24-well plate pre-coated with 1.2 μg/ml polyD lysine (BD Biosciences) with cardiosphere growth medium containing: DMEM F12 (Gibco Invitrogen) supplemented with 2% B27 (Gibco Invitrogen), 80 ng/ml bFGF, 20 ng/ml EGF, 40nmol/L Cardiotropin - 1, 40nmol/L thrombin and 0.1 mmol/L (all from PeproTech) and 2-mercaptoethanol (Gibco Invitrogen). At days 12-14, loosely adherent Csphs were gently collected from the cell culture supernatant and cultured as CDCs. Finally, CDCs were grown from Csphs and expanded until passage 2 (P2). The CDC culture media was the same as for EDCs.

Quantitative PCR

Murine primer sequences were obtained from the PrimerBank website. In order to eliminate any genomic contamination, a BLAST search was carried out in order to confirm the specificity and coverage of exon boundary regions for each primer pair (Table 1). Total RNA was isolated from approximately 10^6 cells using a Qiagen RNA isolation kit following the manufacturer's instructions. cDNA preparation was performed using cDNA reverse transcription kit (Applied Bioscience) from 1μg RNA. Real-time PCR experiments were carried out by SYBR Green Master Mix (Qiagen) and the thermal profile for all qRT-PCR reactions was 95°C for 10 min, followed by 40 cycles of 95°C for 10s and 60°C for 30s using an ABI Fast Real Time PCR System (7900 HT). All samples were analysed in triplicate with three house keeping genes used as internal controls (Gapdh, β-actin and Rps19).

Table1. The list of primers used for qRT-PCR analysis. All primers are from the Primer Bank available at pga.mgh.harvard.edu

Gene	Sequence)5'-3')	Size (bps)	Tm (°C)
Gapdh	F: AACTTTGGCATTGTGGAAGG R: AGAACATCATCCCTGCATCC	132	60
β-actin	F: GGCTGTATTCCCCTCCATCG R: ACATGGCATTGTTACCAACTGG	154	60
Rps-19	F: GCTTGCCTCTAGTGTCC R:TGAGACCAATGAAATCGCCAA	75	60
Sca-1	F: TCAGGAGGCAGCAGTTATTGTG R: CGTGAAGACTTCCTGTTGCCA	160	60
cKit	F: CTCCCCCAACAGTGTATTCAC R: TAGCCCGAAATCGCAAATCTT	90	60
Abcg2	F: GATGAACTCCAGAGCCGTTAGGAC R:AACCTGGCCTTAATGCTATTCTG	169	60
Eng	F: CTGCCAATGCTGTGCGTGAA R: ACTTGGCCTACGACTCCAGCC	191	60
Vegf	F: CTTGTTCAGAGCGGAGAAAGC R: AACGAACGTACTTGCAGAGTG	125	60
Stat3	F: CACCTTGGATTGAGAGTCAAGAC R:AGGAATCGGCTATATTGCTGGT	112	60
Bcl-x	F:TTCGGGATGGAGTAAACTGGG R:CTCCTTGTCTACGCTTTCCAC	77	60

Western blotting

CDCs or EDCs were treated in normoxia or hypoxia for 48 hours before preparing whole cell protein lysates in SDS buffer. Proteins were separated on 10% polyacrylamide gels and transferred onto polyvinylidene fluoride membrane. Then the samples were blocked with 5% powdered milk/TBST and incubated with primary antibody (HIF-1α, Santa Cruz) or β-actin (Sigma). Membranes were incubated with secondary antibody either anti-rabbit HRP in blocking solution for densitometric analysis all samples were assessed ImageQuant TL v2005 software

Immunofluorescence staining and fluorescent activated cell sorting (FACS)

For fluorescent cell staining, cells were blocked with blocking solution (5% goat serum, 1% BSA and 0.5% Tween 20). Then the appropriate primary antibody (Table 2) was added and incubated at 4°C overnight. Following cell wash, the matching secondary antibody (Table 2) was applied and finally mounted with hard set mountant (Vector Laboratories) containing DAPI. For visualisation, ZeissAxio Imager II with apotome was used. For FACS analysis, 10^5 cells in 100μl volume were incubated with an appropriate primary antibody (Table 2). Following the incubation time and cell wash, all tubes were incubated with the appropriate secondary antibodies. Finally, the cells were washed and DAPI (1μg/ml) was added. FACS analysis was performed with LSRII or FACS Canto (BD Biosciences) and the data was analysed by FACSDiVa software. Each analysis was performed with 10^4 events and all viable cells were included in the final data analysis. DAPI staining was used to provide a live/dead cell gate. Separate isotype and negative controls were used in all markers.

Table 2. The list of antibodies used for Immunophenotyping, Immunostaining of EDCs or CDCs and immunohistochemistry staining.

Antibody	Source and catalogue number	Working concentration
Sca-1	Ebioscience (17598181)	1/100
cKit	Ebioscience (171171)	1/100
CD90	BD Pharmingen (105201)	1/100
CD31	BD Pharmingen (102413)	1/100
CD34	BD Pharmingen (128605)	1/100
CD45	BD Pharmingen (103121)	1/100
Flk1	Ebioscience (565821)	1/100
Eng	Ebioscience (171057)	1/100
HIF1-α	Santa Cruz (sc-10790)	1/50
Alexa 594	Invitrogen (A11012)	1/200
Alexa 488 (anti GFP)	Invitrogen (A21311)	1/50
Alexa 647	Invitrogen (A-21247)	1/100
α-SMA Cy3.3	Sigma (C6198)	1/200

Side population studies

EDCs or CDCs were resuspended at the density of 10^6 cells/ml in PBS with 5% FBS. The cells were incubated in 1 μg/ml Hoechst 33342 dye for 60 min at 37°C (light protected), with or without 50 μM verapamil (Sigma). After the incubation time, cells were analysed for Hoechst 33342 (Sigma) dye efflux by LSRII flow cytometric analysis in hypoxic and normoxic samples. Using a UV laser, Hoechst 33342 dye was excited at 350 nm and fluorescent emission was detected through 450nm (Hoechst blue) and 675nm (Hoechst red) filters, respectively.

Enzyme-Linked Immunosorbent Assay (ELISA)

10^5 EDCs or CDCs were seeded per well of a 12-well plate and 1.5 ml of media was added into each well. Cells were incubated in normoxia or hypoxia. At approximately 90% cell confluency, the cell culture medium was removed and centrifuged. VEGF levels in the cell supernatant were measured with a VEGF ELISA kit following the manufacturer's instructions (R & D systems) and the optical density was measured with Stat Fax 2100(Awareness Technology Inc.) at 560 nm.

In vivo angiogenesis

Growth factor reduced Matrigel (BD Biosciences) was thawed at 4°C and kept on ice. Anaesthesia was induced using an anaesthetic chamber (97% O_2/2% isoflurane) for 3 minutes. The flanks were shaved and cleaned with 70% ethanol. EDCs or CDCs derived from CAG-farnesylated-eGFP or C57BL/6 strains were suspended in 600µl matrigel and injected sub-cutaneously into the flank regions. After 10 days, the animals were humanely killed and matrigel plugs were dissected. Plugs were washed and fixed with 0.2% PFA at 4°C/overnight and then incubated with 30% sucrose at 4°C/overnight. Finally, the plugs were frozen by OCT freezing medium and sectioned using Microm HM 560 Cryostat (Thermo Scientific) and the sections were mounted on slides. For micro vessel density (MVD) analysis, matrigel plugs were stained with CD31 antibody as described previously[11]. Briefly, matrigel plug slides were air-dried, washed with PBS and blocked with a blocking solution (5% rabbit serum). The complementary blocking was carried out with Avidin/Biotin buffers (Vector Laboratories) to block unspecific sites. All sections were then incubated with a primary anti-CD31 antibody (BD Pharmingen) at 4°C/overnight. The next day, the slides were washed and incubated with secondary rabbit anti-rat antibody (Vector Laboratories) for 30 minutes at room temperature. All sections were washed again and incubated with ABC reagent for 30 minutes. After washing with PBS, all sections were incubated for 1 minute with the liquid DAB kit (BioGenex) and mounted with histomount (National Diagnostics) following ethanol dehydration. MVD was measured using ImageJ software and the intensity of the staining was normalised against the entire surface area of the matrigel and compared between the groups.

Microscopy

Light microscopy was used to assess cell morphology and growth using a Zeiss Axiovert 200 inverted microscope. For fluorescent-stained sections and Histochemical stained sections, a LeitzDiaplan Fluorescent microscope was used. All images were taken by digital camera and analysed with Image J to measure the staining intensity.

Statistical analysis

SPSS software (version 19, SPSS Inc.) was used to analyse the data. To test the normality, the Shapiro-Wilk test was used and multiple groups of data were analysed by one-way ANOVA followed by Post-Hoc (Tukey test). In all experiments, the paired t-test and p-value of <0.05 were defined as being statistically significant.

Results

Cardiac progenitor cell culture and HIF-1α stabilisation in hypoxic culture of EDCs and CDCs

Cardiac progenitors were obtained from adults C57BL/6 mice hearts and cultured in normoxia or hypoxia as described in (Amirrasouli, 2014)[11]. Figure 1 schematically represents different stages of EDC, Csph and CDC culture.

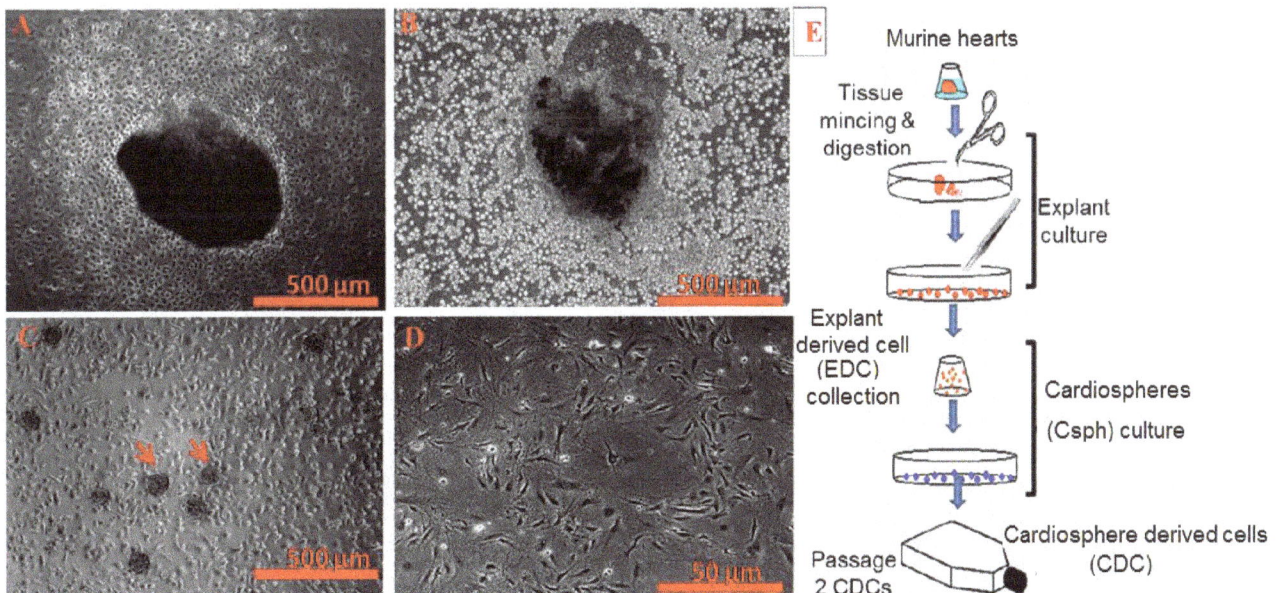

Figure 1. Different stages of cardiac progenitor cell culture. (A) Murine cardiac explant at day 6 of EDCs culture. (B) The same explant at day 14 with migrated phase bright cells and underlying stromal cells (C) Csphs at day 6 (arrows). (D) P2 CDCs, the scale bar is 500µm (A-C) and 50 µm in D. (E) Schematic representation of EDC, Csph and CDC culture. Modified from Amirrasouli 2014[11].

To validate the hypoxic environment, HIF-1α stabilisation in EDCs and CDCs was evaluated by western blot and immunocytochemistry. EDCs and P2 CDCs cultured in normoxia or hypoxia, were analysed based on the stabilisation of the HIF-1α protein (Figure 2). Detailed HIF-1α protein quantification showed that EDCs stabilised HIF-1α twice as much as CDCs upon hypoxic culture induction.

Hypoxia increased the expression of anti-apoptotic markers in EDCs better than CDCs

As the role of Stat3/ Bclx pathway is shown to down regulate

apoptosis *in vitro*[12], propagation of EDCs and CDCs under hypoxia showed a significant increase of Stat3/Bclx expression in comparison to normoxia control group (EDCs; stat3: 5.2 fold and Bclx: 3.9 fold, $p<0.05$), (CDCs; stat3: 2.1 fold and Bclx: 3.7 fold, $p<0.05$)(Figure 3). As EDC culture could take one month, the expression of stat3 was analysed with qRT-PCR at four time points (end of weeks 1 to 4) (Figure 3C). As shown in Figure 3, the mean mRNA level of stat3 marker in EDCs remained constant in hypoxic environment.

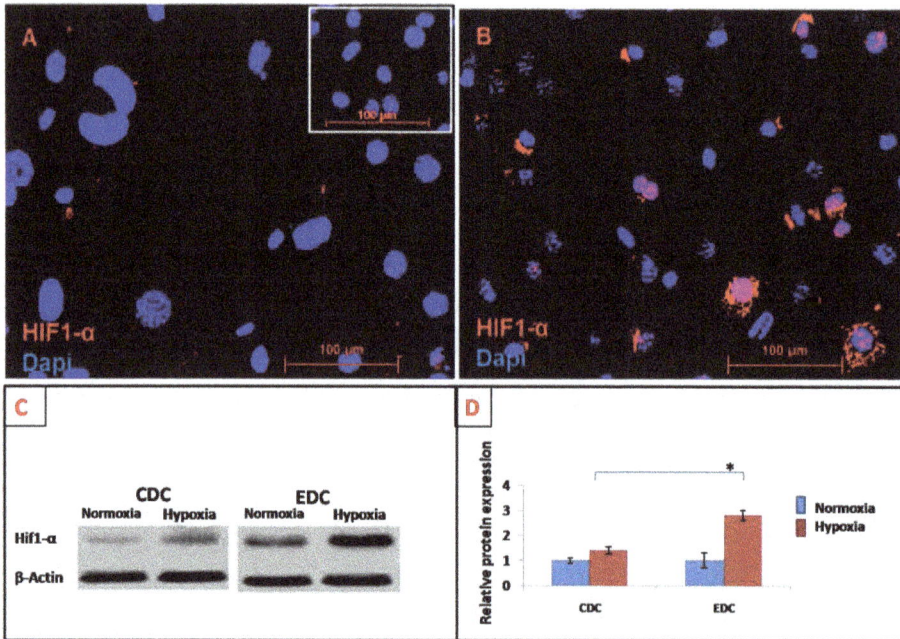

Figure 2. HIF-1α stabilisation in EDCs and P2 CDCs cultured in normoxia or 3%O$_2$. CDCs were stained with anti-HIF-1α specific antibody and detected with an anti-rabbit secondary antibody conjugated with alexa 594 (red). CDCs were cultured in (A) normoxia or (B) hypoxia for 48 hours and DAPI (blue) was used to stain nuclei, 2A and 2B are from[11]. (C) Representative western blot from EDCs or CDCs cultured in normoxia or hypoxia to analyse HIF-1α stabilisation. D) The summary of densitometric analysis of HIF 1-α band intensity in CDCs and EDCs cultured in hypoxia and normoxia relative to β-actin are shown *p<0.05. Scale bar = 100 μm. The inset image in (A) is the negative control (no primary antibody) with the same magnification. Figures (A) and (B) are modified from Amirrasouli 2014[11].

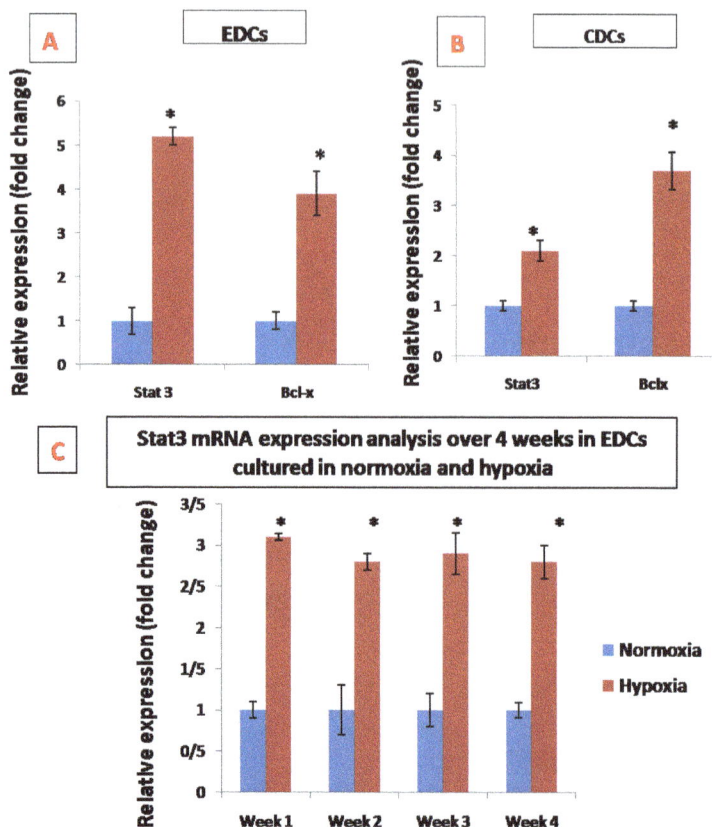

Figure 3. The effect of hypoxia on mRNA expression of anti-apoptotic markers (stat3-Bclx) on EDCs (A) and CDCs (B) compared to normoxia control groups. (C) The analysis of stat3 mRNA level in EDCs cultured in hypoxia 3% O$_2$ and normoxia for 4 weeks. * P<0.05

The effect of hypoxia on EDCs' outgrowth from cardiac explants

It is already shown that hypoxia stimulates cell migration through the perk/atf4/lamp3 pathway[16]. Therefore, to validate the effect of hypoxia on EDCs' migration, we cultured murine cardiac explants from C57BL/6 strain in hypoxia and normoxia for two weeks. The length of cell outgrowth was measured at several points from each explant. The results showed the positive effect of hypoxia on increasing EDCs' outgrowth (1236±48.3 μm in normoxia vs. 2420.7±124μm in hypoxia, p<0.05). However, our initial studies in Newcastle University on Csphs and CDC proliferation in hypoxia did not show any significant difference compared to normoxia counterparts[11]. Figure 4 shows the effect of hypoxia treatment on EDC cultures.

Hypoxia increases the expression of cardiac stem cell and angiogenic markers in EDCs more than CDCs

Using qRT-PCR and FACS, the level of cardiac stem cell (Sca-1, cKit, Abcg2), endothelial (CD31 and CD34) and angiogenic cell markers (VEGF, Eng & Flk1) were analysed in EDCs and CDCs treated with hypoxia or normoxia. At mRNA level (Figure 5A-B), Sca-1 showed the highest expression among stem cell markers in EDCs (6.2-fold, Figure 5A, p<0.05) and CDCs (2.7-fold, figure 5B, p<0.05). Although, cKit mRNA remained unchanged in CDCs (1.3-fold, Figure 5B, p=ns), it showed a significant up-regulation in hypoxia EDCs (3.1-fold, Figure 5A, p=0.05). Hypoxia also increased the level of angiogenic markers (Eng, VEGF) and these enhancements were more evident in EDCs (VEGF: 4.2-fold and Eng: 4.3 fold p<0.05) (Figures 5A and 5B).

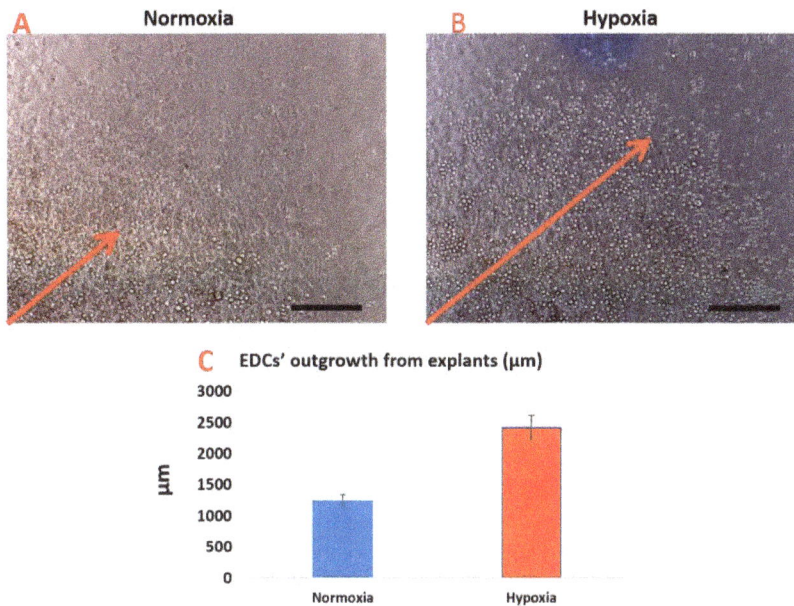

Figure 4. **The effect of hypoxic cell culture on EDCs' outgrowth**. Normoxia (A) and (B) hypoxia. Red arrows are indicating the outgrowth length from the explant. (C) The summary of EDCs' outgrowth compared in normoxia and hypoxia. *p<0.05 Scale bar = 500μm.

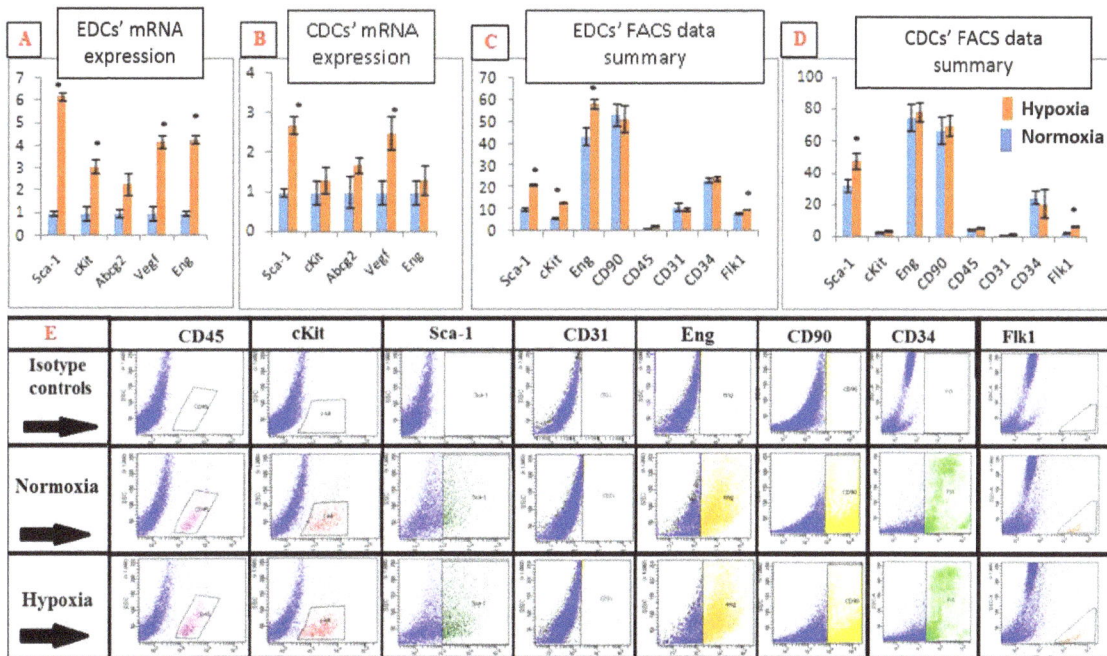

Figure 5. **The effect of hypoxia on EDC and CDC mRNA and cell surface markers**. The comparison of the effect of hypoxia on EDCs mRNA (A), CDCs mRNA (B) cultured in normoxia or hypoxia. Using qRT-PCR the level of stem cell (Sca-1, cKit and Abcg2), angiogenic and endothelial (Vegf and Eng) markers were evaluated in EDCs or CDCs. Protein expression of stem cell (Sca-1, cKit,) Mesenchymal (CD90-Eng), Hematopoietic (CD45), endothelial and angiogenic (CD31, CD34 and Flk1) markers were assessed in EDCs (C) and CDCs (D). Blue and orange bars (A-D) are representing normoxic and hypoxic cell cultures in both qRT-PCR and FACS data respectively. (E) Representative FACS plots form CDC culture, modified from[11]. *p<0.05.

To further evaluate the increase seen in gene expression of EDCs and CDCs, we used flowcytometry in order to validate the results obtained by qRT-PCR. Therefore, the panel of endothelial (Flk1, CD34, CD31), mesenchymal (Eng, CD90), haematopoietic (CD45) and stem cell (Sca-1, cKit) markers were used. Figure 5E shows a representative FACS plots from CDC culture and 5C & D summarise the results as a percentage of positive events for all cell populations analysed in EDCs and CDCs respectively. Although, CDCs cultured in hypoxia showed higher levels of cKit, Eng and CD34, only the level of Sca-1 (32±4 vs 48±5, Figure 5D, p<0.05) and Flk1 (3±0.1 vs 6.8±0.3, figure 5D, p<0.05) reached to significant levels between two groups. Interestingly, in hypoxia EDCs, Sca-1 (10±1 vs 21±0.5, figure 5C, p<0.05) and Flk1 (8±0.2 vs 10.1± 0.1, Figure 5C, p<0.05) levels were significantly higher than their normoxia control groups. The difference in cKit (6±0.5 vs 13.4±0.8, p<0.05) and Eng (43.5±4 vs 58±2, p<0.05) protein expression were also higher in hypoxia EDCs (Figure 5C). More importantly the data showed that a very low

percentage of EDCs or CDCs expressed CD45. Therefore, it is not likely that these cells were originated from hematopoetic tissues. Figure 5 summerises the data from qRT-PCR and FACS experiments, (blue and orange bars are representing normoxic and hypoxic cell culture conditions respectively).

Hypoxia increases the secretion of VEGF in EDCs' supernatant more than in CDCs'

To confirm the up-regulation of VEGF mRNA expression following hypoxia culture, we analysed the level of VEGF in the supernatant of EDCs' and CDCs' with the same cellular density cultured in normoxia or hypoxia. Using ELISA, we observed that hypoxia significantly increased VEGF protein in the supernatant of EDCs' (210±25µg/ml vs 520± 17µg/ml, p<0.001) and CDCs' (128±19µg/ml vs 223 ± 26µg/ml, p<0.001) in comparison with the normoxia counterparts. Interestingly, the level of VEGF was more evident in the supernatant of hypoxia EDCs' (Figure 6).

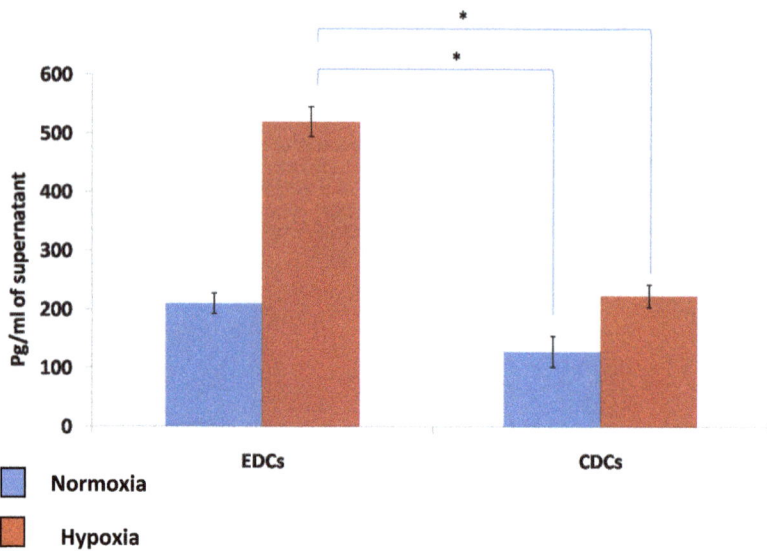

Figure 6.The level of VEGF in the supernatant of EDCs and CDCs cultured in normoxia or hypoxia. The VEGF level was measured with a specific murine VEGF ELISA kit.*p<0.001 Blue and red bars are representing normoxic and hypoxic cell culture conditions.

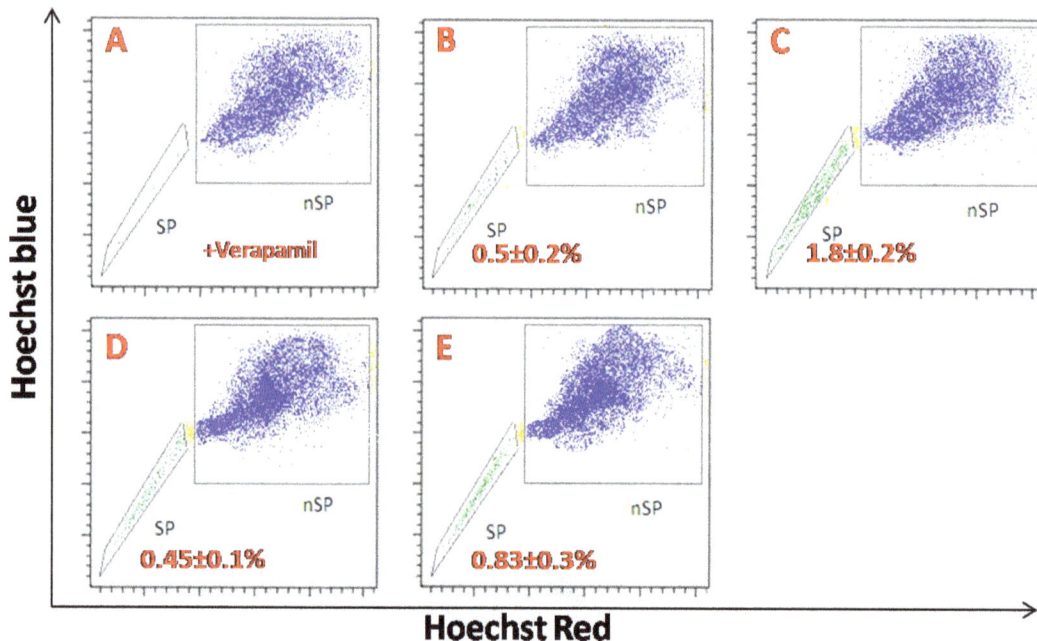

Figure 7: The effect of hypoxia on EDC and CDC, side population percentage. (A) EDCs with Verapamil, (B) EDCs in normoxia, (C) EDCs in hypoxia, (D) CDCs in normoxia and (E) CDCs in hypoxia. p<0.05

The effect of hypoxia on side population cells of EDCs and CDCs

It has been shown that cardiac side population cells contain putative cells with the ability to pump out the dye Hoechst 33342[13]. EDCs or CDCs cultured in hypoxia or normoxia were stained with Hoechst dye and assessed by flowcytometry. When EDCs and CDCs were incubated with 50 µM Verapamil, there were no side population cells in the designated area, indicating that EDCs and CDCs contain some side population cells. The proportions of side population cells in EDCs and CDCs were (0.8±0.2% and 0.45 ±0.1%, p<0.05), respectively. Higher fractions of these cells were observed in hypoxic EDCs and CDCs (1.8±0.2%vs 0.83±0.3%), respectively compared to their normoxia counterparts. The data clearly indicated that EDCs and CDCs contain side population cells and hypoxia increases their quantity (Figure 7).

In vivo angiogenic properties of EDCs and CDCs

Thus far, our data showed that the expression of stem cell (Sca-1,cKit and Abcg2), endothelial and angiogenic markers (Eng, Flk1, Vegf) increased significantly in EDCs and CDCs culture in hypoxia. We also observed that culturing EDCs and CDCs in hypoxia elevates the level of VEGF secreted into their media. Therefore, to assess all these *in vitro* benefits of hypoxic environment, we evaluated EDCs' and CDCs' pro-angiogenic effect (CD31 expression cells) *in vivo* with matrigel plug angiogenesis assay. EDCs and CDCs were derived from CAG-farnesyl-eGFP transgenic mice to enable the tracking of GFP-

labelled cells in the matrigel plugs. This assay does not require surgical procedures and allows for the screening of the angiogenic properties of different cells. Matrigel is an extract of the Engelbreth-Holm-Swarm tumour and contains basement membrane proteins to support vessel formation. In this study (2×10^6) EDCs or CDCs cultured in normoxia or hypoxia were directly injected subcutaneously with growth factor reduced matrigel and after 10 days the effect of EDCs and CDCs on neovascularisation was assessed by detailed quantification of MVD (CD31 positive cells) in the matrigel using histochemistry staining. Comparison of MVD between two groups: normoxia CDCs (nCDC) Figure 8 (A&E), versus hypoxia CDCs (hCDC) Figure 8 (B&F), showed that matrigel plugs with hCDCs had significantly higher MVD levels compared to matrigel plugs with nCDC, (8± 2.4 nCDC vs 14.2± 4.4 hCDC, Figure 8I, P=0.001). Interestingly in EDCs, the hypoxia EDC (hEDC) group, figure 8 (D&H) showed a higher MVD level in comparison with normoxia EDCs (nEDC), Figure 8(C&D). (12.5± 1.8 nEDC/ vs 24.3±2.8 hEDC, Figure 8I, p=0.001). After comparing the angiogenic responses between CDCs and EDCs in both environments, EDCs showed better angiogenesis compared to CDCs. Our previous study at Newcastle University by tracking genetically labelled CDCs showed that very limited numbers of GFP labeled CDCs co-express CD31 (endothelial cell marker- Figure 8J) and α-SMA (smooth muscle marker- Figure 8K). In that we concluded that these cell contribute indirectly to neovessel formation mechanisms and mainly activate paracrine pathways (Figures 8J and 8K)[11].

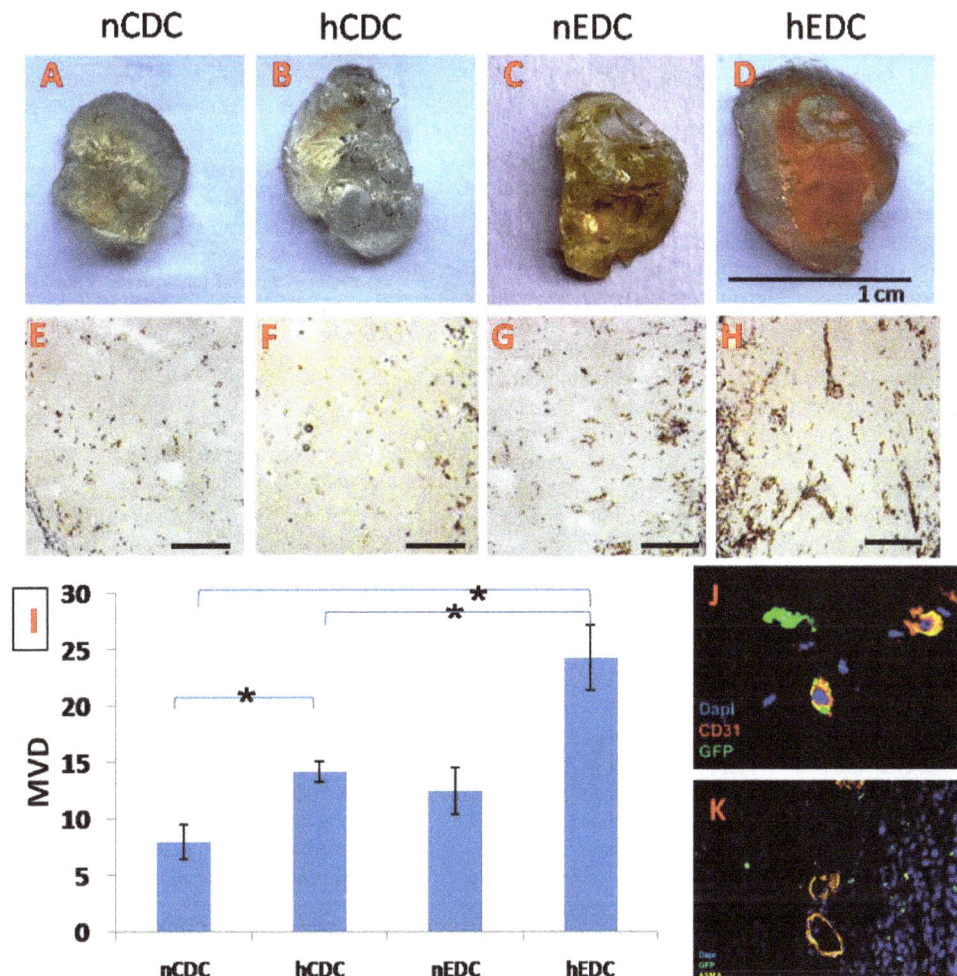

Figure 8: *In vivo* angiogenesis results from EDCs or CDCs cultured in normoxia and hypoxia, following sub-dermal matrigel plug injection. (A&E) matrigel plug from normoxia CDCs, (B&F) Hypoxia CDCs, (C&G) Normoxia EDCS, (D&H) Hypoxia EDCs, (I) The summary of microscopic MVD analysis from matrigel plugs, (J) co-localisation of GFP and CD31 and (K) ASMA in CDCs. J and K are modified from Amirrasouli, 2014[11]. *p=0.001, scale bar (E-H) = 500µm.

Discussion

The aims of this study were to assess the stemness and angiogenic properties of EDCs and CDCs in normoxia and hypoxia. As CDCs and Csphs cultures are time consuming and expensive, here we assessed whether hypoxia preconditioning of EDCs could be used as the ultimate cell therapy method for cardiac repair studies. The novelty of our findings could be summarised as follows: first we showed the positive effect of hypoxia on EDCs outgrowth from cardiac explants, which is quite different from the previous studies[10, 14]. Previous studies used very low O_2 levels (0.1 %)[10], which could be very lethal for stem cells and might not be tolerable for long duration cell cultures such as EDCs. Li et al, (2011) used physiological O_2 (5%)[14], which might not be enough to activate hypoxia mediated pathways in order to enhance their pro-angiogenic and cardiogenic properties. As the final aim of cardiac progenitor cell studies is to provide an optimal cell type for cardiac repair, here we used 3% O_2, which according to Rumsey et al.(1994) recapitulates the O_2 level in the border zone region of the infracted heart[15].This region is the favoured target to deliver candidate cells for cardiac regeneration studies. Therefore if candidate cells are treated with 3% O_2, it is likely that they will be able to tolerate and accommodate themselves more properly than the cells that are treated with different O_2 concentrations.

In vitro studies

Our data showed that hypoxia increased EDC outgrowth significantly (1236 ± 48.3 μm in normoxia vs. 2420.7 ± 124μm in hypoxia, p<0.05) in comparison to normoxia. These data are in agreement with Li et al. (2011) who showed that EDCs grow faster in 5% O_2 than in normoxia. As hypoxia is shown to stimulate cell migration through the perk/atf4/lamp3 pathway[16] it is likely that hypoxia may increase EDC migration out of the explants through the same pathway. Detailed analysis of the cytokines involved in paracrine activities of EDCs could validate this finding. Here, we also showed that hypoxia increased the expression of the Stat3/Bclx pathway, and therefore, it is likely that these cells may be able to live longer than their normoxia control groups and could tolerate the hypoxic environment of the infarct region following cell transplantation. This is in agreement with Yokogami et al.(2013) and Selveniran et al.(2009), who showed the important effect of stat3 in hypoxic environments and the anti-apoptotic features of ovarian cancer cells[17, 18].Analysing the effect of hypoxia on CDC showed that culturing CDCs in hypoxia did not result in any significant difference in CDC proliferation, and this finding is consistent with and van Oorschot et al. (2011), who showed that hypoxic cell culture did not change cardiac progenitor proliferation at earlier stages, however, prolonged hypoxic culture (>6 days) increased cell proliferation and migration significantly[19]. Therefore, we can conclude that the effect of hypoxia on cell proliferation and apoptosis is cell- and context-dependent, and it is also possible to prolong CDC cultures and compare the proliferation rate at their higher passages.

It is already known that cardiac progenitor cells express cardiac stem cell markers such as cKit and Sca-1[20] and the benefit of hypoxic cell culture on human cardiac stem cells has been shown[21]. Our data showed that EDCs cultured in hypoxia, express more stem cell markers than their normoxic counterparts and more than CDCs (Figure 5). Our findings showed that explants contain some progenitor cells that express stem cells and angiogenic factors, including Sca-1, cKit, Abcg2, Eng and Vegf, and if they are cultured in a hypoxic environment, these markers would be expressed more.

Our experiments on cardiac side populations by flowcytometry showed that both cell types (EDCs and CDCs) contain a fraction of side population cells and hypoxia increases these cells significantly ($^{nEDC}0.8 \pm 0.2$ vs $^{hEDC}1.8\pm0.2$/ $^{nCDCs}0.45\pm0.1$ vs $^{hCDC}0.83\pm0.3$, p<0.05). Davis et al. (2010) showed that cardiac explant-derived cells could provide functional benefits equivalent to CDC[1]. In their work, EDCs were assessed by in vitro and in vivo experiments in order to compare their stemness, pro-angiogenic and cardiogenic properties with CDCs[1]. In general, they showed the feasibility of working with EDCs in comparison to CDCs.

In vivo studies

To validate our in vitro findings, we injected EDCs or CDCs derived from CAG-farnesylated-eGFP mice and cultured in normoxia or hypoxia. Then the cells were sub-dermally injected into mouse models and compared their angiogenesis through the quantification of CD31 expressing cells. We utilised 3% O_2 cell culture, a novel hypoxic preconditioning strategy in cardiac progenitor cell culture that is related to the hypoxic environment of the cardiac infarct border zone[15]. This is an important concept because the cardiac region of interest for cell delivery in clinical studies is the border zone. If the candidate cells are cultured with severe hypoxic conditions (0.0 - 0.2% O_2) and then delivered into the border zone, the new environment would be hyperoxic and conversely, if they are preconditioned with physiological O_2 (5-7% O_2), the infarct border zone may be hypoxic. Therefore, either hyperoxic or hypoxic environments could be harmful to the candidate cells and could alter their retention and cardiogenic properties. However, culturing the donor cells with 3% O_2 could mimic very similar conditions of the infarct border zone and could provide a better understanding of their performance.

Our in vivo model of angiogenesis showed that sub-dermal delivery of murine EDCs or CDCs combined with matrigel leads to a significantly enhanced CD31 expression within the matrigel and the EDCs' response was more evident in both normoxia and hypoxia. Previously our immunofluorescence staining with CAG-farnesyl-eGFP transgenic line showed that the majority of eGFP expressing CDCs do not co-localise with CD31-expressing cells, which suggests that the angiogenic response from the injected CDCs is likely to be paracrine (Figures 8J and 8K).

Our in vivo data is confirmed by the in vitro data as we showed that after culturing EDCs and CDCs in hypoxia, the level of cardiac stem cell marker Sca-1 was increased. Sca-1 is shown to be involved in neo-angiogenesis[22] and elevated VEGF expression under the control of HIF1-α from cells in a hypoxic environment is shown to be an early sign of angiogenesis[23]. In addition, the level of VEGF protein in the supernatant of EDCs and CDCs cultured in hypoxia was increased (2.4-fold in EDCs and 1.7-fold in CDCs).

In summary, we have shown that preconditioning of EDCs and CDCs with hypoxia, increases their cardiac stem cell, endothelial sub-populations and enhances their angiogenic capacity in sub-dermal matrigel assay. However, to elucidate the exact mechanisms, it will be important to investigate further the precise role of EDC- or CDC-mediated angiogenesis. More importantly, these findings suggest that sub-dermal injection of EDCs or CDCs act through paracrine mechanisms, and therefore, to understand the exact pathway, it would be advantageous to assess which proteins are ¹nvolved by these cells.

References

1. Davis DR, Kizana E, Terrovitis J, Barth AS, Zhang Y, Smith RR, Miake J, Marbán E. Isolation and expansion of functionally-competent cardiac progenitor cells directly from heart biopsies. J Mol Cell Cardiol.2010; 49 (2), 312-21.
2. Smith RR, Barile L, Cho HC, Leppo MK, Hare JM, Messina E, Giacomello A, Abraham MR, Marbán E. Regenerative potential of cardiosphere-derived cells expanded from percutaneous endomyocardial biopsy specimens. Circulation 2007; 115 (7), 896-908.
3. Reich H, Tseliou E, de Couto G, Angert D, Valle J, Kubota Y, Luthringer D, Mirocha J, Sun B, Smith RR, Marbán L, Marbán E. Repeated transplantation of allogeneic cardiosphere-derived cells boosts therapeutic benefits without immune sensitization in a rat model of myocardial infarction. J Heart Lung Transplant. 2016;35(11):1348-57.
4. Gallet R, de Couto G, Simsolo E, Valle J, Sun B, Liu W, Tseliou E, Zile MR, Marbán E. Cardiosphere-derived cells reverse heart failure with preserved ejection fraction (HFpEF) in rats by decreasing fibrosis and inflammation. JACC Basic Transl Sci 2016; 1 (1-2), 14-28.
5. Zhu HJ, Wang DG, Yan J, Xu J. Up-regulation of microRNA-135a protects against myocardial ischemia/reperfusion injury by decreasing TXNIP expression in diabetic mice. Am J Transl Res 2015; 7 (12), 2661-71.
6. Hosoyama T, Samura M, Kudo T, Nishimoto A, Ueno K, Murata T, Ohama T, Sato K, Mikamo A, Yoshimura K, Li TS, Hamano K. Cardiosphere-derived cell sheet primed with hypoxia improves left ventricular function of chronically infarcted heart. Am J Transl Res 2015; 7 (12), 2738-51.
7. Li Z, Guo X, Guan J. An oxygen release system to augment cardiac progenitor cell survival and differentiation under hypoxic condition. Biomaterials 2012; 33 (25), 5914-23.
8. Tan SC, Carr CA, Yeoh KK, Schofield, CJ, Davies KE, Clarke K. Identification of valid housekeeping genes for quantitative RT-PCR analysis of cardiosphere-derived cells preconditioned under hypoxia or with prolyl-4-hydroxylase inhibitors. Mol Biol Rep 2012; 39 (4), 4857-67.
9. Tan SC, Gomes RS, Yeoh KK, Perbellini F, Malandraki-Miller S, Ambrose L, Heather, LC, Faggian G, Schofield CJ, Davies KE, Clarke K, Carr CA. Preconditioning of Cardiosphere-Derived Cells With Hypoxia or Prolyl-4-Hydroxylase Inhibitors Increases Stemness and Decreases Reliance on Oxidative Metabolism. Cell Transplant 2016; 25 (1), 35-53.
10. Tang YL, Zhu W, Cheng M, Chen L, Zhang J, Sun T, Kishore R, Phillips MI, Losordo DW, Qin G. Hypoxic preconditioning enhances the benefit of cardiac progenitor cell therapy for treatment of myocardial infarction by inducing CXCR4 expression. Circ Res 2009; 104 (10), 1209-16.
11. Amirrasouli MM. Characterisation of cardiosphere derived cells : investigating hypoxic pre-conditioning on pro-angiogenic properties and tracking the cardiac fibroblast component. Thesis (Ph.D.), University of Newcastle Upon Tyne; 2014.
12. Bhattacharya S, Ray RM, Johnson LR. STAT3-mediated transcription of Bcl-2, Mcl-1 and c-IAP2 prevents apoptosis in polyamine-depleted cells. Biochem J 2005; 392 (Pt 2), 335-44.
13. Oyama T, Nagai T, Wada H, Naito AT, Matsuura K, Iwanaga K, Takahashi T, Goto M, Mikami Y, Yasuda N, Akazawa H, Uezumi A, Takeda S, Komuro I. Cardiac side population cells have a potential to migrate and differentiate into cardiomyocytes in vitro and in vivo. J Cell Biol 2007; 176 (3), 329-41.
14. Li TS, Cheng K, Malliaras K, Matsushita N, Sun B, Marbán L, Zhang Y, Marbán E. Expansion of human cardiac stem cells in physiological oxygen improves cell production efficiency and potency for myocardial repair. Cardiovasc Res 2011; 89 (1), 157-65.
15. Rumsey WL, Pawlowski M, Lejavardi N, Wilson DF. Oxygen pressure distribution in the heart in vivo and evaluation of the ischemic "border zone". Am J Physiol 1994; 266 (4 Pt 2), H1676-80.
16. Nagelkerke A, Bussink J, Mujcic H, Wouters BG, Lehmann S, Sweep FC, Span PN. Hypoxia stimulates migration of breast cancer cells via the PERK/ATF4/LAMP3-arm of the unfolded protein response. Breast Cancer Res 2013; 15 (1), R2.
17. Selvendiran K, Bratasz A, Kuppusamy ML, Tazi MF, Rivera BK, Kuppusamy P. Hypoxia induces chemoresistance in ovarian cancer cells by activation of signal transducer and activator of transcription 3. Int J Cancer 2009; 125 (9), 2198-204.
18. Yokogami K, Yamashita S, Takeshima H. Hypoxia-induced decreases in SOCS3 increase STAT3 activation and upregulate VEGF gene expression. Brain Tumor Pathol 2013; 30 (3), 135-43.
19. van Oorschot AA, Smits AM, Pardali E, Doevendans PA, Goumans MJ. Low oxygen tension positively influences cardiomyocyte progenitor cell function. J Cell Mol Med 2011; 15 (12), 2723-34.
20. Meissner K, Heydrich B, Jedlitschky G, Meyer Zu Schwabedissen H, Mosyagin I, Dazert P, Eckel L, Vogelgesang S, Warzok RW, Böhm M, Lehmann C, Wendt M, Cascorbi I, Kroemer HK. The ATP-binding cassette transporter ABCG2 (BCRP), a marker for side population stem cells, is expressed in human heart. J Histochem Cytochem 2006; 54 (2), 215-21.
21. Grayson WL, Zhao F, Bunnell B, Ma T. Hypoxia enhances proliferation and tissue formation of human mesenchymal stem cells. Biochem Biophys Res Commun 2007; 358 (3), 948-53.
22. Kotton DN, Summer RS, Sun X, Ma BY, Fine A. Stem cell antigen-1 expression in the pulmonary vascular endothelium. Am J Physiol Lung Cell Mol Physiol 2003; 284 (6), L990-6.
23. Lin C, McGough R, Aswad B, Block JA, Terek R. Hypoxia induces HIF-1alpha and VEGF expression in chondrosarcoma cells and chondrocytes. J Orthop Res 2004; 22 (6), 1175-81.

Abbreviations

α-SMA	α smooth muscle actin
CDC	Cardiosphere-derived cell
Csphs	Cardiospheres
CDCs	Cardiosphere derived cells
CHD	Coronary heart disease
DAB	3-3"-diaminobenzidine tetrahydrochloride
DMEM	Dulbecco's modified Eagle's medium
EDCs	Explant derived cells
EGF	Epidermal growth factor
ELISA	Enzyme Linked Immunosorbent Assay
Eng	Endoglin
EDTA	Ethylene-diamine-tetra-acetic acid
Flk-1	Foetal liver kinase 1
FACS	Fluorescent activated cell sorting
GFP	Green fluorescent protein
Hif-1α	Hypoxia inducible factor- 1-α
MI	Myocardial infarction
mRNA	Messenger RNA
PBS	Phosphate buffered saline
qRT-PCR	Quantitative reverse transcription polymerase chain reaction
Sca-1	Stem cell antigen
VEGF	Vascular endothelial growth factor

Potential Conflicts of Interests

None

Support / Grants

1) Newcastle Upon Tyne University Overseas Research Scholarship
2) Ghanoon Medical Laboratory Research Grant

Corresponding Authors

Muhammad Mehdi Amirrasouli, Molecular Genetics department, Ghanoon Medical Laboratory, West Hakim highway, Tehran, Iran, Post Code:1473666616. E-mail: amirrasouli@ghanoonmedicallab.com

Long Term Study of Protective Mechanisms of Human Adipose Derived Mesenchymal Stem Cells on Cisplatin Induced Kidney injury in Sprague-Dawley Rats

Elhusseini FM[1,5], Saad M-AAA[2,5], Anber N[3], Elghannam D[4], Sobh M-A[5a], Alsaied A[6], El-dusoky S[6], Sheashaa H[5b], Abdel-Ghaffar H[4], Sobh MA[5b,6]

Background/Aims: Long-term evaluation of cisplatin induced nephrotoxicity and the probable renal protective activities of stem cells are lacking up until now. We evaluated the early and long-term role of human adipose derived mesenchymal stem cells (ADMSCs) in prevention or amelioration of cisplatin induced acute kidney injury (AKI) in Sprague-Dawley rats. For this, we determined the kidney tissue level of oxidative stress markers in conjugation with a renal histopathological scoring system of both acute and chronic renal changes.
Methods: This study used eighty Sprague-Dawley (SD) rats weighing 250-300g. They were assigned into four equal groups (each group n=20): (I) Negative control group, rats injected with single dose of 1 ml normal saline. (II) Positive control cisplatin, rats injected with a single dose of 5 mg/kg I.P in 1 ml saline. (III) Cisplatin and culture media group, rats injected with 0.5 ml of culture media single dose into the tail vein and (IV) Cisplatin and ADMSCs group, rats injected with a single dose of 0.5 ml of culture media containing 5 x10^{6}ADMSCs into the tail vein one day after cisplatin administration. Each main group was further divided according to the timing of sacrifice into four subgroups (each subgroup n=5). Rats in the subgroup A were sacrificed after 4 days; subgroup B were sacrificed after 7 days; subgroup C were sacrificed after 11 days; and subgroup D were sacrificed after 30 days. Before sacrifice, 24 hrs.-urine was collected using a metabolic cage. Renal function was evaluated through blood urea nitrogen (BUN), serum creatinine and creatinine clearance. Kidney tissue homogenate oxidative stress parameters, Malondialdehyde (MDA), Superoxide dismutase (SOD) and Glutathione (GSH) were determined. In addition, histopathological analysis for active injury, regenerative and chronic changes was performed.
Results: ADMSCs were characterized and their capability of differentiation was proved. Cisplatin induced a significant increase in plasma creatinine and tissue MDA and induced a decrease in SOD, GSH and creatinine clearance. ADMSCs attenuated these changes. Cisplatin resulted in prominent histopathological changes in the term of tubular necrosis, atrophy, inflammatory cells infiltration and fibrosis. ADMSCs significantly lowered the injury score at day 4, 7, 11 and 30 with marked regenerative changes starting from day 4 and limited fibrotic score at day 30.
Conclusion: ADMSCs have both protective and regenerative abilities with consequent limitation of the development of renal fibrosis after the cisplatin induced acute tubular necrosis, largely through an anti-oxidative activity.

Key Words: Acute kidney injury in rats, Renal fibrosis, Cisplatin, Adipose mesenchymal stem cells, Oxidative stress markers.

Introduction

Cisplatin is a chemotherapeutic agent largely used for the treatment of many human malignancies. However, nephrotoxicity is one of the serious adverse effects that limit its clinical use. Cisplatin has multiple cellular targets; so blocking its effect on a single target may only offer moderate protection against nephrotoxicity[1]. Hence, to alleviate cisplatin nephrotoxicity a strategy to tackling multiple cellular levels is important. Several potential advantages through cell therapy over specific drugs or growth factors in the treatment of many disorders as AKI have been demonstrated[2, 3].

Mesenchymal stem cells (MSCs) are multi-potent adult stem cells harbouring multi lineage differentiation potential, paracrine and immunosuppressive properties that make MSCs an ideal candidate cell type for immunomodulation and regeneration[4].

Adipose tissue contains different cell types besides adipocytes, including adipose derived mesenchymal stem cells (ADMSCs), which are emerging as cellular therapy tools[5].

Plasticity of ADMSCs and their capability of differentiation into cells of mesodermal origin, such as adipocyte, osteocyte, chondrocyte and myocyte lineages have been demonstrated[6]. In addition to their easy availability as a human source and the absence of ethical restriction, this source has immense clinical importance in regenerative medicine.

Some previous studies have reported the effect of MSCs on cisplatin induced AKI. All of them used a small sample size. One used rat bone marrow MSCs[7] and others used human ADMSCs[8, 9]. The unique feature of our study was the use of large sample size, long-term follow up and assessment of oxidative stress markers levels for evaluating an early protective and late ameliorating effect of ADMSCs on cisplatin induced kidney injury.

Materials and methods

The Local Ethical Committee, Faculty of Medicine and Mansoura University, Egypt approved the experimental protocol.

Author Names in full: Fatma M. Elhusseini[1,5], Mohamed-Ahdy A.A. Saad[2,5], Nahla Anber[3], Doaa Elghannam[4], Mohamed-Ahmed Sobh[5a], Aziza Alsayed[6], Sara El-dusoky[6], Hussein Sheashaa[5b], Hassan Abdel-Ghaffar[4], Mohamed Sobh[5b,6]

[1]Pathology Department, [2]Pharmacology Department, [3]Emergency Hospital, [4]Clinical Pathology, [5a]Zoology-Urology and Nephrology Center, [5b]Urology and Nephrology Center, [6]Medical Experimental Research Center (MERC), Faculty of Medicine, Mansoura University, Mansoura, Egypt.

ADMSC culture

ADMSCs were isolated from human abdominal fat tissue collected during liposuction Surgery at Plastic Surgery Hospital, Faculty of Medicine, Mansoura University, Egypt. All eligible patients or their guardians provided their written informed consent and permission to isolate the MSCs from fat tissues. The culture methods were based on the method of Bunnell *et al.*[10]. The tissue was washed with phosphate-buffered saline (PBS) containing 1% antibiotic–antimycotic solution (Thermo scientific, USA) thrice, until all blood vessels and connective tissue appear liberated. This step was followed by digestion with trypsin (Sigma-Aldrich, USA) 0.125 % at 37 °C with shaking at 100 rpm (3ml for each 1 gm Adipose tissue) for 60 min. The tissue digestion was checked every 15 min and the tissue digestion vessel was shaken vigorously. After digestion, trypsin activity was neutralized by adding equal volume of Dulbecco's modified Eagle's medium (DMEM; Lonza, Verviers, Belgium) containing 10% fetal bovine serum (FBS; Thermo scientific, USA), to the tissue sample. The cell suspension was filtered through 100 µm filters (BD Falcon, USA) for avoiding the solid aggregates. The sample was then centrifuged at 2000 rpm for 5 min at room temperature. The samples were taken out of the centrifuge and shaken vigorously to complete the separation of the stromal cells from the primary adipocytes. The centrifugation step was repeated and the supernatant was removed without disturbing the cells. The pellet was suspended in 1 ml of lysis buffer (Promega, Germany) to lyse the RBCs and then incubated for 10 min. Then the pellet was washed with 10 ml of PBS+1% antibiotic–anti mycotic and centrifuged at 2000 rpm for 5 min. Supernatant was removed and the cell pellet was suspended in DMEM with 20% FBS and 1% antibiotic-anti mycotic solution in 25-cm^2 culture flask and maintained in an incubator supplied with humidified atmosphere of 5% CO_2 at 37°C.

Cell culture

After a day, non-adherent cells were removed by two to three washes with PBS and adherent cells were further cultured in complete medium. The medium was changed every 3 days until the monolayer of adherent cells reached 70-80% confluence. Then, we used trypsinization for cell splitting by employing trypsin-EDTA solution (0. 25%, sigma Aldrich, USA) for passage 1. The number of cells was evaluated using hemocytometer and cellular viability was assessed by the Trypan Blue exclusion test. Each 250-300×10^3 cells were inoculated in a 75 cm^2 culture flask that was incubated at 37°C and 5% CO_2. Cell cultivation was maintained up to the third passage.

Phenotypic analysis with Flow cytometry

Cells were characterized using cell surface mesenchymal markers by fluorescence-activated cell sorting (FACS) analyses. The cells were stained with different fluorescent labeled monoclonal antibodies (mAbs), CD29 and CD90 (eBioscience), CD 13, CD 105, CD34 and 14 mAbs as hematopoietic lineages markers. In brief, 5×10^5 cells (in100 µl PBS/ 0.5% BSA/2mmol/L EDTA) were mixed with 10 µl of the fluorescent labeled mAb and incubated in the dark at 2-8 °C for 30 min. They were then washed twice with PBS containing 2% BSA. The pellet was re-suspended in PBS and analyzed immediately using flow cytometry. The fluorescence intensity of the cells was evaluated by EPICS-XL flow cytometry (Coulter, Miami, FL, USA).

Colony forming unit-fibroblast (CFU-F)

Fibroblast colony growth was evaluated in the primary cells grown on tissue culture in six-well dishes[11]. About 100 cells were plated in 100-mm tissue culture dish (Falcon) in complete culture medium. Cells were incubated for 10–14 days at 37 °C in 5% humidified CO_2,

washed with PBS and fixed in 95% ethanol for 5 minutes, then incubated for 20- 30 minutes at room temperature in 0.5% crystal violet (sigma Aldrich, USA) in 95% ethanol and then the plates were washed twice with distilled H_2O. The plates were dried and the CFU-F units counted.

Differentiation capability of hADMSCs

a) Osteogenic Differentiation:

Passage 3 MSCs were harvested by trypsin digestion as described above. The cells were counted and seeded at a density of 5×10^4 per well in a 6-well plate. Then at 80% confluence, to four of the wells, osteogenesis differentiation media: DMEM supplemented with 10% FBS, 0.1µM dexamethasone, 50µM Ascorbic acid, 10mM β-glycerol phosphate (Sigma-Aldrich, USA) was added. To the other two wells, complete culture media as negative control[12] was added. The media were changed twice per week for 2-3 weeks. The differentiation potential for osteogenesis was assessed by 40 mM Alizarin Red (pH 4.1) after fixation in 10% neutral buffered formalin[13].

b) Adipogenic Differentiation:

Passage 3 MSCs harvested by trypsin digestion as described above were counted and seeded at a density of 10×10^4 per well in a 6-well plate, then at 100% confluence. To four of the wells, adipogenesis differentiation media: DMEM supplemented with 10% FBS, 1µM dexamethasone, 500-µM isobutylmethylxanthine (IBMX) 5µg/ml insulin, 200µM Indomethacin (Sigma-Aldrich, USA) was added. To the other two wells, complete culture media as negative control was added. The media were changed twice per week for 2 weeks[12]. The differentiation potential for adipogenesis and formation of intracellular lipid droplets were assessed by Oil-red-O after fixation in 10% neutral buffered formalin[13].

c) Chondrogenesis Differentiation:

MSCs were harvested and 6×10^5 cells were centrifuged to form a pellet on the bottom of a 15-ml polypropylene tube (Falcon). The micro mass was cultured in 500µl of chondrogenic medium that consisted of 50 µg/ml ascorbic acid 2-phosphate and 1 ng/ml TGF-β1[12] (Sigma). After 3 weeks of culture, cell clumps were harvested, embedded in paraffin, cut into 3-µm sections and stained for glycosaminoglycans using 0.1% safranin O (Sigma).

Detection by Image J analysis

Twenty different digital images corresponding to four different preparations of osteogenic, adipogenic, chondrogenic differentiated cells and undifferentiated controls were analyzed using Image J 1.42 software on an appropriate threshold. Image J can calculate area and pixel value statistics of user-defined selections and intensity threshold objects. It can measure distances and angles. It can create density histograms and line profile plots [14].

Identification of MSCs differentiation to adipocytes by RT-PCR analysis

MSCs differentiation to adipocytes was further demonstrated by Real-time quantitative reverse transcriptase-polymerase chain reaction (RT–PCR) analysis of adipocytic and osteocytic markers expression (Table 1). Total RNA was isolated from MSCs and real-time reverse transcriptase-PCR was performed as described previously[12]. Selective markers and primer sequences were used. Glyceraldehyde-3-phosphate dehydrogenase (GAPDH) was used as an internal standard.

Table 1: Primers for Adipogenic and osteogenic differentiation RT-PCR of human adipose derived mesenchymal stem cells

		Forward Primer	Reverse Primer
1)Adipogenic Genes	Adiponectin	TCCTGCCAGTAACAGGGAAG	GGTTGGCGATTACCCGTTTG
	adipocyte lipid-binding protein (ALBP)	TACCTGGAAACTTGTCTCCAGTGAA	CCATTTCTGCACATGTACCAGGACA
	Lipoprotein Lipase	CTGCTGGCGTAGCAGGAAGT	GCTGGAAAGTGCCTCCATTG
	Lipten	TGACACCAAAACCCTCATCA	TCATTGGCTATCTGCAGCAC
2)Osteogenic Gene	Osteocalcin	ACACTCCTCGCCCTATTG	GATGTGGTCAGCCAACTC

Total RNA extracted from the cultured cells, following the manufacturer's instructions. For adipogenic differentiation, the cells assessed using specific Primers identified in Table 1. The RT-PCR procedure performed using the One Step RT-PCR kit, beginning at 50°C for 30 min and 95°C for 15 min for reverse transcription and then followed by 35 cycles. Each cycle consisted of denaturation at 94°C for 1 min, annealing at 57°C for 1 min, elongation at 72°C for 1 min and the final extension at 72°C for 10 min. The amplified DNA fragments visualized through 2% agarose gel electrophoreses then photographed under UV light.

hADMSCs in basic culture conditions expressed adiponectin and adipocyte lipid-binding protein (ALBP).

Animal Treatment

Male Sprague-Dawley rats (250–300 g) were maintained in a 12:12-h light-/dark cycle in a temperature and humidity- controlled facility. Standard rat chow and water provided. Animal studies were conducted according to the experimental protocol that was approved by the Local Ethical Committee, Faculty of Medicine, Mansoura University. Animals were divided into four equal groups (each group=20). The negative control group received a single injection of saline intraperitoneally. The positive control cisplatin group was given a single intraperitoneal injection of cisplatin (10 mg/kg body wt.) and an equal volume of PBS instead of ADMSCs. The ADMSCs group was given a single injection of ADMSCs (5×10^6 cells) by tail vein. The cisplatin and ADMSCs group received single dose cisplatin and only one dose ADMSCs given at day 1 after cisplatin injection. For long term study on the protective effect of ADMSC against cisplatin AKI, each main group was further divided according to the timing of sacrifice, into four equal subgroups (each subgroup n=5). Subgroup A sacrificed after 4 days; subgroup B sacrificed after 7 days; subgroup C sacrificed after 11 days and subgroup D sacrificed after 30 days. Before sacrifice, 24 hrs.-urine was collected using a metabolic cage. Rats were sacrificed using an over dose of thiopental. Blood samples were collected from the heart immediately centrifuged at approximately 3000 g for 5 min., and then taken for biochemical measurements. The kidneys were removed for histological evaluation.

Assessment of renal function

Serum samples were examined for blood urea nitrogen (BUN), serum creatinine, creatinine clearance using Diamond Diagnostics (Egypt) standard diagnostic kits.

Assessment of Oxidative stress markers

Kidney tissue homogenate was used for assessment of MDA, SOD, and GSH, using Biodiagnostic Co. (Egypt) for all the groups and subgroups.

Renal histology and damage scoring

The left kidney was perfused in a retrograde fashion through the abdominal aorta using saline 0.9% until complete clearance of the perfusion fluid and then 10% neutral buffered formalin for in situ fixation. Renal samples were coded and processed for light microscopic examination. Histopathological changes were analyzed in the different regions of the kidney (cortex, outer strip of outer medulla "OSOM", inner strip of outer medulla "ISOM" and inner medulla using H&E, periodic acid- Schiff (PAS) reagent and Masson trichrome stains according to a new scoring system *(submitted for publication).*

Active injury changes

These include necrotic tubules and interstitial infiltration by inflammatory cells. Necrotic tubules were scored according to the number of necrotic tubules counted/high power field (HPF) and scored to 1, 2, 3 and 4 corresponding to 1-3, 4-5, 6-10 and >10 necrotic tubules / HPF. The inflammatory cells were scored as 1, 2, 3 corresponding to mild, moderate & severe. The maximum score of active injury is 7.

Regenerative changes

These include presence of mitosis, solid cellular sheets between the tubules, intraluminal cellular proliferation forming solid tubules, tubules lined with large vesicular nuclei and tubules lined by cells having hyperchromatic prominent nuclei and little cytoplasm giving the luminal border a festooned appearance. Each of the solid cellular sheets and solid tubules was counted as 1-2, 3-5 and > 5 / HPF were scored as 1, 2 and 3 respectively. Mitosis was scored as 1, 2 and 3 corresponding to 1-2, 3-5 and > 5 /10 HPF. Tubules with large vesicular nuclei and tubules with basophilic prominent nuclei got score 1, when present and got score 0, if absent. The maximum score of regeneration was 11.

Chronic changes

These include atrophic tubules with flat lining, casts, and thick basement membrane and interstitial fibrosis. The maximum chronicity score was 7; where the number of atrophic tubules /HPF of 1-5, 6-10 and > 10 were scored 1, 2 and 3 respectively. In addition, the percentages of interstitial fibrosis / HPF of 25, 25-50, 50-75 and more than 75 % got scores of 1, 2, 3 and 4 respectively.

Statistical analysis

Data was analyzed using SPSS version 16. Variables were tested for normality of distribution using Kolmogrov-Smirnov test. Both the biochemical and the morphological results were non-parametric. Kruskal-Wallis test was used for comparison. The results are presented as mean± SD. P≤0.05 was considered statistically significant.

Results

Isolation and characterization of human ADMSCs

Human ADMSCs were isolated from human fat tissue that was obtained from abdominal fat of liposuction surgery. Attachment of spindle-shaped cells to tissue culture plastic flask was observed after 1 day of culture of the ADMSCs. After 5 days, spindle-shaped cells reached 80% confluency. Morphology of cells changed gradually with the increase in passage number. Cells became more flat-shaped with increase in passage number (Figure 1A).

Colony forming unit- fibroblast (CFU-F)

CFU-F assay was a suitable tool for evaluating the proliferation and colonogenic capacity of the cells (3rd passage) expanded in culture. The colony number of 100 ADMSCs per 100-mm tissue culture dish was 38 ± 1 (Figure 1 B&C). The ADMSCs isolated from human adipose tissue used in our experiments, were plastic-adherent and capable of extensive proliferation when maintained in their standard culture conditions.

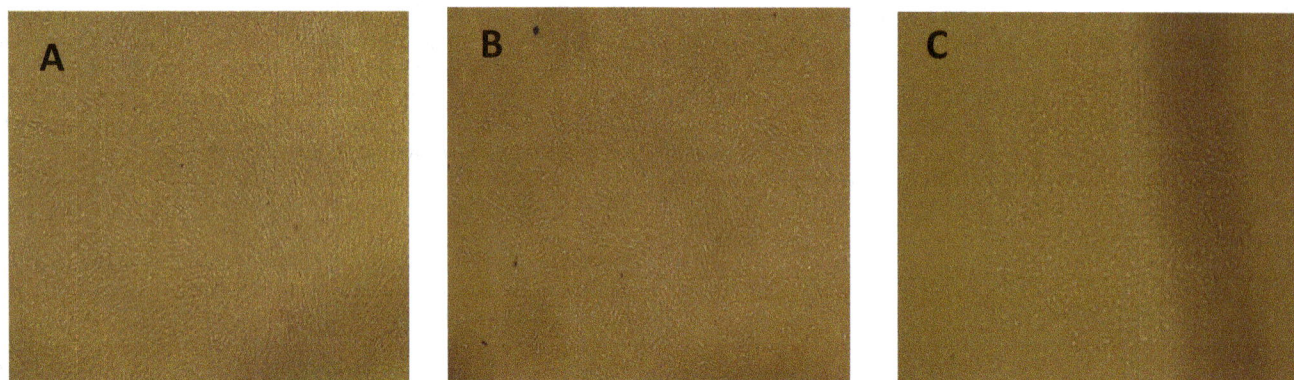

Figure (1). *Characterization of human adipose- derived mesenchymal cells (AD-MSCs). (A): Under an inverse microscopy (magnification × 200) cultured mesenchymal stem cell (MSCs) derived from human adipose tissue at passage three were morphologically defined by the fibroblast–like appearance. (B) & (C) Colony forming unit- fibroblast (CFU-F): Photomicrographs of human adipose tissue derived mesenchymal stem cell (MSCs) after one week of culture grew in colonies that contained heterogeneous small spindle-shaped fibroblastoid cells and more rounded cells {A and B original magnification × 100}*

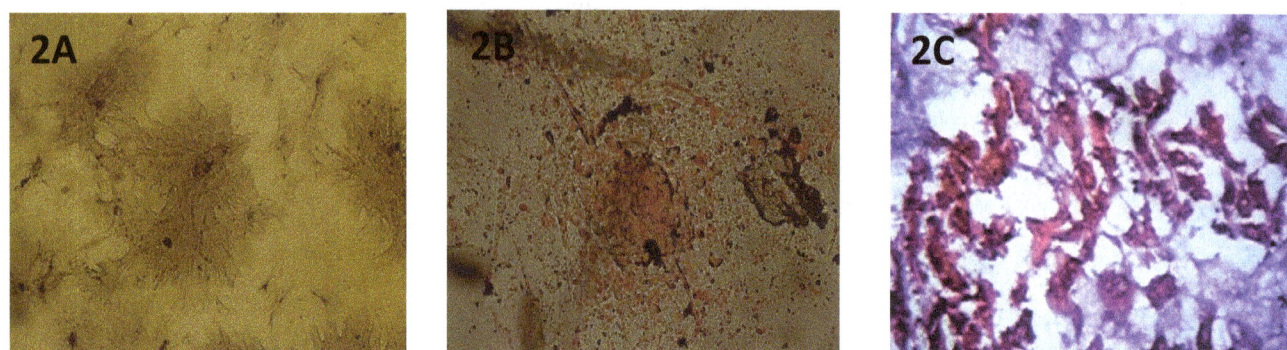

Figure 2: *hADMSCs differentiation capability. Photomicrographs of mesenchymal stem cells (MSC) derived from human adipose tissue showing differentiative potential. (A) Osteogenic differentiation indicated by the formation of calcium-rich hydroxyapatite detected with Alizarin red and appear as irregular red –orange {magnification × 200}. (B) Adipogenic differentiation apparent after 1 week of incubation with adipogenic induction medium. Between the culture periods of 3±2 weeks, almost all cells contained numerous Oil Red O-positive lipid droplets (C) Chondrogenic differentiation apparent after 1 week of incubation with chondrogenic induction medium. Between the culture periods of 3±2 weeks, almost all cells contained numerous glycosaminoglycans.*

Differentiation capability of hADMSCs

Distinct culture conditions demonstrated the pluripotency of ADMSCs. They enabled cells to differentiate into osteoblasts, adipoblasts and chondroblasts. According to Image J analysis and spectrophotometric analysis, Image J analysis of differentiated vs. undifferentiated cells resulted in fold increase of ADMSCs for each type of cells; 3.4±0.5 for osteoblasts, 2.6±0.7 for adipoblasts and 3.3±0.6 for chondroblasts (Figure 2 A, B & C respectively).

Immunophenotypic characterization (RT- PCR)

In Adipogenic culture conditions a transcription factor was identified (Figure 3). Figure 3A shows amplification plot of leptin expression at 4,7,14 days. ADMSCs expressed lipoprotein lipase (Figure 3B), leptin (Figure 3C) and adiponectin (Figure 3D) as demonstrated by Gel electrophoresis. For osteocytic gene markers expression, under human adipose osteogenesis culture conditions ADMSCs expressed osteocalcin at different time intervals of 4, 7, 14 and 21 days (Figure 4).

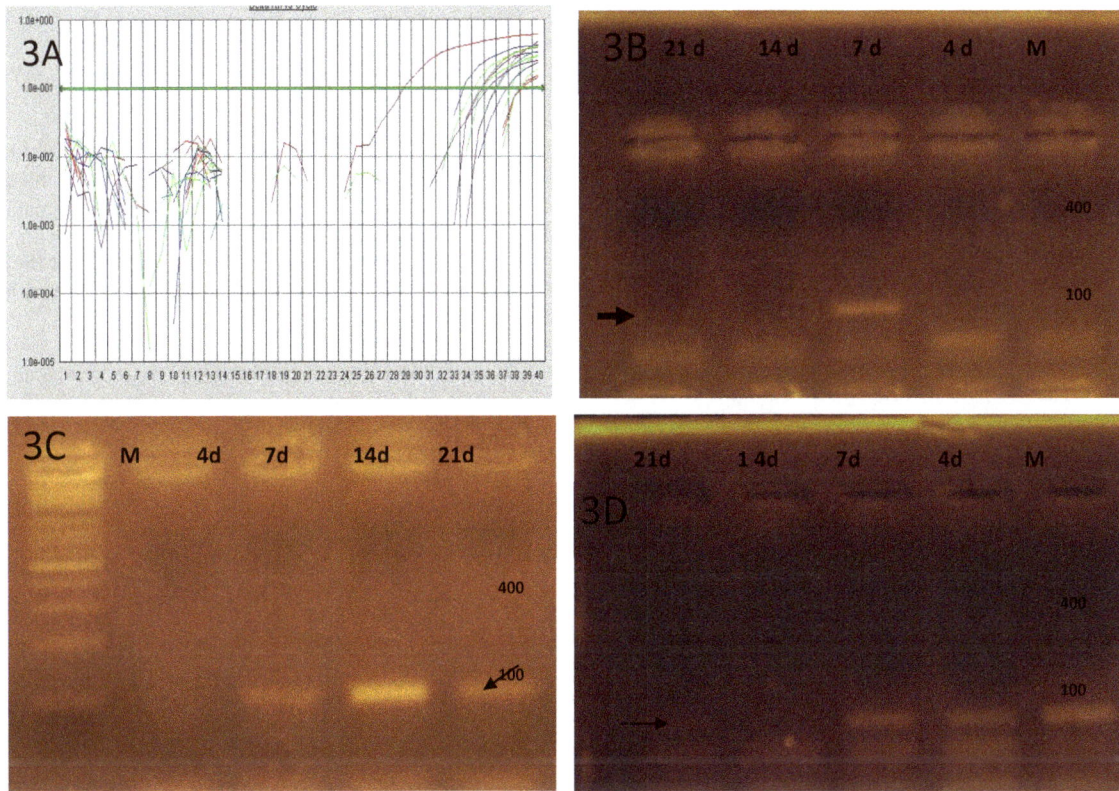

Figure3: ADMSCs differentiation demonstrated adipogenic differentiation by RT-PCR analysis of genes markers expression; (A) Amplification Plot of adipocytic marker gene (Leptin) at 4, 7, 14, 21 days. (B) Agarose gel electrophoresis showing positive expression of lipoprotein lipase at day 7 by RT- PCR. (C) Agarose gel electrophoresis showing positive expression of leptin at day 7, 14, 21 by RT- PCR. (D) Agarose gel electrophoresis showing positive expression of adiponectin

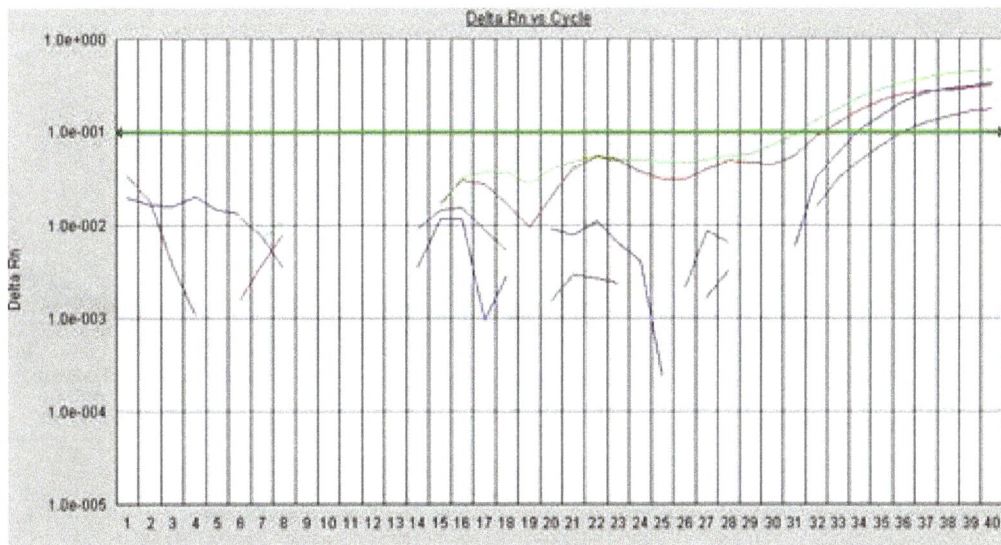

Figure4: ADMSCs differentiation demonstrated osteogenic differentiation by RT-PCR analysis of genes markers expression; Amplification Plot of osteogenic marker gene (osteocalcin) at 4, 7, 14, 21 days.

Phenotypic analysis

We carried on further characterization of ADMSCs. Fluorescence-activated cells confirmed the endogenous expression of the most important surface markers for MSCs; CD90, CD29, CD105 and CD13. On the other hand, those rarely expressed CD34 and CD14 showed negative results (Figure 5).

ADMSCs' protective effect against renal impairment caused by cisplatin

Evaluated by serum creatinine, BUN and creatinine clearance (Table 2). I.P injection of 5 mg/kg cisplatin induced significant increases in serum creatinine and BUN, which peaked at days 4 and 7 and declined at days 11.

They stabilized at the 30th day to values slightly higher than baseline. Meanwhile, intravenous injection of 5×10^5 MSC on day 1 after receiving cisplatin strongly protected renal function at days 4, 7, 11 and 30 as reflected by significantly lower serum creatinine and BUN values in comparison to cisplatin-treated rats that were given fresh culture media intravenously. Figure 6A indicates the long-term protective effect of ADMSCs on kidney function in term of creatinine clearance.

ADMSCs effect on oxidative stress caused by cisplatin: (Table2).

Cisplatin increased renal tissue MDA detectable at days 4, 7, 11 and 30. Intravenous injection of 5×10^6 MSC into the rats on day 1 after receiving cisplatin induced significant decrease in MDA measured at days 4, 7, 11 and 30 when compared with cisplatin-injected rats treated with fresh culture media via tail vein. ADMSCs increased significantly, the renal tissue homogenate GSH and SOD levels content which was demonstrated in MSCs group at all intervals when compared to the non-treated groups. Figure 6B indicates the protective effect of ADMSCs on kidney function in the term of MDA on the long term.

ADMSCs reduced renal injury caused by cisplatin on long-term study

Evaluated by H&E that was performed on the kidney sections. Regenerative changes were found as early as the 4th day in addition to less tubular necrosis and atrophy than in cisplatin injected rats (Group I) and cisplatin injected rats treated with culture media through tail vein (Group III). Moreover, the ADMSCs continued to offer protection to renal tissue and ameliorate renal injury until the 30th day.

The detailed histological changes were observed in kidney tissue samples at the different time intervals (Figure 7 A & B) (Table 3):

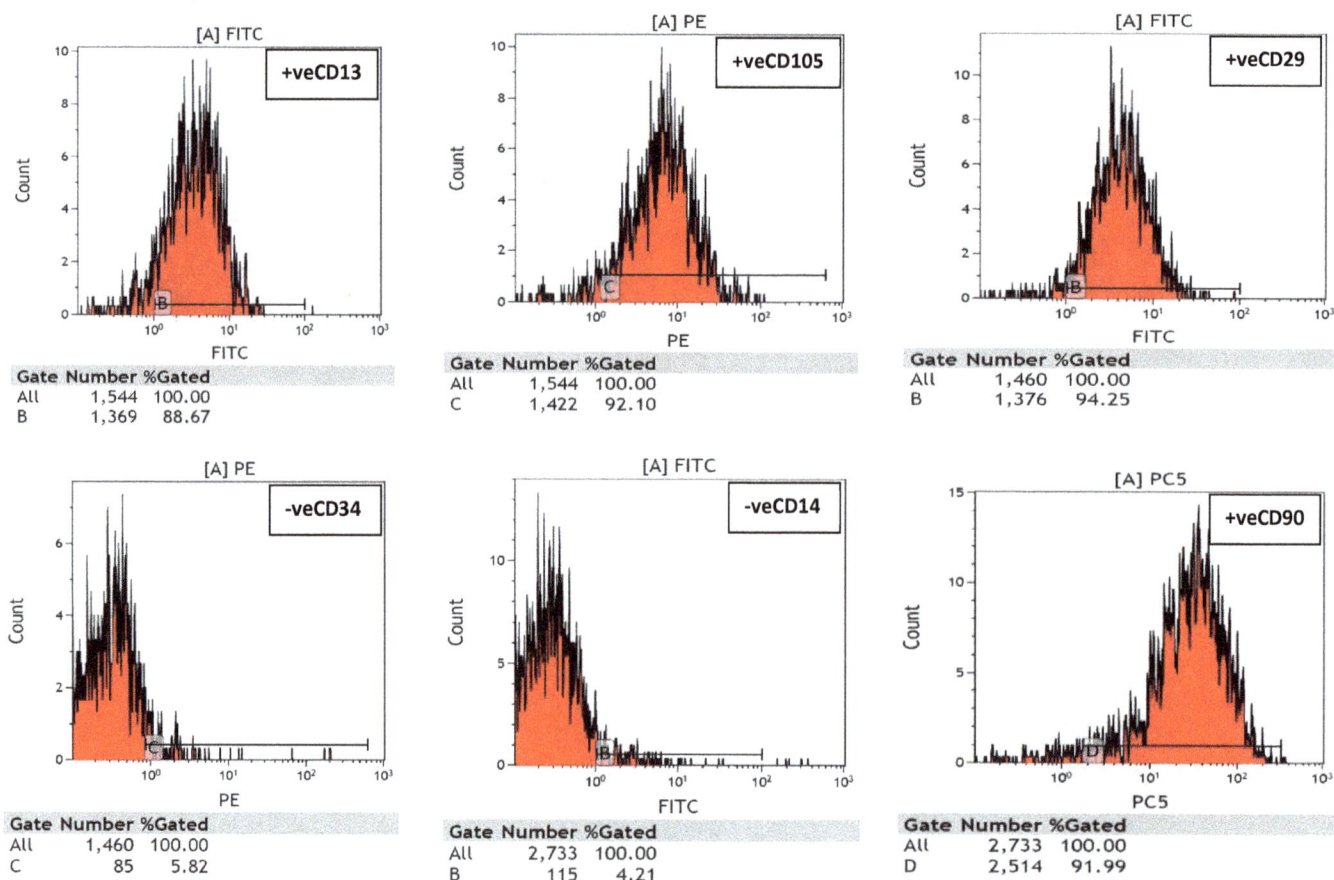

Figure 5: *Flow cytometry analysis of surface markers on cultured human adipose tissue mesenchymal stem cells revealed that their expression of surface antigens such as CD29 (94%), CD 90 (92%), CD 105 (92%) and CD13 (89%). (Passage 4:8) was strongly positive; but CD14 (4%) and CD34 (6%) was negative.*

Table 2: ADMSCs' effects on renal function and tissue oxidative stress markers level in cisplatin- induced nephrotoxicity on long term. (mean ± SD)

	Control	Cisplatin	Cisplatin+C.Medium	Cisplatin+ SCs
S. Creatinine(mg/dl)				
Day 4	0.47±0.11	1.92±0.04*	1.89±0.12*	1.02±0.11*°
Day 7	0.48±0.13	1.61±0.06*‡	1.62±0.04*‡	0.85±0.11*°‡
Day 11	0.48±0.18	0.97±0.14*‡†	0.98±0.18*‡†	0.70±0.08*°‡
Day 30	0.43±0.11	0.76±0.04*‡†	0.79±0.05*‡†	0.56±0.07*°‡†
Cr.Clearance(ml/min./100gm)				
Day 4	1.600±0.860	0.007±0.002*	0.008±0.002*	0.017±0.009*°
Day 7	1.600±0.760	0.014±0.001*‡	0.012±0.003*‡	0.045±0.012*°‡
Day 11	1.600±0.790	0.054±0.016*‡†	0.056±0.020*‡†	0.650±0.117*°‡†
Day 30	1.600±0.350	0.340±0.240*‡†•	0.360±0.320*‡†•	0.860±0.243*°‡†
S.BUN(mg/dl)				
Day 4	054.36±03.31	266.70±08.70*	265.30±08.60*	097.80±07.67*°
Day 7	053.39±04.51	228.70±18.00*‡	236.00±15.00*‡	076.40±04.30*°‡
Day 11	054.43±03.91	137.40±14.70*‡†	138.60±16.30*‡†	068.34±04.60*°‡†
Day 30	054.55±03.62	111.46±11.50*‡†•	112.58±08.40*‡†•	068.34±04.60*°‡†
MDA tissue (nmol/gm)				
Day 4	14.50±3.43	67.40±3.40*	69.50±4.80*	34.20±8.54*°
Day 7	14.50±3.89	65.10±4.54*	63.20±3.87*	25.40±2.86*°‡
Day 11	14.60±2.56	34.10±4.70*‡†	37.20±4.60*‡†	17.30±3.82°‡†
Day 30	14.50±2.46	32.80±5.10*‡†	33.20±5.40*‡†	16.32±3.65°‡†
Tissue GSH (mmol/gm)				
Day 4	5.36±0.17	0.26±0.03*	0.27±0.05*	0.77±0.03*°
Day 7	5.38±1.15	0.53±0.04*‡	0.56±0.05*‡	2.56±0.05*°‡
Day 11	5.35±0.18	1.38±0.42*‡†	1.35±0.35*‡†	3.53±0.21*°‡†
Day 30	5.39±0.35	1.92±0.04*‡†•	1.95±0.08*‡†•	4.12±0.22*°‡†•
Tissue SOD U/gm)				
Day 4	20.86±1.24	3.25±0.64*	3.70±0.65*	6.85±0.52*°
Day 7	20.82±1.64	6.24±0.57*‡	6.46±0.62*‡	10.67±0.38*°‡
Day 11	20.78±1.28	9.96±0.30*‡†	9.94±0.52*‡†	15.62±0.43*°‡†
Day 30	20.73±0.84	15.24±0.46*‡†•	15.43±0.52*‡†•	18.67±0.42°‡†•

Significant difference compared to corresponding * control, ° cisplatin groups

Significant difference compared to intra-group day4‡, day7†, day11• by Kruskal-Wallis test at P≤0.05

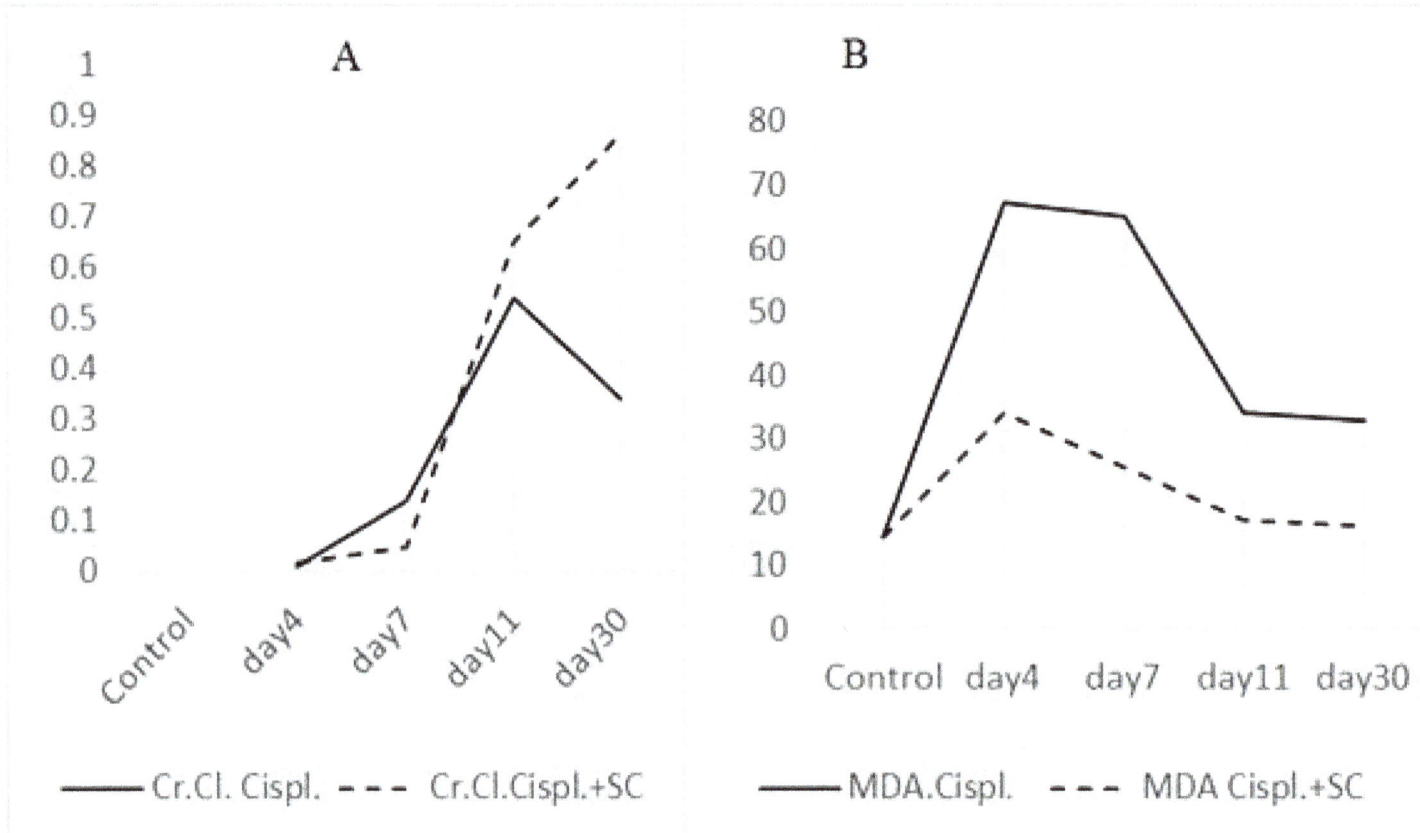

Figure 6: ADMSCs effect on A] creatinine clearance and on B] renal tissue MAD level in cisplatin induced AKI at different time intervals.

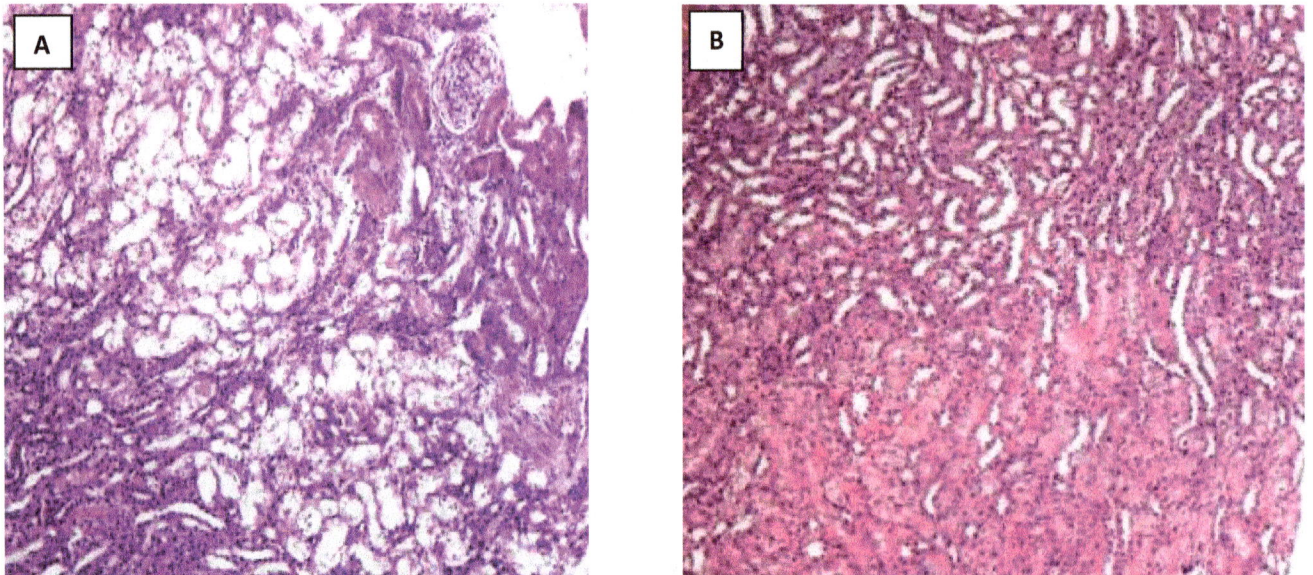

*Figure 7: Long-term ADMSCS effects on Renal **Histopathology and Scoring** in cisplatin- induced nephrotoxicity (mean ± SD).: Day 4 A) Sections taken from cisplatin injected rats (group I) after 4 days revealed marked necrotic and degenerative changes in the OSOM where the tubules are dilated with thin denuded lining epithelium. Degenerative changes with apoptosis and shedding of tubular cells in about 90% of the tubules. Mild regenerative changes were also detected in OSOM in the form of some regenerating tubules (5%) lined by large cells with prominent nucleoli and with occasional mitotic figures. No solid sheets were detected .B) In ADMSCs injected group VI, less degenerative changes with less complete tubular necrosis. Regenerative changes were markedly detected in the OSOM in the form of many regenerating tubules (70-80%) lined by large cells with large hyperchromatic active nuclei with few solid sheets (less than 1/20 HPF). (HX&E× 100}.*

Table 3: ADMSCs effect on acute renal injury, regenerative and chronicity scores in the outer stripe of the outer medulla of rat kidney after cisplatin (n = 5 in each group for each time subgroup; mean ± SD)

	Control	Cispl.	Cispl.+ C.Medium	Cispl.+ ADMSC
Necrotic tub.				
4	0.0±0.0	12.6±2.1*	8.4±1.7*	3.9±0.3*°
7	0.0±0.0	8.6±1.3*‡	8.3±1.5*	4.6±0.4*°
11	0.0±0.0	7.4±1.8*‡	7.5±2.2*	2.6±0.2*°‡†
30	0.0±0.0	4.7±0.1*‡†•	2.4±0.3*‡†•	1.0±0.6*°‡†•
Inflam. cells				
4	0.0±0.0	8.8±1.3*	8.4±1.6*	1.8±0.2*°
7	0.0±0.0)	8.4±1.6*	8.3±1.9*	1.5±0.3*°
11	0.0±0.0	8.5±1.1*	8.1±1.5*	0.0±0.0°‡†
30	0.0±0.0	4.7±0.2*‡†•	4.4±0.3*‡†•	0.0±0.0°‡†
Reg. Tub.				
4	0.0±0.0	0.0±0.0	0.0±0.0	1.2±0.2*°
7	0.0±0.0	0.0±0.0	0.0±0.0	2.7±0.2*°‡
11	0.0±0.0	0.0±0.0	0.0±0.0	7.5±1.6*°‡†
30	0.0±0.0	1.4±0.2*‡†•	1.6±0.3*‡†•	7.4±2.9*°‡†
Mitosis				
4	0.0±0.0	0.0±0.0	0.0±0.0	2.2±0.8*°
7	0.0±0.0	0.0±0.0	0.0±0.0	3.7±0.2*°‡
11	0.0±0.0)	1.7±0.2*‡†	1.5±0.3*‡†	4.5±0.3*°‡†
30	0.0±0.0	1.7±0.2*‡†	1.5±0.2*‡†	4.9±0.9*°‡†
Solid Sheets				
4	0.0±0.0	0.0±0.0	0.0±0.0	2.8±0.8*°
7	0.0±0.0	0.0±0.0	0.0±0.0	4.8±0.6*°‡
11	0.0±0.0	0.0±0.0	0.0±0.0	5.7±0.5*°‡
30	0.0±0.0	1.3±0.2*‡†•	1.4±0.4*‡†•	6.9±2.8*°‡
Int. Fibrosis				
4	0.0±0.0	0.0±0.0	0.0±0.0	0.0±0.0
7	0.0±0.0)	23.7±0.91*‡	23.1±1.4*‡	4.6±0.3*°‡
11	0.0±0.0	34.2±1.3*‡†	32.8±2.3*‡†	11.9±1.8*°‡†
30	0.0±0.0)	47.6±2.6*‡†•	43.7±2.7*‡†•	17.8±1.7*°‡†•
Atrophic Tub.				
4	0.0±0.0	13.3±2.3*	12.5±1.4*	6.5±0.3*°
7	0.0±0.0	12.7±1.2*	12.5±1.3*	4.7±0.4*°‡
11	0.0±0.0	12.4±0.8*	12.3±0.6*	3.8±1.8*°‡
30	0.0±0.0	4.4±0.2*‡†•	4.6±0.2*‡†•	2.8±0.6*°‡†

Significant difference compared to corresponding * control, ° cisplatin groups &
Significant difference compared to intragroup day4‡, day7†, day11• by Kruskal-Wallis test at P≤0.05

<u>Day 4:</u>

Sections taken from cisplatin-injected rats (Group II) and cisplatin-injected rats treated with culture media through tail vein (Group III) after 4 days revealed marked degenerative changes mainly in OSOM. It varied from tubular cell vacuolar degeneration, up to complete tubular necrosis with apoptosis and shedding of tubular cells in about 90% of the tubules. Mild regenerative changes were also detected in OSOM in the form of some regenerating tubules (5%) lined by large cells with prominent nucleoli and with occasional mitotic figures. No solid sheets were detected.

In ADMSCs injected group VI, regenerative changes were markedly detected in the OSOM and ISOM in the form of many regenerating tubules (70-80%) lined by large cells with large hyperchromatic active nuclei with few solid sheets (less than 1/20 HPF).

<u>Day 7:</u>

Sections from cisplatin injected (Group II) and cisplatin-injected rats treated with culture media through tail vein (Group III) on 7th day showed pathological features mainly in the OSOM in the form of combined degenerative and regenerative changes. The degenerative changes predominated representing about 90% of all studied fields in this group. They varied from tubular cell vacuolar degeneration up to complete tubular necrosis with pyknosis and shedding of tubular cells. The regenerative changes detected in about 20% of all fields examined in the group, varied from tubular cell enlargement, mitosis and interstitial solid sheet formation.

Sections obtained from cisplatin-injected rats and ADMSCs (Group VI) sacrificed on the 7th day showed less marked degenerative changes in OSOM. The degenerative changes varied from tubular cell vacuolar degeneration, up to complete tubular necrosis with apoptosis and shedding of tubular cells in about 60-70% of the tubules.

Regenerative changes detected in both outer and inner medulla were in the form of many interstitial solid sheets (12/10 HPF) and tubules lined by large cells with prominent nucleoli with occasional mitosis.

<u>Day 11:</u>

Kidney sections obtained from cisplatin-injected rats (Group II) and cisplatin-injected rats injected with culture media through tail vein (Group III) on the 11th day revealed that the degenerative changes were more marked. The degenerative changes varied from tubular cell vacuolar degeneration, upto complete tubular necrosis with apoptosis and shedding of tubular cells in more than 80 - 90% of the tubules. In addition, there was mild interstitial round cell infiltrate. Regenerative changes were also detected and varied from tubular cell enlargement with regenerative atypia, mitosis and interstitial solid sheets (5/10 HPF).

Kidney sections obtained from cisplatin-injected rats treated with ADMSCs via tail vein (Group VI) and sacrificed on the 11th day revealed necrotic tubules (about 1 tubule /HPFs) with epithelial shedding and tubular dilatation. Regenerative changes were detected in the form of solid sheets having prominent bulging nuclei (about 1/10 HPFs), mitosis (less than 1/10HPFs) and regenerating tubules were detected in one rat of the group. The interstitium was the seat of focal round cell infiltration in one rat.

<u>Day 30:</u>

Sections obtained on day 30 from cisplatin-injected rats (Group II) and cisplatin injected and treated with culture media through tail vein (Group III) revealed occasional regenerating large tubules in the OSOM lined by large cells with prominent nucleoli and occasional mitotic figures (1/10HPFs). There was mild peritubular and perivascular fibrosis (about 5-10% of all fields).

Sections from kidney samples obtained from cisplatin-injected rats

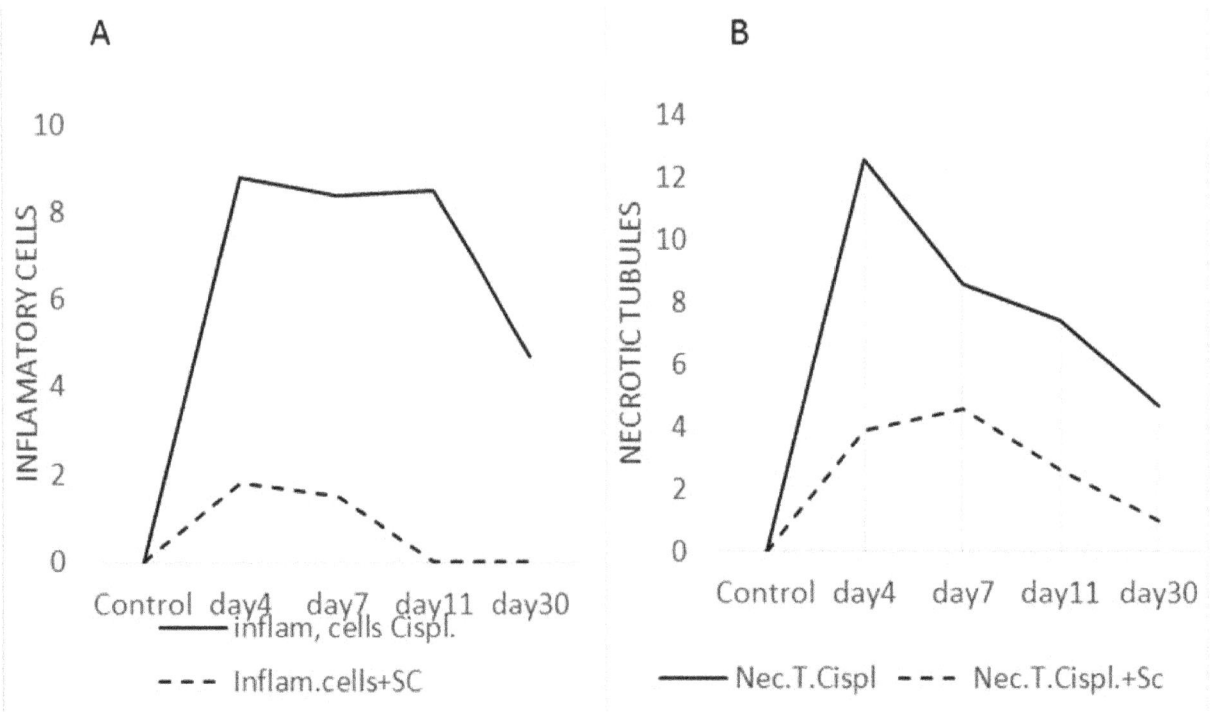

Figure 8: ADMSCs protective effect for renal tubules from cisplatin induced AKI at different time intervals. Histological changes observed in kidney tissue samples at different time intervals identified the variation in (A) inflammatory cell infiltration, (B) Necrotic tubules.

treated with ADMSCs via tail vein (Group VI) and sacrificed on the 30th day showed significantly less chronicity in regard to the tubular atrophy and the renal fibrosis, when compared with the cisplatin groups. The effect of ADMSCs on renal structure in term of inflammatory cell infiltration and on the necrotic tubules indicate their long-term protective activity (Figure 8 A & B).

Discussion

Several human malignancies are largely managed with cisplatin. However, in the setting of nephrotoxicity, which is one of the serious side effects of cisplatin, its clinical use as a chemotherapeutic agent is largely limited. Cisplatin acts on multiple cellular targets and hence, blocking its effect on a single target may only offer partial protection against nephrotoxicity[1].

Although the clinical management of AKI patients has significantly improved in recent years, we still lack specific therapies to enhance kidney repair. Recovery after acute injury is critical for patient morbidity and mortality in the hospital setting[16]. The emerging field of regenerative medicine is progressing rapidly and supported by a large number of studies which have demonstrated the capacity of stem cells to substitute for the damaged or lost differentiated cells in various organs and tissues[17-22].

Few studies have discussed the use of cord blood and bone marrow MSCs for the management of AKI models[23-25]. In addition, the ability of adipose tissue derived stromal cells to ameliorate the AKI induced via cisplatin has been reported[26].

Reviewing the literature, some published studies have reported the impact of MSCs on cisplatin induced AKI[7-9]. Shaohua and Dongcheng's study in 2013[7] was based on rat BMMSCs, while Weique et al. 2015[8] and Kim et al. 2015[9] studies were based on human ADMSCs. The latter reported that ADMSCs exert a paracrine protective effect on cisplatin nephrotoxicity and suggested that human ADMSCs might be a new therapeutic approach for patients with acute kidney injury. Many points distinguish our work from these studies as follows; (1) all of the previous studies evaluated the protective effect of MSCs only for a short duration (only the acute effect for 3 to 5 days of cisplatin induced AKI). While our work, in addition to evaluating the short duration effect, has evaluated the long term protective effect (the chronic effect) (2) the sample size used in those studies was noticeably small while our work included a large sample size, (3) these studies identified renal protective effect of MSCs only using biochemical renal function analyses and renal histology. An important parameter in our work, was the assessment of the oxidative stress in kidney tissue for evaluating the ADMSCs' protective effect (4) In addition, through scoring of different histopathological findings, this study tried to evaluate both the protective and the regenerative activities of ADMSCs by correlating them to the biochemical parameters.

The damaging effect of cisplatin on the kidney comprises of complex interrelated sequence of events eventually resulting in both apoptosis and necrosis of the renal cells[1]. Thus, an ideal modality to manage cisplatin nephrotoxicity should work by multiple mechanisms.

The aim of our study was to address the role of ADMSCs in AKI secondary to cisplatin administration where 80 rats were divided into four equal groups: positive control (cisplatin injected); negative control (saline injected group); (cisplatin injected and culture media treated) and (cisplatin injected and ADMSCs treated) group.

Moreover, in each group, rats' were subgrouped based on day of sacrifice on day 4, day 7, day 11 and day 30 to study the evolution of ADMSCs activity on the acute injury, regenerative activity and the tissue chronicity events induced by cisplatin separately. In our study, the use of ADMSCs was capable of ameliorating renal dysfunction; as demonstrated by improvement of serum creatinine, creatinine clearance and improvement of the histological indices of injury in the renal cortex and outer medulla.

ADMSCs rapidly ameliorated and protected the kidneys in-group IV starting from day 4 (Figure 8). Regeneration of the tubular cells under the influence of ADMSCs cannot explain the recovery. There was markedly less necrotic changes in spite of only 1/20 HPF interstitial solid sheets. The possible explanation could be through the paracrine effect of the ADMSCs as previously demonstrated by numerous studies, which have shown that organ protection by administered stem cells is primarily due to paracrine mechanisms rather than the replacement of damaged cells by differentiated stem cells[27-31].

Other workers studying the ADMSCs role in cisplatin induced AKI[8,9] have reached to the same conclusion. They suggested that ADMSCs might exert beneficial paracrine actions on the injured kidney by releasing biologically active factors where they used a culture media from cultured ADMSCs. Co-culturing ADMSCs or culture media of ADMSCs with proximal renal tubular cells, protected cultured human renal proximal tubular cells from cisplatin toxicity[25].

Reactive oxygen species are important mediators exerting toxic effects on various organs including the kidney where Chin et al. [29] concluded that ADMSCs administration minimized the AKI through suppression of the inflammatory response and the oxidative stress. This possible mechanism of renal protection was also demonstrated in our study where the use of ADMSCs partially suppressed oxidative stress and lipid peroxidation as reflected by decrease in the level of Malondialdehyde. Concomitantly ADMSCs increased superoxide dismutase and glutathione reductase in the renal tissue.

Our data indicate the ability of ADMSCs to protect against an advanced acute tubular necrosis as that detected in the control positive group of cisplatin. In addition, in spite of an early single dose of ADMSCs, this group of rats had developed a significant regenerative activity extending until day 30 with limited fibrotic activity. These observations raise the importance of latter booster doses of ADMSCs.

Interestingly, ADMSCs treated group of rats' showed highly important parallel improvement in renal tissue oxidative stress markers with the acute injury morphological scores (Table2; Figure 6B) better than with the creatinine clearance (Figure 6A) when compared with the control positive group. This improvement was of many folds with GSH as compared with the cisplatin group, indicating a key role of GSH in protecting against cisplatin induced acute tubular necrosis. The latter finding raises the question about the molecular mechanism of ADMSCs in promoting GSH. In addition, the early-administered single dose of ADMSCs seems to exercise long-term beneficial activity. This observation needs further exploration in regard to the probable interaction between the exogenously administered stem cells and the endogenous stem cells.

In conclusion, ADMSCs represent an easy practical source of stem cells. They have both protective and regenerative activities with consequent limitation of the development of renal fibrosis on top of the cisplatin induced acute tubular necrosis. Proposed anti-oxidative activity mediated through GSH activity promotion has an important role. The chronicity of the histopathological scoring indicates a promising advantage for a late booster dose of ADMSCs.

References

1. Pabla N, Dong Z. Cisplatin nephrotoxicity: mechanisms and renoprotective strategies. Kidney Int 2008; 73 (9): 994–1007.

2. Herrera MB, Bussolati B, Bruno S, Fonsato V, Romanazzi GM, Camussi G. Mesenchymal stem cells contribute to the renal repair of acute tubular epithelial injury. Int J Mol Med 2004; 14 (6): 1035–41.

3. Kunter U, Rong S, Djuric Z, Boor P, Müller-Newen G, Yu D, Floege J. Transplanted mesenchymal stem cells accelerate glomerular healing in experimental glomerulonephritis. J Am Soc Nephrol 2006; 17 (8): 2202–12.

4. Ling SI Y, LiZhao Y, Hao HJ, BingFu X, Han WD. MSCs: Biological characteristics, clinical applications and their outstanding concerns. Ageing Research Reviews 2011; 10(1): 93-103.

5. Bassi G, Pacelli L, Carusone R, ZanoncelloJasmina, Krampera M. Adipose-derived stromal cells (ASCs). Transfusion and Apheresis Science 2012; 47 (2): 193–8.

6. Zuk PA. Stem cell research has only just begun. Science 2001; 293(5528):211–12.

7. Shaohua QI, Dongcheng WU. Bone marrow-derived mesenchymal stem cells protect against cisplatin-induced acute kidney injury in rats by inhibiting cell apoptosis. International Journal of Molecular Medicine 2013; 32 (6): 1262-72.

8. Weiqi Yao, Qinyong HU, Yuhong MA, Wenping Xiong, Tingting WU, Jun CAO, Dongcheng WU. Human adipose-derived mesenchymal stem cells repair cisplatin-induced acute kidney injury through anti-apoptotic pathways. Exp Ther Med. 2015;10(2):468-476.

9. Kim JH, Park DJ, Yun JC, Jung MH, Yeo HD, Kim HJ, Kim DW, Yang JI, Lee GW, Jeong SH, Roh GS, Chang SH. Human adipose tissue-derived mesenchymal stem cells protect kidneys from cisplatin nephrotoxicityin rats. Am J Physiol Renal Physiol. 2012; 1; 302(9):F1141-50.

10. Bunnell BA, Flaat M, Gagliardi C, Patel B, Ripoll C. Adipose-derived stem cells: isolation, expansion and differentiation. Methods 2008; 45(2):115-20.

11. Phinney DG, Kopen G, Isaacson RL &Prockop DJ. Plastic adherent stromal cells from the bone marrow of commonly used strains of inbred mice: variations in yield, growth, and differentiation. J Cell Biochem 1999; 72(4):570–85.

12. Rombouts WJ, Ploemacher RE. Primary murine MSC show highly efficient homing to the bone marrow but lose homing ability following culture. Leukemia 2003; 17(1): 160–70.

13. Peister A, Mellad JA, Larson BL, Hall BM, Gibson LF, Prockop DJ. Adult stem cells from bone marrow (MSCs) isolated from different strains of inbred mice vary in surface epitopes, rates of proliferation, and differentiation potential. Blood 2004; 103(5): 1662-68.

14. Collins TJ. Image J for microscopy. BioTechniques 2007; 43 (1 Suppl): 25–30.

15. Van Roeyen CR, Ostendorf T, Denecke B, Bokemeyer D, Behrmann I, Strutz F, Lichenstein HS, LaRochelle WJ, Pena CE, Chaudhuri A, Floege J. Biological responses to PDGF-BB versus PDGF-DD in human mesangial cells. Kidney Int. 2006; 69(8) 1393–1402.

16. Bussolati B, Tetta C, Camussi G. Contribution of Stem Cells to Kidney Repair Am J Nephrol 2008;28(5):813–22.

17. Donovan P, Gearhart J. The end of the beginning for pluripotent stem cells. Nature 2001; 414: 92–97.

18. Goodell M. Stem-cell 'plasticity': befuddled by the muddle. Curr Opin Hematol 2003; 10(3): 208–13.

19. Herzog E, Chai L, Krause D. Plasticity of marrow-derived stem cells. Blood 2003; 102(10): 3483–93.

20. Weissman I. Stem cells: units of development, units of regeneration, and units of evolution. Cell 2000; 100(1): 157–68.

21. Erpicum P, Detry O, Weekers L, Bonvoisin C, Lechanteur C, Briquet A,Yves Beguin Y, Krzesinski J-M, Jouret F. Mesenchymal stromal cell therapy in conditions of renal ischaemia/reperfusion. Nephrol Dial Transplant. 2014; 29(8):1487-93.

22. Zou X, Zhang G, Cheng Z, Yin D, Du T, Ju G, Miao S, Liu G, Lu M, Zhu Y. Microvesicles derived from human Wharton's Jelly: mesenchymal stromal cells ameliorate renal ischemia-reperfusion injury in rats by suppressing CX3CL1. Stem Cell Research & Therapy 2014, 5(2):40-53.

23. Morigi M, Imberti B, Zoja C, Corna D, Tomasoni S, Abbate M, Rottoli D, Angioletti S, Benigni A, Perico N, Alison M, Remuzzi G. Mesenchymal stem cells are renotropic, helping to repair the kidney and improve function in acute renal failure. J Am Soc Nephrol 2004; 15(7): 1794–1804.

24. Morigi M, Introna M, Imberti B, Corna D, Abbate M, Rota C, Rottoli D, Benigni A, Perico N, Zoja C, Rambaldi A, Remuzzi A, Remuzzi G. Human bone marrow-mesenchymal stem cells accelerate recovery of acute renal injury and prolong survival in mice. Stem Cells 2008; 26(8): 2075–82.

25. Morigi M, Rota C, Montemurro T, Montelatici E, Lo Cicero V, Imberti B, Abbate M, Zoja C, Cassis P, Longaretti L, Rebulla P, Introna M, Capelli C, Benigni A, Remuzzi G, Lazzari L. Life-sparing effect of human cord blood-mesenchymal stem cells in experimental acute kidney injury. Stem Cells 2010; 28(3): 513–22.

26. Bi B, Schmitt R, Israilova M, Nishio H, Cantley LG. Stromal cells protect against acute tubular injury via an endocrine effect. Am Soc Nephrol 2007; 18(9): 2486–96.

27. Gnecchi M, He H, Liang OD, Melo LG, Morello F, Mu H, Noiseux N, Zhang L, Pratt RE, Ingwall JS, Dzau VJ. Paracrine action accounts for marked protection of ischemic heart by Akt-modified mesenchymal stem cells. Nat Med 2005; 11(4): 367–68.

28. Kinnaird T, Stabile E, Burnett MS, Lee CW, Barr S, Fuchs S, Epstein SE. Marrow-derived stromal cells express genes encoding a broad spectrum of arteriogenic cytokines and promote in vitro and in vivo arteriogenesis through paracrine mechanisms. Circ Res 2004; 94(5): 678–85.

29. Kinnaird T, Stabile E, Burnett MS, Shou M, Lee CW, Barr S, Fuchs S, Epstein SE. Local delivery of marrow-derived stromal cells augments collateral perfusion through paracrine mechanisms. Circulation 2004; 109(12): 1543–49.

30. Togel F, Hu Z, Weiss K, Isaac J, Lange C, Westenfelder C. Administered mesenchymal stem cells protect against ischemic acute renal failure through differentiation-independent mechanisms. Am J Physiol Renal Physiol 2005; 289(1): F29-30.

31. Chen YT, Sun CK, Lin YC, Chang LT, Chen YL, Tsai TH, Chung SY, Chua S, Kao YH, Yen CH, Shao PL, Chang KC, Leu S, Yip HK. Adipose-derived mesenchymal stem cell protects kidneys against ischemia-reperfusion injury through suppressing oxidative stress and inflammatory reaction. J Transl Med. 2011; 9:51.

Abbreviations

h-ADMSCs	: Human-Adipose Derived Mesenchymal Stem Cells
AKI	: Acute Kidney Injury
BUN	: Blood Urea Nitrogen
MDA	: Malondialdehyde
SOD	: Superoxide dismutase
GSH	: Reduced Glutathione
PBS	: Phosphate-Buffered Saline
DMEM	: Dulbecco's Modified Eagle's Medium
FBS	: Fetal Bovine Serum
FACS	: Fluorescence-Activated Cell Sorting
CFU-F	: Colony Forming Unit-Fibroblast
RT–PCR	: Real-Time quantitative Reverse Transcriptase-Polymerase Chain Reaction
ALBP	: Adipocyte Lipid-Binding Protein
OSOM	: Outer Strip of Outer Medulla
ISOM	: Inner Strip of Outer Medulla

Potential Conflicts of Interests

None

Acknowledgements

This work was supported by Science and Technology Development Fund (STDF), grant number 1061, Ministry of Scientific Research, Egypt.

Corresponding Author

Mohamed-Ahdy A.A. Saad, Faculty of Medicine, Mansoura University, Mansoura, Egypt; E-mail: ahady2007@yahoo.com

17

Re-Defining Stem Cell-Cardiomyocyte Interactions: Focusing on the Paracrine Effector Approach

Mahapatra S[1], Martin D[1], Gallicano GI[1]

Stem cell research for treating or curing ischemic heart disease has, till date, culminated in three basic approaches: the use of induced pluripotent stem cell (iPSC) technology; reprogramming cardiac fibroblasts; and cardiovascular progenitor cell regeneration. As each approach has been shown to have its advantages and disadvantages, exploiting the advantages while minimizing the disadvantages has been a challenge. Using human germline pluripotent stem cells (hgPSCs) along with a modified version of a relatively novel cell-expansion culture methodology to induce quick, indefinite expansion of normally slow growing hgPSCs, it was possible to emphasize the advantages of all three approaches. We consistently found that unipotent germline stem cells, when removed from their niche and cultured in the correct medium, expressed endogenously, pluripotency genes, which induced them to become hgPSCs. These cells are then capable of producing cell types from all three germ layers. Upon differentiation into cardiac lineages, our data consistently showed that they not only expressed cardiac genes, but also expressed cardiac-promoting paracrine factors. Taking these data a step further, we found that hgPSC-derived cardiac cells could integrate into cardiac tissue *in vivo*. Note, while the work presented here was based on testes-derived hgPSCs, data from other laboratories have shown that ovaries contain very similar types of stem cells that can give rise to hgPSCs. As a result, hgPSCs should be considered a viable option for eventual use in patients, male or female, with ischemic heart disease

Key Words: Cardiomyocytes, Paracrine factors, Human germline pluripotent stem cells, Cardiogenesis, Cardiac repair, Neuregulin, Embryonic stem cells, Adult stem cells, Heart disease

Introduction

After a half century of focused research, heart disease remains a leading cause of death in developed nations. Although advancements in research have led to numerous breakthroughs and progress for treating cardiovascular disease, in many respects, we are still only scratching the surface of innovative ideas for reducing cardiac-related deaths. A significant problem remaining to be solved is identifying the parameters and/or inductive signals that are necessary for repairing heart muscle damaged by ischemia. To solve this problem, decades of research have led to three primary areas of investigation: The potential use of induced pluripotent stem cell (iPSCs) technology, direct reprogramming of surviving cardiac fibroblasts, and regeneration of endogenous cardiovascular progenitor cells[1, 2]. The first approach using iPSCs has shown promise *in vitro*; however, problems remain for their use *in vivo* such as teratoma formation, genetic instability, and accumulation of mitochondrial DNA mutations in iPSCs from elderly patients, which would most likely be the largest demographic needing iPSC-therapy[3, 4]. In contrast, the latter two regenerative approaches have recently gained interest due to their paracrine-inducing abilities for restoring cardiac function[1, 5-9]; however, the methodologies and protocols for inducing cardiac regeneration continue to vary widely.

Clinical trials that test the efficacy of transplanted adult stem cells (ASCs) within ischemic heart tissue have been common practice for nearly a decade; however, outcomes have not provided definitive clinical applications for patients. One explanation for the investigative ambiguity stems from the many different types of ASCs that have been pursued for transplantation. For example, adult epidermal stem cells are different than adult mesenchymal bone marrow stem cells with respect to gene expression, physiology, and origin. As a result, when introduced into the cardiac niche, the different types of ASCs present unanticipated variations. Consequently, finding a stem cell population that is the most suitable for treating cardiac ischemia remains an important endeavor.

Some of the more successful stem cell trials have been those that utilize both direct and indirect mechanisms to help induce cardiac repair[2, 10]. Stem cells that are differentiated into cardiomyocytes *in vitro* (or *in vivo*) can integrate and adhere upon transplantation with endogenous cardiac cells *via* gap junctions (e.g., connexin 43 gap junction proteins). Cellular adhesion can then exert direct physiological interaction/repair. Some stem cells can also secrete paracrine factors that indirectly affect surrounding tissue to 'regenerate' or inhibit apoptosis[5, 9, 11-13]. Debate has arisen, though, concerning which of these approaches is best for clinical use. For example, direct physiological interaction where stem cell-derived cardiomyocytes physically 'beat' can result in positive or negative outcomes for patients. If stem cell-derived cardiomyocytes are electrically connected to the heart muscle, ventricular force can be significantly restored[14-16]. However, if that electrical connection is not complete, transplanted cardiomyocytes that beat can cause detrimental arrhythmias and decreased ventricular force. Alternatively, stem cells that do not beat, but do secrete paracrine factors that can effect surrounding healthy cardiac tissue, have become a strong investigative mechanism for repairing ischemic tissue.

Previously we, and others as well, presented evidence that germline stem cells when removed from their niche acquire the

Author Names in full: Samiksha Mahapatra[1], Dianna Martin[1], G. Ian Gallicano[1]

[1] *Department of Biochemistry and Molecular Biology, Georgetown University Medical Center, 3900 Reservoir Rd, Washington, DC, USA*

ability to differentiate into cell types from all three germ layers (ectoderm, mesoderm, and endoderm)[17-21]. Others have since confirmed this work; however, testing their application within a cardiac setting has not been thoroughly analyzed.

Our hypothesis is straightforward. We postulate that germline stem cells when removed from their niche begin to express factors redefining their stemness from unipotent (able to make sperm or eggs) to pluripotent. These redefined cells, known as germline pluripotent stem cells (hgPSCs), can then be induced to form paracrine effector-yielding cardiac cells. At first, our data provided constant, clear evidence that hgPSCs could be induced to form cardiomyocytes; however, we encountered a consistent obstacle with our initial approach; hgPSCs grew very slowly. Expansion of cells from dish to dish took months and it was concluded that their growth curve could significantly impede their use *in vivo*. Thus, to solve this problem, we modified a novel technological cell culture advancement that had been shown to promote certain cell types to acquire or maintain 'stemness' while simultaneously pushing them into the cell cycle[22]. This approach had not been reported in the literature for expanding hgPSCs. Our initial observations after subjecting hgPSCs to this novel culturing technology resulted in data leading us to generate a secondary hypothesis; that hgPSCs could be 'quickly' and indefinitely expanded to enrich their population, followed by their differentiation into cardiomyocytes. After testing our hypotheses, the data revealed that cardiomyocytes generated from hgPSCs acquired the ability to positively influence cardiac tissue.

Methods and Materials

Gene names and abbreviations

Table 1 provides a reference list of abbreviations for the genes and proteins that were analyzed.

Isolation and culture of SSCs from human testes

Testes were acquired from the Washington Regional Transplant Community (WRTC) with permission from the next of kin. The *tunica albica* was removed and the seminiferous tubules were cut into 1g tissue samples and either stored in liquid nitrogen or used fresh[18].

Frozen tissue samples were transferred to a 120ml container with 40ml ice-cold DMEM/F12 (Life Technologies Cat #11320082) + Antibiotic- Antimycotic (Life Technologies Cat #15240062), and washed twice. After washing in the medium, 2-3ml of the medium was left in the 120ml container (on ice) where the sample tissue is sliced by sterile scissors. The tissue was transferred into a 50ml tube with an additional 40ml ice-cold DMEM/F12 + Antibiotic-Antimycotic. The tissue was allowed to sediment for 2-5 minutes and supernatant is removed. A 10ml enzyme solution of 1x Hank's Balanced Salt Solution (HBSS) (Life Technologies Cat #14025076) was prepared with 2.5 mg/ml Collagenase Type IV (Life Technologies Cat #17104019), 1.25 mg/ml Dispase (Life Technologies Cat #17105041), vortex and filter through 0.22μm syringe filter (MidSci Cat #TP99722). The solution is added to the tissue sediment. The enzyme solution along with the tissue sediment was incubated 30mins in a 37℃ water bath with 100rpm shaking. Afterwards, the enzyme was removed and re-suspended in 10ml human embryonic stem cell (hESC) medium (500ml DMEM/F12, 20% knockout serum replacement (Life Technologies Cat #A3181502), 0.1mM beta-mercaptoethanol (Life Technologies Cat #21985023), 5ml Non-essential amino acids (100X) (Life Technologies Cat #11140050), L-glutamine (100X) (Life Technologies Cat #25030081), and Antibiotic-Antimycotic. A 40μm mesh filter (Sigma Aldrich Cat #22363547) was placed atop of a 50ml tube and the supernatant and sample were slowly filtered through it to extract spermatogonial cells.

The filtered tissue sample was then centrifuged (1000rpm/5min). The supernatant was removed, and re-suspended in fresh 6ml hESC medium. The medium and sample were then seeded into a 6-well tissue culture plate along with 3.5μl of 10ng/ml Recombinant human GDNF (Life Technologies Cat #PHC7045) and the plate was placed into a 34℃ and 5% CO2 incubator and cultured for 4 days.

Originally, we coated plates with gelatin (Sigma Aldrich Cat #Z707910); however, we later found that hgPSCs could grow virtually the same in uncoated TPP tissue culture plates (Sigma Inc. #92006).

Production of hESLCs from SSCs

After isolation, SSCs were cultured in hESC medium along with 3.5μl of GDNF for 4 days to stimulate growth and colony formation. They were incubated at 37℃ and 5% CO₂. Media was changed every other day. After the 4th day of incubation, the hESC medium plus GDNF was replaced with hESC medium supplemented with 10 ng/ml fibroblast growth factor (bFGF) (Peprotech Cat #100-18C-10UG). Colonies must be cultured for at least 10 days to form hgPSCs[18].

hgPSC culture in modified GE médium

hgPSCs were expanded in germline expansion medium (GEM: Complete DMEM high glucose (500ml) supplemented with 10% human serum (Sigma Aldrich Cat #H4522) and 100X Pen/Strep (Life Technologies Cat #11995040), (100X) Ham's F12 nutrient mixture (Life Technologies Cat #1165054), 0.13μg/ml Hydrocortisone (Sigma Aldrich Cat #H0888-10G), EGF (Life Technologies Cat #PHG0313), 5mg/ml Insulin (Sigma Aldrich Cat #91077C-1G), 11.7μM Cholera Toxin (Sigma Aldrich Cat #C8052-5MG), 10mg/ml Gentamicin (Life Technologies Cat #15710072)) containing 5mM ROCK inhibitor (Y-27632) (Axxora Inc Cat #ALX-270-333-M005) for 7-10 days[22]. *Note: We did not use the J2 cell component found in the protocol by Suprynowicz et al[22]. We also replaced fetal bovine serum with human serum to remove all animal products. The ROCK inhibitor assists in the increased proliferation of hgPSCs to enhance colony population for later differentiation into cardiomyocytes[23].*

Reestablishing hgPSCs from expansion in GEM

After expansion, GEM was replaced with hESC medium containing bFGF. This medium was replaced every other day. Colonies spontaneously and consistently formed within 5-10 days.

Differentiation of hgPSCs into cardiac lineages

Un-expanded or previously expanded hgPSCs were cultured in hESC medium and 0.25μM Cardiogenol-C Hydrochloride (Sigma Aldrich Cat #C4866-5MG) for 10 days. After differentiation, the media was replaced into complete DMEM medium supplemented with 20% human serum. This medium was considered post- differentiation medium where the cardiac clusters could be cultured for up to 30 days.

Confocal analysis

Colonies were isolated using Dumont #5 forceps and fixed in 4% paraformaldehyde for 1 hour, followed by permeabilization with 1% Triton-X-100 for 30 minutes. After two washes in PBS, areas were blocked with 2% BSA in PBS and 1% Tween 20. Primary (1:100) and secondary (1:800) antibodies were diluted in blocking solution, and colonies were incubated with each antibody for 1 hour at 37˚ C or overnight at 4°C. In the final step, colonies were moved directly from secondary antibody into a DAPI solution at 2μg/mL. Colonies were then mounted onto slides with anti-fade and sealed with

Table 1: Gene names and functions

SSC GENE CANDIDATES	Abbreviation	BP Size	Published function	Refs
G protein coupled receptor 125	GPR125	136BPS	Canidate marker for human and mouse SSCs. Multiple functions in different tissues.	[32, 61]
GDNF family receptor 1 alpha	GFR1α	163BPS	Canidate marker for human and mouse SSCs.	[32, 61]
Stage-specific antibody-4	SSEA-4	359nps	Expressed in specific cells of the seminiferous basal membrane. Canidate marker for human and mouse SSCs.	[47, 48, 51]
hESC GENES	**Abbreviation**	**BP Size**	**Published function**	**Refs**
SRY (Sex Determining Region Y)-Box 2	SOX2	153bps	Transcriptional regulator of somatic cell reprogramming; helps maintain pluripotency.	[21, 62-64]
Octamer-Binding Transcription Factor 3/4	OCT3/4	117bps	Plays the central role in pluripotency.	[21, 65, 66]
LIN28 Homolog A	LIN 28A	128bps	Regulates stemness and self renewal capacity in human and mouse pluripotent stem cells.	[21, 67, 68]
Homeobox Transcription Factor Nanog	NANOG	200bps	Required for final states of pluripotency.	[69, 70]
Kruppel-like factor 4	KLF-4	143 bps	Essential for ESC maintenance and self-renewal capacity.	[21, 71, 72]
Cluster of differentiation 73	CD73	219bps	Essential stemness marker for human somatic cells.	[34]
EARLY CARDIAC GENES	**Abbreviation**	**BP Size**	**Published function**	**Refs**
Activated Leukocyte Cell Adhesion Molecule	ALCAM	388bps	Surface marker for early cardiomyocytes	[73]
Cardiac Helicase Activated MEF2C protein	CHAMP	200bps	Cardiac transcription factor expressed specifically in postnatal and embryonic cardiomyocytes.	[40]
T-Box Transcription Factor 18	TBX18	112bps	It is critical for early sino atrial node (SAN) specification (pacemaker cells).	[74]
DIFFERENTIATED CARDIAC GENES	**Abbreviation**	**BP Size**	**Published function**	**Refs**
Atrial Natriuretic Peptide	ANP	204bps	Cardiac hormone that regulates blood pressure, vasodilation, natriuresis, and diuresis.	[75]
NK2 homeobox 5	NKX2.5	215bps	Cardiac transcription factor responsible for heart formation and development.	[76]
Cardiac Troponin-I	CTNI	335bps	Key regulatory protein associated with the thin filament, inhibits actomyosin interactions at diastolic levels of intracellular Ca2+.	[77]
Cardiac Troponin-T	CTNT	217bps	Fixation of troponin complex on the actin filament and also participitates in muscle contraction	[78]
Myosin heavy chain	MHC	542bps	Molecular motor of the heart that generates motion by coupling its ATPase activity to its cyclic interaction with actin.	[26, 79]
Myosin light chain 2A	MLC2A	270bps	Atrial marker expressed during devlopment and adulthood. Also regulates heart contraction along with MLC 2V.	[80, 81]
Myosin light chain 2V	MLC2V	380bps	Ventricular marker during human heart development and in adulthood	[80, 81]
Myocyte Enhancer Factor 2C	ISL-1	127bps	a LIM homeodomain transcription factor expressed in majority of cells in both right ventricle and atria of the heart. ISL1 is also responsible for survival, proliferation, and migration of cardiac progenitor cells.	[82-84]
PARACRINE FACTORS	**Abbreviation**	**BP Size**	**Published function**	**Refs**
Vascular Endothelial growth factor-A	VEGFA	280bps	Promotes vasculo-and angiogenesis in myocardium and cardiomyocyte proliferation. Also helps regenerates mycoardium.	[1, 11, 39, 85, 86]
Insulin-like growth factor	IGF-1	372bps	Switch macrophages from pro-inflammatory to anti-inflammatory phenotype both in vitro and vivo. Also promotes resident stem mobilization and cardiac lineage commitment.	[1, 11, 39, 85, 86]
Stromal derived factor-1	SDF-1	250bps	Promotes repair and regeneration by recruiting circulating progenitor cells to the injured site. Also secreted by cardiac stem cells.	[1, 11, 39, 85, 86]
Connective tiddue growth factor	CTGF	237bps	Acts as a cofactor for other growth factor that promotes fibrosis and wound healing by enhancing ECM protein synthesis.	[1, 11, 39, 85, 86]
Endothelin-1	END-1	270bps	Vasoactive peptide secreted by the endothelium required for cardiomyocyte survival. It decreases susceptibility to TNF-mediated apoptosis; secreted from cardiomyocytes under mechanical stress.	[1, 11, 39, 85, 86]
Angio-associated migratory protein	AAMP	283bps	Associated with angiogenesis, endothelial tube formation, and migration of endothelial cells. It may also regulate smooth muscle cell migration via the RhoA pathway.	[1, 11, 39, 85, 86]
Neuregulin-1	NRG-1	203bps	Activates ErbB2 receptor present on differentiated cardiomyocytes and promotes cardiomyocyte proliferation.	[1, 11, 39, 85, 86]
Indoleamine 2,3-dioxygenase	IDO	222 bps	Inhibits T-cell and NK cell proliferation, cytotoxicity, cytokine production; also mediates T-cell apoptosis.	[1, 11, 39, 85, 86]
TERATOMA GENES	**Abbreviation**	**BP Size**	**Published Function**	**Refs**
Dead end gene	DND1	271 bps	It is an RNA-binding protein that suppresses teratoma growth	**[38]**
P18 Cyclin dependent kinase Inhibitor	p18 INK4C CDKI	270 bps	It is responsible for growth of EBs and is known as a suppressor of teratoma formation. Also a negative regulator of cell cycle.	**[37,38]**
P19 Cyclin dependent kinase Inhibitor	P19 CDKI	441 bps	Negative regulator of cell cycle and a suppressor of teratoma formation	**[37,38]**

coverslips. Confocal images of colonies were taken on an Olympus Fluoview 500 Laser Scanning Microscope (Olympus America Inc., Melville, NY) using the accompanying Fluoview image acquisition and analysis software (version 4.3). Cells within areas were imaged using a 1.3 numerical aperture, 40X Olympus objective. Primary Antibodies: Sox2 [488nm] (Goat; Santacruz SC #17320), Nanog [594nm] (Mouse; Abcam ab 62734), Oct 4 [647nm] (Mouse; Santacruz SC 5279) and Lin28 [647nm] (Rabbit; Cell Signaling A177 Cat #3978S). Secondary Antibodies: Donkey-anti-mouse Alexa fluor 647 nm (Abcam Cat # ab150107), Donkey-anti-rabbit Alexa fluor 594 nm (Abcam Cat #ab150076) and Donkey-anti-goat Alexa fluor 488 nm (Abcam Cat #ab150129)

Embryo and heart tube procurement and cell fusion

Female FVB mice were gonadotropin primed. E9.5 Embryos were collected from the uterine horns using Dumont #5 forceps to tease away fetal membranes; a modified version of previously described protocols[24, 25]. Embryos were transferred to organ culture dishes (No. 3037, Falcon Inc., Lincoln Park, NJ). Beating hearts were isolated using two Dumont #5 forceps, one to spread the head away from the tail of the embryo, the other forceps was used to snip the heart from the body at the most caudal and rostral ends of the heart. Fetal hearts were then placed into a well of a 96 well plate and incubated at 37°C and 5% CO2. Hearts could beat for 72-96 hrs without distortion of morphology.

Mature Cardiomyocyte colonies were transiently transfected with uncut 5ul of cMHC-GFP DNA for 24 hours in 6-well dishes using Lipofectamine transfection kit (Life Technologies Cat #L3000001). cMHC-GFP (a kind gift from Dr. Eugene Kolossov[26]) transfected colonies were picked using a 10μl pipette tip and placed into a holding well containing differentiation medium (above). They were then seeded into crevasses of fetal hearts using hand-drawn glass needle attached to a mouth pipette. Excess GFP-positive colonies were laid on top of beating fetal hearts. The 96 well plate was then incubated at 37°C and 5% CO2 for 48hrs.

Fetal hearts and colonies were analyzed first using a Leica stereoscope equipped with a fluorescent light source to globally identify areas of GFP within heart tissue. Those that appeared positive were fixed in 4% paraformaldehyde (Electron Microscopy Sciences Cat# 15714-S) for 2 hrs and then quenched in 1% glycine/PBS for 30min. Fetal hearts were then permeabilized with 1% Triton-X-100 for 2hrs. After three 30min washes in PBS, hearts were blocked with 2% BSA in PBS and 1% Tween 20. Primary CNX43 antibody (Rabbit Cell Signaling Cat #3512) and secondary antibodies (Peroxidase Affinipure Donkey Anti-Rabbit- Cat #711-035-152, Jackson Immunoresearch Labs) were diluted in blocking solution 1:100 and 1:800 respectively, and hearts were incubated with each antibody overnight 4° C. In the final step, hearts were moved directly from secondary antibody and incubated in a DAPI (Cat #D1306, ThermoFisher Scientific) solution at 2μg/mL. Hearts were then mounted onto slides with anti-fade and sealed with coverslips. Confocal images of colonies were taken on an Olympus Fluoview 500 Laser Scanning Microscope (See above).

Western Blot analysis

Isolated undifferentiated or differentiated colonies (each comprised of ~1 x 10³ cells) were immediately placed into sample buffer (62.5 mM Tris-HCl, pH 6.8, 2% SDS w/v, 1mM β-mercaptoethanol, 10% glycerol)[27]. Samples were placed into a 95 degrees heat block for 5 min and then loaded onto 4-20% gradient polyacrylamide gels (BioRad Inc. Cat #4561094) with molecular weight markers (Biorad Inc Cat #1610374) and separated by SDS-PAGE. Proteins were transferred to PVDF membrane and blocked with blocking reagent (5% dry milk [Bio Rad Cat #170-6404] in PBS, pH 7.4, with 0.1%

Tween 20) at room temperature. The blots were challenged with primary antibody at dilutions of 1/500-1/1000 in block overnight at 4°C, followed by washing 3 times with PBST (1x PBS + 0.1% Tween 20) at room temperature and challenge with appropriate secondary antibody (1/5,000-1/10,000) conjugated to horseradish peroxidase (Jackson Laboratories) for 2 hours followed by washing 3 times with 1X PBST at room temperature. The blot was then visualized under chemiluminescence in an ECL Imager (Thermo Scientific) using Clarity Western ECL Substrate (Bio Rad Cat #170- 5061). Primary Antibody- Desmin (Rabbit) (Cat #5332P, Cell Signaling). Secondary Antibody- Peroxidase Affinipure Donkey Anti-Rabbit (Cat #711-035-152, Jackson Immunoresearch Labs)

RT-PCR analyses

For each stage of stem cell development, colonies were picked and mRNA was extracted using the miRNeasy Mini Kit (QIAGEN® cat. No. 217004). cDNA was generated via the iScript cDNA synthesis kit (BioRad Cat #1708890) using a 20μl mixture (5x Supermix (4μl), 5x iScript reverse transcriptase (1μl), Nuclease-free water (5μl), and RNA template (10μl). RT-PCR analysis was performed by using a 22μl mixture (MyTaq Supermix (BIOLINE PCR Kit®) 12μl, Forward (2μl) and Reverse (2μl) primers, (2μl) Nuclease-free water, (4ul) cDNA template). These experiments were conducted at a melting temperature of 56°C and for 40 PCR cycles. No RT control was performed using Maxima H Minus First Strand cDNA Synthesis Kit (Thermo Fisher Scientific Cat #K1651). Primer pairs for each gene are listed in Table 2.

Detection of secreted proteins

Paracrine factors secreted into the medium were detected by two methods. First, ~150 cardiac differentiated colonies were grown in 1ml of differentiation medium (containing serum replacement instead of human serum). Media was then isolated at 12hrs, 24hrs, and 48hrs and frozen. Antibodies to specific paracrine factors were then added to the thawed medium along with 10ml of protease inhibitor cocktail (Sigma Aldrich Cat #P8340) overnight at 4° C with rocking. The next day, magnetic beads (10μl) coated with g-protein (Life Technologies Cat #10003D) were added directly to the medium containing the primary antibodies. The slurry mixed for 2 hrs at 4° C. Using a magnet, the beads were washed 5x with PBS. Sample buffer was added to the beads, which were then heated at 95°C for 5 min. 15μl of each time-point sample was added to a lane of a 4-20% polyacrylamide gel and the subjected to SDS-PAGE. The resultant gel was silver-stained (Bio Rad Cat #1610449) to observe the bands.

The second method, ethanol precipitation of proteins [modified from[28-30]], was used to analyze proteins that were either too close to the molecular weight of the antibody heavy chain or was not compatible with Immunoprecipitation (I.P). In this case, 1ml samples of media taken at 12, 24, and 48hrs were subjected to four volumes of 100% ethanol and precipitated overnight at -80°C. The next day the samples were centrifuged at 14,000rpm for 5 min and the supernatant was discarded. The remaining pellet was allowed to dry for 30min-1hr after which sample buffer was added and heated to 95°C for 5 min. 15μl of each time-point sample was added to a lane of a 4-20% polyacrylamide gel and the subjected to SDS-PAGE. The gel was then used for Western Blot analysis to detect the paracrine factors.

ELISA

TGFB secreted into the medium was detected by Human TGF beta 1 Platinum ELISA kit (Cat # BMS249-4, Life Technologies, Inc). Medium cultured in differentiated cardiomyocytes at 0h, 12h, 24h and 48h were tested along with TGFB standards (31pg/ml-2000pg/ml) at 450nm. A standard curve for TGF beta was plotted

Table 2: Primer Sequences

CARDIOMYOCYTE PRIMER SEQUENCES (5'-3')	
SSC GENE CANDIDATES	Abbreviation
F- AAAGCTTGGCGCAGATGTGA R- TTGCCACGGCATTGGTAAGA	GPR125
F- TTTACCAACTGCCAGCCAGA R- TGTTGCTGCAGTCACACCAT	GFR1α
F- GAGAAGCTGTTCCAGATAGTGC R- CTCAGGGTACATGAAATGGTGG	SSEA-4

hESC GENES	Abbreviation
F- ATGTACAACATGATGGAGACGG R- CCACACCATGAAGGCATTCA	SOX2
F- TTTGCCAAGCTCCTGAAGCA R- AAAGCGGCAGATGGTCGTTT	OCT3/4
F- GAGCATGCAGAAGCGCAGATCAAA R- TATGGCTGATGCTCTGGCAGAAGT	LIN 28A
F- TCAGAGACAGAAATACCTCAGC R- AGGAAGAGTAAAGGCTGGGG	NANOG
F- TTCAACCTGGCGGACATCAA R- TTCAGCACGAACTTGCCCAT	KLF-4
F- GTATTGCCCTTTGGAGGCAC R- AGGGTCATAACTGGGCACTC	CD73

EARLY CARDIAC GENES	Abbreviation
F- TTCCAGAACACGATGAGGCA R- ACCTGTGACAGCTTGGTAGA	ALCAM
F- AAGGTGTCTAGTAAGACAGCAG R- ATCATTTTGCCTAGCCCACC	CHAMP
F- ATGCATTCTGGCGACCATCA R- ACGCCATTCCCAGTACCTTG	TBX18

DIFFERENTIATED CARDIAC GENES	Abbreviation
F- AGTGGATTGCTCCTTGACGA R- GGGCACGACCTCATCTTCTA	ANP
F- ACCCTAGAGCCGAAAAGAAAG R- GCCGCACAGTAATGGTAAGG	NKX2.5
F- AAGATCTCCGCCTCGAGAAA R- GCAGAGATCCTCACTCTCCG	CTNI
F- CTTTGATGAGAGACGTCGGG R-CTTCCCACTTTTCCGCTCTG	CTNT
F- GGGGACAGTGGTAAAAGCAA R- TCCCTGCGTTCCACTATCTT	MHC
F- GAGTTCAAAGAAGCCTTCAGC R- ATCCTTGTTCACCACCCCTT	MLC2A
F- GGTGCTGAAGGCTGATTACG R- TTGGAACATGGCCTCTGGAT	MLC2V
F- CTGTGGGCTGTTCACCAACT R- GCCGCAACCAACACATAGG	ISL-1

PARACRINE FACTORS	Abbreviation
F- GGGCAGAATCATCACGAAGT R- TGTTGTGCTGTAGGAAGCTC	VEGFA
F- GAGCCTGCGCAATGGAATAA R- ATACCCTGTGGGCTTGTTGA	IGF-1
F- TCAACACTCCAAACTGTGCC R- AGCAAGTGAACTGTGGTCCAT	SDF-1
F- CGACTGGAAGACACGTTTGG R- TTTGGGAGTACGGATGCACT	CTGF
F- CACAACAGAGCCAACAGAGTC R- TCCAGGTGGCAGAAGTAGAC	END-1
F- AGAGTGAGTCCAACTCGGTG R- AGGGCAAAGTCCAGGATCTC	AAMP
F- GGAGCATATGTGTCTTCAGCTAC R- AAGCTGGCCATTACGTAGTTTTG	NRG-1

TERATOMA GENES	Abbreviation
F- AAGCGGGATTGTGAGCTGTG R- TGAAGGTCATCATCAGGCGG	DND 1
F- AAAATGGGGGCGGGTTTTTC R-CGCTCCCAGTGACAGTTTCT	P18 CDKI
F- CGGCGAGGAGGAGGGAG R- GTCCCTGCGATGGAGATCAG	P19 CDKI

GENES EXPRESSED BY ALL EMBRYONIC GERM LAYERS	Abbreviation
F- TGCCCAGTTTGTTC R- ACATCTCCTCTGCAACAGTGCTCA	AFP
F- AGCCATTCCGTAGTGCCATC R- CAGAAGTGTCGCCTCGAAGT	BMP4
F- CAGGAGAAACAGGGCCTACAG R- GCACAGGTGTCTCAAGGGTA	NES

using OD values from standards. Concentration of circulating TGFB of each time point was calculated from the standard curve and then multiplied by a dilution factor of 30 (samples were diluted 1:30 prior to experiment). The negative controls in this experiment were ES media cultured at 0h. Concentration of TGFB was normalized to 0h ES media. Final concentrations in media cultured in cardiomyocytes at the different time points were plotted against normalized values to 0h ES using a bar graph.

Statistical analyses.

Standard error of the means were calculated from N > 3, which were then analyzed by student t tests. A p < 0.05 or better was considered significant.

Results

Identifying the source cell from testis

Recent investigations have demonstrated that when isolated and cultured in the proper medium, germline stem cells can be induced to form cell/tissue from all three germ layers (i.e., ectoderm, mesoderm, and endoderm)[18-20, 31].

Identifying the stem cells within the human testes that give rise to hgPSCs has been somewhat elusive. To begin identifying this stem cell population, we first generated single cell suspensions assaying them for clonal expansion, which is accepted as a primary characteristic of stem cells. We used this approach first because, particularly in humans, a molecular or cellular target for identifying the actual stem cell population within the testes remains a debated topic in the literature. Consequently, we initially used cell size as a marker for isolating and identifying this population of stem cells. Figure 1 shows typical examples of isolated single cells, while Figure 2A shows the milieu of different sizes of cells enzymatically isolated from human testes tissue[18]. Using a hand-drawn glass pipette connected to a plastic filtered mouth suctioning tip, small (<5-7µm), medium (~8-12µm), and large (>12-20µm) cells were placed one by one into wells of a 96 well plate (Figure 1). As a reference, a typical, single mouse ESC cell expanded into a colony very quickly after plating (Figure 1A). Different cells isolated from the human testis (Figure 1B) did not all expand *in vitro*. After 10-14 days of culture, only medium-sized cells grew into colonies capable of being differentiated and expressing markers from the three embryonic germ layers (Figure 1 C-F). Although the table in figure 1G reports that only 32% of medium-sized cells actually grew into distinctive colonies identical to that seen in Figure 1E, we concluded that this methodology was useful for confirming that a specific sub-population of cells within the SSC--enriched fraction could grow clonally and generate cells from all three germ layers.

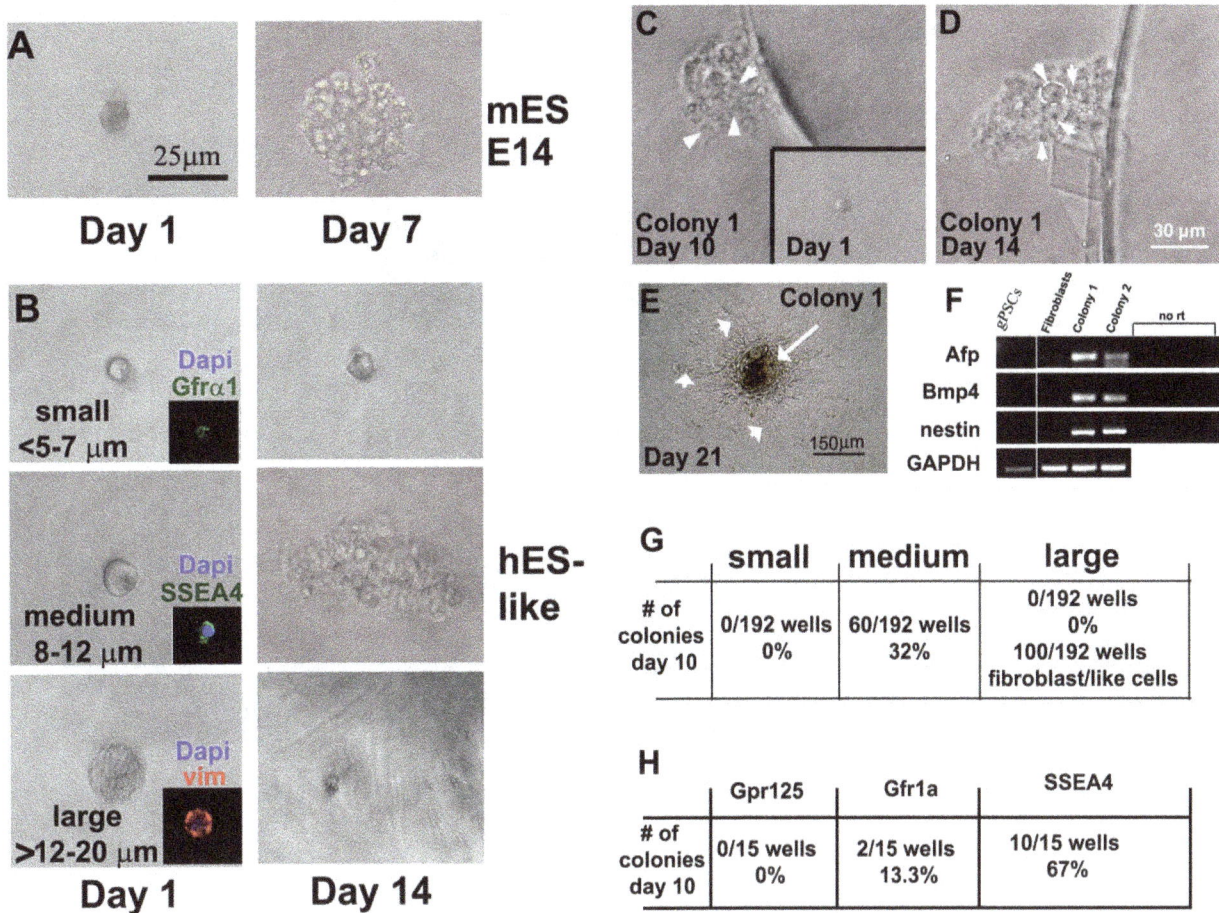

Figure 1: Identifying the stem cell within testes that gives rise to clonal hgPSCs. A) Acting as a positive control, a single mouse E14 strain embryonic stem cell gives rise to a colony within 7 days of culture. B) After enzymatic digestion and filtration of human testes tissue, distinctive size differences among cells were clearly evident. Small (<5-7µm), medium (~8-12µm), and large (>12-20µm) cells were isolated using a mouth pipette and placed into a well of a 96 well plate. After 14 days of incubation wells were assessed for clonal growth. Only medium size cells produced colonies. C-F) Removing bFGF from the hESC medium to induce differentiation by 10 and 14 days, respectively. Arrowheads in C and D point to individual cells within a colony, while the white circle in D outlines one cell within the colony. By ~21 days of differentiation, RT-PCR showed expression of genes from all three germ layers; Alpha fetal protein (AFP-Endoderm), Bone morphogenic protein 4 (Bmp4-mesoderm), and Nestin (neuroectoderm). However, hgPSCs did not express any of the genes from all three germ layers. GAPDH was our RT-PCR control gene. E) A central mass of differentiated cells (Arrow) are surrounded by fibroblasts, which do not show expression of these three specific genes (arrowheads in E and fibroblasts in F). G) Table quantifies colony formation from the three sizes of cells. F and insets in B) Using antibodies directed against previously explored SSC markers, SSEA4 but not Gpr125 or Gfr1α identified the cells that produced colonies of hgPSCs. SSEA4 positive cells are 8-12µm in diameter, while Gfr1α are much smaller. The large cells were mostly vimentin positive most likely representing Sertoli cells.

To apply a more rigorous approach for identifying which cell type could grow clonally into colonies of hgPSCs, we relied on data from many independent laboratories that had previously analyzed candidate markers for SSCs (publications found in[32]). Different laboratories had previously analyzed candidate genes as markers for the testicular stem cells pinpointing SSEA4, GFR1α and GPR125 as putative SSC markers [publications found in[32]]. To confirm or refute clonal growth of cells expressing each marker, we isolated immunofluorescently tagged cells from a testicular isolate using the same mouth pipette procedure as above, again placing each cell into its own well in a 96 well plate. Cells were labeled with primary antibodies directed against SSEA4, GFR1α, GPR125, or vimentin[32], followed by fluorescently labeled secondary antibodies. The insets in Figure 1 show examples of fluorescent single cells within each well. Interestingly, SSEA4+ cells not only formed colonies, they were the same size as the medium cells previously seen to form colonies. Conversely, Gfrα1+ cells were much smaller and did not form colonies while the larger cells were only able to divide a few times in culture and resembled fibroblasts. Most of the larger cells were vimentin positive suggesting they were Sertoli cells or cells from the lamina propria. As a result, these data confirmed that SSEA4+ cells are most likely the hgPSCs that acquire the ability to not only grow clonally when isolated from the testes and

grown in a specified hESC medium, but also form cells/tissues from all three germ layers.

hgPSC colony-derived cardiac-lineage cells express cardioprotective paracrine factors

One approach that is gaining momentum for improving cardiac function after ischemic injury is the delivery of paracrine factors that can reprogram or induce repair of existing cardiac tissue. To identify if hgPSCs could be induced to form cardiac cells that secrete cardioprotective paracrine factors, we subjected them to a protocol used for human ESCs documented by[33], followed by assaying by gene expression analysis using RT-PCR.

The procedure begins with 1g pieces of human testes tissue. Individual tissue samples are thawed and the SSC-enriched fraction is isolated using the protocol from[18]. Each sample yields ~500 hgPSC colonies. SSCs undergo de-differentiation to form hgPSCs when cultured in hESC medium for 10 days. Distinct hgPSC colonies begin to form after 2-3 days and each Yamanaka factor (Sox2, Oct4, Lin28, Klf4) as well as other stemness factors, nanog and CD73, are expressed (Figure 2B). CD73 represents a marker for newly described endogenous plastic somatic cells (ePSCs; [34] Figure 2B).

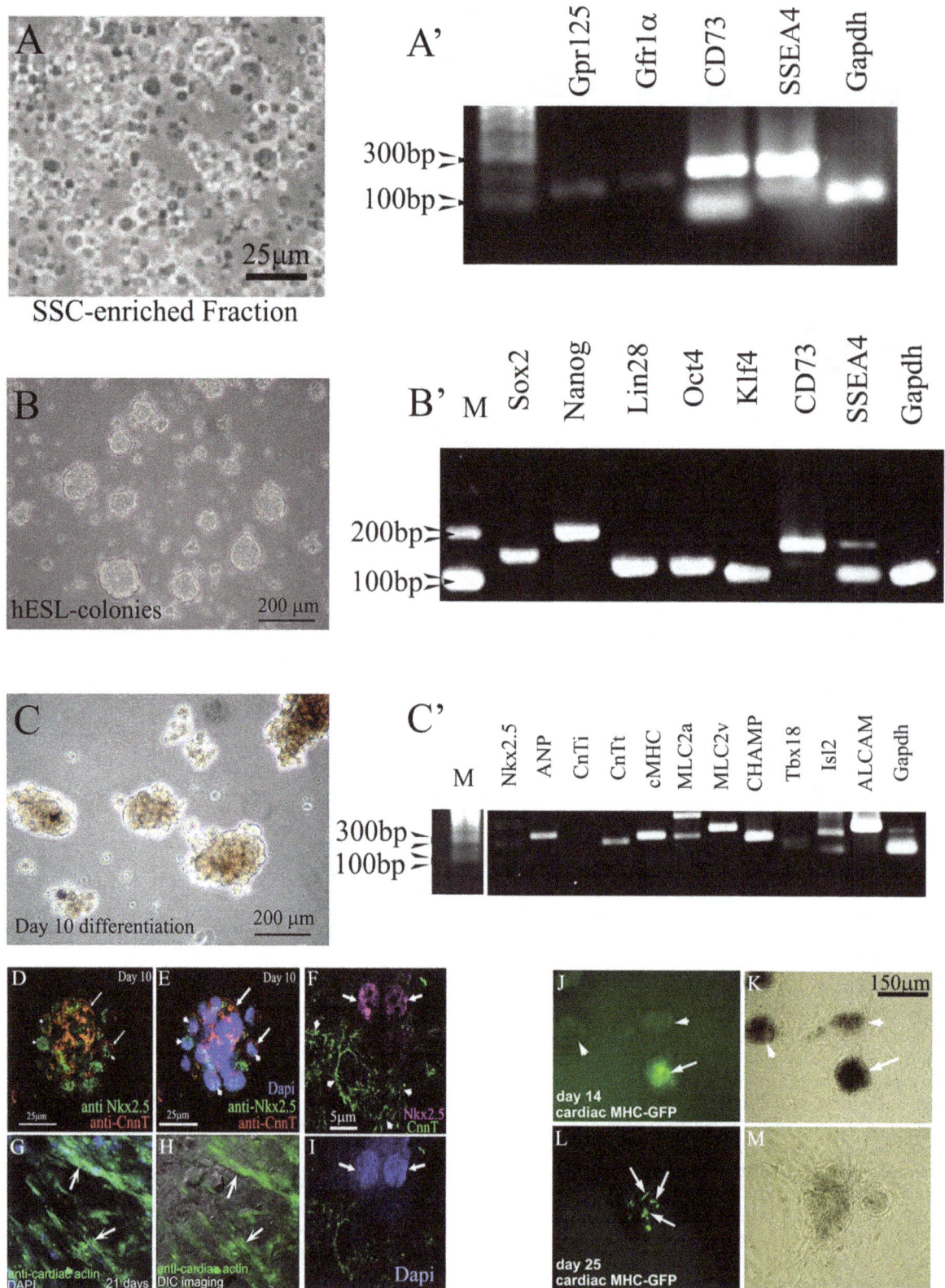

Figure 2. *Cardiac lineages can be produced from hgPSCs. A). Cells of the SSC-enriched fraction are cultured in medium containing GDNF for four days. The fraction is full of cells positive for various SSC markers including SSEA4. B) After four days, the medium is switched to a basic hESC medium containing bFGF and serum replacement. Cells are incubated for at least 10 days, after which rt-PCR shows evidence of all four Yamanaka factors plus nanog and CD73. C) Switching hESC medium for cardiac differentiation medium results in growth and morphologically darker looking colonies. RT-PCR shows expression of 9 out of 10 cardiac genes within 10 days of differentiation. D-I) Confocal analyses show protein expression of specific cardiac genes including nuclear staining of Nkx2.5 (F arrows). Arrows in D and E point to areas positive for cardiac troponin (cTNT), while arrowheads point to nuclear Nkx2.5 staining. Dapi staining in E identifies the nuclei. Arrows in G and H point to distinct filaments of cardiac actin. The DIC image in H reveals the actin fibers within healthy cells. J-M) Transfection of colonies with a cMHC-GFP further confirms cardiac gene expression. Arrow in J points to a GFP positive colony. Arrowheads point to untransfected colonies. These untransfected colonies serve as an internal control ruling out autofluorescence. L) Arrows point to cells within the colony expressing cMHC-GFP. K and M) Phase contrast views show healthy colonies.*

All are detected in colonies after 10-14 days in culture. It is important to note that unlike iPSCs, which need exogenous expression of Yamanaka factors, these same factors are endogenously expressed and regulated in hgPSCs. Upon differentiation of hgPSC colonies, expression of cardiac genes is usually detected ~10 days of culture (Figure 2C). Confocal microscopy verified distinct cardiac protein expression (Figure 2D-I), while transient transfection with a cardiac MHC-promoter reporter construct confirmed induction of the cardiac lineage (Figure 2J-L).

To test the ability of hgPSC-derived cardiac cells to express cardio-protective paracrine factors, we utilized the cMHC-GFP construct to pick cardiac-lineage colonies from the surrounding fibroblast-like cells. We then assayed for cardio-protective paracrine factor expression[1, 6]. Strong gene expression of each paracrine factor was detected (Figure 3A), while protein expression for two paracrine proteins in particular, IGF-1 and NRG1, was also very strong (Figure 3B-D). Expression of IGF-1 and NRG-1 has recently been shown to be important for inducing surrounding healthy cardiac tissue to both proliferate and differentiate into the ischemic region[1, 6]. NRG-1 is of special interest because of its potential for translation into the clinic for treating infarcts[1]. These data reveal that expression of paracrine factors is relatively robust within hgPSC-derived cardiac lineage cells after 21 days of differentiation. To our knowledge, this is the first evidence that hgPSC-induced cardiac lineage cells express these factors.

Differentiated hGPSCs show loss of pluripotency and teratoma formation

For quality-control issues, it was important to confirm that hGPSCs lost their ability to form teratomas. First, using RT-PCR, we verified that virtually all of the pluripotency genes were down regulated (Figure 3E); however, there was weak expression of Nanog and CD73 in cardiomyocytes. Through literature search, we found that Nanog can be expressed in the myocardium of rats[35] and CD73 is needed for successful differentiation into cardiomyocytes[36] (Figure 3E). Equally as important to identifying loss of pluripotency was identifying molecularly, the ability (or loss of) of these cells to form teratomas. The RT-PCR data in Figure 3F clearly show expression of three genes, DND1 and p19 CDKI and p18ink4C in hGPSCs–derived cardiomycoytes[37]. The expression of these genes are consistent with the *loss* of teratoma formation in hGPSCs and cardiomyocytes[37, 38]. As a result, cardiomyocytes differentiated from hGPSCs are molecularly incapable of forming teratomas. We also performed a no- RT control on p18[INK4C] primers because they sit on one exon and observed that there was no genomic DNA contamination in both hgPSCs and cardiomyocytes (data not shown).

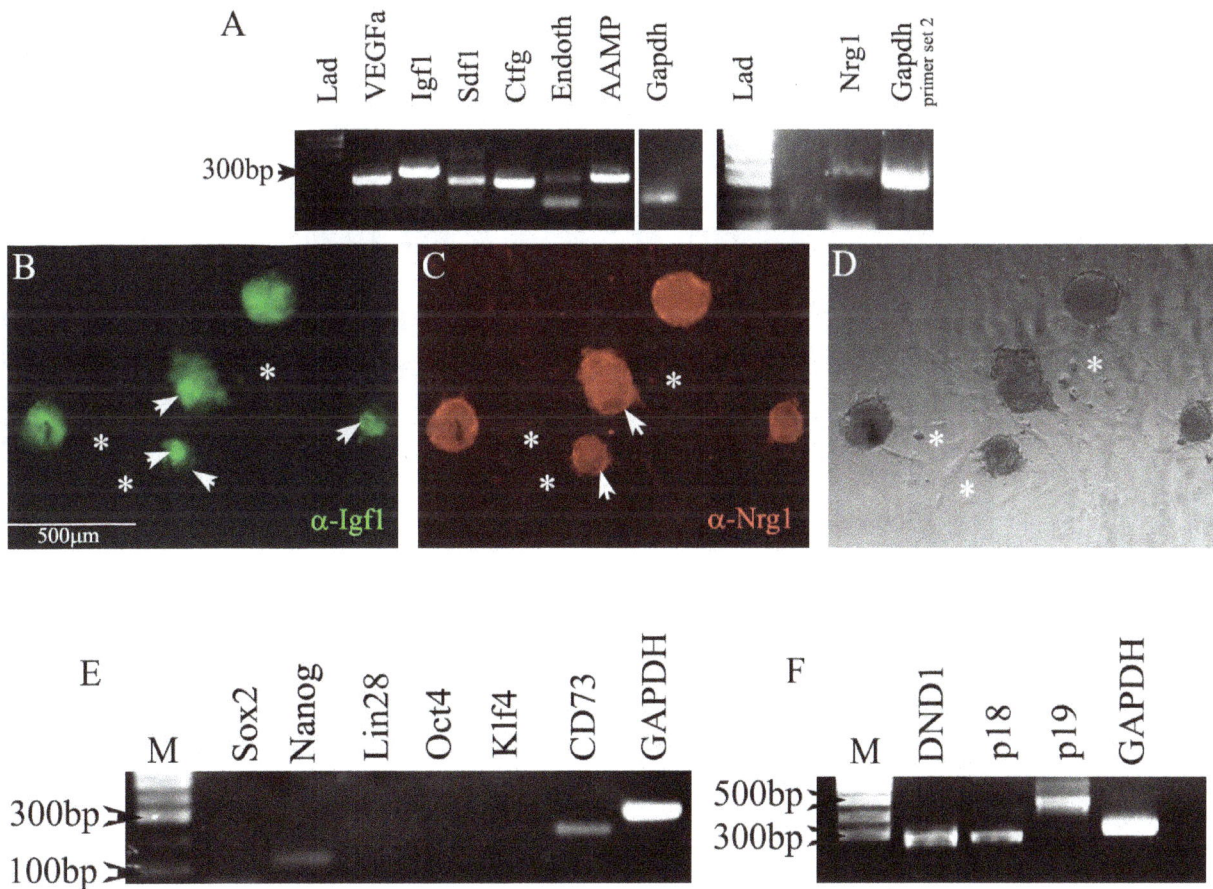

Figure 3. *Differentiation of cardiac colonies beyond day10 results in colonies that express pro-cardiac regenerative paracrine factors. A) Rt-PCR shows expression of seven pro-cardiac regenerative paracrine factors. B-D) Immunofluorescent and DIC analyses using antibodies directed against IGF-1 and NRG-1 show colonies staining positive for both paracrine factors. Arrowheads in B and C point to regions of variable staining within colonies. Asterisks highlight fibroblasts that can emanate from colonies. They show no fluorescent staining. E) Expression of most pluripotency genes is below the level of detection in differentiated colonies. Nanog and CD73 are expressed; however, nanog expression has been reported at low levels by [35] and CD73 expression has been reported as necessary for cardiac development[37]. F) Genes known to inhibit teratoma formation are expressed in hgPSC-derived cardiomyocytes. They are also expressed in hGPSCs (data not shown).*

Quick, efficient expansion of hgPSCs using hgPSC expansion medium (GEM)

The data preceding figure 4 were acquired from primary hgPSCs and cardiac cells differentiated directly from primary hgPSC colonies. However, we found that while hgPSC-derived cardiac cells showed much promise for eventual cardiac repair, it was somewhat painstaking to accumulate the amount of cells that would be needed for injection into a patient. Months were needed to generate enough biological material from 1g biopsy-sized pieces of testes. As a result, we modified a cellular reprogramming technique by[22] and applied it to hgPSCs to determine if we could expand the hgPSC population more quickly (and using no animal components) when compared to conventional expansion protocols.

Figure 4 illustrates the process of germ cell expansion and subsequent re-establishment of hgPSCs, followed by their differentiation into cardiac lineages. By day 10 in GEM, the cells within colonies took on a cobble-stone appearance typical of previous reports[22]. While in GEM, these cells could be expanded indefinitely and quickly; that is, one colony placed in a 96 well plate would typically be split into two wells of a 96 well plate within 7 days. Comparing expansion rates of primary hgPSCs to expanded hgPSCs grown in GEM from two patients, we found that upon re-establishment in hESC medium, ~4X more colonies were obtained by the fourth passage when compared to primary hgPSCs grown in conventional culture medium. More importantly, it took 30 days less time to expand hgPSCs in GEM compared to primary hgPSCs grown in conventional medium (Figure 5; Table 3). We have expanded hgPSCs in GEM at least 20X. Re-establishing hgPSC colonies is accomplished by replacing GEM with hESC medium. Usually within ten days of culture, gene expression patterns match primary hgPSCs including the expression of all Yamanaka factors, nano([34]; Figure 4F). Confocal microscopy of colonies provided further evidence that these cells retained pluripotent markers (Figure 4G).

These re-established hgPSC colonies could then be differentiated down the cardiac pathway resulting in an expression pattern of paracrine factors similar to that observed in cardiac cells differentiated from primary hgPSCs (Figure 4H, I). As a result, we conclude that re-established cardiac colonies are virtually identical to cardiac colonies generated from fresh primary hgPSCs.

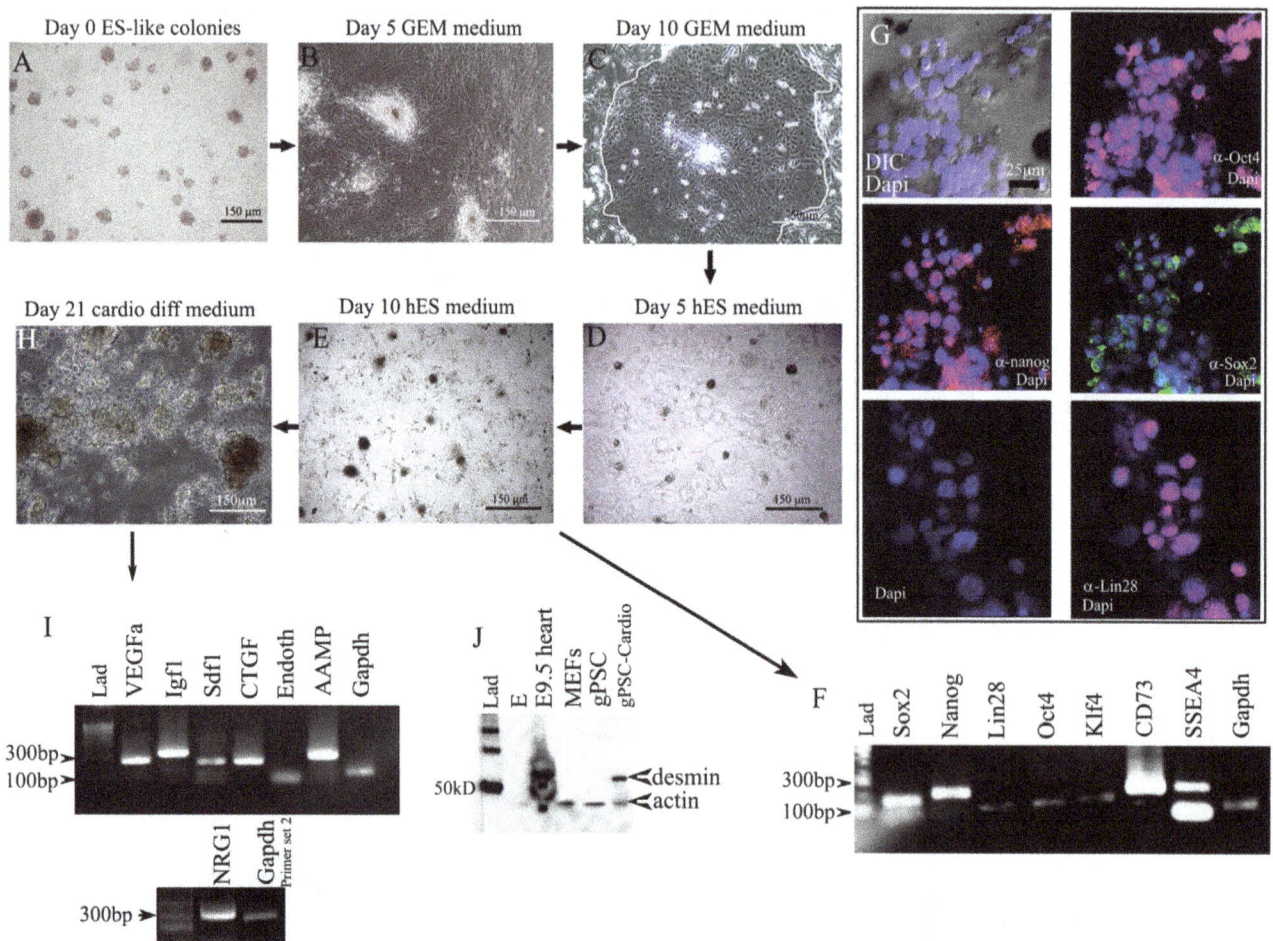

Figure 4. *Culturing hgPSC colonies in GEM allows for their rapid expansion without the loss of stemness. A) hgPSC colonies grown in hESC medium lose their colony structure beginning ~5days post switching to GEM (B). By day 10, most colonies become individual layers of cobble-stone shaped cells (C-white outline shows region of cobblestone pattern of cells), which can be expanded indefinitely. Switching GEM for hESC medium, colonies begin to re-form within 5 days (D), and by day 10 hgPSC colonies fully return (E). F-G) Rt-PCR shows that these colonies express all the same stem cell factors prior to expansion, which is confirmed by confocal microscopy. Nuclear staining of Oct4 (647 nm- Far red), Nanog (594 nm/ Rhodamine- Red), Sox2 (488nm/FITC- Green), and Lin28 (647 nm- Far red) is prevalent (G). H) 21 days post differentiation, large dark colonies form, which are all positive for paracrine factor gene expression (I). J) Western Blot analysis of the colonies shows they are positive for the cardiac intermediate filament desmin similar to the mouse heart. Undifferentiated gPSCs are negative for desmin as are mouse embryonic fibroblasts (MEFs).*

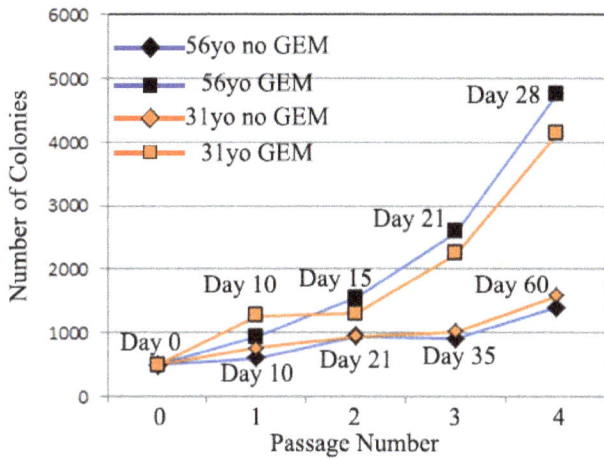

Figure 5. 500 hgPSC colonies were expanded by traditional conditions (i.e., by trypsinization and passaging 1:2) or they were expanded 1:2 in GEM. Comparing two different patients, no marked difference was observed until the second and third passages where GEM-grown hgPSCs grew ~2X faster than conventional growth. By the fourth passage, GEM-grown colonies re-generated close to 4X more colonies when compared to conventional growth and passaging. More importantly, those ~4x more colonies were obtained in almost half the time.

Paracrine factors are secreted by re-established cardiac colonies

While it was important to show that cardiomyocytes derived from hgPSCs expressed cardiac and paracrine factor genes (see Table 1 for paracrine factor list and functions), it was further necessary to identify their physiological ability to secrete those paracrine factors. A consensus of at least six paracrine 'effects' categories has been endorsed within the literature[1, 11, 39, 40] (see Table 1). These categories include (Survival, proliferation, immune cells, remodeling, vascularization, and CPC activation). Secretion of paracrine factors would mean they can affect surrounding tissue.

To detect secretion, two different methods were employed. First, after culturing day 21-differentiated cardiomyocytes for 0hrs, 12hrs, 24hrs and 48hrs, the entire compliment of medium (1.0 ml) from each time point was directly tested by immunoprecipitation (IP) using antibodies to specific paracrine factors, followed by antibody isolation using magnetic protein G-coated beads. The pull-down products were subjected to SDS-PAGE, followed by silver stain of the gels. This highly sensitive approach revealed VEGFA, CTGF, IGF-1, and TGFβ all increasing in concentration over a 48hr period of incubation (Figure 6).

Table 3: Comparing expansion rates of primary hgPSCs to expanded hgPSCs grown in GEM

Passage #	56yo Patient 1 — Number of gPSC colonies — NO Conditional Reprogramming Medium (No GEM)																Time
P0	500																Day 0
P1	380								320								Day 10
P2	280				220				235				215				Day 21
P3	113		163		89		108		123		93		105		113		Day 35
P4	85	94	101	96	58	73	80	93	103	94	76	89	88	91	87	92	Day 60
Total # of colonies	1,400																

Passage #	56yo Patient 1 — Number of gPSC colonies — Expanded in Conditional Reprogramming Medium (+ GEM)																Time
P0	500																Day 0
P1	455								476								Day 10
P2	387				358				396				403				Day 15
P3	308		310		303		317		302		287		363		397		Day 21
P4	302	275	280	285	295	283	301	275	267	258	275	285	355	310	365	352	Day 28
Total # of colonies	4,763																

Passage #	31yo Patient 2 — Number of gPSC colonies — NO Conditional Reprogramming Medium (No GEM)																Time
P0	500																Day 0
P1	385								380								Day 10
P2	286				222				205				235				Day 21
P3	133		114		113		124		143		127		118		147		Day 35
P4	101	102	88	98	84	88	104	102	110	113	95	101	95	87	115	103	Day 60
Total # of colonies	1,587																

Passage #	31yo Patient 2 — Number of gPSC colonies — Expanded in Conditional Reprogramming Medium (+ GEM)																Time
P0	500																Day 0
P1	489								478								Day 10
P2	287				318				337				306				Day 15
P3	221		247		276		285		307		315		287		305		Day 21
P4	205	210	222	230	245	237	275	245	301	275	303	289	275	263	300	268	Day 28
Total # of colonies	4,143																

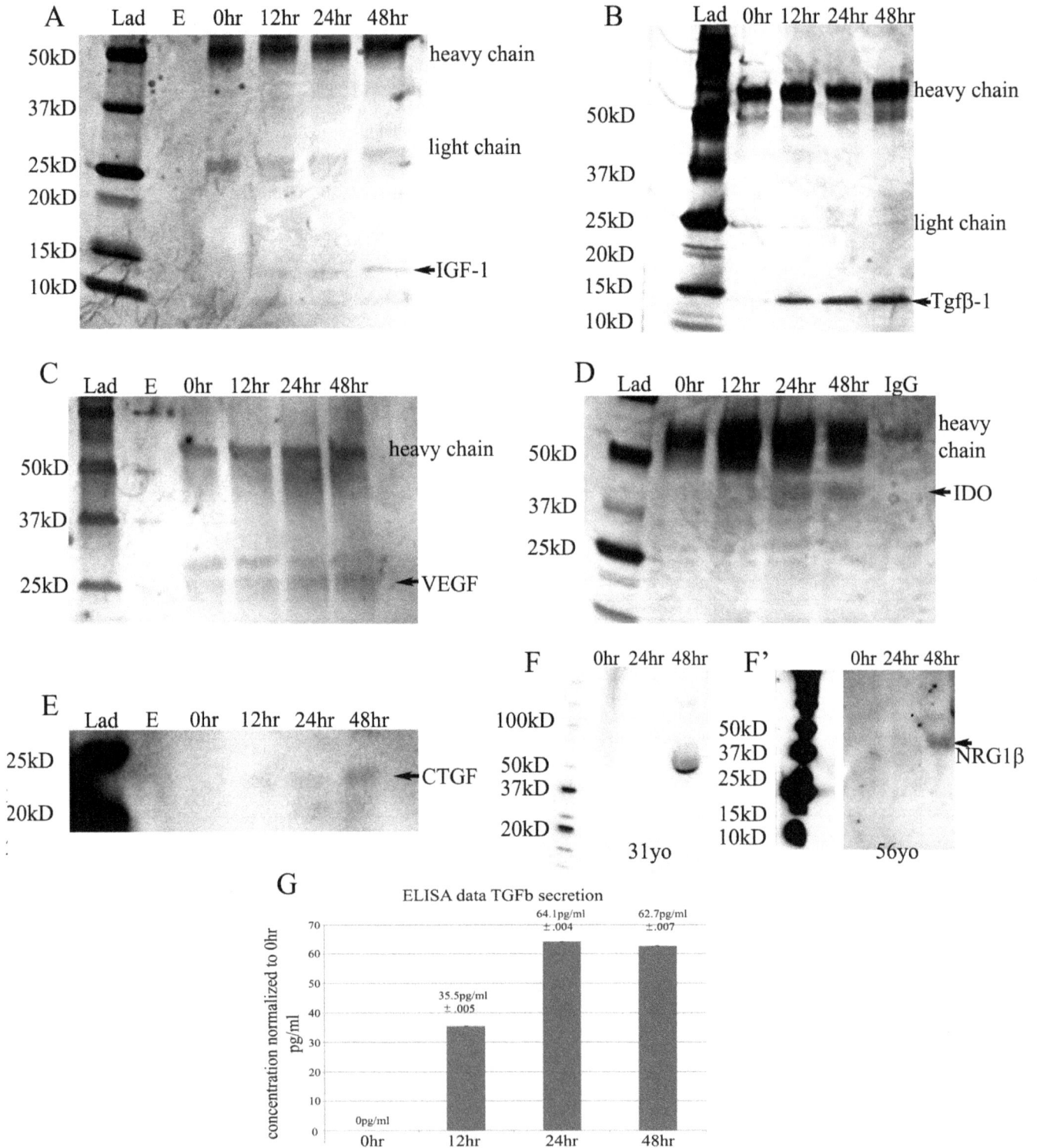

Figure 6. *Immunoprecipitation (I.P.) and Western Blot analysis of culture medium shows that paracrine factors are secreted from hgPSC-derived cardiac colonies. A) Silver stained SDS-PAGE gel detected IGF-1 by IP after 12hrs of culture, increasing in intensity through 48hrs of culture. B). Silver staining shows TGFb secretion within 12hrs becoming more intense after 48hrs. C) VEGF is detectable by about 24hrs of culture. D) Western analysis of CTGF secretion is detected within 24hrs while NRG-1 secretion (E-F) is detected after 48hrs of culture. Cardiac differentiation of hgPSCs from two patients are shown for Nrg1. All IP experiments were run with a lane containing IgG alone to identify the heavy and light chain bands. 2µl from all samples were analyzed using a nano-drop ND-8000 (Thermo Fisher Inc.) to normalize protein concentrations. G) ELISA bar graph data shows quantitative amounts of TGFβ secretion detected within 12-48 hours of culture. ELISA data confirm the silver stained SDS PAGE gels, which detected a similar secretion pattern as found in the ELISA.*

The second method we used to detect secreted proteins involved precipitation of proteins from the medium using 4 volumes of ice cold ethanol (as published in[28-30]), then separating them by SDS-PAGE, and probing by Western blot using antibodies directed against each paracrine factor (Figure 6E and F). This Western blot approach was employed primarily where the antibodies had not been tested for applications such as I.P. Here, we found that CTGF and NRG-1 were secreted into the medium by 24-48hrs. When combined, these data provided strong evidence that hgPSC-derived cardiomyocytes secrete paracrine factors known to be proangiogenic and procardiogeneic[1, 6, 41].

It is difficult to quantify these data because secreted "housekeeping" genes are not well characterized for these cells; however, we do know that the lower level of protein detection for silver stained gels is in the ~ 1-10ng range. In an attempt to confirm and quantify what we observed from our silver stain data, we analyzed media by ELISA (Figure 6G). Since, sensitivity of both ELISA and silver stain are similar (0.1-10ng of protein), the ELISA data confirmed what we observed in the silver stains; TGFβ is secreted within the 1-10ng/ml range within 48 hrs of culture. More specifically, our silver stain results showed that from 10μl of sample media loaded into each well, ~5.0 x 10^5 cells secrete paracrine factors in the 1-10ng/ml range by 48 hrs of culture. Figure 6G illustrates ELISA data showing a gradual increase of TGFβ from 0h to 24h, with very little change in secretion between 24h and 48h of incubation. According to Beck et al[42], the active form of TGFβ can last for over a day after which it is subjected to various types of degradation. This observation by Beck et al[42] may

be the reason for the slight decrease we see at 48 hours compared to 24 hours as some of the TGFβ might have started to degrade by 48 hours. Most importantly, however, is that these TGFβ ELISA data confirm the silver stain results. The concentration of each paracrine factor is well within range for effecting of surrounding tissues (Figure 6). These data are the first to show that hgPSC-derived cardiac cells not only express, but also secrete cardio-protective paracrine effectors.

hgPSC-derived cardiomyocytes can integrate to beating cardiac tissue in vivo

We next wanted to determine if hgPSC-derived cardiomyocytes could fuse with beating heart tissue. Many different animal models have been utilized, with rodent hearts being the most prevalently used model system, to demonstrate infiltration and integration-ability of various types of stem cells within cardiac tissue[14, 43]. One problem with rodent model systems for human stem cell research, however, is that the normal beat-rate for mouse hearts can vary between 400-600 beats/minute. The dramatic difference between human cardiac cells and rodent hearts has been reported to create incompatible physiological variances that can skew results[14]. As a result, we chose the mouse fetal heart as a 'better', more physiologically compatible model system for transplanting cardiac-specific, GFP-labeled, hgPSC-derived cardiomyocytes (Figure 2 and 7). This model system is better than adult cardiac model systems because the mouse fetal heart beats at ~60-70 beats/min, which is very similar physiologically to the human heart.

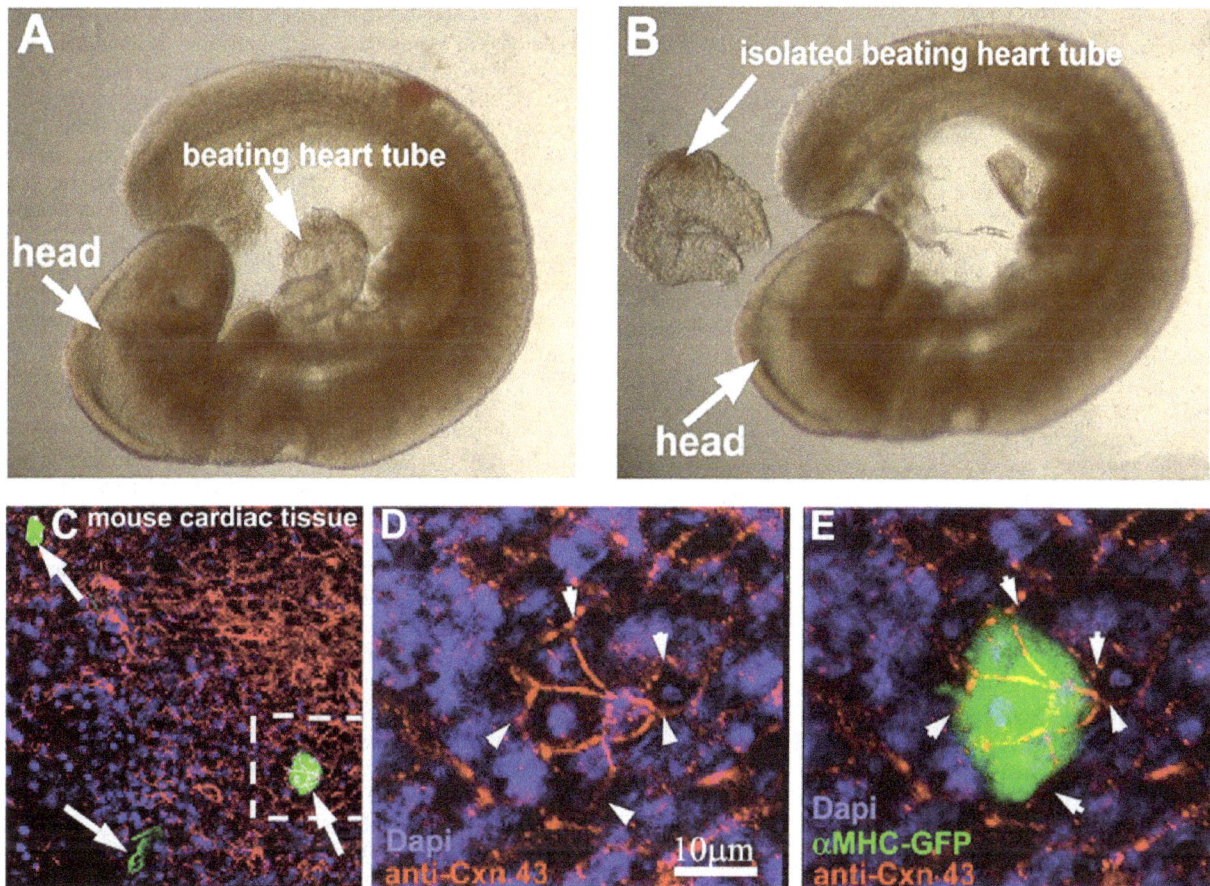

Figure 7. *hgPSC-derived cardiac colonies can fuse with beating cardiac tissue. **A-B**) E9.5 fetal hearts were isolated from mouse embryos using Dumont #5 forceps. 10-15 fetal hearts were placed in one well of a 96 well plate and cMHC-GFP positive colonies were mouth pipetted into crevasses within the beating heart or simply overlaid onto the hearts. 24 hours later, hearts were analyzed live using a Leica stereoscope equipped with fluorescence. Hearts containing green areas were then fixed, stained for CNX43, and Dapi and visualized by confocal microscopy. **C**) Multiple GFP-positive regions were evident (arrows). **D-E**) Higher magnification clearly showed GFP positive cells fused to cardiac tissue via gap junctions (Arrowheads) on the same focal plane as surround heart tissue.*

cMHC-GFP-positive hgPSC-derived cardiac colonies were physically isolated by mouth pipette using a Leica Fluorescent stereoscope. GFP+ Colonies were then pipetted into tight crevices within the heart tube so that they could not fall away from the beating heart tube. Each well of the 96 well plate contained 10-15 fetal hearts, which forced virtually all loose cardiac colonies to remain in close contact with cardiac tissue. After 48hrs of incubation, fetal hearts were observed live using the same fluorescent stereoscope to identify GFP(+) areas. Upon detection, fetal hearts were fixed in 3.0% formaldehyde for 2hrs, followed by processing for immunofluorescence using an antibody for the cardiac gap junction protein Connexin43 (CNX43). Multiple areas of GFP labeled cells were visibly co-stained with the gap junction protein CNX43 providing evidence that the hgPSC-derived cardiac cells directly fused with the mouse cardiac tissue. Fusion of GFP labeled cells was observed in 8 out of the 10 fetal hearts.

Discussion

Although optimism remains for investigating stem cells for treating or curing cardiovascular disease, much disparity remains among the various published approaches and results. Here, we show three novel outcomes that could lead to the production and delivery of paracrine factors known to induce and improve cardiac function in ischemically injured heart muscle[1, 8, 9, 13]. First, we show that hgPSC-derived cardiac cells express and secrete pro-cardiac regenerative paracrine factors. Secondly, the expansion of hgPSCs can be markedly amplified when cultured in GEM using human serum (no animal products); and thirdly, the data provide strong evidence that hgPSC-derived cardiomyocytes can physically incorporate into the cardiac niche.

Since the initial findings that a germ-line stem cell could 'revert' to a state that resembled hESCs/hiPSCs both genotypically and phenotypically, understanding their biology and therapeutic potentials has been consistently investigated by various laboratories[1, 18, 20, 31, 44]. Defining the 'stemness' of germ-line stem cells has been debated[45]; however, the most recent study from the Skutella laboratory has provided the best evidence yet as to their true identity[31]. They reported that hgPSCs are adult stem cells, but they share a gene expression profile that is related to, but not identical to true pluripotent stem cells. Perhaps the most important finding in [31] was the confirmation of hgPSC colony plasticity as they were shown to attain the ability to differentiate into cells of all three germ layers[17, 18, 31, 32, 46]. From a swath of previously identified 'potential' SSC markers, the elegant studies from two independent laboratories pinpointed SSEA4 as a strong candidate marker for the testicular stem cells that might be giving rise to hgPSCs. Interestingly, these data somewhat contradicted data from other laboratories who had previously suggested Gfr1α and Gpr125 as candidate SSC markers [publications found in[32]]. In light of this controversy, research on human testes using various methodologies including magnetic-activated cell sorting [MACS[47], indirect immunofluorescence[48], and FACS[49]] provided the evidence that SSEA4+ cells were most likely the best candidates that, when cultured in hESC medium, could progressively expressed pluripotent factors and subsequently generate cells from all three germ layers. Closer inspection of those studied showed that they did not clearly identify the ability of SSEA4+ cells to grow clonally into hgPSC colonies.

Here, we confirmed that hgPSCs do endogenously express all of the pluripotent Yamanaka factors plus newly identified others (Nanog and CD73) known to be important for stemness (This study [18]) and that they are readily down-regulated once differentiation commences. Thus, once differentiated, hgPSCs show virtually no risk of teratoma formation in vivo. In fact, closer inspection of reports where teratoma formation was specifically analyzed after injection of naked hgPSCs

into nude mice revealed that tens of millions of hgPSCs over a month were needed to generate a tiny nodule containing multiple cell types[18]. This result was in stark contrast to the teratomas that formed within three weeks from mere thousands of ESCs injected into the opposing hind flank of the same nude mice. It is these types of observations, when taken together, that keep hgPSC research relevant.

Upon differentiation of hgPSCs, similar to hESC and hiPSC-derived cardiac cells[15, 50, 51], we found that hgPSC-derived cardiac cells varied with respect to atrial/ventricle gene expression representing a mixed population of cardiac cells; however, one aspect that was not shared was spontaneous beating. Cardiac cells derived from human hESCs and hiPSCs consistently show rhythmic beating; however, hgPSC-derived cardiac cells did not. Initially, we were discouraged by this non-beating phenotype; however, recent revelations within the literature led us to pursue the alternative, paracrine effector, and regenerative pathway.

For years, numerous investigations have tapped into the 'beating' phenotype for potentially repairing ischemically damaged heart muscle. In fact, some adult stem cell (ASC) work has shown promise as ejection fractions slightly improve after beating ASC-derived cardiomyocytes are injected into infarcted heart muscle. However, one major detriment with many ASC-cardiac repair studies is the potential for arrhythmias as stem cell-derived cardiomyocytes, in many cases, can beat at their own pace. As a result, instead of matching stem cell/cardiac tissue electrophysiology, a paradigm shift towards cardiac tissue regeneration mediated either directly or indirectly by paracrine factors has been proposed as more beneficial. We originally showed that hgPSCs could express a small cohort of cardiac genes representing differentiation[18]; however, in depth analyses of these cells for potential cardiac repair was not assessed in[18]. There have been hundreds of studies investigating if and how ASCs as well as ESCs and iPSCs function to repair ischemic cardiac tissue (reviewed by[2, 7]). Some of those studies have resulted in clinical trials; however, the varying outcomes of those trials have not led to their routine clinical use because the best mechanism for translating their potential in vivo remains debated. On one hand, generating cardiomyocytes with the ability to electrically couple within the ischemic region of the heart has resulted in some, albeit good, evidence showing attenuation of left ventricular (LV) remodeling and improved LV systolic function[40, 52, 53]. In addition, data from non-human primates and large mammals have also shown neovascularization upon stem cell injection[50, 54]. On the other hand, much of the data where matching stem cell/heart electrophysiology was a focus of the study, stem cells were found to generate a diverse set of mature and immature atrial, ventricle, and even sinusoidal cells periodically resulting in arrhythmic islands of beating cells[50, 54]. As a result, although the electrophysiology avenue of research remains ardently investigated among many different types of stem cells, it was exciting to find that the differentiation potential of hgPSC-derived cardiomyocytes included expression and secretion of key paracrine factors known to be pro-growth and pro-differentiation [1, 9].

A consensus of at least six paracrine 'effects' categories has been endorsed within the literature[1, 11, 39, 40]. Analyzing the SSEA+, medium-size hgPSC-derived cardiomyocytes revealed that they expressed and secreted paracrine factors from all six paracrine 'effects' categories. Genes including VEGFA (representing vascularization and remodeling), NRG1 (proliferation and vascularization), IGF1 (survival, proliferation, and suppression of immune response), TGFβ (Immune regulation, remodeling), and SDF1 (vascularization and CPC activation) all were not only expressed, but also secreted into the media at or near nanogram/ml levels. As a result, the data presented here provide evidence that hgPSC-derived cardiomyocytes can either directly or indirectly influence cardiac tissue via paracrine effects.

Although identifying expression and secretion of paracrine factors was an important step in determining the ability of hgPSC-derived cardiac cells for potential use *in vivo*, it was also important to identify their ability to integrate into cardiac tissue. Without integration into cardiac tissue, delivery of paracrine effectors would be impaired or highly unlikely. The model system we employed to identify integration took into consideration both successes and failures identified by many investigations[11, 39, 51, 55]. For example, injecting undifferentiated adult stem cells or differentiated hESCs/hiPSCs into infarcted rodent hearts has resulted in widely varying reports from improved cardiac function to little or no attenuation[7, 15, 55]. Efficacy of integration into the cardiac niche was one characteristic dictating their successes or failures. Shared gap junctions characteristically represent good integration[56, 57]; however, even if gap junctions are readily observed between endogenous and exogenous cells, problems can still arise including arrhythmias. Arrhythmic beating can result from injected cells 'beating' on their own and/or because they cannot match the beat-rate of the injected heart[7]. Rodent hearts can beat >400 beats/min. A human heart beating that fast would be considered undergoing tachycardia. On the contrary, because embryonic hearts beat at ~70 beats/min, we determined they would serve as a better model system for identifying the integration ability of hgPSC-derived cardiac cells into a cardiac niche. hgPSC-derived cardiac cells expressing a cardiac promoter-driven GFP reporter gene along with immunofluorescent staining of the endogenously expressed cardiomyocyte gap junction protein CNX43 clearly showed multiple areas of integration. As a result, these data provide good evidence justifying further, more detailed investigations of hgPSC-derived cardiac cells for use in cardiac repair, perhaps within a non-human primate model.

None of these data would have been possible, though, if we had not had enough hgPSC-derived cardiac cells to work with. Soon after we began work on the data presented here, a novel technology was published for growing primary epithelial cells indefinitely[22]. That work astonishingly, yet elegantly showed that a small tracheal biopsy could be grown indefinitely in a specifically defined medium (>40 passages), followed by complete re-establishment of all cell types within the trachea when transferred back to a media promoting tracheal development. Their medium was composed of a DMEM/Hams F12 mix (1:1) containing a ROCK inhibitor *and* 25% J2 cell conditioned medium. We found that hgPSCs grew very quickly in the medium defined by[22]. About 100 colonies would grow to confluency in a 6 well dish within ~5 days and could then be passaged indefinitely; however, we did encounter a problem in about 50% of our experiments. The cells would fill with small, dark vacuoles that would eventually kill the cells. As a result, we tried growing cells in medium using various combinations of the components specified in[22]. We found that growing hgPSCs in medium containing a ROCK inhibitor *without* the J2 component did not alter their ability to expand indefinitely. We also substituted animal serum with human serum to remove all animal products. Consequently, these two changes were substantial enough to warrant renaming our medium to 'hgPSC expansion medium' (GEM) to quell any confusion. So far we have reached ~20 passages of hgPSCs using GEM while not losing the ability to re-establish colonies positive for all Yamanaka factors, CD73 and Nanog.

Conclusion

With this technique in hand, generating cells for experimental analysis has become much more efficient. We also believe this technique could speed up the time needed for treating patients from months to weeks. The resulting re-established hgPSCs also re-attained their differentiation potential as they not only expressed the same cardiac marker set tested in primary hgPSC-derived cardiac cells, but also the same set of paracrine factors. We believe the data presented here could eventually, truly help patients with heart disease. An important fact to note is that the work presented here is not male-centric.

Evidence from the Tilly laboratory has revealed the existence of gPSCs within the ovary[58, 59]. Patients suffering from ischemic heart injury could be subjected to a testes/ovary biopsy (could be done in an IVF clinic). The biopsy is then given to the scientist for isolating SSCs/OSCs (isolated from the biopsy) and subsequent de-differentiation into hgPSCs. Indefinite expansion of hgPSCs in GEM would be followed by re-establishment into hgPSCs, and then differentiation into paracrine factor yielding cardiomyocytes. These cells would be sent back to the medical doctor who would then inject them back into the patient. Some of the expanded hgPSCs in GEM could be frozen down for future treatment (in case the same patient comes back for treatment again).

While we are planning to expand this work into the ovary to identify the potential of female hgPSCs for treating or curing heart disease in women, we also do not want to rule out the research being pursued on very small embryonic-like stem cells (VSELs). It was recently suggested that VSELs might share similarities with gPSCs with respect to their capacity to restore spermatogenesis in mice [60]. Whether VSELs and gPSCs are one in the same remains to be determined. If they are based on the data presented here, both should be pursued with vigor to help treat or cure heart disease.

References

1. Hodgkinson CP, Bareja A, Gomez JA, Dzau VJ. Emerging Concepts in Paracrine Mechanisms in Regenerative Cardiovascular Medicine and Biology. Circ Res. 2016;118(1):95-107.
2. Trivedi P, Tray N, Nguyen T, Nigam N, Gallicano GI. Mesenchymal stem cell therapy for treatment of cardiovascular disease: helping people sooner or later. Stem Cells Dev. 2010 ;19(7):1109-20.
3. Kang E, Wang X, Tippner-Hedges R, Ma H, Folmes CD, Gutierrez NM, Lee Y, Van Dyken C, Ahmed R, Li Y, Koski A, Hayama T, Luo S, Harding CO, Amato P, Jensen J, Battaglia D, Lee D, Wu D, Terzic A, Wolf DP, Huang T, Mitalipov S. Age-Related Accumulation of Somatic Mitochondrial DNA Mutations in Adult-Derived Human iPSCs.Cell Stem Cell. 2016 May 5;18(5):625-36.
4. Kang E, Wu J, Gutierrez NM, Koski A, Tippner-Hedges R, Agaronyan K, Platero-Luengo A, Martinez-Redondo P, Ma H, Lee Y, Hayama T, Van Dyken C, Wang X,Luo S, Ahmed R, Li Y, Ji D, Kayali R, Cinnioglu C, Olson S, Jensen J, Battaglia D, Lee D, Wu D, Huang T, Wolf DP, Temiakov D, Belmonte JC, Amato P, Mitalipov S. Mitochondrial replacement in human oocytes carrying pathogenic mitochondrial DNA mutations. Nature. 2016 Dec 8;540(7632):270-275.
5. Cote GM, Sawyer DB, Chabner BA. ERBB2 inhibition and heart failure. N Engl J Med. 2012;367(22):2150-3.
6. Gnecchi M, Zhang Z, Ni A, Dzau VJ. Paracrine mechanisms in adult stem cell signaling and therapy. Circ Res. 2008;103(11):1204-19.
7. Madonna R, Van Laake LW, Davidson SM, Engel FB, Hausenloy DJ, Lecour S, Leor J, Perrino C, Schulz R, Ytrehus K, Landmesser U, Mummery CL, Janssens S, Willerson J, Eschenhagen T, Ferdinandy P, Sluijter JP. Position Paper of the European Society of Cardiology Working Group Cellular Biology of the Heart: cell-based therapies for myocardial repair and regeneration in ischemic heart disease and heart failure. Eur Heart J. 2016 ;37(23):1789-98.
8. Uemura R, Xu M, Ahmad N, Ashraf M. Bone marrow stem cells prevent left ventricular remodeling of ischemic heart through paracrine signaling. Circ Res. 2006;98(11):1414-21.
9. Yi BA, Mummery CL, Chien KR. Direct cardiomyocyte reprogramming: a new direction for cardiovascular regenerative medicine. Cold Spring Harb Perspect Med. 2013;3(9):a014050.
10. Shiba Y, Fernandes S, Zhu WZ, Filice D, Muskheli V, Kim J, Palpant NJ, Gantz J, Moyes KW, Reinecke H, Van Biber B, Dardas T, Mignone JL, Izawa A, Hanna R, Viswanathan M, Gold JD, Kotlikoff MI, Sarvazyan N, Kay MW, Murry CE, Laflamme MA. Human ES-cell-derived cardiomyocytes electrically couple and suppress arrhythmias in injured hearts. Nature. 2012;489(7415):322-5.

11. Braun T, Dimmeler S. Breaking the silence: stimulating proliferation of adult cardiomyocytes. Dev Cell. 2009 Aug;17(2):151-3.

12. Dimmeler S, Zeiher AM, Schneider MD. Unchain my heart: the scientific foundations of cardiac repair. J Clin Invest. 2005 ;115(3):572-83.

13. Gnecchi M, He H, Liang OD, Melo LG, Morello F, Mu H, Noiseux N, Zhang L, Pratt RE, Ingwall JS, Dzau VJ. Paracrine action accounts for marked protection of ischemic heart by Akt-modified mesenchymal stem cells. Nat Med. 2005;11(4):367-8.

14. Garbern JC, Mummery CL, Lee RT. Model systems for cardiovascular regenerative biology. Cold Spring Harb Perspect Med. 2013;3(4):a014019.

15. van Laake LW, Passier R, Doevendans PA, Mummery CL. Human embryonic stem cell-derived cardiomyocytes and cardiac repair in rodents. Circ Res. 2008;102(9):1008-10.

16. Veerman CC, Kosmidis G, Mummery CL, Casini S, Verkerk AO, Bellin M. Immaturity of human stem-cell-derived cardiomyocytes in culture: fatal flaw or soluble problem? Stem Cells Dev. 2015;24(9):1035-52.

17. Cooke PS, Simon L, Nanjappa MK, Medrano TI, Berry SE. Plasticity of spermatogonial stem cells. Asian J Androl. 2015;17(3):355-9.

18. Golestaneh N, Kokkinaki M, Pant D, Jiang J, DeStefano D, Fernandez-Bueno C, Rone JD, Haddad BR, Gallicano GI, Dym M. Pluripotent stem cells derived from adult human testes. Stem Cells Dev. 2009;18(8):1115-26.

19. Kossack N, Meneses J, Shefi S, Nguyen HN, Chavez S, Nicholas C, Gromoll J, Turek PJ, Reijo-Pera RA. Isolation and characterization of pluripotent human spermatogonial stem cell-derived cells. Stem Cells. 2009;27(1):138-49.

20. Mizrak SC, Chikhovskaya JV, Sadri-Ardekani H, van Daalen S, Korver CM, Hovingh SE, Roepers-Gajadien HL, Raya A, Fluiter K, de Reijke TM, de la Rosette JJ, Knegt AC, Belmonte JC, van der Veen F, de Rooij DG, Repping S, van Pelt AM. Embryonic stem cell-like cells derived from adult human testis. Hum Reprod. 2010 ;25(1):158-67.

21. Takahashi K, Tanabe K, Ohnuki M, Narita M, Ichisaka T, Tomoda K, Yamanaka S. Induction of pluripotent stem cells from adult human fibroblasts by defined factors. Cell. 2007;131(5):861-72.

22. Suprynowicz FA, Upadhyay G, Krawczyk E, Kramer SC, Hebert JD, Liu X, Yuan H, Cheluvaraju C, Clapp PW, Boucher RC Jr, Kamonjoh CM, Randell SH, Schlegel R. Conditionally reprogrammed cells represent a stem-like state of adult epithelial cells. Proc Natl Acad Sci U S A. 2012 Dec 4;109(49):20035-40.

23. Liu X, Krawczyk E, Suprynowicz FA, Palechor-Ceron N, Yuan H, Dakic A, Simic V, Zheng YL, Sripadhan P, Chen C, Lu J, Hou TW, Choudhury S, Kallakury B, Tang DG, Darling T, Thangapazham R, Timofeeva O, Dritschilo A, Randell SH, Albanese C, Agarwal S, Schlegel R. Conditional reprogramming and long-term expansion of normal and tumor cells from human biospecimens. Nat Protoc. 2017;12(2):439-451.

24. Gallicano GI, Kouklis P, Bauer C, Yin M, Vasioukhin V, Degenstein L, Fuchs E. Desmoplakin is required early in development for assembly of desmosomes and cytoskeletal linkage. J Cell Biol. 1998;143(7):2009-22.

25. Gallicano GI, Bauer C, Fuchs E. Rescuing desmoplakin function in extra-embryonic ectoderm reveals the importance of this protein in embryonic heart, neuroepithelium, skin and vasculature. Development. 2001;128(6):929-41.

26. Kolossov E, Bostani T, Roell W, Breitbach M, Pillekamp F, Nygren JM, Sasse P, Rubenchik O, Fries JW, Wenzel D, Geisen C, Xia Y, Lu Z, Duan Y, Kettenhofen R, Jovinge S, Bloch W, Bohlen H, Welz A, Hescheler J, Jacobsen SE, Fleischmann BK. Engraftment of engineered ES cell-derived cardiomyocytes but not BM cells restores contractile function to the infarcted myocardium. J Exp Med. 2006;203(10):2315-27.

27. Laemmli UK. Cleavage of structural proteins during the assembly of the head of bacteriophage T4. Nature. 1970;227(5259):680-5.

28. Capco DG, Gallicano GI, McGaughey RW, Downing KH, Larabell CA. Cytoskeletal sheets of mammalian eggs and embryos: a lattice-like network of intermediate filaments. Cell Motil Cytoskeleton. 1993;24(2):85-99.

29. Gallicano GI, McGaughey RW, Capco DG. Cytoskeletal sheets appear as universal components of mammalian eggs. J Exp Zool. 1992;263(2):194-203.

30. Gallicano GI, McGaughey RW, Capco DG. Cytoskeleton of the mouse egg and embryo: reorganization of planar elements. Cell Motil Cytoskeleton.1991;18(2):143-54.

31. Conrad S, Azizi H, Hatami M, Kubista M, Bonin M, Hennenlotter J, Sievert KD, Skutella T. Expression of Genes Related to Germ Cell Lineage and Pluripotency in Single Cells and Colonies of Human Adult Germ Stem Cells. Stem Cells Int. 2016;2016:8582526.

32. Dym M, Kokkinaki M, He Z. Spermatogonial stem cells: mouse and human comparisons. Birth Defects Res C Embryo Today. 2009;87(1):27-34.

33. Wu X, Ding S, Ding Q, Gray NS, Schultz PG. Small molecules that induce cardiomyogenesis in embryonic stem cells. J Am Chem Soc. 2004;126(6):1590-1.

34. Pan D, Roy S, Gascard P, Zhao J, Chen-Tanyolac C, Tlsty TD. SOX2, OCT3/4 and NANOG expression and cellular plasticity in rare human somatic cells requires CD73. Cell Signal. 2016;28(12):1923-1932.

35. Land SC, Walker DJ, Du Q, Jovanović A. Cardioprotective SUR2A promotes stem cell properties of cardiomyocytes. Int J Cardiol. 2013;168(5):5090-2.

36. Li Q, Qi LJ, Guo ZK, Li H, Zuo HB, Li NN. CD73+ adipose-derived mesenchymal stem cells possess higher potential to differentiate into cardiomyocytes in vitro. J Mol Histol. 2013;44(4):411-22.

37. Li Y, Pal R, Sung LY, Feng H, Miao W, Cheng SY, Tian C, Cheng T. An opposite effect of the CDK inhibitor, p18(INK4c) on embryonic stem cells compared with tumor and adult stem cells. PLoS One. 2012;7(9):e45212.

38. Takashima S, Hirose M, Ogonuki N, Ebisuya M, Inoue K, Kanatsu-Shinohara M, Tanaka T, Nishida E, Ogura A, Shinohara T. Regulation of pluripotency in male germline stem cells by Dmrt1. Genes Dev. 2013;27(18):1949-58.

39. Bersell K, Arab S, Haring B, Kühn B. Neuregulin1/ErbB4 signaling induces cardiomyocyte proliferation and repair of heart injury. Cell. 2009;138(2):257-70.

40. Liu ZP, Nakagawa O, Nakagawa M, Yanagisawa H, Passier R, Richardson JA, Srivastava D, Olson EN. CHAMP, a novel cardiac-specific helicase regulated by MEF2C. Dev Biol. 2001;234(2):497-509.

41. Zacchigna S, Giacca M. Extra- and intracellular factors regulating cardiomyocyte proliferation in postnatal life. Cardiovasc Res. 2014;102(2):312-20.

42. Beck LS, DeGuzman L, Lee WP, Xu Y, Siegel MW, Amento EP. One systemic administration of transforming growth factor-beta 1 reverses age- or glucocorticoid-impaired wound healing. J Clin Invest. 1993;92(6):2841-9.

43. Fraidenraich D, Stillwell E, Romero E, Wilkes D, Manova K, Basson CT, Benezra R. Rescue of cardiac defects in id knockout embryos by injection of embryonic stem cells. Science. 2004;306(5694):247-52.

44. Yamada M, De Chiara L, Seandel M. Spermatogonial Stem Cells: Implications for Genetic Disorders and Prevention. Stem Cells Dev. 2016.

45. Ko K, Reinhardt P, Tapia N, Schneider RK, Araúzo-Bravo MJ, Han DW, Greber B, Kim J, Kliesch S, Zenke M, Schöler HR. Brief report: evaluating the potential of putative pluripotent cells derived from human testis. Stem Cells. 2011;29(8):1304-9.

46. Kanatsu-Shinohara M, Takashima S, Ishii K, Shinohara T. Dynamic changes in EPCAM expression during spermatogonial stem cell differentiation in the mouse testis. PLoS One. 2011;6(8):e23663.

47. Kokkinaki M, Djourabtchi A, Golestaneh N. Long-term Culture of Human SSEA-4 Positive Spermatogonial Stem Cells (SSCs). J Stem Cell Res Ther. 2011;2(2). pii: 2488.

48. Altman E, Yango P, Moustafa R, Smith JF, Klatsky PC, Tran ND. Characterization of human spermatogonial stem cell markers in fetal, pediatric, and adult testicular tissues. Reproduction. 2014;148(4):417-27.

49. Smith JF, Yango P, Altman E, Choudhry S, Poelzl A, Zamah AM, Rosen M, Klatsky PC, Tran ND. Testicular niche required for human spermatogonial stem cell expansion. Stem Cells Transl Med. 2014;3(9):1043-54.

50. Chong JJ, Murry CE. Cardiac regeneration using pluripotent stem cells--progression to large animal models. Stem Cell Res. 2014 ;13(3 Pt B):654-65.

51. Luan NT, Sharma N, Kim SW, Ha PT, Hong YH, Oh SJ, Jeong DK. Characterization and cardiac differentiation of chicken spermatogonial stem cells. Anim Reprod Sci. 2014 Dec 30;151(3-4):244-55.

52. Cai J, Yi FF, Yang XC, Lin GS, Jiang H, Wang T, Xia Z. Transplantation of embryonic stem cell-derived cardiomyocytes improves cardiac function in infarcted rat hearts. Cytotherapy. 2007;9(3):283-91.

53. Caspi O, Huber I, Kehat I, Habib M, Arbel G, Gepstein A, Yankelson L, Aronson D, Beyar R, Gepstein L.Transplantation of human embryonic stem cell-derived cardiomyocytes improves myocardial performance in infarcted rat hearts. J Am Coll Cardiol. 2007;50 (6):1884-93.

54. Chong JJ, Yang X, Don CW, Minami E, Liu YW, Weyers JJ, Mahoney WM, Van Biber B, Cook SM, Palpant NJ, Gantz JA, Fugate JA, Muskheli V, Gough GM, Vogel KW, Astley CA, Hotchkiss CE, Baldessari A, Pabon L, Reinecke H, Gill EA, Nelson V, Kiem HP, Laflamme MA, Murry CE. Human embryonic-stem-cell-derived cardiomyocytes regenerate non-human primate hearts. Nature. 2014;510(7504):273-7.

55. Ellison GM, Vicinanza C, Smith AJ, Aquila I, Leone A, Waring CD, Henning BJ, Stirparo GG, Papait R, Scarfò M, Agosti V, Viglietto G, Condorelli G, Indolfi C, Ottolenghi S, Torella D, Nadal-Ginard B. Adult c-kit(pos) cardiac stem cells are necessary and sufficient for functional cardiac regeneration and repair. Cell. 2013;154(4):827-42.

56. Lundy SD, Murphy SA, Dupras SK, Dai J, Murry CE, Laflamme MA, Regnier M.Cell-based delivery of dATP via gap junctions enhances cardiac contractility. J Mol Cell Cardiol. 2014;72:350-9.

57. Mihic A, Li J, Miyagi Y, Gagliardi M, Li SH, Zu J, Weisel RD, Keller G, Li RK. The effect of cyclic stretch on maturation and 3D tissue formation of human embryonic stem cell-derived cardiomyocytes. Biomaterials. 2014;35(9):2798-808.

58. Navaroli DM, Tilly JL, Woods DC. Isolation of Mammalian Oogonial Stem Cells by Antibody-Based Fluorescence-Activated Cell Sorting. Methods Mol Biol. 2016;1457:253-68.

59. White YA, Woods DC, Takai Y, Ishihara O, Seki H, Tilly JL. Oocyte formation by mitotically active germ cells purified from ovaries of reproductive-age women. Nat Med. 2012;18(3):413-21.

60. Anand S, Patel H, Bhartiya D. Chemoablated mouse seminiferous tubular cells enriched for very small embryonic-like stem cells undergo spontaneous spermatogenesis in vitro. Reprod Biol Endocrinol. 2015 Apr 18;13:33

61. He Z, Kokkinaki M, Jiang J, Dobrinski I, Dym M. Isolation, characterization, and culture of human spermatogonia. Biol Reprod. 2010;82(2):363-72.

62. Liu S, Bou G, Sun R, Guo S, Xue B, Wei R, Cooney AJ, Liu Z. Sox2 is the faithful marker for pluripotency in pig: evidence from embryonic studies. Dev Dyn. 2015;244(4):619-27.

63. White MD, Angiolini JF, Alvarez YD, Kaur G, Zhao ZW, Mocskos E, Bruno L, Bissiere S, Levi V, Plachta N. Long-Lived Binding of Sox2 to DNA Predicts Cell Fate in the Four-Cell Mouse Embryo. Cell. 2016;165(1):75-87.

64. Foshay KM, Gallicano GI. Regulation of Sox2 by STAT3 initiates commitment to the neural precursor cell fate. Stem Cells Dev. 2008;17(2):269-78.

65. Chen J, Chen X, Li M, Liu X, Gao Y, Kou X, Zhao Y, Zheng W, Zhang X, Huo Y, Chen C, Wu Y, Wang H, Jiang C, Gao S. Hierarchical Oct4 Binding in Concert with Primed Epigenetic Rearrangements during Somatic Cell Reprogramming. Cell Rep. 2016;14(6):1540-1554.

66. Goolam M, Scialdone A, Graham SJL, Macaulay IC, Jedrusik A, Hupalowska A, Voet T, Marioni JC, Zernicka-Goetz M. Heterogeneity in Oct4 and Sox2 Targets Biases Cell Fate in 4-Cell Mouse Embryos. Cell. 2016;165(1):61-74.

67. Shyh-Chang N, Daley GQ. Lin28: primal regulator of growth and metabolism in stem cells. Cell Stem Cell. 2013;12(4):395-406.

68. Shyh-Chang N, Zhu H, Yvanka de Soysa T, Shinoda G, Seligson MT, Tsanov KM, Nguyen L, Asara JM, Cantley LC, Daley GQ. Lin28 enhances tissue repair by reprogramming cellular metabolism. Cell. 2013;155(4):778-92.

69. Silva J, Nichols J, Theunissen TW, Guo G, van Oosten AL, Barrandon O, Wray J, Yamanaka S, Chambers I, Smith A. Nanog is the gateway to the pluripotent ground state. Cell. 2009;138(4):722-37.

70. Em S, Kataria M, Shah F, Yadav PS. A comparative study on efficiency of adult fibroblasts and amniotic fluid-derived stem cells as donor cells for production of hand-made cloned buffalo (Bubalus bubalis) embryos. Cytotechnology. 2016;68(4):593-608.

71. Fang L, Zhang J, Zhang H, Yang X, Jin X, Zhang L, Skalnik DG, Jin Y, Zhang Y, Huang X, Li J, Wong J. H3K4 Methyltransferase Set1a Is A Key Oct4 Coactivator Essential for Generation of Oct4 Positive Inner Cell Mass. Stem Cells. 2016;34(3):565-80.

72. Zhang P, Andrianakos R, Yang Y, Liu C, Lu W. Kruppel-like factor 4 (Klf4) prevents embryonic stem (ES) cell differentiation by regulating Nanog gene expression. J Biol Chem. 2010;285(12):9180-9.

73. Hirata H, Murakami Y, Miyamoto Y, Tosaka M, Inoue K, Nagahashi A, Jakt LM, Asahara T, Iwata H, Sawa Y, Kawamata S. ALCAM (CD166) is a surface marker for early murine cardiomyocytes. Cells Tissues Organs. 2006;184(3-4):172-80.

74. Kapoor N, Liang W, Marbán E, Cho HC. Direct conversion of quiescent cardiomyocytes to pacemaker cells by expression of Tbx18. Nat Biotechnol. 2013;31(1):54-62.

75. Temsah R, Nemer M. GATA factors and transcriptional regulation of cardiac natriuretic peptide genes. Regul Pept. 2005;128(3):177-85.

76. Kodama H, Inoue T, Watanabe R, Yasuoka H, Kawakami Y, Ogawa S, Ikeda Y, Mikoshiba K, Kuwana M. Cardiomyogenic potential of mesenchymal progenitors derived from human circulating CD14+ monocytes. Stem Cells Dev. 2005;14(6):676-86.

77. Saito T, Kuang JQ, Lin CC, Chiu RC. Transcoronary implantation of bone marrow stromal cells ameliorates cardiac function after myocardial infarction. J Thorac Cardiovasc Surg. 2003;126(1):114-23.

78. Bin Z, Sheng LG, Gang ZC, Hong J, Jun C, Bo Y, Hui S. Efficient cardiomyocyte differentiation of embryonic stem cells by bone morphogenetic protein-2 combined with visceral endoderm-like cells. Cell Biol Int. 2006;30(10):769-76.\

79. Krenz M, Sanbe A, Bouyer-Dalloz F, Gulick J, Klevitsky R, Hewett TE, Osinska HE, Lorenz JN, Brosseau C, Federico A, Alpert NR, Warshaw DM, Perryman MB, Helmke SM, Robbins J. Analysis of myosin heavy chain functionality in the heart. J Biol Chem. 2003;278(19):17466-74.

80. Mobley S, Shookhof JM, Foshay K, Park M, Gallicano GI. PKG and PKC Are Down-Regulated during Cardiomyocyte Differentiation from Embryonic Stem Cells: Manipulation of These Pathways Enhances Cardiomyocyte Production. Stem Cells Int. 2010;2010:701212.

81. Zhao P, Ise H, Hongo M,Ota M, Konishi I, Nikaido T.Human amniotic mesenchymal cells have some characteristics of cardiomyocytes. Transplantation. 2005;79(5):528-35.

82. Barnes RM, Harris IS, Jaehnig EJ, Sauls K, Sinha T, Rojas A, Schachterle W, McCulley DJ, Norris RA, Black BL. MEF2C regulates outflow tract alignment and transcriptional control of Tdgf1. Development. 2016;143(5):774-9.

83. Palazzolo G, Quattrocelli M, Toelen J, Dominici R, Anastasia L, Tettamenti G, Barthelemy I, Blot S, Gijsbers R, Cassano M, Sampaolesi M. Cardiac Niche Influences the Direct Reprogramming of Canine Fibroblasts into Cardiomyocyte-Like Cells. Stem Cells Int. 2016;2016:4969430.

84. Cai CL, Liang X, Shi Y, Chu PH, Pfaff SL, Chen J, Evans S. Isl1 identifies a cardiac progenitor population that proliferates prior to differentiation and contributes a majority of cells to the heart. Dev Cell. 2003;5(6):877-89.

85. Baraniak PR, McDevitt TC. Stem cell paracrine actions and tissue regeneration.Regen Med. 2010;5(1):121-43.

86. Lui KO, Zangi L, Chien KR. Cardiovascular regenerative therapeutics via synthetic paracrine factor modified mRNA. Stem Cell Res. 2014;13(3 PtB):693-704.

Abbreviations

GPR125	G protein coupled receptor 125
GFR1α	GDNF family receptor 1 alpha
SSEA-4	Stage-specific antibody-4
SOX2	SRY (Sex Determining Region Y)- Box 2
OCT3/4	Octamer-Binding Transcription Factor ¾
LIN 28A	LIN28 Homolog A
KLF-4	Kruppel-like factor 4s
CD73	Cluster of differentiation 73
ALCAM	Activated Leukocyte Cell Adhesion Molecule
CHAMP	Cardiac Helicase Activated MEF2C protein
TBX18	T-Box Transcription Factor 18
ANP	Atrial Natriuretic Peptide
NKX2.5	NK2 homeobox 5
CTNI	Cardiac Troponin I
CTNT	Cardiac Troponin T
MHC	Myosin heavy chain
MLC2A	Myosin light chain 2A
MLC2V	Myosin light chain 2V
ISL-1	Myocyte Enhancer Factor 2C
VEGFA	Vascular Endothelial
IGF-1	Insulin-like growth factor
SDF-1	Stromal derived factor-1
CTGF	Connective tiddue growth factor
END-1	Endothelin-1
AAMP	Angio-associated migratory protein
NRG-1	Neuregulin-1
IDO	Indoleamine 2,3-dioxygenase
AFP	Alpha Fetal Protein
BMP4	Bone Morphogenic protein
NES	Nestin

Potential Conflicts of Interests

None

Acknowledgments

We would like to acknowledge Vaughn E. Gallicano for repeating key I.P. experiments. VEG is in the 8th grade at Mark Twain Middle school. His interest in this project partially fulfilled Fairfax County School District mandatory volunteer requirements.

Support/ Grants

Sponsored in part by The Appleby Foundation and the Partners in Research, Georgetown University Medical Center

Corresponding Author

G. Ian Gallicano, Department of Biochemistry and Molecular & Cellular Biology, Georgetown University Medical Center, 3900 Reservoir Rd. NW, Room NE203, Washington, DC 20007, Email: gig@georgetown.edu

18

Proliferation, migration and differentiation potential of human mesenchymal progenitor cells derived from osteoarthritic subchondral cancellous bone

Krüger JP[1#], Enz A[2#], Hondke S[1], Wichelhaus A[2], Endres M[1], Mittlmeier T[2]

Abstract

Background: For regenerative therapies in the orthopedic field, one prerequisite for therapeutic success in the treatment of cartilage defects is the potential of body's own cells to migrate, proliferate and differentiate into functional cells. While this has been demonstrated for mesenchymal stem and progenitor cells (MPC) from healthy tissue sources, the potential of cells from degenerative conditions is unclear. In this study the regenerative potential of MPC derived from subchondral cancellous bone with diagnosed osteoarthritis is evaluated *in vitro*.
Methods: OaMPC isolated from bone chips of three individual patients with Kellgren grade 3 osteoarthritis were characterized by analysis of cell surface antigen pattern. Cell proliferation was evaluated by doubling time and population doubling rate. Cell migration was assessed using a multi-well migration assay. Multi-lineage potential was evaluated by histological staining of adipogenic, osteogenic and chondrogenic markers. In addition, chondrogenic differentiation was verified by qPCR.
Results: OaMPC showed a stable proliferation and a typical surface antigen pattern known from mesenchymal stem cells. Cell migration of oaMPC can be induced by human blood serum. OaMPC were capable of adipogenic, osteogenic and chondrogenic differentiation comparable to MPC derived from healthy conditions.
Conclusion: OaMPC derived from knee joints affected by osteoarthritic conditions showed regeneration potential regarding migration, proliferation and chondrogenic differentiation. This suggests that oaMPC are able to contribute to cartilage repair tissue formation.

Key Words: Osteoarthritis, Stem cells, Cartilage, Migration, Differentiation

Introduction

To date, the self-healing capacity of the human body is one of the most important sources for regenerative medicine. The aim is to rehabilitate malfunctioned cells and to regenerate parts of tissues or organs. A new generation of cell-free scaffolds, aiming at focal traumatic cartilage defects, should support the body's self-renewal. Articular cartilage is frequently damaged as a result of trauma and degenerative joint diseases. Different cartilage regeneration strategies and techniques are used in today's clinical practice. Simple and often used techniques are the abrasion technique and the microfracture technique where mesenchymal stem and progenitor cells are used for regeneration approaches. Other regenerative strategies are the osteochondral transfer and the autologous chondrocyte implantation[1]. One concept among others is based on the well-known microfracture technique combined with an implant composed of e.g., resorbable polyglycolic acid combined with hyaluronan and a blood derivate[2] to cover the cartilage defect. A possible source of self-renewal results from migrated progenitor cells since these cells are able to differentiate and synthesize a cartilage repair tissue[3]. The microfracture technique enables the influx of mesenchymal stem and progenitor cells into the cartilage defect[4]. Especially the migration, proliferation and differentiation potential of these cells are necessary for cartilage regeneration[3,5,6] as the progenitor cells are attracted to the right place and support repair tissue formation. But, several pathological conditions such as rheumatoid arthritis or osteoarthritis (OA) may affect these cells. In a healthy joint the synovia covers the joint cavity and regulates the transport of nutrients and other molecules between the joint cavity and the adjacent tissue[7]. In joints affected by OA, the synovial membrane becomes hyperplastic due to the proliferation of genuine synovial cells such as synovial fibroblasts resulting in a massive infiltration of inflammatory cells[8]. Today, OA is attributed to diseases of articular cartilage. The current concept of OA involves the entire joint organ, including the articular cartilage, subchondral bones, ligaments, joint capsule, menisci and synovial membrane[9]. OA has always been classified as a non-inflammatory arthritis. However, increasing evidence has shown that inflammation occurs as cytokines and matrix metalloproteinases are released into the joint. This leads to the imbalance between inflammatory mediators and proteinase inhibitors compared to healthy individuals[10]. It is obvious that cartilage degradation and inflammatory surrounding of OA create a completely different environment, e.g., compared to traumatic defects. But, chondrogenesis of osteoarthritic chondrocytes proved that the chondrogenic capacity *in vitro* is not significantly affected by OA[11]. Furthermore, it was shown that synovial fluid from donors with OA does not have a negative influence on chondrogenesis[1,12] and stimulates cell migration[13] of mesenchymal progenitor cells (MPC).

Author Names in full: Jan Philipp Krüger[1#], Andreas Enz[2#], Sylvia Hondke[1], Alice Wichelhaus[2], Michaela Endres[1], Thomas Mittlmeier[2]

[1]TransTissue Technologies GmbH, 10117 Berlin, Germany, [2]Department of Trauma, Hand and Reconstructive Surgery, Universitätsmedizin Rostock, 18057 Rostock, Germany

# Authors contributed equally to the work

The regeneration potential of MPC from an osteoarthritic environment is still unknown. Therefore, the aim of this study was to characterize the proliferation, migration and differentiation potential of MPC derived from osteoarthritic subchondral cancellous bone, in order to prove if oaMPC are a suitable cell source for autologous matrix-induced chondrogenesis (aMIC).

Method

Isolation of osteoarthritic mesenchymal progenitor cells derived from osteoarthritic cortico-cancellous bone

Mesenchymal progenitor cells (oaMPC) were isolated from bone chips from knee joints of three individual OA patients (Table 1) with Kellgren-Lawrence grade 3 (Figure 1). In brief, the chips were cut in small fragments and washed with Hank´s saline solution (Merck, Germany). Bone fragments were digested for 4 hours with 7,680U collagenase XI (Sigma-Aldrich, USA). Afterwards, the fragments were transferred into culture flasks (Primaria, Becton & Dickinson, USA) and cultured with DMEM (Dulbecco's Modified Eagle Medium) containing 10% human serum (German Red Cross, Germany), 100U/ml penicillin, 100μg/ml streptomycin, 200nM L-glutamine, 100μg/ml gentamycin, 0.1μg/ml amphotericin (all Biochrom) and 2ng/ml FGF-2 (Peprotech, Germany) at 37°C and 5% CO_2. The medium was changed every 2-3 days. After the cells reached 80-90% confluence they were detached with trypsin-EDTA/PBS (1:1 v/v) (Merck) and seeded with a cell density of 8,000 cells/cm². The study was approved by the ethics committee of the Bavarian State Chamber of Medicine (#12045).

Migration Assay of oaMPC

To characterize the migration potential of oaMPC (n=3 donors), a 96 multi-well migration assay (Neuro Probe, USA) was used. In brief, human serum in concentrations of 5% and 10% diluted with DMEM containing 0.1% human serum (German Red Cross), 100U penicillin and 100μg/ml streptomycin (Merck) was added into the lower wells of the multi-well plate and covered with a polycarbonate membrane (pore size of 8μm). DMEM containing 0.1% human serum served as control. In the upper compartment of each well 30,000 oaMPC in DMEM containing 0.1% human serum was given. The assay was performed in triplicates. The assay was incubated at 37°C and 5% CO_2 for 20 hours. Afterwards, the membrane was fixed with methanol/acetone (1:1 v/v) for 5 minutes. Remaining oaMPC on top of the membrane were carefully wiped off and cells underneath the membrane were visualized using a Hemacolor staining kit (Merck-Millipore, Germany). Migrated cells were enumerated microscopically by counting the number of stained cells in four representative fields using ImageJ software (National Institutes of Health, USA) and extrapolated to the complete well area.

Growths kinetics of oaMPC

To determine the growth kinetic of oaMPC, cells of each individual patient (n=3) were seeded in T25 culture flasks with a density of

10,000 cells/cm² and cultivated for four days with DMEM containing 10% human serum, 100U/ml penicillin, 100μg/ml streptomycin, 200nM L-glutamine, 100μg/ml gentamycin, 0.1μg/ml amphotericin and 2ng/ml FGF-2 at 37°C and 5% CO_2. After four days of cultivation, vital cells were detached and counted with trypan blue and seeded again with the same cell density of 10,000 cells/cm². All in all, cells were cultivated from passage 1 to 7. For each passage the proliferation factor was determined and the cell doubling time (t_d) and the population doubling rate (n) were calculated as follows.

$$t_d = \frac{\ln 2}{specific\ growth\ rate\ (\mu)}$$

$$n = \frac{\log \frac{initial\ cell\ number}{terminal\ cell\ number}}{\log 2}$$

Flow cytometric analysis of oaMPC

OaMPC (250,000 cells, passage 3) of 3 donors were washed with PBS/0.5% BSA and incubated with mouse anti-human conjugated antibody fluorescent CD14-phycoerythrin (PE), CD34-PE, CD44-fluorescein isothiocyanate (FITC), CD45-FITC, CD73-PE, CD90-FITC, CD105-FITC or CD166-PE (All Becton & Dickinson, USA)

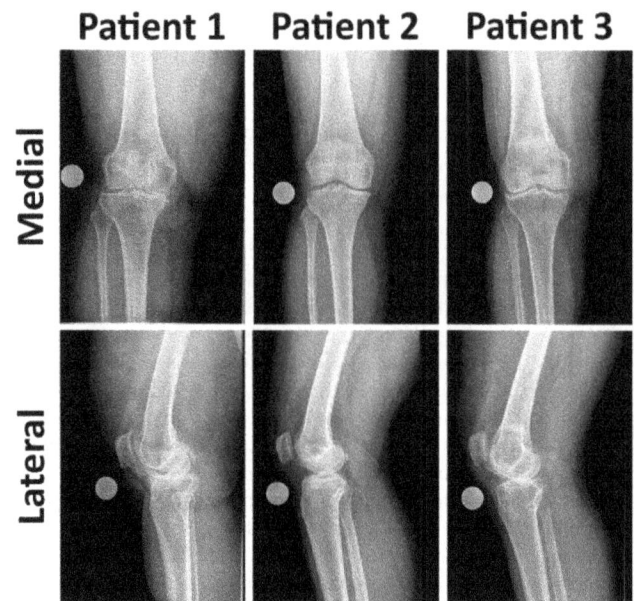

Figure 1: *Medial and lateral x-ray images of the right knee form all three patients included in this study (all Kellgren and Lawrence score of 3).*

Table 1: Patient characterization

	Patient 1	Patient 2	Patient 3
Age	61 years	50 years	60 years
Gender	female	female	female
Medical history	Primary gonarthrosis right knee	Primary gonarthrosis right knee	Primary gonarthrosis right knee
Synovia	Hypertrophic	Hypertrophic	Hypertrophic
Knee replacement	Total endoprosthesis of the knee joint	Total endoprosthesis of the knee joint	Total endoprosthesis of the knee joint
Kellgren-Lawrence score	**3**	**3**	**3**

For 15 minutes on ice. After incubation oaMPC were washed by adding 1ml buffer (PBS with 0.5% BSA), centrifuged at 400x*g* for 10 minutes at 4°C and resuspended in 500µL buffer. The analyses were performed using FACS Calibur (Becton & Dickinson). Dead cells were excluded from analyses using propidium iodide (PI) and CD34 stained cells were used as isotype control.

Differentiation of oaMPC along adipogenic, osteogenic and chondrogenic lineage

To show multi-lineage differentiation potential of oaMPC, cells of 3 individual patients were differentiated into adipogenic, osteogenic and chondrogenic lineage.

For adipogenic and osteogenic differentiation oaMPC (passage 3) were plated with a density of 10,000 cells/well in 6-well cell culture plates (Becton & Dickinson). To induce adipogenic differentiation oaMPC were stimulated with DMEM (Merck) containing 10% human serum (German Red Cross), 100U/ml penicillin and 100µg/ml streptomycin (all Merck), 1µM dexamethasone, 0.2mM indomethacin, 0.5mM 3-isobutyl-1-methyl-xanthine (IBMX) (all Sigma-Aldrich) and 0.01mg/ml insulin (Novo Nordisk, Denmark) for 21 days. In this process, oaMPC were stimulated for 3 days alternating with a non-stimulated period of 2 days. Non-stimulated controls were cultured without dexamethasone, indomethacin, IBMX and insulin.

For osteogenic differentiation, confluent oaMPC cultures were stimulated with DMEM containing 10% human serum, 100U/ml penicillin, 100µg/ml streptomycin, 0.01µM dexamethasone, 0.05mM ascorbic acid-2-phosphate (Sigma-Aldrich) and 10mM β-glycerolphosphate (Sigma-Aldrich) for 28 days. Non-stimulated controls were cultured without dexamethasone, ascorbic acid-2-phosphate and β-glycerolphosphate.

For chondrogenic differentiation high-density pellet cultures (250,000 oaMPC per pellet) were formed by centrifugation at 130x*g* for 10 minutes. Chondrogenesis was induced by adding 10ng/ml transforming growth factor-beta3 (TGFB3) (Peprotech) to DMEM (high glucose) containing 100U/ml of penicillin and 100µg/ml streptomycin (all Merck), 1% (v/v) insulin-transferrin-sodium selenite (ITS+1), 0.1µM dexamethasone, 1mM sodium pyruvate, 0.17mM ascorbic acid-2-phosphate, 0.35mM L-proline (all Sigma-Aldrich). Non-stimulated controls were cultured without TGFB3. The pellets were cultivated for 21 days and the medium was changed every 2-3 days.

Histological and immunohistochemical staining of oaMPC

Intracellular lipid vacuoles in adipogenic cultures were visualized using Oil Red O staining (Sigma-Aldrich). Osteogenic differentiation was detected by staining of mineralized matrix components according to von Kossa. For detection of extracellular matrix deposition indicating chondrogenic differentiation, cryosections (6µm; n=3 cell pellets, n=3 sections per cell pellet for n=3 donor) were prepared and proteoglycan synthesis was visualized by alcian blue and safranin O staining. Collagen type II formation was visualized by incubation with rabbit anti-human type II collagen antibody (Acris, Germany) for 40 min. Colorimetrical detection was performed using 3-amino-9-ethylcarbazole (EnVision++; Dako, Denmark) following a counterstaining with hematoxylin (Merck-Millipore).

Quantitative histomorphometric analysis was performed using the Adobe Photoshop Software CS6 as described[14]. In brief, a standard color was defined that represents the particular color of the specific staining. The tools "magic wand" and "select similar" were used to select areas of that particular color. The amount of stained pixels in relation to the total amount of pixels of the section gave the percentage of the positively stained area for proteoglycans or collagen type II, respectively.

Gene expression analysis of oaMPC

To evaluate the gene expression of typical chondrogenic marker genes, total RNA from 20 oaMPC pellet cultures per group was isolated at day 21 as described previously[15]. Subsequently, 3µg of total RNA was reversely transcribed with the iScript cDNA Synthesis Kit according to the manufacturer's instructions (BioRad, Germany). The relative expression level of the housekeeping gene glyceraldehyde-3-phosphate dehydrogenase (GAPDH) was used to normalize the samples. Real-time RT-PCR using i-Cycler PCR System (BioRad) was performed with 1µL of each cDNA sample in triplicates using the SYBR green PCR Core Kit (Applied Biosystems, USA). Relative quantification of gene expression was performed and is given as percentage of the GAPDH product.

Statistical analysis

Statistical analysis was performed using SigmaStat 3.5 (Systat Software GmbH, Germany). The Anderson-Darling test was used to determine normal distribution of data. Subsequently, one way analysis of variance with the *post hoc* analysis according to the Student-Newman-Keuls-Test was used. P-values less than 0.05 were considered statistically significant.

Results

Growths kinetics of oaMPC

OaMPC of 3 donors were expanded up to passage 7. Absolute cell counts from passage 1 to 7 were normalized to oaMPC growth of 250,000 initially seeded cells to calculate the cell doubling time (t_d) and the population doubling rate (n). The cell doubling time ranged from 3.67 to 3.99 days, and the population doubling rate was 8.09 ± 0.57.

Migration potential of oaMPC

The migration assay was performed to determine the migration potential of oaMPC stimulated with human serum (HS). In the presence of 0.1% HS 2,100 up to 2,500 oaMPC migrated through the pores of the membrane (Figure 2). Stimulation of oaMPC with 5% HS resulted in a migration of 7,500 up to 10,300 cells and 10% HS stimulated the migration of 6,300 up to 10,400 cells (Figure 2). Compared to oaMPC stimulated with 0.1% HS, the number of migrated cells was significantly increased (*p≤0.0004) by stimulation with 5% and 10% HS for all 3 donors (Figure 2).

Cell surface antigen pattern of oaMPC

The immuno-phenotype of oaMPC of 3 patients was determined by flowcytometrical analyses (Figure 3). All oaMPC (n=3), which were derived from osteoarthritic cancellous bone chips, were homogenously positive for CD44 (mean 99.96% ± 0.0003%), CD73 (mean 99.88% ± 0.0006%), CD90 (mean 99.52% ± 0.006%), CD105 (mean 90.35% ± 0.04%) and CD166 (mean 99.29% ± 0.004%). Additionally, oaMPC did not present CD14 (mean 0.02% ± 0.0002%), CD34 (mean 0.01% ± 0.0001%) and CD45 (mean 0.23% ± 0.004%) (Table 2).

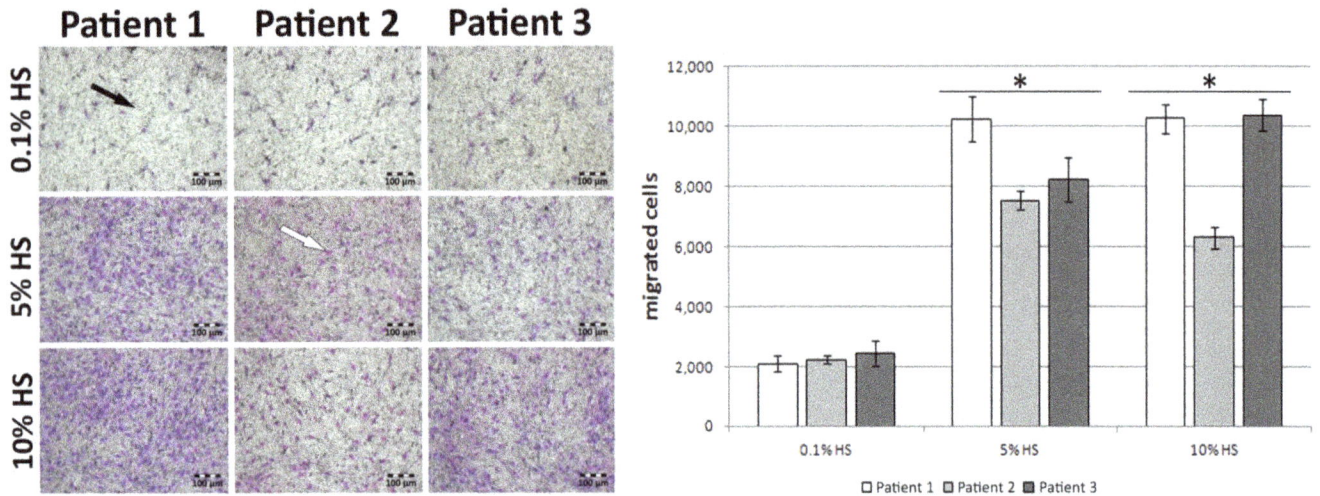

Figure 2: Medium with 5% or 10% human serum (HS) significantly (*p≤0.0004) stimulated the migration of osteoarthritic mesenchymal progenitor cells (black arrow indicates a membrane pore and white arrow indicates a migrated cell) compared to 0.1% HS. The bars show the mean (n=3 triplicates) and the 95% CI.

Table 2: Flowcytometric analysis of oaMPC

	CD14	CD34	CD44	CD45	CD73	CD90	CD105	CD166
Patient 1	0.01%	0.01%	99.98%	0.01%	99.90%	98.83%	88.29%	98.83%
Patient 2	0.01%	0.01%	99.93%	0.01%	99.81%	99.97%	87.63%	99.71%
Patient 3	0.05%	0.00%	99.99%	0.66%	99.93%	99.77%	95.14%	99.35%

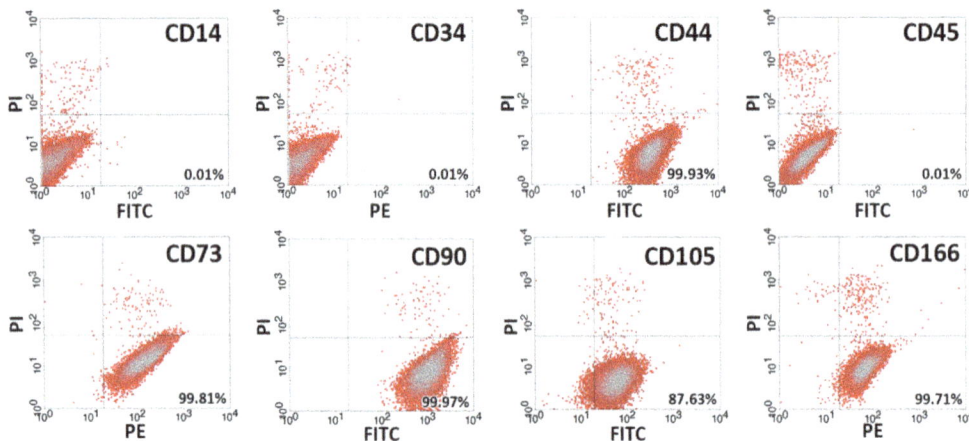

Figure 3: Flowcytometrical analyses of cell surface antigen pattern for one representative patient.

Differentiation potential of oaMPC

The potential of oaMPC to undergo adipogenic and osteogenic differentiation was documented by the visualization of lipid vesicles by Oil Red O staining and of matrix mineralization by von Kossa staining. At day 21, Oil Red O staining showed that lipid-filled vesicles were presented in oaMPC stimulated with adipogenic supplements. In non-induced oaMPC no lipid vesicles were detectable (Figure 4). At day 28, von Kossa staining showed a brown stained matrix in oaMPC stimulated with osteogenic supplements with only slight staining in the non-induced controls (Figure 4).

After 28 days of culture in high-density pellets, oaMPC showed a chondrogenic differentiation upon stimulation with TGFB3, while no signs of chondrogenesis were observed in non-induced controls (Figure 5). Proteoglycans as assessed by alcian blue staining were evident in pellets stimulated with TGFB3 and weakly in non-induced oaMPC pellets. Safranin O stained sulfated proteoglycans were detectable in oaMPC pellets induced with TGFB3, while non-induced samples were negative. Collagen type II was found in pellets cultured

with TGFB3 but not in non-induced oaMPC pellets.

Histomorphometric quantification (n=9; 3 sections per patient) (Figure 5) showed a significant (*p<0.0003) increase of proteoglycans visualized by alcian blue staining in oaMPC pellet cultures induced with TGFB3 from day 7 (mean 42.1% ± 12.1%) to day 21 (mean 74.3% ± 10.2%). The non-induced oaMPC pellet cultures showed an increasing concentration of proteoglycans (but not significant) from day 7 (mean 10.5% ± 5.1%) to day 21 (mean 31.0% ± 13.0%). Quantification of sulfated proteoglycans (safranin O staining) showed a significant (*p<0.0002) increase of proteoglycan-rich areas in pellets stimulated with TGFB3 from day 7 (mean 11.7% ± 4.2%) to day 21 (mean 77.4% ± 4.9%). In contrast, non-induced oaMPC pellet cultures showed almost no proteoglycan-rich areas at day 7, day 14 and day 21 (mean 0.01% to 0.1%). Collagen type II was present and significantly (p*<0.0002) increased in oaMPC pellet cultures induced with TGFB3 from day 14 (mean 46.8% ± 8.2%) to day 21 (mean 59.9% ± 6.3%) compared to non-induced oaMPC pellet cultures from day 14 (mean 1.9% ± 1.1%) to day 21 (mean 2.7% ± 1.1%).

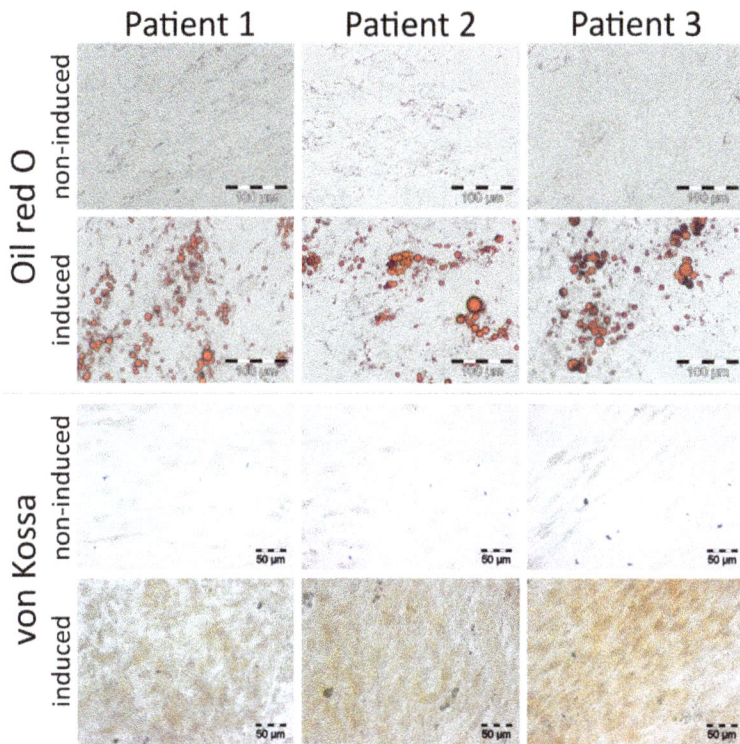

Figure 4: Oil Red O staining showed the presence of lipid vacuoles in adipogenic induced osteoarthritic mesenchymal progenitor cells (oaMPC) at day 21. Von Kossa staining of matrix mineralization showed a brown stained matrix in osteogenic induced oaMPC at day 28.

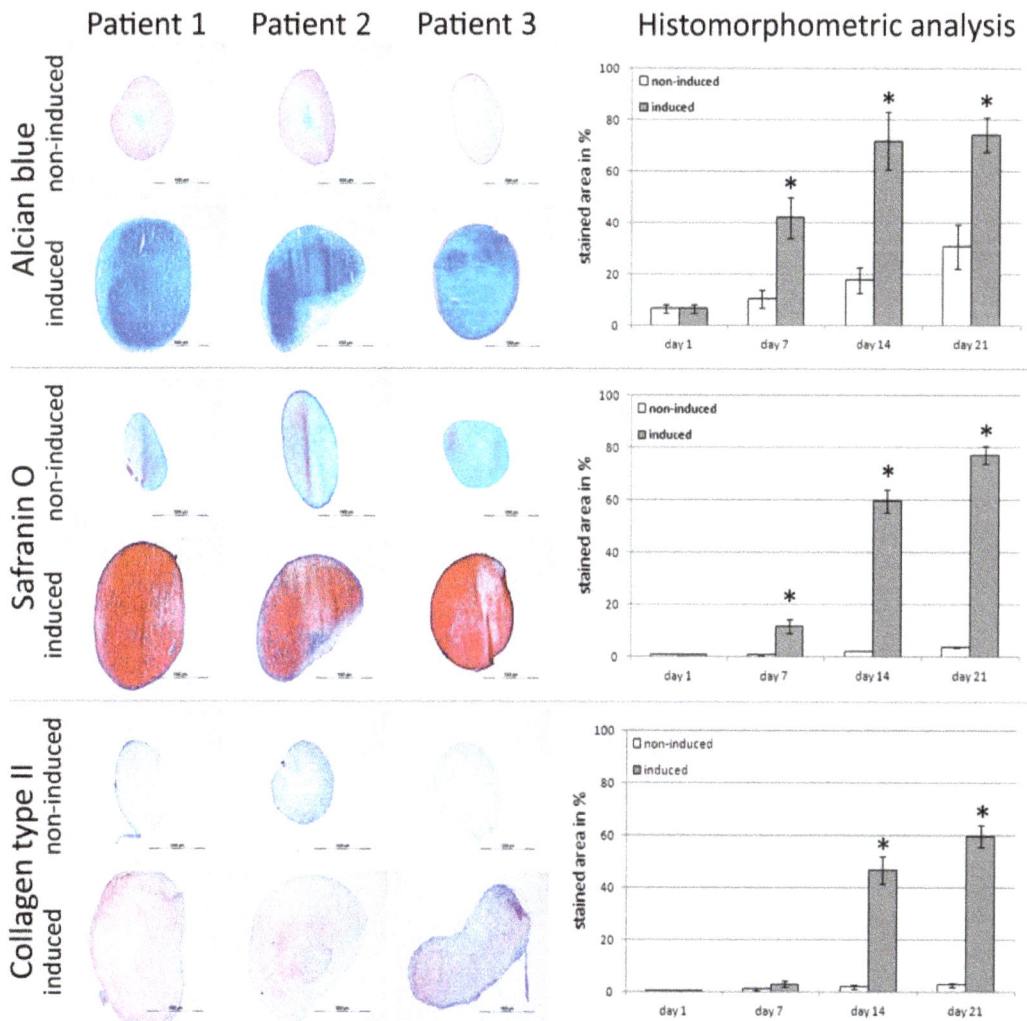

Figure 5: Osteoarthritic mesenchymal progenitor cells (oaMPC) induced with TGFB3 showed a significant (*p<0.0003) increased formation of proteoglycans and collagen type II after 21 days compared to non-induced oaMPC. The bars show the mean (n=9; 3 sections/pellet/donor) and the 95% CI.

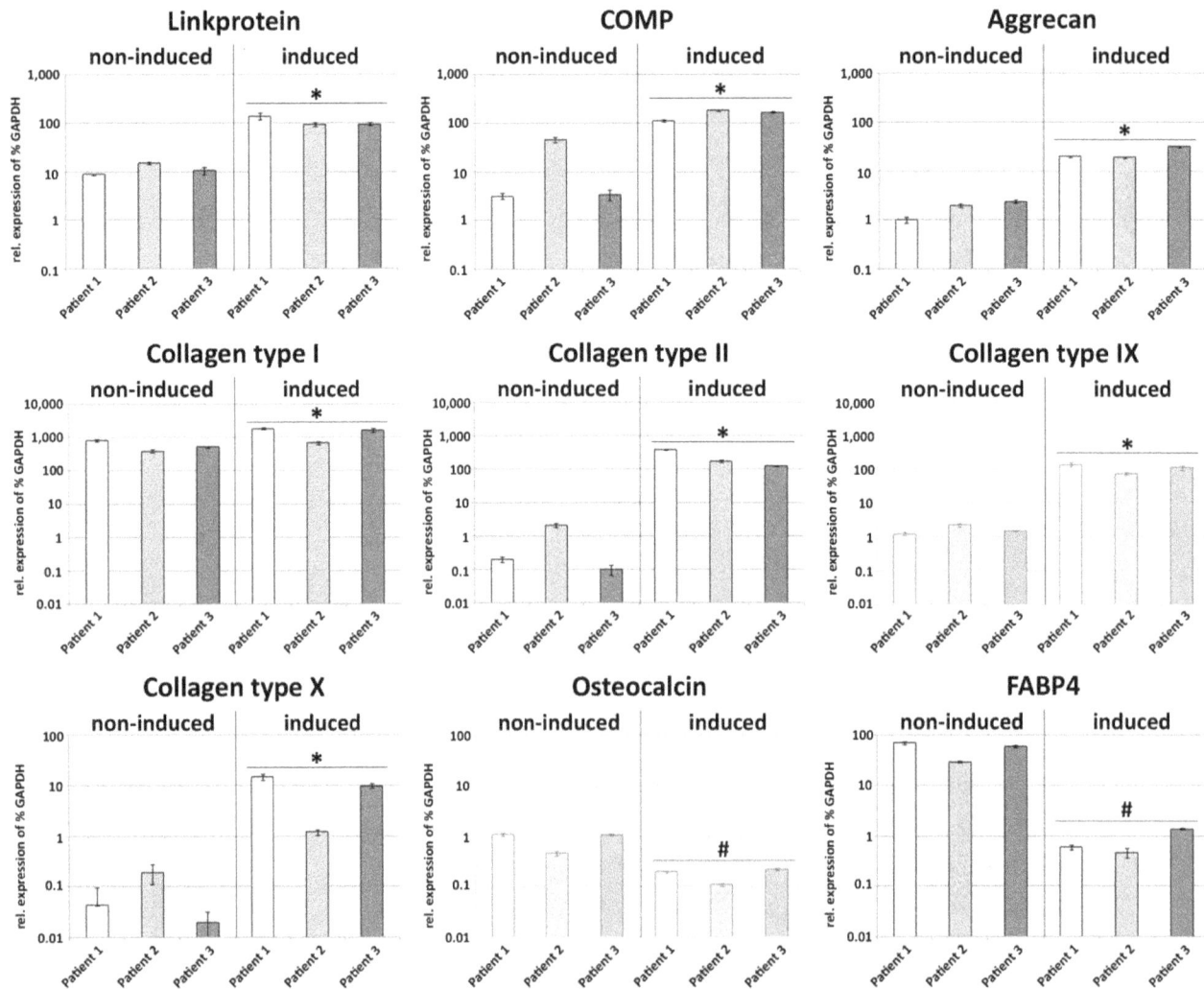

Figure 6: *Chondrogenic development of osteoarthritic mesenchymal progenitor cells (oaMPC) was analyzed by gene expression analysis of typical chondrogenic marker genes. The bars show the mean (n=3 triplicates) and the 95% CI. Significantly (p<0.0012) *induced or #decreased gene expression compared to non-induced oaMPC. COMP - cartilage oligomeric matrix protein, FABP4 - fatty acid binding protein-4*

Gene expression analysis of oaMPC

To confirm chondrogenic differentiation of oaMPC (n=3), semi-quantitative gene expression of typical cartilage marker were analyzed at day 21 (Figure 6). Treatment of oaMPC pellet cultures with TGFB3 significantly (*p<0.0012) induced the expression of the chondrogenic marker genes link-protein (mean 100 times), cartilage oligomeric matrix protein (COMP, mean 10 times), aggrecan (mean 13 times), collagen type II (mean 230 times) and collagen type IX (mean 50 times), compared to non-induced oaMPC pellet cultures. Collagen type I, a gene which is more associated with fibrous tissue development showed an induction (mean 3 times). To evaluate osteogenic or adipogenic differentiation of oaMPC pellet cultures, gene expression analyses of selected osteogenic and adipogenic markers were performed at day 21. Pellet cultures of oaMPC induced with TGFB3 showed a significant (*p<0.0002) increase of collagen type X (mean 85 times). In contrast, the gene expression level of osteocalcin was significantly decreased (#p<0.0003) in oaMPC cultures treated with TGFB3 (mean 5 times) compared to non-induced cultures. At day 21, oaMPC cultures induced with TGFB3 showed a significant (#p<0.0001) decrease in expression level of fatty acid binding protein-4 (FABP4, mean 65 times) compared to non-induced pellet cultures.

Discussion

In our study, we demonstrated that human osteoarthritic mesenchymal progenitor cells (oaMPC) have the ability to migrate, proliferate and differentiate along the adipogenic, osteogenic and chondrogenic lineage. OaMPC did not lose their migration potential *in vitro* in response to the osteoarthritic disorder. These findings are in line with previous experiments with mesenchymal stem and progenitor cells from healthy donors[5]. Additionally, the growth kinetics for oaMPC showed a stable proliferation and there were no differences between the respective population doubling times and population doubling rates of the three patients. In contrast, the population doubling rate of MPC without an inflammatory environment is twofold higher[16]. But, a reduced proliferation capacity is described for chondrocytes as well as for mesenchymal stem and progenitor cells from patients with osteoarthritis[17,18]. It is conceivable that the reduced proliferation capacity of oaMPC is a consequence of the osteoarthritic disorder. For verification of the progenitor cell character, oaMPC were analyzed by flowcytometrical analyses of typical surface antigen known from MPC. A change of phenotype or a less presentation of surface antigens is not mentionable in comparison to healthy MPC[1,16]. Furthermore, oaMPC were differentiated along the adipogenic, osteogenic and chondrogenic lineage. A previous study suggested a reduced adipogenic differentiation potential for osteoarthritic mesenchymal stem and progenitor cells from patients who received a total hip or total knee replacement[18], which could not be confirmed by our results. Osteogenic induced oaMPC showed a less calcified matrix by von Kossa staining, but it is not possible to conclude that the osteoarthritic disorder is responsible for the insufficient mineralization of the extracellular matrix. Other differentiation studies with MPC demonstrated various results showing insufficient mineralization of the formed matrix after 28 days of cultivation[3] as well as a highly calcified matrix after 18 days of cultivation[1]. Therefore, it is not clear if the insufficiently calcified matrix is a result of the influence of the degenerative disease or a normal appearance during osteogenesis of MPC/oaMPC. Sections of chondrogenic induced high-density oaMPC pellet cultures demonstrated a proteoglycan-rich extracellular matrix. In contrast to the uniformly stained TGFB3 induced oaMPC pellets, the non-induced controls showed marginal proteoglycan-rich matrix, which indicates a TGFB3-mediated chondrogenesis. Nevertheless, in non-induced controls marginal deposition of proteoglycans is evident that can be explained by the influence of the 3D arrangement[19] which is also known to induce or at least support chondrogenesis. The results on protein level are in line with the results obtained by gene expression analysis of typical chondrogenic marker genes. There are no notable differences of protein or gene expression results compared to MPC[3]. However, a significant increase of collagen type I expression by oaMPC compared to MPC without an inflammatory environment could be noticed[3]. That may lead to the assumption that the chondrogenic induced oaMPC pellet cultures form fibrocartilaginous tissue or a hybrid of hyaline and fibrous cartilage depending on the co-presence of collagen type II[19,20]. However, our current study has some limitations. This *in vitro* study does not reflect the *in vivo* situation and cannot predict effects or activities of an inflammatory environment *in vivo*. Due to limited donor tissue availability, we included only female tissue donors of the same age group in this study. However, it is described that two times more females are affected by gonarthrosis than men[21]. Possible gender specific differences in the chondrogenic regeneration potential have to be analyzed in clinical studies and cannot be predicted from our results. Taking into account that the *in vivo* environment of cartilage in osteoarthritis (OA) is affected by several pathological conditions such as a hyperplastic synovial membrane and a massive infiltration of inflammatory cells, the clinical outcome of regenerative approaches (e.g., autologous matrix induced chondrogenesis (aMIC)) is not predictable. Under normal conditions the cartilage matrix is subjected to a dynamic remodeling process in which low levels of degradative and synthesizing enzyme activities are balanced, so that natural turnover of cartilage is maintained[22]. In advanced OA, cartilage matrix degrading enzymes are overexpressed shifting the balance to an increased degradation that might result in the loss of collagen and proteoglycans from the cartilage matrix[1]. First case series showed good results in patients suffering from beginning articular degeneration and early degenerative cartilage defects one and five years after microfracture and aMIC procedure using a resorbable polyglycolic acid (PGA) implant[23,24]. From our results we suggest that oaMPC have the potential to undergo chondrogenic differentiation and might be useful as autologous source for regenerative therapies, but the etiology of inflammatory environment or abnormal mechanics need to be eliminated before[25]. Nevertheless, clinical studies need to be undertaken to show whether oaMPC are able to develop sufficient repair tissue for cartilage defect treatment.

In conclusion, it is possible to say that MPC from patients with osteoarthritis present a comparable phenotypic antigen pattern and the potential of migration, proliferation, and multi-lineage differentiation along chondrogenesis, adipogenesis and osteogenesis to MPC from healthy patients.

References

1. Krüger JP, Endres M, Neumann K, Stuhlmuller B, Morawietz L, Haupl T, Kaps C. Chondrogenic differentiation of human subchondral progenitor cells is affected by synovial fluid from donors with osteoarthritis or rheumatoid arthritis. J Orthop Surg Res. 2012;7:10.

2. Erggelet C, Neumann K, Endres M, Haberstroh K, Sittinger M, Kaps C. Regeneration of ovine articular cartilage defects by cell-free polymer-based implants. Biomaterials. 2007;28(36):5570-5580.

3. Neumann K, Dehne T, Endres M, Erggelet C, Kaps C, Ringe J, Sittinger M. Chondrogenic differentiation capacity of human mesenchymal progenitor cells derived from subchondral cortico-spongious bone. J Orthop Res. 2008;26(11):1449-1456.

4. Steadman JR, Briggs KK, Rodrigo JJ, Kocher MS, Gill TJ, Rodkey WG. Outcomes of microfracture for traumatic chondral defects of the knee: average 11-year follow-up. Arthroscopy. 2003;19(5):477-484.

5. Kruger JP, Hondke S, Endres M, Pruss A, Siclari A, Kaps C. Human platelet-rich plasma stimulates migration and chondrogenic differentiation of human subchondral progenitor cells. J Orthop Res. 2012;30(6):845-852.

6. Kreuz PC, Kruger JP, Metzlaff S, Freymann U, Endres M, Pruss A, Petersen W, Kaps C. Platelet-Rich Plasma Preparation Types Show Impact on Chondrogenic Differentiation, Migration, and Proliferation of Human Subchondral Mesenchymal Progenitor Cells. Arthroscopy. 2015 ;31(10):1951-1961.

7. Schmid FR, Ogata RI. The composition and examination of synovial fluid. J Prosthet Dent. 1967;18(5):449-457.

8. Kraan MC, Versendaal H, Jonker M, Bresnihan B, Post WJ, t Hart BA, Breedveld FC, Tak PP. Asymptomatic synovitis precedes clinically manifest arthritis. Arthritis Rheum. 1998;41(8):1481-1488.

9. Braun HJ, Gold GE. Diagnosis of osteoarthritis: imaging. Bone. 2012;51(2):278-288.

10. Murphy G, Knäuper V, Atkinson S, Butler G, English W, Hutton M, Stracke J, Clark I. Matrix metalloproteinases in arthritic disease. Arthritis Res. 2002;4 Suppl 3:S39-49.

11. Dehne T, Karlsson C, Ringe J, Sittinger M, Lindahl A. Chondrogenic differentiation potential of osteoarthritic chondrocytes and their possible use in matrix-associated autologous chondrocyte transplantation. Arthritis Res Ther. 2009;11(5):R133.

12. Krüger JP, Endres M, Neumann K, Haupl T, Erggelet C, Kaps C. Chondrogenic differentiation of human subchondral progenitor cells is impaired by rheumatoid arthritis synovial fluid. J Orthop Res. 2010;28(6):819-827.

13. Endres M, Neumann K, Haupl T, Erggelet C, Ringe J, Sittinger M, Kaps C. Synovial fluid recruits human mesenchymal progenitors from subchondral spongious bone marrow. J Orthop Res. 2007;25(10):1299-1307.

14. Kruger JP, Machens I, Lahner M, Endres M, Kaps C. Initial boost release of transforming growth factor-beta3 and chondrogenesis by freeze-dried bioactive polymer scaffolds. Ann Biomed Eng. 2014 ;42(12):2562-2576.

15. Chomczynski P. A reagent for the single-step simultaneous isolation of RNA, DNA and proteins from cell and tissue samples. Biotechniques. 1993;15(3):532-534, 536-537.

16. Tuli R, Tuli S, Nandi S, Wang ML, Alexander PG, Haleem-Smith H, Hozack WJ, Manner PA, Danielson KG, Tuan RS. Characterization of multipotential mesenchymal progenitor cells derived from human trabecular bone. Stem Cells. 2003;21(6):681-693.

17. Aigner T, Kurz B, Fukui N, Sandell L. Roles of chondrocytes in the pathogenesis of osteoarthritis. Curr Opin Rheumatol. 2002;14(5):578-584.

18. Murphy JM, Dixon K, Beck S, Fabian D, Feldman A, Barry F. Reduced chondrogenic and adipogenic activity of mesenchymal stem cells from patients with advanced osteoarthritis. Arthritis Rheum. 2002;46(3):704-713.

19. Richter W. Mesenchymal stem cells and cartilage in situ regeneration. J Intern Med. 2009;266(4):390-405.

20. Kaul G, Cucchiarini M, Remberger K, Kohn D, Madry H. Failed cartilage repair for early osteoarthritis defects: a biochemical, histological and immunohistochemical analysis of the repair tissue

after treatment with marrow-stimulation techniques. Knee Surg Sports Traumatol Arthrosc. 2012;20(11):2315-2324.

21. Glyn-Jones S, Palmer AJ, Agricola R, Price AJ, Vincent TL, Weinans H, Carr AJ. Osteoarthritis. Lancet. 2015;386(9991):376-387.

22. Goldring MB, Tsuchimochi K, Ijiri K. The control of chondrogenesis. J Cell Biochem. 2006;97(1):33-44.

23. Siclari A, Mascaro G, Gentili C, Cancedda R, Boux E. A cell-free scaffold-based cartilage repair provides improved function hyaline-like repair at one year. Clin Orthop Relat Res. 2012 ;470(3):910-919.

24. Siclari A, Mascaro G, Kaps C, Boux E. A 5-year follow-up after cartilage repair in the knee using a platelet-rich plasma-immersed polymer-based implant. Open Orthop J. 2014;8:346-354.

25. Hogenmiller MS, Lozada CJ. An update on osteoarthritis therapeutics. Curr Opin Rheumatol. 2006;18(3):256-260.

Abbreviations

CI:	Confidence interval
COMP:	Cartilage oligomeric matrix protein
DMEM:	Dulbecco's Modified Eagle Medium
FABP4:	Fatty acid binding protein-4
FITC:	Fluorescein isothiocyanate
HS:	Human serum
IBMX:	3-isobutyl-1-methyl-xanthine
ITS+1:	Insulin-transferrin-sodium selenite
MPC:	Mesenchymal progenitor cells
oaMPC:	Mesenchymal progenitor cells derived from osteoarthritic tissue
PE:	Phycoerythrin
PI:	Propidium iodide
TGFB3:	Transforming growth factor-beta3

Potential Conflicts of Interests

Authors Krüger, Hondke & Endres are employees of TransTissue Technologies GmbH, Germany.

Acknowledgements

The authors thank Annina Wanzek and Samuel Vetterlein for their excellent technical assistance.

Corresponding Author

Michaela Endres, TransTissue Technologies GmbH Charitéplatz 1, 10117 Berlin, Germany; Email: michaela.endres@transtissue.com

19

Cardiomyogenic Heterogeneity of Clonal Subpopulations of Human Bone Marrow Mesenchymal Stem Cells

Tripathy NK[#1], Rizvi SHM[#1], Singh SP[1], Garikpati VNS [1], Nityanand S[1]

Abstract

We have evaluated the cardiomyogenic potential of clonal populations of human bone marrow mesenchymal stem cells (BM-MSC). Four rapidly proliferating clones of BM-MSC were obtained from the BM of a healthy donor which were then treated with 5-azacytidine and evaluated for the expression of GATA-4, NKx-2.5, FOG-2, TDGF-1, β-MHC, MEF2D and NPPA genes and cTnT, Desmin and β-MHC proteins. Of the four clones (i) Clone-1 had high expression of GATA-4 (1.89 fold ($p<0.05$), Nkx2.5 (2.29 fold; $p<0.05$), FOG2 (2.76 fold; $p<0.05$), TDGF1 (6.97 fold, $p<0.005$), βMHC (10.22 fold; $p<0.005$), MEF-2D (1.91 fold; $p<0.005$) and NPPA (1.65 fold; $p<0.005$); (ii) clone-2 had up-regulation of Nkx2.5 (1.98 fold; $p<0.05$) but down-regulation of rest of the genes; (iii) clone-3 had up-regulation of Nkx2.5 (2.11 fold; $p<0.05$), TDGF1 (1.88 fold; $p<0.05$), MEF-2D (1.30 fold; $p<0.05$) and NPPA (1.21 fold; $p<0.05$), down regulation of GATA-4 and Fog-2 but no change in βMHC gene; and (iv) clone-4 had up-regulation of MEF-2D (1.17 fold; $p<0.05$) and down regulation of GATA-4, Nkx2.5 but no change in other genes compared to untreated cells of the clones. At the protein level, clone-1 expressed cTnT, Desmin, and βMHC; clone-2 Desmin only while clones-3 and 4 each expressed cTnT, Desmin, and βMHC. Our data shows that BM-MSC are a heterogenous population of stem cells with sub-populations exhibiting a marked difference in the expression of cardiac markers both at gene and protein levels. This highlights that administering selected sub-populations of BM-MSC with a cardiomyogenic potential may be more efficacious than whole population of cells for cardiac regeneration.

Key Words: Human bone marrow mesenchymal stem cells, Clonal subpopulations, Cardiac heterogeneity

Introduction

Bone marrow-derived mesenchymal stem cells (BM-MSC) are being widely explored for cardiac regenerative therapy[1-3], based on their ability to differentiate into cardiomyocytes *in vitro* and in the damaged myocardium *in vivo*[4-6]. In addition, their secretome is also reported to contribute to the therapeutic effects by paracrine mechanisms[7, 8]. However, BM-MSC based cell therapy has not been able to reach an optimal clinical translation stage in cardiac regeneration because of variable therapeutic effects in different pre-clinical and clinical studies[9-11]. One of the factors could be variability in the MSC population used for therapy.

For several years BM-MSC have been considered to be a homogenous population of stem cells with a uniform multipotent differentiation potential. It is only recently that data is emerging on subpopulations of BM-MSC with varying biochemical, metabolic and functional characteristics[12-14]. Thus, our hypothesis was that there may be cardiac heterogeneity amongst sub-populations of MSC and infusing populations with optimal cardiomyogenic potential would have a bearing in cardiac regeneration.

Therefore, the aim of the present study was to evaluate cardiomyogenic heterogeneity of BM-MSC by analyzing expression of cardiomyogenic genes and cardiac structural proteins in 5-azacitidine treated single cell-derived clonal sub-populations of human BM-MSC.

Materials and Methods

The BM-MSC were isolated, cultured and characterized as described earlier[11]. Briefly, after obtaining informed consent, approximately 10 ml of bone marrow aspirate from iliac crest of a healthy volunteer was collected into heparinized tube. The mononuclear cells obtained from the aspirate by density gradient centrifugation were cultured in 25 cm^2 flasks (BD Biosciences, USA) at 37^{0}C in 5% CO_2 using 5 ml of complete culture media consisting of α-MEM, 1% glutamax, 16.5% fetal bovine serum, 100 U/ml penicillin and 100 g/ml streptomycin (all from Gibco, Thermo Fisher Scientific, USA). After 48 hours, non-adherent cells were removed and medium was replaced. When culture reached 70-80% confluency, adherent cells were harvested using 0.05% trypsin (Gibco) and the cells were re-plated. Finally, 2nd passage cells were subject to limiting dilution assay to generate single cell derived clones.

Osteogenic and Adipogenic Differentiation:

The BM-MSC were treated with osteogenic medium consisting of DMEM medium (Gibco) containing 10% FBS (Hyclone, GE lifesciences, USA), 1 mM dexamethasone, 10 mg/mL glyceraldehydes 3-phosphate, and 0.1 mM ascorbic acid (osteogenesis kit, Chemicon, Merck's life science, Germany).

Author Names in full: Naresh Kumar Tripathy[#1], Syed Husain Mustafa Rizvi[#1], Saurabh Pratap Singh[1], Venkata Naga Srikanth Garikpati[1], Soniya Nityanand[1]

[1]Stem Cell Research Facility, Department of Hematology, Sanjay Gandhi Post-Graduate Institute of Medical Sciences (SGPGIMS), Raebareli Road, Lucknow-226014, India

# Both authors contributed equally to the work

After 21 days, the cells were fixed with 4% paraformaldehyde and stained with alizarin red stain to visualize mineralization. For adipogenic differentiation, BM-MSC were treated with adipogenic medium consisting of DMEM medium (Gibco) containing 10% FBS (Hyclone), 500 mM IBMX, 1 mM dexamethasone, 10 mg/mL insulin, and 100 mM indomethacin (adipogenesis kit, Chemicon). After 18 days, the cells were fixed and stained with oil red O stain to visualize the fat droplets in the cells.

Flow-cytometry

The phenotype of BM-MSC and their clones was analyzed by two color flow cytometry using flourescein isothiocyanate (FITC)) conjugated CD34, CD45 and HLA-DR and phycoerythrin (PE) conjugated CD73, CD90 and CD105 monoclonal antibodies (all from AbD Serotec, Bio-Rad, USA). The flow-cytometer used was FACS-calibur (BD Biosciences) and data analysis was done using FACS express software.

Limiting Dilution Assay

Single cell-derived BM-MSC clones were generated by limiting dilution method[15]. Briefly, 2nd passage BM-MSC were plated into four, 96 well tissue-culture plates at a density of 0.5 cells per well, each well contained 50 µl fresh complete culture media and 50 µl MSC conditioned media. To ensure single cell-derived clones of BM-MSC, this method of limiting dilution was used as out of two consecutive wells only one well had a single cell while the other well had no cell. After 24 hours of culture under standard conditions each well was investigated under microscope and wells that contained single cell were marked. Every 2nd day 50µl media was removed from

each well and made up to 100 µl with 50µl fresh complete culture media. After 8-10 days the sub-confluent cultures were harvested by trypsinization and transferred to six well tissue culture plates (BD Biosciences) and finally the cultures were maintained in 25 cm² flasks for further experiments.

Real Time Quantitative PCR:

BM-MSC clones were treated with 5-azacytidine and total RNA of the cells was isolated with RNA AQUEOUS KIT (Ambion, Thermo Fisher Scientific, USA) and reverse-transcribed into cDNA with High Capacity cDNA Reverse Transcription kit (Applied Biosystems, Thermo Fisher Scientific, USA). Quantitative real-time PCR was performed using LightCycler 480 Roche, USA. Real time assays were done with HotStart-IT SYBR Green qPCR Master Mix (USb, Thermo Fisher Scientific, USA) according to manufacturer's protocol. PCR amplification were performed at 94°C for 1 min followed by 40 cycles of 94°C for 15 seconds, 56°C for 30 seconds 72°C for 1 min. Melting curve was obtained by incubating the reactions at 94°C for 5 sec, 65°C for 1 min, and continuous at 94°C. Each PCR was performed in triplicate to ensure the reproducibility of the results. Dissociation reactions were performed to confirm that all the primer sets were giving only single product. Results were expressed relative to the housekeeping gene glyceraldehyde 3 phosphate dehydrogenase (GAPDH). Oligonucleotides used as primers (From MWG Bangalore, India) in this study are given in Table 1. The relative quantitative value of target gene, normalized to an endogenous control GAPDH (housekeeping) gene and relative to a calibrator (control), is expressed as 2-$\Delta\Delta$Ct (-fold difference), where ΔCt = (Ct of target genes – Ct of endogenous control gene (GAPDH), and $\Delta\Delta$Ct = (ΔCt of samples for target gene) – (ΔCt of calibrator for the target gene).

Table-1: List of primers

Name	Sequence	Accession number
GATA4 Forward GATA4 Reverse	GCT CCT TCA GGC AGT GAG AG CTG TGC CCG TAG TGA GAT GA	NM_002052.3
Nkx2.5 Forward Nkx2.5 Reverse	CTTCAAGCCAGAGGCCTACG CCGCCTCTGTCTTCTTCAGC	NM_004387.3
FOG-2 Forward FOG-2 Reverse	GCTTCTATTTTGCCCACAGC CTTCTCTTTGCCTCCCACTG	NM_012082.3
TDGF1 Forward TDGF1 Reverse	GGATACCTGGCCTTCAGAG CGCACATCGTGCTCACAGTT	NM_003212.2
βMyHC Forward βMyHC Reverse	GAGC CTCC AGAG TTTG CTGA AGGA TTGG CACG GACT GCGT CATC	NM_000257.2 for MYH7 NM_002471.2 for MYH6
GAPDH Forward GAPDH Reverse	GA TTT GGT CGT ATT GGG TCC ACG ACG TAC TCA GC	NM_002046.3

Immunofluorescence

The cells were grown on poly-L-lysine coated cover slips in 12 well tissue culture plates (BD Biosciences), and then treated with complete culture medium containing 10μM 5-azacytidine (Sigma-Aldrich, Merck's Life Science, Germany). Control cells were treated with complete medium alone. After incubating for 24 h, the experimental and control cells were washed twice with PBS (Gibco) and further incubated in complete culture medium. The medium was changed every three days and the experiment was terminated at 21 days after 5-azacytidine treatment. Cells were fixed in 4% paraformaldehyde (Sigma-Aldrich), permeabilized with 0.1% triton X (Sigma-Aldrich), non-specific binding sites were blocked with 5% sheep serum (Hyclone) and 0.1% triton X in PBS. Thereafter, primary antibodies against beta myosin heavy chain (bMHC) (1:100 dilution), cardiac troponin T (cTnT) (1:100 dilution) (all from Abcam, UK) and desmin (AbD Serotec) were added. Hoechst 2.5mg/μl (Sigma-Aldrich) in PBS was added to stain nucleus. The cells were observed under fluorescent microscope (Nikon, Japan).

Statistical analysis

All experiments were performed for a minimum of three times and results have been presented as mean ± SE. Statistical analysis was performed using SPSS 14.0 statistical package (SPSS Inc., USA).

Statistical significance of the results was determined using student t-Test. Differences were considered statistically significant at (*$p < 0.05$).

Results

BM-MSC

The primary cultures of BM-MSC had fibroblastoid morphology, expressed CD73, CD90, and CD105 but had no expression of CD34, CD45 and HLA-DR. On treatment with   lineage-specific induction medium they differentiated into adipogenic and osteogenic lineages, as evidenced by Oil red-O and Alizarin red staining, respectively (Figure 1).

BM-MSC Clones

The limiting dilution of primary culture BM-MSC yielded a total of nine clones out of which only four clones exhibited rapid growth and survived till sixth passage in culture. All these rapidly growing clones had comparable expression of mesenchymal markers CD73, CD90, CD105 but no expression of CC34, CD45 and CD105 (Figure 2A). These clones were subsequently analyzed for evaluation of their cardiomyogenic potency.

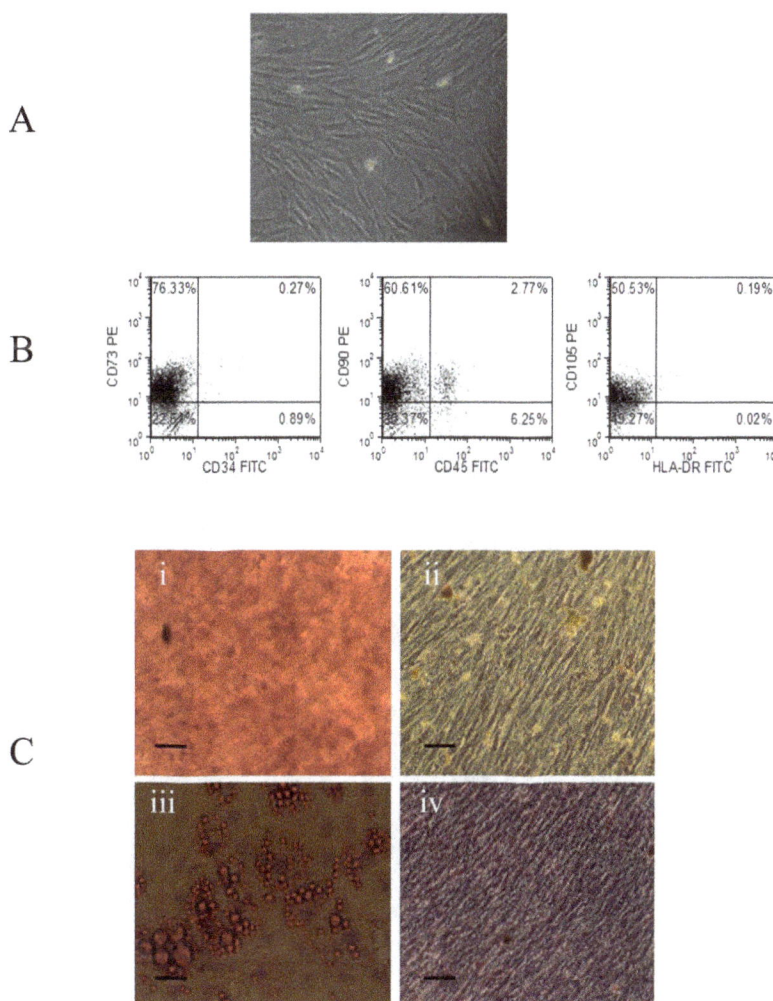

Figure 1:
(A) Photomicrograph of BM-MSC showing fibroblastoid morphology (10X).
(B) Flow cytometric dot plots showing CD73, CD90, CD105 positive and CD34, CD45 and HLA-DR negative phenotype of BM-MSC.
(C) Alizarin Red staining of BM-MSC showing osteogenic differentiation of (i) induction medium treated and (ii) control cells. Oil-Red-O staining of BM-MSC showing adipogenic differentiation of (iii) induction medium treated cells; (iv) control cells (10X).

A

B

C

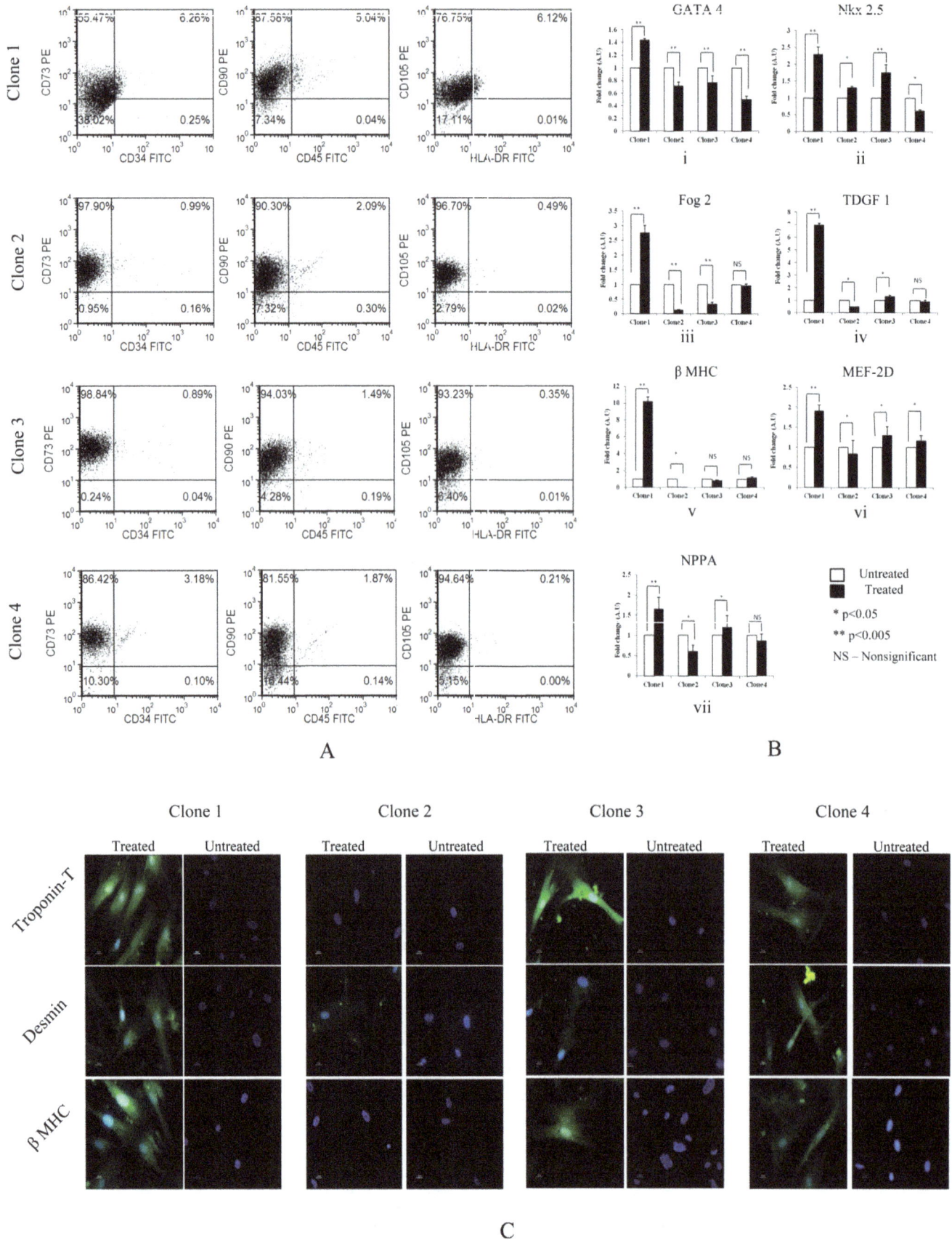

Figure 2:
(A) Flow cytometric dot plots showing that BM-MSC clones have a CD73, CD90, CD105 positive and CD34, CD45 and HLA-DR negative phenotype.
(B) Expression of cardiomyogenic genes; (i) GATA4, (ii) NKx2.5, (iii) FOG2, (iv) TDGF1, (v) βMHC, (vi) MEF-2D and (vii) NPPA by 5-azacytidine treated human BM-MSC clones. All values were normalized to glyceraldehyde-3-phosphate dehydrogenase (GAPDH) and expressed as mean ± SE of three independent experiments. *p<0.05 and ** p<0.005.
(C) Immunofluorescence staining of cardiac specific proteins viz. Cardiac Tropnin-T (cTnT , desmin, and beta-myosin heavy chain (β-MHC), in 5-azacytidine treated human BM-MSC clones viewed under phase contrast microscope (40X).

Cardiomyogenic genes in BM-MSC clones

The expression of cardiomyogenic genes in the four rapidly growing BM-MSC clones obtained was as follows. The clone-1 had significantly increased expression of GATA4 (1.89 fold (p<0.05), Nkx2.5 (2.29fold; p<0.05), FOG2 (2.76fold; p<0.05), TDGF1 (6.97fold, p<0.005), βMHC (10.22 fold; p<0.005), MEF-2D (1.91 fold; p<0.005) and NPPA (1.65 fold; p<0.005) as compared to its untreated cells taken as control. The clone-2 had increased expression only of Nkx2.5 (1.98 fold; p<0.05) but down-regulation of GATA4, FOG2, TDGF1, βMHC, MEF-2D and NPPA genes as compared to its control. Clone-3 had increased expression of Nkx2.5 (2.11 fold; p<0.05), TDGF (1.88 fold; p<0.05), MEF-2D (1.30 fold; p<0.05) and NPPA (1.21 fold; p<0.05), down regulation of GATA4 and Fog2 but no difference in the expression of β-MHC as compared to its control. The clone-4 had up-regulation of MEF-2D (1.17 fold; p<0.05) and down-regulated expression of GATA4 and Nkx2.5 but no difference in the expression levels of TDGF1, FOG2, βMHC and NPPA genes as compared to its control (Figure 2B).

Cardiomyogenic proteins in BM-MSC clones

The expression of cardiac structural proteins in the four rapidly growing BM-MSC clones obtained was as follows. The Clone-1 stained positive for all the three cardiac structural proteins namely cTnT, Desmin and βMHC. The clone-2 was positive for Desmin but lacked expression of cTnT and βMHC proteins. Clone-3 and clone-4, each was positive for cTnT, Desmin and βMHC proteins. The untreated cells of these clones which were taken as control had no staining for any of these proteins (Figure 2C).

Discussion

The present study reports that human BM-MSC consist of different subpopulations of stem cells having variable degree of cardiomyogenic potency as revealed by expression of GATA-4, Nkx2.5, FOG2, TDGF1 and βMHC cardiomyogenic genes and cTnT, Desmin and βMHC cardiac structural proteins in 5-azacytidine pre-treated single cell derived BM-MSC clones. The study also shows that only a small fraction of whole population of BM-MSC possesses optimal cardiomyogenic potency at gene and protein levels.

We have established single cell-derived clonal subpopulations of BM-MSC from the bone marrow aspirate of a single donor to evaluate cardiomyogenic potency of individual clones of whole population of BM-MSC. All these clones expressed comparable level of mesenchymal specific markers showing a homogenous population of cells. However, following cardiomyogenic induction with 5-azacytidine, we observed a highly variable pattern of cardiac gene expression in these clones. The clone-1 had up-regulation of all the five cardiac genes studied namely GATA-4, Nkx2.5, FOG2, TDGF1 and βMHC; clone-2 had up-regulation of only Nkx2.5 but down-regulation of rest of the genes; clone-3 had up-regulation of Nkx2.5 and TDGF1 while down regulation of GATA4 and Fog2 but no change in β-MHC; and clone-4 had down-regulation of GATA4 and Nkx2.5 but no change in rest of the cardiac genes. This heterogeneity of cardiac gene expression in our BM-MSC clones is consistent with the data of a recent study reporting differential expression of osteogenic genes osteocalcin, RUNX2, and osterix in different clonal subpopulations of equine BM-MSC[16]. The differentiation of stem cells into functional cardiomyocytes requires a combinatorial action of multiple transcription factors including GATA-4, Nkx2.5, FOG2, TDGF-1 and β-MHC [17, 18]. Of these GATA-4 functions as a master transcription factor and a critical regulator for induction of other cardiac genes in stem cells and their differentiation into cardiomyocytes [19, 20]. Moreover, the GATA-4 deficient stem cells are reported not to differentiate into cardiomyocytes[21].

Thus, in the light of these studies, it is likely that clone-1 expressing GATA-4 and other cardiac genes may be fully programmed towards cardiomyogenic lineage. The remaining clones which had down-regulation of GATA-4 had either down-regulation or no up-regulation of most of the cardiac genes studied and thus may have partial or no programming towards cardiac lineage.

We also evaluated expression of cardiac structural proteins cTnT, Desmin and βMHC in the 5-azactidine treated BM-MSC clones. Clone-1 similar to its gene profile expressed all the three cardiac proteins cTnT, Desmin and βMHC. Clone-2 was positive only for Desmin which was also matching with its gene expression profile showing up-regulation of only one gene. However, it was surprising to note that clone-3 which exhibited up-regulation of Nkx2.5 and TDGF1 genes only and clone-4 with up-regulation of none of the cardiac genes studied, also stained positive for cTnT, Desmin and βMHC proteins. Although the reason for expression of cardiac structural proteins in these clones having poor cardiomyogenic genetic programming, is not clear but since both of these subpopulations had no up-regulation of GATA-4, which is essential for terminal differentiation and survival of stem cells[20, 21], these cells may represent partially differentiated or progenitor cardiac cells undergoing apoptosis.

In addition, we analyzed gene expression of NPPA and MEF2D representing functional and structural markers of mature cardiomyocytes, respectively. It was observed that similar to other cardiac genes, the cardiomyocytic cells differentiated from clone -1 had a high expression of NPPA and MEF2D indicating their functional and structural maturity.

From our data it emerges that only a small fraction of BM-MSC express complete repertoire of cardiac genes and proteins. This corroborates with a recent study which showed that on 5-azacytidine induction only eight of twenty-four MSC clones expressed cardiac specific markers and exhibited electrophysiological properties typical of functional cardiomyocytes, while the rest of the clones with low cardiac markers did not display electrophysiological features, and thus less than 30% of MSC contributed to functional cardiomyocytic differentiation[22]. Similarly, a single clonal population of human BM-MSC which expressed high levels of cardiac markers on cardiomyogenic induction was shown to have a greater beneficial effect in cardiac repair in rats than whole population of BM-MSC and thus indicating further that only a small fraction of BM-MSC has cardiomyogenic potential[23]. This cardiomyogenic heterogeneity in BM-MSC may be responsible for the non-congruent results of preclinical studies and clinical trials reported in the literature over the past decade[24].

We investigated BM-MSC obtained from a single donor, since donor to donor variation is a major contributor to differences in the biologic properties of BM-MSC[25] and we wanted to avoid any donor specific variation in the cardiomyogenic potency of these stem cells. However, this data needs to be further confirmed by using a cohort of subjects and evaluating the efficacy of different clonal subpopulations in a suitable experimental model of myocardial infarction.

Conclusion

In summary, our data shows that human BM-MSC exhibit cardiomyogenic heterogeneity and only a small fraction of these stem cells express the complete panel of the studied cardiac markers both at the gene and protein level. This highlights that for cardiac regeneration, therapy with sub-populations of BM-MSC with a cardiomyogenic potential may be more optimal than whole population of BM-MSC.

References

1. Williams AR, Hare JM. Mesenchymal stem cells: biology, pathophysiology, translational findings, and therapeutic implications for cardiac disease. Circ Res. 2011;109(8):923-40.
2. Chou SH, Lin SZ, Kuo WW, Pai P, Lin JY, Lai CH, Kuo CH, Lin KH, Tsai FJ, Huang CY. Mesenchymal stem cell insights: prospects in cardiovascular therapy. Cell Transplant. 2014;23(4-5):513-29.
3. Karantalis V, Hare JM. Use of mesenchymal stem cells for therapy of cardiac disease. Circ Res. 2015;116(8):1413-30.
4. Toma C, Pittenger MF, Cahill KS, Byrne BJ, Kessler PD. Human mesenchymal stem cells differentiate to a cardiomyocyte phenotype in the adult murine heart. Circulation. 2002;105(1):93-8.
5. Piryaei A, Soleimani M, Heidari MH, Saheli M, Rohani R, Almasieh M. Ultrastructural maturation of human bone marrow mesenchymal stem cells-derived cardiomyocytes under alternative induction of 5-azacytidine. Cell Biol Int. 2015;39(5):519-30.
6. Quevedo HC, Hatzistergos KE, Oskouei BN, Feigenbaum GS, Rodriguez JE, Valdes D, Pattany PM, Zambrano JP, Hu Q, McNiece I, Heldman AW, Hare JM. Allogeneic mesenchymal stem cells restore cardiac function in chronic ischemic cardiomyopathy via trilineage differentiating capacity. Proc Natl Acad Sci U S A. 2009;106(33):14022-7.
7. Duran JM, Makarewich CA, Sharp TE, Starosta T, Zhu F, Hoffman NE, Chiba Y, Madesh M, Berretta RM, Kubo H, Houser SR. Bone-derived stem cells repair the heart after myocardial infarction through transdifferentiation and paracrine signaling mechanisms. Circ Res. 2013;113(5):539-52.
8. Gallina C, Turinetto V, Giachino C. A New Paradigm in Cardiac Regeneration:The Mesenchymal Stem Cell Secretome. Stem Cells Int. 2015;2015:765846.
9. Mazo M, Araña M, Pelacho B, Prosper F. Mesenchymal stem cells and cardiovascular disease: a bench to bedside roadmap. Stem Cells Int. 2012;2012:175979.
10. Telukuntla KS, Suncion VY, Schulman IH, Hare JM. The advancing field of cell-based therapy: insights and lessons from clinical trials. J Am Heart Assoc. 2013;2(5):e000338.
11. Singh SP, Tripathy NK, Nityanand S. Comparison of phenotypic markers and neural differentiation potential of multipotent adult progenitor cells and mesenchymal stem cells. World J Stem Cells. 2013;5(2):53-60.
12. Phinney DG. Functional heterogeneity of mesenchymal stem cells: implications for cell therapy. J Cell Biochem. 2012;113(9):2806-12.
13. Phinney DG. Biochemical heterogeneity of mesenchymal stem cell populations: clues to their therapeutic efficacy. Cell Cycle. 2007;6(23):2884-9.
14. Liu Y, Muñoz N, Bunnell BA, Logan TM, Ma T. Density-Dependent Metabolic Heterogeneity in Human Mesenchymal Stem Cells. Stem Cells. 2015 ;33(11):3368-81.
15. Fedr R, Pernicová Z, Slabáková E, Straková N, Bouchal J, Grepl M, Kozubík A, Souček K. Automatic cell cloning assay for determining the clonogenic capacity of cancer and cancer stem-like cells. Cytometry A. 2013;83(5):472-82.
16. Radtke CL, Nino-Fong R, Rodriguez-Lecompte JC, Esparza Gonzalez BP, Stryhn H, McDuffee LA. Osteogenic potential of sorted equine mesenchymal stem cell subpopulations. Can J Vet Res. 2015;79(2):101-8.
17. Wu WS, Lai FJ. Detecting Cooperativity between Transcription Factors Based on Functional Coherence and Similarity of Their Target Gene Sets. PLoS One. 2016;11(9):e0162931.
18. Nemer G, Nemer M. Regulation of heart development and function through combinatorial interactions of transcription factors. Ann Med. 2001;33(9):604-10.
19. Charron F, Paradis P, Bronchain O, Nemer G, Nemer M. Cooperative interaction between GATA-4 and GATA-6 regulates myocardial gene expression. Mol Cell Biol.1999;19(6):4355-65.
20. Grépin C, Nemer G, Nemer M. Enhanced cardiogenesis in embryonic stem cells overexpressing the GATA-4 transcription factor. Development. 1997;124(12):2387-95.
21. Grépin C, Robitaille L, Antakly T, Nemer M. Inhibition of transcription factor GATA-4 expression blocks in vitro cardiac muscle differentiation. Mol Cell Biol. 1995;15(8):4095-102.
22. Wei F, Wang T, Liu J, Du Y, Ma A. The subpopulation of mesenchymal stem cells that differentiate toward cardiomyocytes is cardiac progenitor cells. Exp Cell Res. 2011;317(18):2661-70.
23. Zhang S, Ge J, Sun A, Xu D, Qian J, Lin J, Zhao Y, Hu H, Li Y, Wang K, Zou Y. Comparison of various kinds of bone marrow stem cells for the repair of infarcted myocardium: single clonally purified non-hematopoietic mesenchymal stem cells serve as a superior source. J Cell Biochem. 2006;99(4):1132-47.
24. Singh A, Singh A, Sen D. Mesenchymal stem cells in cardiac regeneration: a detailed progress report of the last 6 years (2010-2015). Stem Cell Res Ther. 2016;7(1):82.
25. Katsara O, Mahaira LG, Iliopoulou EG, Moustaki A, Antsaklis A, Loutradis D, Stefanidis K, Baxevanis CN, Papamichail M, Perez SA. Effects of donor age, gender, and in vitro cellular aging on the phenotypic, functional, and molecular characteristics of mouse bone marrow-derived mesenchymal stem cells. Stem Cells Dev. 2011;20(9):1549-61.

Abbreviations

β MHC:	Beta Myosin Heavy Chain
cTnT:	Cardiac Troponin T
FOG-2:	Family of GATA member 2
GATA-4:	GATA binding protein 4
HLA:	Human Leukocyte Antigen
IBMX:	3-Isobutyl-1-methylxanthine
MEF-2D:	Myocyte-specific Enhancer Factor 2D
NKX2-5:	NK2 transcription factor related, locus 5
NPPA:	Natriuretic Peptide A
RUNX2:	Runt-related transcription factor 2
TDGF1:	Teratocarcinoma-Derived Growth Factor 1

Potential Conflicts of Interests

None

Acknowledgements

This work was supported by an extramural grant entitled "*Mesenchymal Stem Cell Therapy in Myocardial Infarction, Stroke, Renal Failure and Diabetes*" (BT/PR6519/MED/14/826/2005) sanctioned by Department of Biotechnology, Government of India, to Dr S Nityanand.

Corresponding Author

Soniya Nityanand, Prof & Head, Dept. of Hematology, Sanjay Gandhi Post Graduate Institute of Medical Sciences, Raebareli Road.Lucknow -226014, UP, India. E-mail: soniya_nityanand@yahoo.co.in

20

Generation of dopamine neuronal-like cells from induced neural precursors derived from adult human cells by non-viral expression of lineage factors

Playne R[1], Jones KS[1], Connor B[1]

Abstract

Reprogramming technology holds great promise for the study and treatment of Parkinson's disease (PD) as patient-specific ventral midbrain dopamine (vmDA) neurons can be generated. This should facilitate the investigation of early changes occurring during PD pathogenesis, permitting the identification of new drug targets and providing a platform for drug screening. To date, most studies using reprogramming technology to study PD have employed induced pluripotent stem cells. Research into PD using direct reprogramming has been limited due to an inability to generate high yields of authentic human vmDA neurons. Nevertheless, direct reprogramming offers a number of advantages, and development of this technology is warranted. Previous reports have indicated that induced neural precursors (iNPs) derived from adult human fibroblasts by lineage factor-mediated direct reprogramming can give rise to dopamine neurons expressing tyrosine hydroxylase (TH+). Using normal adult human fibroblasts, the present study aimed to extend these findings and determine the capacity of iNPs for generating vmDA neurons, with the aim of utilising this technology for the future study of PD. While iNPs expressed late vmDA fate markers such as NURR1 and PITX3, critical early regional markers LMX1A, FOXA2 and EN1 were not expressed. Upon differentiation, iNPs gave rise to dopamine neuronal-like cells expressing TUJ1, TH, AADC, DAT, VMAT2 and GIRK2. To induce an authentic A9 phenotype, a series of experiments investigated temporal exposure to patterning factors. Exposure to SHH-C24II, purmorphamine, CHIR99021 and/or FGF8b during or after reprogramming was insufficient to induce expression of early vmDA regional markers. Addition of LMX1A/FOXA2 to the transfection cocktail did not induce a sustained vmDA iNP phenotype. This study reports for the first time that iNPs derived from healthy adult human cells by non-viral expression of lineage factors can give rise to dopamine neuronal-like cells. Direct-to-iNP reprogramming could be a suitable strategy for modelling PD in vitro using aged donor-derived cells.

Key Words: Induced neural precursor cells; Dopamine neurons; Direct reprogramming; Adult human fibroblasts; Parkinson's disease

Introduction

Cell reprogramming technology offers exciting prospects for studying and treating Parkinson's disease (PD)[1]. Human foetal mesencephalic tissue transplants have provided proof-of-principle that stem cell therapies hold promise for treating PD[2]. Cell reprogramming technology permits autologous or HLA-matched cell transplants, circumventing the requirement for immunosuppression and avoiding ethical issues related to using large amounts of foetal tissue. Another important application for cell reprogramming is disease modelling. The ability to generate patient-specific ventral midbrain dopamine (vmDA) neurons permits the investigation of early changes occurring during PD pathogenesis, the identification of new drug targets, and provides a platform for screening therapeutic compounds.

Reprogramming to an induced pluripotent stem cell (iPSC) fate is a popular method to derive human neurons. As iPSC technology was preceded by years of mouse and human embryonic stem cell work, existing protocols for deriving neuronal subtypes such as vmDA neurons are advanced[3, 4]. Induced pluripotent stem cells provide an indefinitely expandable cell source that is not restricted to a particular lineage. However, producing and validating iPSC clones is a lengthy process, taking 4 – 6 months to generate functional neurons from a starting population of fibroblasts[5]. Additionally, by reverting adult cells to an embryonic state, markers of age are erased, posing a problem for modelling age-related diseases[6]. For use in cell-based therapies, the potential presence of residual pluripotent cells in differentiated cultures poses a threat of tumour formation.

By contrast, direct-to-neuronal reprogramming technology is at an earlier stage of development. This technology is faster and more efficient than iPSC reprogramming, generating functional human induced neural (iN) cells within 1 – 3 weeks[7, 8]. As cells are not rejuvenated, age-related aspects of PD may be more readily studied in vitro. While mature iN cells are not suitable for transplantation therapy, the possibility of reprogramming in vivo[9, 10] may offer advantages to cell-based therapies, such as avoiding an immune response, a higher efficiency of neuronal generation, and a lower probability of tumour formation. However, for in vitro applications, direct-to-neuronal reprogramming generates a limited supply of post-mitotic neurons and for studies aiming to examine PD-related developmental changes in dopamine neurons, iN cells are not suitable. To date, the generation of authentic human vmDA iN cells from adult cells has not been described[1].

Author Names in full: Rebecca Playne[1], Kathryn Jones[1], Bronwen Connor[1]

[1]Department of Pharmacology & Clinical Pharmacology, Centre for Brain Research, Faculty of Medical and Health Sciences, University of Auckland, Auckland, New Zealand

Direct reprogramming to induced neural stem cells/precursors (iNSC/iNPs) offers an intermediate strategy, where proliferative cells may be obtained in a faster process than iPSC reprogramming, generating iNSC/iNPs within 1 – 4 weeks, with additional time required for differentiation[5]. The three strategies for direct-to-iNSC/iNP reprogramming are to use pluripotency factors, lineage specific factors and/or chemicals[1]. Direct reprogramming using pluripotency factors may not be 'direct', but similar to iPSC reprogramming, inducing a transient state of pluripotency[11, 12]. Chromosomal abnormalities are more frequent in pluripotent factor-than lineage factor-reprogrammed iNSC/iNPs, which may increase the probability of tumour formation[13]. By using pluripotency factors, iNSC/iNPs may be rejuvenated, as observed with iPSC reprogramming. The mechanism underlying lineage factor-mediated direct-to-iNSC/iNP reprogramming has not been examined in detail, and as many different combinations of genes have been reported, mechanisms and stages of development may differ between protocols[1].

Reprogramming to an iNSC/iNP fate represents a promising strategy for generating neuronal lineages from somatic cells. A handful of studies have reported the generation of dopamine neurons from adult human pluripotent factor-reprogrammed iNSC/iNPs[14-17] (for a full review, see[1]). Several studies have reported generating dopamine neurons from human foetal or post-natal cells via lineage factor-mediated reprogramming[18-20], yet only two have generated tyrosine hydroxylase (TH+) cells from adult human donors[21, 22]. Further examination into the dopaminergic phenotype of TH+ cells generated from adult donors *via* this method has not been reported. Although reprogramming is less efficient in aged donor cells than younger cells[23], successful modelling of age-related diseases like PD will rely on using adult cells as a source for generating dopamine neurons. Finally, it is essential to confirm that directly reprogrammed dopamine neurons represent an authentic ventral midbrain A9 phenotype prior to PD modelling.

A method to reprogram adult human fibroblasts to an iNP fate by non-viral *SOX2/PAX6* transfection has been developed in our laboratory[21]. Using non-viral methods of gene introduction reduces the chance of insertional mutagenesis which may be important for downstream applications. This method gives rise to TH+/NSE+ cells from adult human fibroblasts[21]. Based on the potential advantages of direct-to-iNSC/iNP reprogramming, the present study aimed to extend our previous work and determine the capacity of iNPs for generating dopamine neurons from adult human fibroblasts. Healthy donor cells were selected for optimising this protocol, with a view to utilising this technology for the study of PD in donor-derived cells.

Materials & Methods

Cell culture

Adult human fibroblast cells from healthy donors (n = 3), aged 39 – 56 years, were sourced from Cell Applications, Inc. No substantial differences were observed between cell lines throughout the study. Plasmid transfections were carried out using Lipofectamine LTX, Plus reagent (Invitrogen) and plasmid constructs at a ratio 3:1:1 (v/v/w) as per[24]. The plasmids contained cDNAs encoding human *SOX2,* human *PAX6,* mouse *LMX1A* and/or mouse *FOXA2,* and were used at 1.6 – 2.5 µg/plasmid/well (6-well format). The vectors pLV.PGK.mLmx1a and pLV.PGK.mFoxa2 were a gift from Malin Parmar, Lund University (Addgene plasmids #33013 and #33014)[25]. Transfection was confirmed by concurrent transfection with plasmids expressing fluorescent protein, and/or performing immunocytochemistry on cells fixed 1 – 3 days post-transfection.

Three days after transfection, cells were transferred to reprogramming medium containing Neurobasal-A medium (Gibco), 1 mM valproic

acid (Sigma), 0.3% D-(+)-Glucose (Sigma), 1x Penicillin-Streptomycin-Glutamine (Gibco), 1x B27 supplement with retinoic acid (Gibco), 20 ng/ml EGF (Peprotech), 2 µg/ml Heparin (Sigma), with 25 ng/ml midkine (Peprotech) supplemented until day 17 – 21 post-transfection. Media was supplemented with 20 – 500 ng/ml SHH-C24II (R&D Systems), 0.7 – 3 µM CHIR99021 (Stemgent or Miltenyi Biotec), 2 µM purmorphamine (Stemgent) and/or 100 ng/ml FGF8b (Peprotech), as indicated.

To differentiate iNPs, cells were cultured in basal differentiation media containing Neurobasal-A medium (Gibco), 0.3% D-(+)-Glucose (Sigma), 1x Penicillin-Streptomycin-Glutamine (Gibco), 1x B27 supplement without retinoic acid (Gibco) and 1x N2 supplement (Gibco). Patterning media was supplemented with 200 ng/ml SHH-C24II (Peprotech) and 100 ng/ml FGF8b (Peprotech). Maturation media was supplemented with 20 ng/ml BDNF (Creative Biomart or Peprotech), 20 ng/ml GDNF (Merck Millipore or Peprotech), 1 ng/ml TGFβ3 (Peprotech), 500 µM dibutyryl cAMP (Sigma) and 200 µM L-ascorbic acid (Sigma). Cells were differentiated for up to one week in Patterning media and up to four weeks in Maturation media.

Quantitative real-time PCR

RNA was isolated using the Nucleospin RNA kit (Macherey-Nagel) and reverse transcription was conducted using SuperScript III First-Strand Synthesis (Invitrogen), with an equivalent amount of RNA per sample. Three independent duplex qPCR reactions were performed for each sample using the TaqMan system (Applied Biosystems) with ribosomal 18S rRNA as the internal standard and an equivalent of 4 ng mRNA per reaction. Analysis was performed using the comparative Ct ($\Delta\Delta$Ct) method[26].

Immunocytochemistry

The following primary antibodies were used: AADC (Millipore/AB1569), ASCL1 (Millipore/AB5696), DAT (Abcam/AB5990), FOXA2 (Santa Cruz/SC-6554), FOXG1 (Abcam/AB18259), GIRK2 (Abcam/AB30738), KI67 (DAKO/M7240), LMX1A (Millipore/AB10533), NESTIN (Abcam/AB22035), NGN2 (R&D Systems/MAB3314), NURR1 (Santa Cruz/SC-990), SOX1 (Millipore/AB15766), SOX2 (R&D Systems/MAB2018), TH (Millipore/MAB5280), TH (Millipore/AB152), TUJ1 (Biolegend/801202), VMAT2 (Millipore/AB1598P). Fluorescent imaging was performed on a Nikon Eclipse TE2000U microscope with an Optronics Microfire camera or Photometrics Evolve EMCCD camera. Phase contrast images were taken on the Nikon Eclipse TS100 microscope with a Nikon Digital Sight DS-U1 camera. For cell quantification experiments, the investigator was blinded to the condition during image acquisition and counting.

Results

SOX2/PAX6-iNPs show temporal changes in the expression of genes related to vmDA development

To give rise to dopamine neurons, it was reasoned that iNPs would need to express genes implicated in the development of vmDA neurons *in vivo*. To investigate this, a time course experiment examining the expression of a range of neural stem, progenitor and regional markers was performed during *SOX2/PAX6*-reprogramming, focussing on genes involved in vmDA development (Figure 1A; Study One). Over the course of reprogramming, and particularly after the first passage (day 31), cells transitioned from extended, polarised fibroblast morphologies to epithelial-like morphologies, with regular dimensions and cells growing in discrete patches (Figure 1B). In addition, floating and semi-adherent clusters of cells reminiscent of neurospheres were observed.

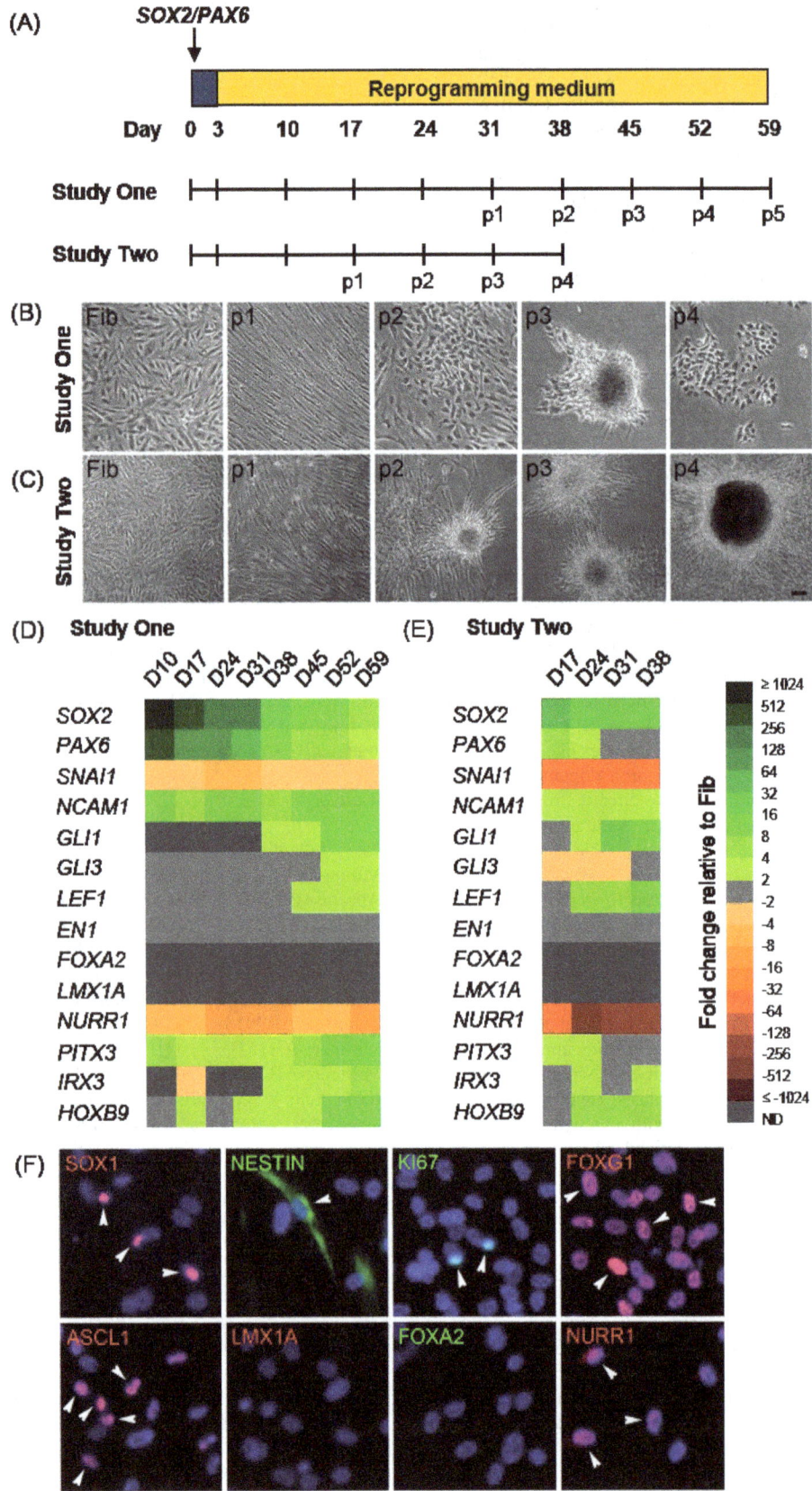

Figure 1: *Characterisation of SOX2/PAX6-iNPs. (A) Schematic detailing experimental outline for Studies One and Two. Weekly passaging was commenced at day 31 (Study One) or day 17 (Study Two) post-transfection. (B) – (C) Phase contrast images of fibroblasts (Fib) reprogramming into iNPs over time. Scale bar: 100 μm. (D) – (E) Heat map depicting gene expression in iNPs over time as fold changes relative to fibroblasts. ND: not detected. (F) Expression of neural progenitor and regional markers in p4 SOX2/PAX6-iNPs. Arrowheads indicate some cells with positive staining. Scale bar: 50 μm.*

Gene expression analysis (Figure 1D) found that *SOX2* and *PAX6* expression subsided over time, but remained elevated relative to fibroblasts. The fibroblast marker *SNAI1* was downregulated while the neural marker *NCAM1* was upregulated relative to fibroblasts. *GLI1*, *GLI3* and *LEF1*, which are downstream targets and effectors of SHH and WNT signalling, were upregulated later during reprogramming. Importantly, the early vmDA regional markers *EN1*, *FOXA2* and *LMX1A* were not upregulated by reprogramming, while the late vmDA marker *NURR1* was downregulated and *PITX3* was upregulated relative to fibroblasts.

In Study One, the expression of a number of genes was upregulated late during reprogramming after the commencement of weekly passaging. Study Two sought to determine if weekly passaging could be commenced earlier to reduce the duration of reprogramming (Figure 1A). Changes in cell morphologies were observed earlier (Figure 1C), and similar patterns of gene expression were seen at earlier time points (Figure 1E).

Protein expression of neural precursor and regional markers in *SOX2/PAX6*-iNPs was examined (Figure 1F). Widespread expression of the anterior marker FOXG1 was found, with heterogeneous expression of SOX1, NESTIN, NURR1, KI67 and ASCL1. The vmDA progenitor markers LMX1A and FOXA2 were not observed.

SOX2/PAX6-iNPs show minimal response to timed exposure to patterning molecules

Studies One and Two found that *SOX2/PAX6*-iNPs upregulated *GLI1* and *LEF1* towards the end of reprogramming. These genes are involved in SHH and WNT signal transduction, and indicate that *SOX2/PAX6*-iNPs may respond to patterning molecules. To determine if *SOX2/PAX6*-iNPs would differentiate into dopamine neurons in response to commonly used patterning and maturation cues, cells were differentiated by applying BDNF, GDNF, TGFβ3, dcAMP and ascorbic acid, as a maturation medium, with or without a preceding period of patterning by SHH-C24II (SHH) and FGF8b (Figure 2A). A population of differentiated cells co-expressed TUJ1 with TH or AADC, and TH+ cells also expressed AADC, GIRK2, VMAT2 and DAT (Figure 2B). Quantification revealed that the addition of SHH/FGF8 had no effect on the yields of TUJ1+, TH+/TUJ1+ or AADC+/TUJ1+ cells (Figure 2C). Overall the yields of TUJ1+ cells co-expressing TH or AADC were low ($\leq 2.1\%$ of all cells), however the proportion of TUJ1+ cells that co-expressed TH or AADC was at least 24.9% (Figure 2D).

Pluripotent stem cell studies have indicated that early exposure to potent SHH and WNT signalling is critical to pattern differentiating neural progenitors towards an authentic vmDA fate[3, 4, 27, 28]. Established *SOX2/PAX6*-iNPs may be too mature to respond to SHH/FGF8 patterning. We, therefore, investigated if exposure to SHH, or the Smoothened agonist purmorphamine (PUR), with WNT signalling by the GSK3β inhibitor CHIR99021 (CHIR) during reprogramming could induce expression of vmDA markers in iNPs (Figure 3A). Cells were exposed to these patterning conditions from the first passage onwards (Study Four), for the full duration of reprogramming (Study Five), or until the start of weekly passaging (Study Six). At p3, cells exposed to SHH/CHIR or PUR/CHIR for the last phase or the full duration of reprogramming showed upregulated *GLI1* relative to unpatterned control iNPs (Figure 3B). Late patterning induced downregulation of *NURR1* and *PITX3*, whereas patterning for the full duration of reprogramming upregulated both *NURR1* and *PITX3* (Figure 3B). Nevertheless, *FOXA2*, *LMX1A* and *EN1* were unchanged by exposure to patterning molecules during reprogramming (Figure 3B). Importantly, exposure to patterning molecules for the full duration of reprogramming caused cellular

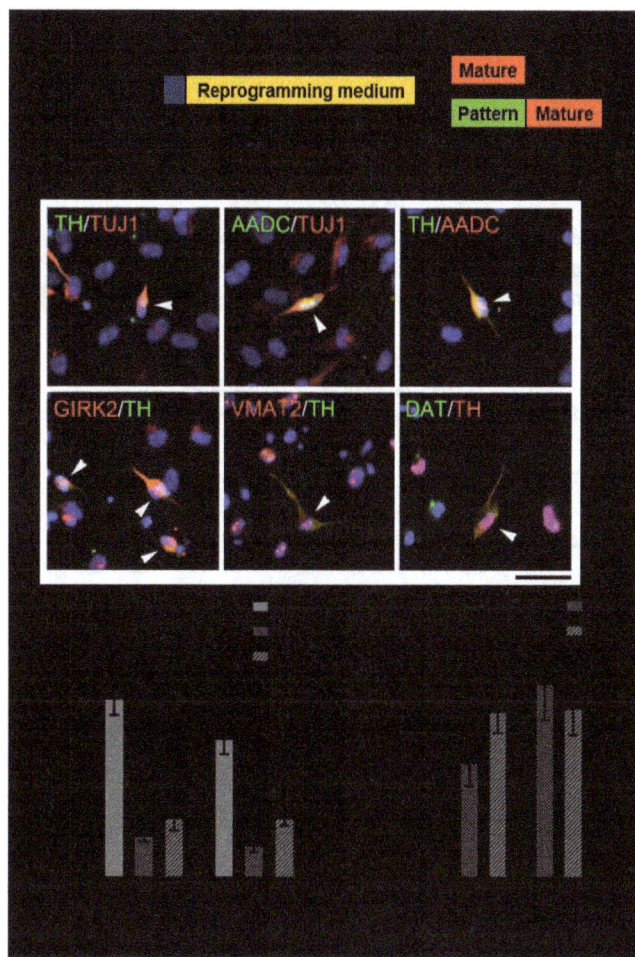

Figure 2: *Determining the dopaminergic differentiation capacity of SOX2/PAX6-iNPs. (A) Schematic detailing experimental outline for Study Three. (B) Expression of dopaminergic markers in cultures differentiated with Patterning and Maturation media. Arrowheads indicate cells with positive staining. Scale bar: 50 µm. (C) Quantification of TUJ1+, TUJ1+/TH+ and TUJ1+/AADC+ cells in differentiated iNP cultures. Data are presented as mean ± SEM, n = 16 - 32 fields of view from two independent cell lines (number of cells counted per condition ≥ 2519). Unpaired t-tests revealed no effect of SHH/FGF8 patterning on yields of TUJ1+, TH+/TUJ1+ or AADC+/TUJ1+ cells. (D) Quantification of TH+ and AADC+ cells out of TUJ1 in differentiated iNP cultures. Data are presented as mean ± SEM, n = 16 fields of view from two independent cell lines (number of cells counted per condition ≥ 2519). Unpaired t-tests revealed no effect of SHH/FGF8 patterning on yields of TH+ or AADC+ cells.*

toxicity, and this precluded further examination of the differentiation capacity of these cells. It was reasoned that early, restricted exposure to patterning factors might be sufficient to induce similar changes in vmDA gene expression without causing cellular toxicity (Study Six). However, few sustained changes in gene expression were observed when cells were exposed to SHH/CHIR or PUR/CHIR for the first period of reprogramming only. Differentiation of cells in Study Six found that PUR/CHIR-patterned iNPs died upon exposure to maturation medium (Figure 3C), while SHH/CHIR-patterning had no effect on TUJ1+ or TH+ cell yields (not shown).

SOX2 alone produces iNPs under standard reprogramming conditions

PAX6 is an anterior neuroectodermal marker that is not expressed in the ventral mesencephalon, the region where vmDA neurons arise[29,30]. Several studies have demonstrated that to pattern differentiating pluripotent stem cells to a floor plate fate, PAX6 induction must be avoided by early potent ventralisation[28, 31]. *SOX2*-iNPs have been generated from rodent and human foetal cells when combined with a feeder layer or a cocktail of small

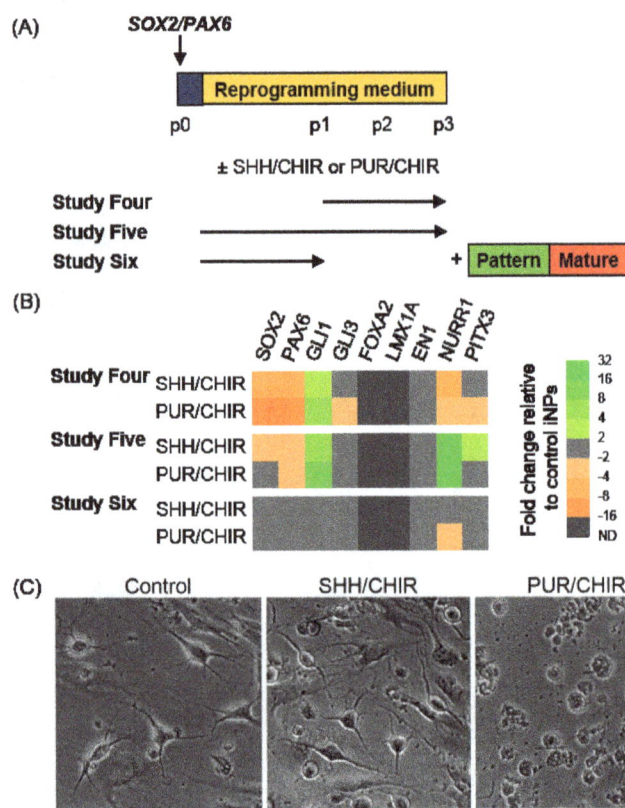

Figure 3: *Investigating the effect of exposure to patterning molecules during SOX2/PAX6-mediated reprogramming. (A) Schematic detailing experimental outline for Studies Four – Six. SHH: 200 ng/ml SHH-C24II, PUR: 2 μM purmorphamine, CHIR: 0.7 μM CHIR99021. (B) Heat map depicting gene expression in iNPs at p3 as fold changes relative to control SOX2/PAX6-iNPs cultured under standard reprogramming conditions. (C) Phase contrast images of differentiated iNP cultures from Study Six after one week in Patterning media and one week in Maturation media .Scale bar: 50 μm.*

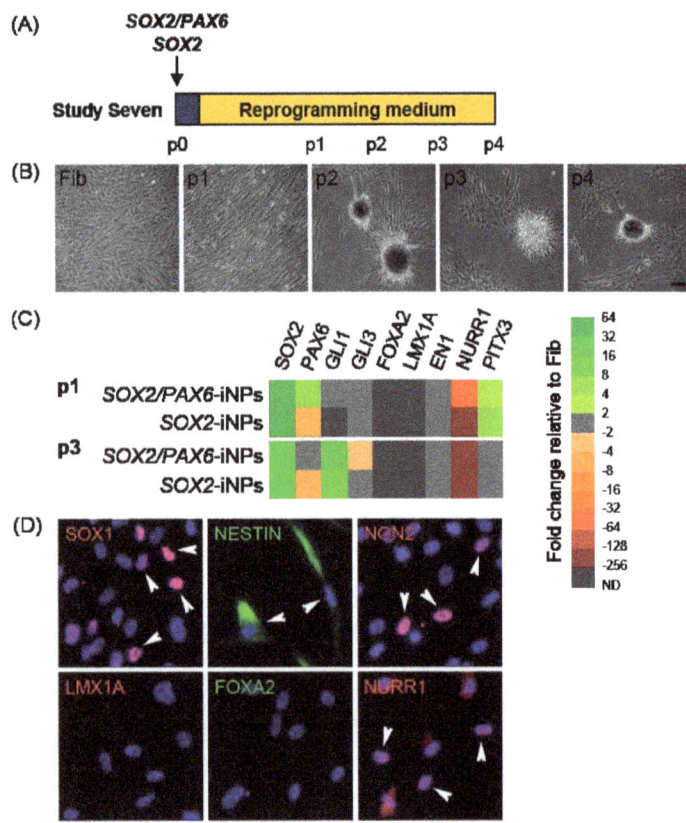

Figure 4: *Characterisation of SOX2-iNPs. (A) Schematic detailing experimental outline for Study Seven. Weekly passaging was commenced at day 17 post-transfection. (B) Phase contrast images of SOX2-iNPs over the course of reprogramming. Scale bar: 100 μm. (C) Heat map depicting gene expression in SOX2/PAX6- and SOX2-iNPs at p1 and p3 as fold changes relative to fibroblasts. (D) Expression of neural progenitor and regional markers in p4 SOX2-iNPs. Arrowheads indicate some cells with positive staining. Scale bar: 50 μm.*

molecules[32, 33]. To determine if *SOX2* alone could induce an iNP fate in adult fibroblasts under our direct reprogramming conditions, Study Seven investigated reprogramming fibroblasts by *SOX2* transfection with standard culture conditions (Figure 4A). Similar changes in cellular morphologies during reprogramming were observed in *SOX2*-iNPs as in *SOX2/PAX6*-iNPs (Figure 4B). Gene expression analysis revealed similar profiles between *SOX2/PAX6*-iNPs and *SOX2*-iNPs (Figure 4C). At the protein level, *SOX2*-iNPs expressed SOX1, NESTIN, NGN2 and NURR1, but as observed in *SOX2/PAX6*-iNPs, there was no expression of either LMX1A or FOXA2 (Figure 4D).

SOX2-iNPs show minimal response to early exposure to SHH/CHIR

As *SOX2*-iNPs could be generated without *PAX6* transfection, it was of interest to determine if these cells would respond to patterning cues. The concentration of 0.7 μM CHIR used to pattern differentiating pluripotent stem cells to a midbrain fate as described in a previous study[4] may require optimisation for this system, due to potentially varying degrees of endogenous WNT signalling[34]. To determine if *SOX2*-iNPs could respond to SHH/CHIR-patterning, cells were exposed to early SHH in conjunction with CHIR at 0.7, 1.5 or 3 μM for the first period of reprogramming (Figure 5A). Patterning *SOX2/PAX6*-iNPs at this point did not induce lasting changes in vmDA gene expression in Study Six, however the responsiveness of *SOX2*-iNPs to patterning cues may be altered in the absence of *PAX6*

expression. Additionally, pluripotent stem cell studies indicate that early patterning is essential[3, 4, 28, 31], and prolonged exposure to patterning molecules induced toxicity in Study Five. Transcriptional analysis found few changes in gene expression compared to unpatterned *SOX2*-iNPs, three weeks after withdrawal of patterning factors (Figure 5B). *GLI1* and *LEF1* were upregulated by higher concentrations of CHIR (1.5 or 3 μM). However no changes in vmDA gene expression or differentiation capacity was observed as a result of early SHH/CHIR-patterning (Figure 5B, C).

Addition of LMX1A and FOXA2 has little effect on vmDA identity in iNPs

As media components were not sufficient to induce early vmDA genes in iNPs, we investigated whether the addition of *LMX1A* and *FOXA2* was able to promote a vmDA phenotype. Fibroblasts were transfected with *SOX2*, *SOX2/PAX6*, *SOX2/LMX1A* or *SOX2/LMX1A/FOXA2* and cultured under standard reprogramming conditions (Figure 6A). While expression of the transgenes was observed following transfection by immunocytochemistry (Figure 6B) and qPCR (not shown), at p3 iNPs did not show endogenous expression of either *LMX1A* or *FOXA2* (Figure 6C). Furthermore, upon differentiation, there was no change in the yields of TUJ1+ or TH+/TUJ1+ cells compared to *SOX2/PAX6*- or *SOX2*-iNPs (Figure 6D).

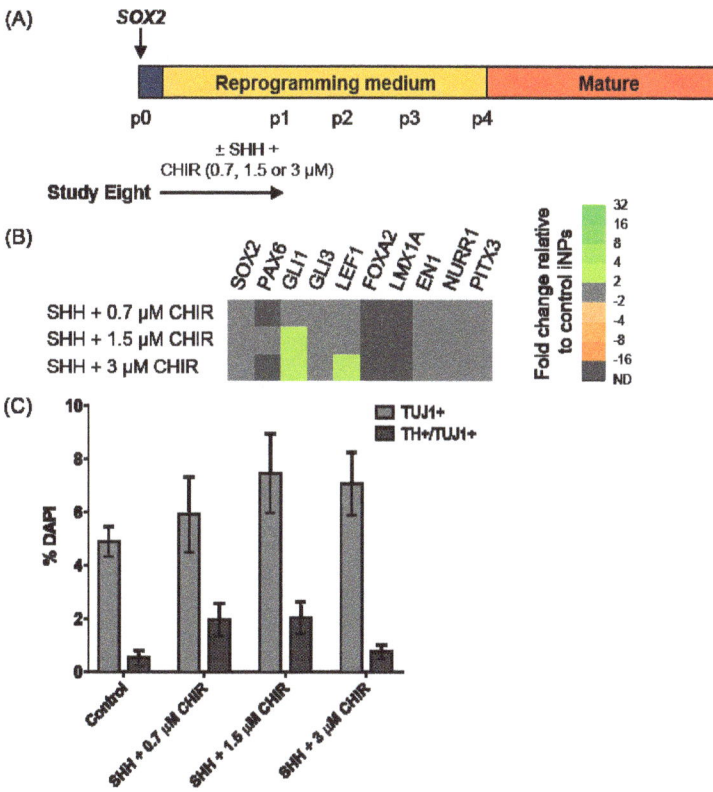

Figure 5: *Investigating the effect of exposure to patterning molecules during SOX2-mediated reprogramming. (A) Schematic detailing experimental outline for Study Eight. (B) Heat map depicting gene expression in iNPs as fold changes relative to control SOX2-iNPs cultured under standard reprogramming conditions. (C) Quantification of TUJ1+ and TUJ1+/TH+ cells in differentiated iNP cultures. Data are presented as mean ± SEM, n = 8 fields of view from one cell line (number of cells counted per condition ≥ 819). An ordinary one-way ANOVA revealed no effect of SHH/CHIR patterning on yields of TUJ1+ or TH+/TUJ1+ cells.*

Figure 6: *Investigating the effect of adding vmDA transgenes during reprogramming. (A) Schematic detailing experimental outline for Study Nine. Cells were cultured in standard reprogramming medium. (B) Immunocytochemistry at three days post-transfection confirms transfection of plasmids. Scale bar: 50 μm. (C) Heat map depicting gene expression in iNPs as fold changes relative to fibroblasts. (D) Quantification of TUJ1+ and TUJ1+/TH+ cells in differentiated iNP cultures. Data are presented as mean ± SEM, n = 6 – 13 fields of view from one cell line (number of cells counted per condition ≥ 738). An ordinary one-way ANOVA revealed no effect of the transfection factor combination on yields of TUJ1+ or TH+/TUJ1+ cells.*

Previous studies have indicated that for exogenous *LMX1A* to exert its effect, SHH exposure is required[35, 36]. Therefore fibroblasts were transfected with *SOX2/LMX1A* or *SOX2/LMX1A/FOXA2* and reprogrammed with early SHH/CHIR patterning, after which point CHIR was withdrawn and SHH concentration was dropped to 20 ng/ml (Figure 7A). The literature is mixed as to the requirement for FGF8 exposure to induce a vmDA fate[3, 4, 27, 37-39], however, it was reasoned that it was unlikely to be detrimental to the acquisition of a vmDA fate, so FGF8 was added for the full duration of reprogramming. Under these patterning conditions, we still did not observe the induction of endogenous *LMX1A* or *FOXA2*, and the expression of other vmDA genes such as *EN1*, *NURR1* and *PITX3* was unchanged relative to unpatterned iNPs (Figure 7B). Upon differentiation, SHH/CHIR/FGF8-patterned iNPs gave rise to higher yields of TUJ1+ cells than unpatterned iNPs (Figure 7C). The yields of AADC+/TUJ1+ cells were modestly increased in *SOX2/LMX1A*-iNPs by SHH/CHIR/FGF8-patterning, however, this was not observed in *SOX2/LMX1A/FOXA2*-iNPs, nor was a difference observed in TH+/TUJ1+ cell yields (Figure 7C).

Finally, to determine if the increased TUJ1+ and AADC+/TUJ1+ cell yields were the result of FGF8 or the result of combining *LMX1A* with patterning conditions, cells were reprogrammed with *SOX2/LMX1A* and cultured under the same patterning conditions with or without FGF8 (Figure 8A). Additionally, to determine if stronger

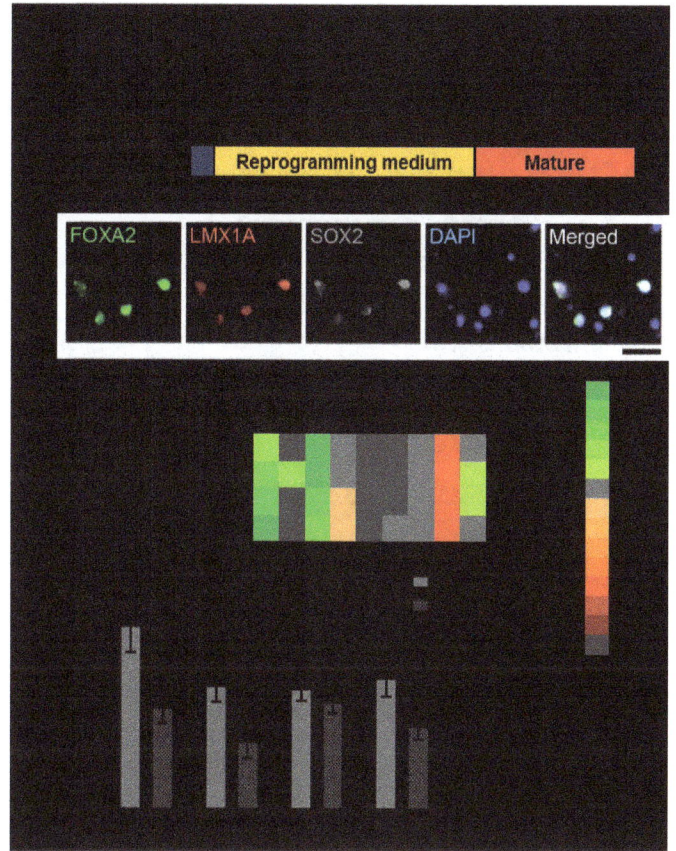

ventralisation could induce a vmDA fate, these conditions were examined with a high SHH concentration (high; 500 ng/ml) or the standard concentration (med; 200 ng/ml). Gene expression analysis showed no upregulation of endogenous vmDA markers in *SOX2/LMX1A*-iNPs (Figure 8B). Upon differentiation, both conditions cultured with FGF8 showed significantly increased yields of TUJ1+ cells compared to cells cultured in control reprogramming medium, or patterning media without FGF8, regardless of the concentration of SHH (Figure 8C). There was no significant effect of patterning on TH+/TUJ1+ and AADC+/TUJ1+ cell yields.

Discussion

This study aimed to generate vmDA neurons from adult human cells using lineage factor-mediated direct-to-iNP reprogramming. The expression of a range of vmDA markers was examined in *SOX2/PAX6*-iNPs, and it was found that iNPs expressed *PITX3* and NURR1. Additionally, iNPs could be differentiated into neuronal-like cells that expressed a range of dopaminergic markers, including TH, AADC, DAT, VMAT2 and GIRK2. This is the first report to describe the potential for adult human somatic cells to be converted into dopamine neurons *via* non-viral lineage factor-mediated direct-to-iNSC/iNP reprogramming. Previous studies have reported the generation of TH+ cells from adult human cells without further characterisation of a vmDA identity[21, 22].

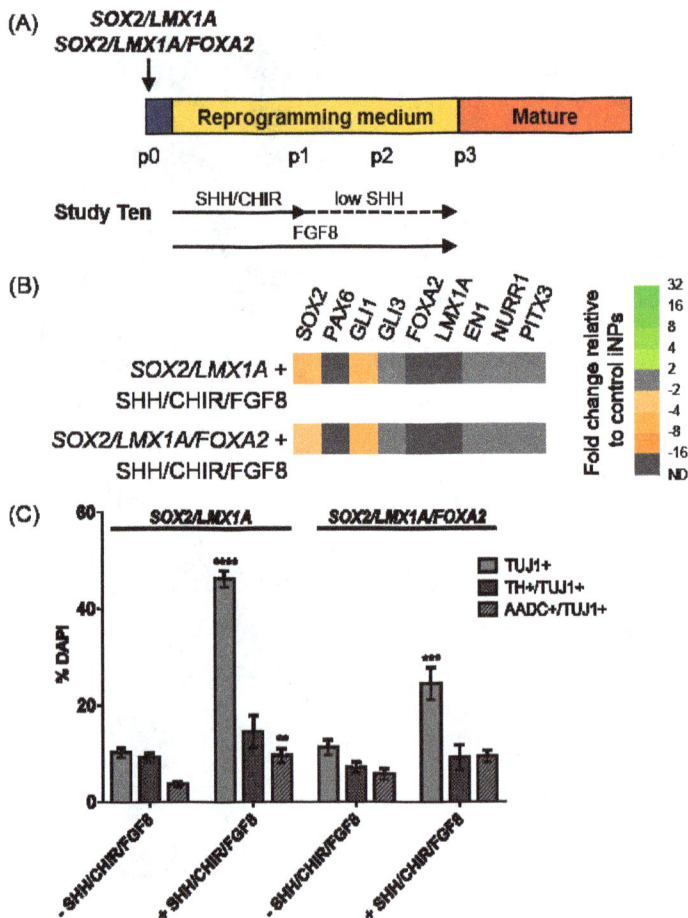

Figure 7: *Investigating the effect of combining vmDA transgenes with patterning molecules during reprogramming.(A) Schematic detailing experimental outline for Study Ten. Standard SHH concentration was 200 ng/ml, low SHH was 20 ng/ml. (B) Heat map depicting gene expression in iNPs as fold changes relative to iNPs generated with the same transgene combinations but reprogrammed in the absence of patterning cues. (C) Quantification of TUJ1+, TUJ1+/TH+ and TUJ1+/AADC+ cells in differentiated iNP cultures. Data are presented as mean ± SEM, n = 6 – 13 fields of view from one cell line (number of cells counted per condition ≥ 1559). Unpaired t-tests were performed to compare the effect of patterning with SHH/CHIR/FGF8 on differentiation yields.*

Figure 8: *Investigating the effect of FGF8 and SHH concentration during SOX2/LMX1A-mediated reprogramming. (A) Schematic detailing experimental outline for Study Eleven. High SHH concentration was 500 ng/ml, med SHH was 200 ng/ml, low SHH was 20 ng/ml. (B) Heat map depicting gene expression in iNPs at p3 as fold changes relative to SOX2/LMX1A-iNPs reprogrammed standard reprogramming medium. (C) Quantification of TUJ1+, TUJ1+/TH+ and TUJ1+/AADC+ cells in differentiated iNP cultures. Data are presented as mean ± SEM, n = 16 – 33 fields of view from one cell line (number of cells counted per condition ≥ 3066). An ordinary one way ANOVA was performed for each stain, with Tukey's multiple comparison test. Comparisons are as follows: to control iNPs (*), to med SHH/CHIR-patterned iNPs (#) or to high SHH/CHIR-patterned iNPs ($).*

As authentic A9 dopamine neurons are required for downstream applications, further optimisation of the generation of vmDA neurons was examined in healthy cells (Figure 9). While expression of many late vmDA markers was observed (NURR1, PITX3, TH, AADC, DAT, VMAT2 and GIRK2), the acquisition of a correct vmDA identity would be expected to be accompanied by the presence of early, sustained regional markers such as FOXA2, LMX1A/B, EN1 and CORIN, as well as enhanced dopaminergic differentiation. Exposure to patterning molecules is important for differentiating neural stem/precursor cells to adopt desired regional fates. SHH/FGF8 exposure to established *SOX2/PAX6*-iNPs did not enhance dopaminergic differentiation, and exposure to patterning molecules during reprogramming was insufficient to induce a true vmDA iNP fate. As PAX6 is detrimental to the generation of an authentic vmDA identity, *PAX6* was removed, and iNPs comparable to *SOX2/PAX6*-iNPs were generated from *SOX2*-transfected cells, consistent with previous studies[32, 33]. Nonetheless, exposure of patterning molecules to *SOX2*-iNPs still did not induce a true vmDA fate. Over expression of genes involved in the specification of a

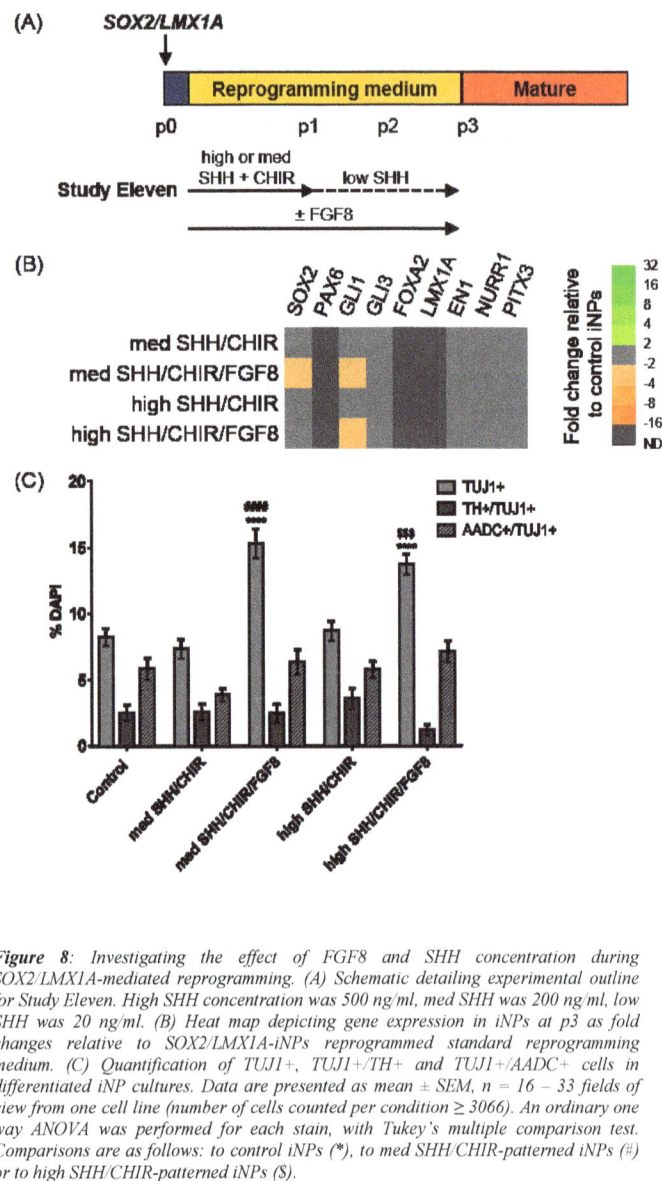

vmDA fate has been widely used in stem cell and fate conversion studies. However, the addition of exogenous *LMX1A/FOXA2* with or without patterning molecules did not induce a vmDA fate in iNPs. Exposure to FGF8b for the full duration of reprogramming increased the yield of TUJ1+ cells following differentiation, however, this effect was not specific for dopaminergic neurons. Overall, while these strategies did not induce an authentic vmDA fate in iNPs derived from adult human cells, these results are consistent with other lineage factor-mediated direct reprogramming studies[18, 38, 40, 41].

Using pluripotent factor-mediated reprogramming, rodent vmDA iNPs have been generated by adding CHIR99021, SHH, FGF8 and JI1 during reprogramming[42]. Another pluripotent factor-mediated reprogramming study derived vmDA iNSCs from adult human fibroblasts by exposure to a low concentration of SHH and FGF8[17], however the requirement for SHH/FGF8 was not examined. The success of this strategy probably lies in the fact that

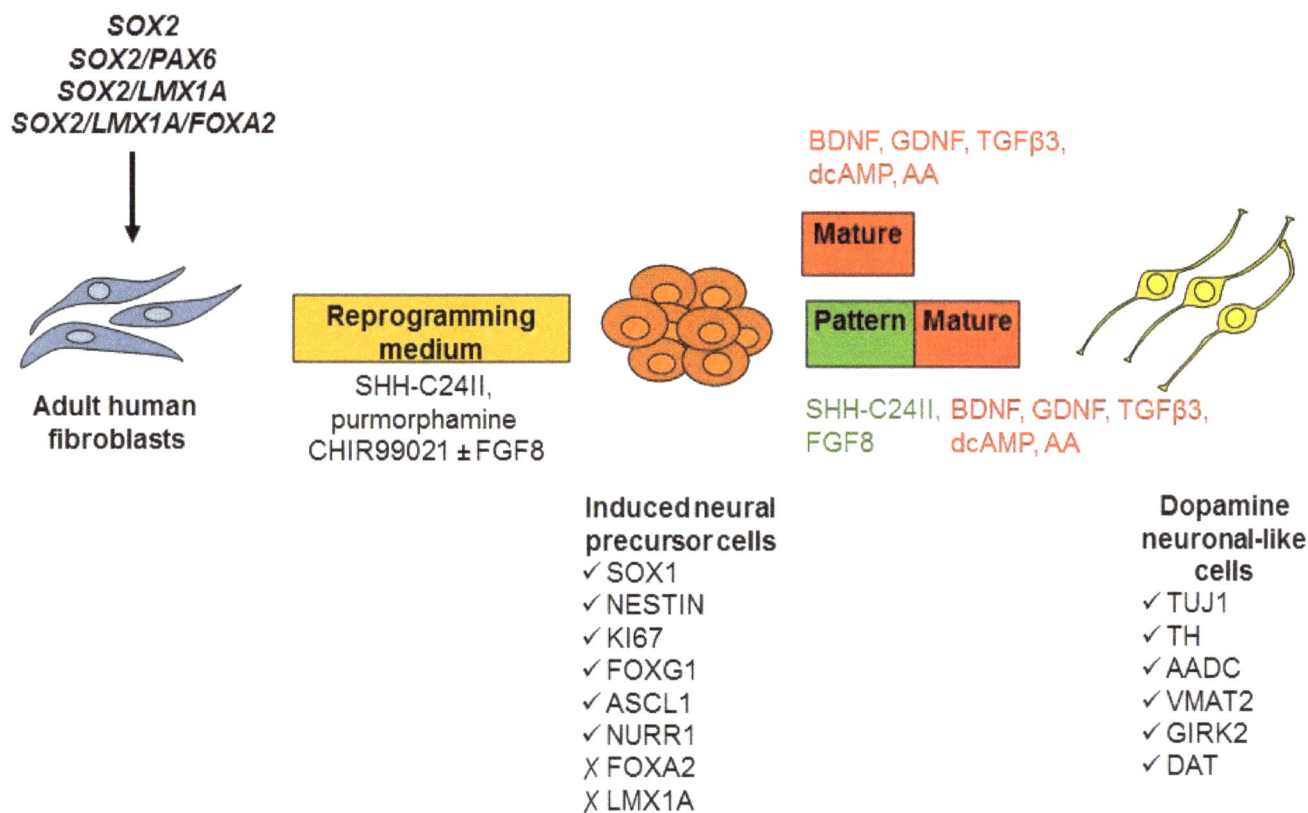

Figure 9: *Schematic overview of the experimental processes trialled to optimise the generation of vmDA neurons from human iNPs. Transfection of adult human fibroblasts with SOX2 and PAX6 followed by culture in reprogramming medium generates iNP cells that express SOX1, NESTIN, FOXG1, ASCL1 and NURR1, and can be differentiated into dopamine-like neurons positive for TH, AADC, VMAT2, GIRK2 and DAT. In order to enhance the yield and induce an authentic vmDA identity of these cells, a range of neural and dopaminergic lineage transgenes were trialled coupled with exposure to the patterning factors SHH-C24II, purmorphamine, CHIR99021 and/or FGF8 during reprogramming. The effect of exposure to the patterning factors SHH-C24II and FGF8 during the early stage of differentiation to promote a vmDA fate was also investigated. AA = ascorbic acid.*

the iNSCs were at a very primitive stage of development. LIF-dependent neural stem cells have been reported to express mesencephalic genes[43], however, iNSCs showed pluripotent characteristics and could be converted into iPSCs[17]. The reliance on pluripotency factors for reprogramming raises the question as to whether these cells are directly reprogrammed without passing through a pluripotent stage [11, 12]. If iNSCs transition through a state of pluripotency, then they do not reflect true direct reprogramming, and may be more akin to pluripotent stem cells.

Amongst the lineage factor-mediated direct-to-iNSC/iNP reprogramming studies, the precise requirements for patterning factors have not been thoroughly examined. Correlating with the findings in Study Three, a mouse iNP study reported that established iNPs did not respond to SHH/FGF8, however, addition of these molecules to the reprogramming media was not examined, and overexpression of *FOXA2* with or without *LMX1A* was required to induce vmDA genes[40]. Another rodent iNP study found that when lineage factor-reprogrammed iNPs were treated with FGF8 during reprogramming, very low numbers of TH+/TUJ1+ cells were generated, and *NURR1/FOXA2* overexpression was required to improve TH yields and induce vmDA markers[38, 41]. Due to the differences in rodent and human development, methods for fate specification in rodent cells may not be directly applicable to human cells.

Only one other study has attempted to generate vmDA iNPs by lineage factor-mediated reprogramming in human cells[18]. This group took a similar approach to the present study, adding CHIR99021 and purmorphamine to the reprogramming medium during non-viral

SOX2-mediated reprogramming of human post-natal fibroblasts[18, 33]. The requirement of these small molecules was not reported, only the effect of a cocktail of small molecules[33] or the effect of the addition of LMX1A[18]. Furthermore, the authenticity of the vmDA fate of iNPs generated by this method is unclear; while iNPs expressed SOX2, LMX1A and FOXA2, PAX6 was also expressed, suggesting that iNPs do not represent authentic vmDA progenitors[18]. Additionally, the long-term maintenance of a vmDA iNP fate in the absence of exogenous LMX1A was not shown, and the yields of TH+ neurons were not reported[18].

Currently, the derivation of authentic vmDA iNPs from adult human cells *via* lineage factor-mediated direct reprogramming remains elusive. In the present study, the addition of *LMX1A/FOXA2* to the reprogramming cocktail, with or without exposure to patterning factors, did not induce a vmDA progenitor fate. The transient nature of plasmid transfection may mean that transgenes are not expressed for sufficient time to initiate endogenous vmDA-related gene expression programs, or that any changes induced by *LMX1A/FOXA2* are not sustained in the long-term. While the use of transiently expressed, non-integrating vectors presents advantages for clinical translation, this strategy may be insufficient for generating vmDA progenitors from adult human fibroblasts, which are more difficult to reprogram than younger cells[23]. Future work could investigate the use of alternative gene expression systems, such as lentiviruses, stabilised RNA or Sendai viruses. Sustained, widespread transgene expression combined with patterning molecules may be effective at inducing a vmDA progenitor fate in directly reprogrammed adult human iNPs. Recent chemical reprogramming studies suggest that reprogramming efficiency could be improved by targeting certain pathways, such as the SHH, FGF2 pathways; inhibition of cellular senescence, autophagy, Rho/ROCK, TGFβ and GSK3β signalling pathways; the use of additional epigenetic modifiers; and hypoxia and/or antioxidant use[44-48].

The present study drew from patterning strategies employed in pluripotent stem cells to reprogram to a vmDA iNP fate. However, direct reprogramming, especially in adult cells, may require more powerful cues to induce desired fates. vmDA progenitors arise early in development, prior to the formation of the neuroectoderm. Future studies should, therefore, specifically aim to generate midbrain floor plate progenitors, rather than attempt to adapt methods for generating neuroepithelial-like precursors. This might be achieved through the use of potent SHH signalling and/or sustained *GLI1* or *FOXA2* overexpression[49], along with WNT1 signalling and/or *LMX1A* overexpression. However, signalling through these pathways was examined in the present study and found to be insufficient. Additional chemical components may be required to not only improve reprogramming efficiency, but also to induce the correct regional fate. Default anterior neuroectoderm specification might be targeted by blocking DKK1 expression[31]. Signalling through the p38 MAPK and JAK2/STAT3 pathways has recently been implicated in floor plate specification from human pluripotent stem cells[50].

Conclusion

Direct-to-iNSC/iNP reprogramming is a relatively new technology that offers a number of potential advantages over iPSCs and iN cells for the study and treatment of PD. This study has demonstrated for the first time that healthy adult human fibroblasts can be reprogrammed by non-viral lineage factor-mediated reprogramming into iNPs, capable of giving rise to dopamine neuronal-like cells. However, the expression of early vmDA regional markers was not seen in iNPs. Exposure to patterning molecules and/or vmDA transgenes was insufficient to induce an authentic vmDA fate in iNPs. Nevertheless, this study indicates that direct-to-iNSC/iNP reprogramming by lineage factors may be suitable for modelling PD *in vitro* using aged donor-derived cells. Future studies may improve the vmDA fate of derived cells by optimising gene expression systems and investigating the effect of chemical agents on reprogramming.

References

1. Playne R, Connor B. Understanding Parkinson's Disease through the Use of Cell Reprogramming. Stem Cell Rev. 2017;13(2):151-69.
2. Barker RA, Drouin-Ouellet J, Parmar M. Cell-based therapies for Parkinson disease—past insights and future potential. Nat Rev Neurol. 2015;11(9):492-503.
3. Kriks S, Shim JW, Piao J, Ganat YM, Wakeman DR, Xie Z, Carrillo-Reid L, Auyeung G, Antonacci C, Buch A, Yang L, Beal MF, Surmeier DJ, Kordower JH, Tabar V, Studer L. Dopamine neurons derived from human ES cells efficiently engraft in animal models of Parkinson's disease. Nature. 2011;480(7378):547-51.
4. Kirkeby A, Grealish S, Wolf DA, Nelander J, Wood J, Lundblad M, Lindvall O, Parmar M. Generation of regionally specified neural progenitors and functional neurons from human embryonic stem cells under defined conditions. Cell Rep. 2012;1(6):703-14.
5. Mertens J, Marchetto MC, Bardy C, Gage FH. Evaluating cell reprogramming, differentiation and conversion technologies in neuroscience. Nat Rev Neurosci.2016;17(7):424-37.
6. Miller JD, Ganat YM, Kishinevsky S, Bowman RL, Liu B, Tu EY, Mandal PK, Vera E, Shim JW, Kriks S, Taldone T, Fusaki N, Tomishima MJ, Krainc D, Milner TA, Rossi DJ, Studer L. Human iPSC-based modeling of late-onset disease via progerin-induced aging. Cell Stem Cell. 2013;13(6):691-705.
7. Pang ZP, Yang N, Vierbuchen T, Ostermeier A, Fuentes DR, Yang TQ, Citri A, Sebastiano V, Marro S, Südhof TC, Wernig M. Induction of human neuronal cells by defined transcription factors. Nature. 2011;476(7359):220-3.
8. Liu ML, Zang T, Zou Y, Chang JC, Gibson JR, Huber KM, Zhang CL. Small molecules enable neurogenin 2 to efficiently convert human fibroblasts into cholinergic neurons. Nat Commun. 2013;4:2183.
9. Guo Z, Zhang L, Wu Z, Chen Y, Wang F, Chen G. In vivo direct reprogramming of reactive glial cells into functional neurons after brain injury and in an Alzheimer's disease model. Cell Stem Cell. 2014;14(2):188-202.
10. Torper O, Ottosson DR, Pereira M, Lau S, Cardoso T, Grealish S, Parmar M. In Vivo Reprogramming of Striatal NG2 Glia into Functional Neurons that Integrate into Local Host Circuitry. Cell Rep. 2015;12(3):474-81.
11. Maza I, Caspi I, Zviran A, Chomsky E, Rais Y, Viukov S, Geula S, Buenrostro JD, Weinberger L, Krupalnik V, Hanna S, Zerbib M, Dutton JR, Greenleaf WJ, Massarwa R, Novershtern N, Hanna JH. Transient acquisition of pluripotency during somatic cell transdifferentiation with iPSC reprogramming factors. Nat Biotechnol. 2015;33(7):769-74.
12. Bar-Nur O, Verheul C, Sommer AG, Brumbaugh J, Schwarz BA, Lipchina I, Huebner AJ, Mostoslavsky G, Hochedlinger K. Lineage conversion induced by pluripotency factors involves transient passage through an iPSC stage. Nat Biotechnol. 2015;33(7):761-8.
13. Weissbein U, Ben-David U, Benvenisty N. Virtual karyotyping reveals greater chromosomal stability in neural cells derived by transdifferentiation than those from stem cells. Cell Stem Cell. 2014;15(6):687-91.
14. Wang L, Wang L, Huang W, Su H, Xue Y, Su Z, Liao B, Wang H, Bao X, Qin D, He J, Wu W, So KF, Pan G, Pei D. Generation of integration-free neural progenitor cells from cells in human urine. Nat Methods. 2013;10(1):84-9.
15. Lu J, Liu H, Huang CT, Chen H, Du Z, Liu Y, Sherafat MA, Zhang SC. Generation of integration-free and region-specific neural progenitors from primate fibroblasts. Cell Rep. 2013;3(5):1580-91.
16. Zhu S, Ambasudhan R, Sun W, Kim HJ, Talantova M, Wang X, Zhang M, Zhang Y, Laurent T, Parker J, Kim HS, Zaremba JD, Saleem S, Sanz-Blasco S, Masliah E, McKercher SR, Cho YS, Lipton SA, Kim J, Ding S. Small molecules enable OCT4-mediated direct reprogramming into expandable human neural stem cells. Cell Res. 2014;24(1):126-9.
17. Miura T, Sugawara T, Fukuda A, Tamoto R, Kawasaki T, Umezawa A, Akutsu H. Generation of primitive neural stem cells from human fibroblasts using a defined set of factors. Biol Open. 2015;4(11):1595-607.
18. Mirakhori F, Zeynali B, Rassouli H, Salekdeh GH, Baharvand H. Direct conversion of human fibroblasts into dopaminergic neural progenitor-like cells using TAT-mediated protein transduction of recombinant factors. Biochem Biophys Res Commun. 2015;459(4):655-61.
19. Zou Q, Yan Q, Zhong J, Wang K, Sun H, Yi X, Lai L. Direct conversion of human fibroblasts into neuronal restricted progenitors. J Biol Chem. 2014;289(8):5250-60.
20. Shahbazi E, Moradi S, Nemati S, Satarian L, Basiri M, Gourabi H, Zare Mehrjardi N, Günther P, Lampert A, Händler K, Hatay FF, Schmidt D, Molcanyi M, Hescheler J, Schultze JL, Saric T, Baharvand H. Conversion of Human Fibroblasts to Stably Self-Renewing Neural Stem Cells with a Single Zinc-Finger Transcription Factor. Stem Cell Reports. 2016;6(4):539-51.
21. Maucksch C, Firmin E, Butler-Munro C, Montgomery J, Dottori M, Connor B. Non-Viral Generation of Neural Precursor-like Cells from Adult Human Fibroblasts. J Stem Cells Regen Med. 2012;8(3):162-70.
22. Yu KR, Shin JH, Kim JJ, Koog MG, Lee JY, Choi SW, Kim HS, Seo Y, Lee S, Shin TH, Jee MK, Kim DW, Jung SJ, Shin S, Han DW, Kang KS. Rapid and Efficient Direct Conversion of Human Adult Somatic Cells into Neural Stem Cells by HMGA2/let-7b. Cell Rep. 2015. pii: S2211-1247(14)01067-5

23. Trokovic R, Weltner J, Noisa P, Raivio T, Otonkoski T. Combined negative effect of donor age and time in culture on the reprogramming efficiency into induced pluripotent stem cells. Stem Cell Res. 2015;15(1):254-62.

24. Connor B, Firmin E, Maucksch C, Liu R, Playne R, Jones K, Dottori M. Direct Conversion of Adult Human Fibroblasts into Induced Neural Precursor Cells by Non-Viral Transfection. Protoc Exch. 2015. doi 10.1038/protex.2015.034

25. Pfisterer U, Kirkeby A, Torper O, Wood J, Nelander J, Dufour A, Björklund A, Lindvall O, Jakobsson J, Parmar M. Direct conversion of human fibroblasts to dopaminergic neurons. Proc Natl Acad Sci U S A. 2011;108(25):10343-8.

26. Livak KJ,. Schmittgen TD. Analysis of relative gene expression data using real-time quantitative PCR and the 2−ΔΔCT method. Methods 2001. 25(4): p. 402-08.

27. Xi J, Liu Y, Liu H, Chen H, Emborg ME, Zhang SC. Specification of midbrain dopamine neurons from primate pluripotent stem cells. Stem Cells. 2012;30(8):1655-63.

28. Denham M, Bye C, Leung J, Conley BJ, Thompson LH, Dottori M. Glycogen synthase kinase 3β and activin/nodal inhibition in human embryonic stem cells induces a pre-neuroepithelial state that is required for specification to a floor plate cell lineage. Stem Cells. 2012;30(11):2400-11.

29. Vitalis T, Cases O, Engelkamp D, Verney C, Price DJ. Defect of tyrosine hydroxylase-immunoreactive neurons in the brains of mice lacking the transcription factor Pax6. J Neurosci. 2000;20(17):6501-16.

30. Kirkeby A, Parmar M. Building authentic midbrain dopaminergic neurons from stem cells - lessons from development. Transl Neurosci, 2012. 3(4): p. 314-19.

31. Fasano CA, Chambers SM, Lee G, Tomishima MJ, Studer L. Efficient derivation of functional floor plate tissue from human embryonic stem cells. Cell Stem Cell. 2010;6(4):336-47.

32. Ring KL, Tong LM, Balestra ME, Javier R, Andrews-Zwilling Y, Li G, Walker D, Zhang WR, Kreitzer AC, Huang Y. Direct reprogramming of mouse and human fibroblasts into multipotent neural stem cells with a single factor. Cell Stem Cell. 2012;11(1):100-9.

33. Mirakhori F, Zeynali B, Rassouli H, Shahbazi E, Hashemizadeh S, Kiani S, Salekdeh GH, Baharvand H. Induction of Neural Progenitor-Like Cells from Human Fibroblasts via a Genetic Material-Free Approach. PLoS One. 2015;10(8):e0135479.

34. Moya N, Cutts J, Gaasterland T, Willert K, Brafman DA. Endogenous WNT signaling regulates hPSC-derived neural progenitor cell heterogeneity and specifies their regional identity. Stem Cell Reports. 2014;3(6):1015-28.

35. Andersson E, Tryggvason U, Deng Q, Friling S, Alekseenko Z, Robert B, Perlmann T, Ericson J. Identification of intrinsic determinants of midbrain dopamine neurons. Cell. 2006;124(2):393-405.

36. Panman L, Andersson E, Alekseenko Z, Hedlund E, Kee N, Mong J, Uhde CW, Deng Q, Sandberg R, Stanton LW, Ericson J, Perlmann T. Transcription factor-induced lineage selection of stem-cell-derived neural progenitor cells. Cell Stem Cell. 2011;8(6):663-75.

37. Cooper O, Hargus G, Deleidi M, Blak A, Osborn T, Marlow E, Lee K, Levy A, Perez-Torres E, Yow A, Isacson O. Differentiation of human ES and Parkinson's disease iPS cells into ventral midbrain dopaminergic neurons requires a high activity form of SHH, FGF8a and specific regionalization by retinoic acid. Mol Cell Neurosci. 2010;45(3):258-66.

38. Lim MS, Lee SY, Park CH. FGF8 is Essential for Functionality of Induced Neural Precursor Cell-derived Dopaminergic Neurons. Int J Stem Cells. 2015;8(2):228-34.

39. Kirkeby A, Nolbrant S, Tiklova K, Heuer A, Kee N, Cardoso T, Ottosson DR, Lelos MJ, Rifes P, Dunnett SB, Grealish S, Perlmann T, Parmar M. Predictive Markers Guide Differentiation to Improve Graft Outcome in Clinical Translation of hESC-Based Therapy for Parkinson's Disease. Cell Stem Cell. 2017;20(1):135-48.

40. Tian C, Li Y, Huang Y, Wang Y, Chen D, Liu J, Deng X, Sun L, Anderson K, Qi X, Li Y, Mosley RL, Chen X, Huang J, Zheng JC. Selective Generation of Dopaminergic Precursors from Mouse Fibroblasts by Direct Lineage Conversion. Sci Rep. 2015;5:12622.

41. Lim MS, Chang MY, Kim SM, Yi SH, Suh-Kim H, Jung SJ, Kim MJ, Kim JH, Lee YS, Lee SY, Kim DW, Lee SH, Park CH. Generation of Dopamine Neurons from Rodent Fibroblasts through the Expandable Neural Precursor Cell Stage. J Biol Chem. 2015;290(28):17401-14.

42. Kim HS, Kim J, Jo Y, Jeon D, Cho YS. Direct lineage reprogramming of mouse fibroblasts to functional midbrain dopaminergic neuronal progenitors. Stem Cell Res. 2014;12(1):60-8.

43. Li W, Sun W, Zhang Y, Wei W, Ambasudhan R, Xia P, Talantova M, Lin T, Kim J, Wang X, Kim WR, Lipton SA, Zhang K, Ding S. Rapid induction and long-term self-renewal of primitive neural precursors from human embryonic stem cells by small molecule inhibitors. Proc Natl Acad Sci U S A. 2011;108(20):8299-304.

44. Li Y, Zhang Q, Yin X, Yang W, Du Y, Hou P, Ge J, Liu C, Zhang W, Zhang X, Wu Y, Li H, Liu K, Wu C, Song Z, Zhao Y, Shi Y, Deng H. Generation of iPSCs from mouse fibroblasts with a single gene, Oct4, and small molecules. Cell Res. 2011;21(1):196-204.

45. Cheng L, Hu W, Qiu B, Zhao J, Yu Y, Guan W, Wang M, Yang W, Pei G. Generation of neural progenitor cells by chemical cocktails and hypoxia. Cell Res. 2014;24(6):665-79.

46. Hu W, Qiu B, Guan W, Wang Q, Wang M, Li W, Gao L, Shen L, Huang Y, Xie G, Zhao H, Jin Y, Tang B, Yu Y, Zhao J, Pei G. Direct Conversion of Normal and Alzheimer's Disease Human Fibroblasts into Neuronal Cells by Small Molecules. Cell Stem Cell. 2015;17(2):204-12.

47. Zhang M, Lin YH, Sun YJ, Zhu S, Zheng J, Liu K, Cao N, Li K, Huang Y, Ding S. Pharmacological Reprogramming of Fibroblasts into Neural Stem Cells by Signaling-Directed Transcriptional Activation. Cell Stem Cell. 2016;18(5):653-67.

48. Zheng J, Choi KA, Kang PJ, Hyeon S, Kwon S, Moon JH, Hwang I, Kim YI, Kim YS, Yoon BS, Park G, Lee J, Hong S, You S. A combination of small molecules directly reprograms mouse fibroblasts into neural stem cells. Biochem Biophys Res Commun. 2016;476(1):42-8.

49. Denham M, Thompson LH, Leung J, Pébay A, Björklund A, Dottori M. Gli1 is an inducing factor in generating floor plate progenitor cells from human embryonic stem cells. Stem Cells. 2010;28(10):1805-15.

50. Chi L, Fan B, Zhang K, Du Y, Liu Z, Fang Y, Chen Z, Ren X, Xu X, Jiang C, Li S, Ma L, Gao L, Liu L, Zhang X. Targeted Differentiation of Regional Ventral Neuroprogenitors and Related Neuronal Subtypes from Human Pluripotent Stem Cells. Stem Cell Reports. 2016;7(5):941-54.

Abbreviations

PD	Parkinson's disease
vmDA	Ventral midbrain dopamine neuron
iNP	Induced neural precursor cell
TH	Tyrosine hydroxylase
FGF8b	Fibroblast growth factor 8b
iPSC	Induced pluripotent stem cell
iN	Induced neuron
iNSC	Induced neural stem cell
NSE	Neuron specific enolase
EGF	Epidermal growth factor
SHH	Sonic hedgehog
BDNF	Brain-derived neurotrophic factor
GDNF	Glial-derived neurotrophic factor
TGFβ3	Transforming growth factor β3
AADC	Aromatic L-amino acid decarboxylase
VMAT2	Vesicular monoamine transporter 2
DAT	Dopamine transporter
TUJ1	Beta-3 tubulin
PUR	Purmorphamine
CHIR	CHIR99021

Potential Conflicts of Interests

None

Acknowledgements

Neurological Foundation of New Zealand

Corresponding Author

Bronwen Connor, Dept of Pharmacology & Clinical Pharmacology, Centre for Brain Research, FMHS, University of Auckland, Private Bag 90219, Auckland 1142, New Zealand; Email: b.connor@auckland.ac.nz

Permissions

The contributors of this book come from diverse backgrounds, making this book a truly international effort. This book will bring forth new frontiers with its revolutionizing research information and detailed analysis of the nascent developments around the world.

We would like to thank all the contributing authors for lending their expertise to make the book truly unique. They have played a crucial role in the development of this book. Without their invaluable contributions this book wouldn't have been possible. They have made vital efforts to compile up to date information on the varied aspects of this subject to make this book a valuable addition to the collection of many professionals and students.

This book was conceptualized with the vision of imparting up-to-date information and advanced data in this field. To ensure the same, a matchless editorial board was set up. Every individual on the board went through rigorous rounds of assessment to prove their worth. After which they invested a large part of their time researching and compiling the most relevant data for our readers.

The editorial board has been involved in producing this book since its inception. They have spent rigorous hours researching and exploring the diverse topics which have resulted in the successful publishing of this book. They have passed on their knowledge of decades through this book. To expedite this challenging task, the publisher supported the team at every step. A small team of assistant editors was also appointed to further simplify the editing procedure and attain best results for the readers.

Apart from the editorial board, the designing team has also invested a significant amount of their time in understanding the subject and creating the most relevant covers. They scrutinized every image to scout for the most suitable representation of the subject and create an appropriate cover for the book.

The publishing team has been an ardent support to the editorial, designing and production team. Their endless efforts to recruit the best for this project, has resulted in the accomplishment of this book. They are a veteran in the field of academics and their pool of knowledge is as vast as their experience in printing. Their expertise and guidance has proved useful at every step. Their uncompromising quality standards have made this book an exceptional effort. Their encouragement from time to time has been an inspiration for everyone.

The publisher and the editorial board hope that this book will prove to be a valuable piece of knowledge for researchers, students, practitioners and scholars across the globe.

List of Contributors

Stephany Cares Huber, José Luiz Rosenberis Cunha Júnior, Silmara Montalvão, Letícia Queiroz da Silva, Aline Urban Paffaro, Francesca Aparecida Ramos da Silva, Bruno Lima Rodrigues, José Fabio Santos Duarte Lana and Joyce Maria Annichinno-Bizzacchi
Hemocentro, Haemostasis Laboratory, State University of Campinas UNICAMP, Brazil

Hayam Hussein, Jennifer Dulin, Lauren Smanik, Mohamed Azab and Alicia L. Bertone
Department of Veterinary Clinical Sciences, College of Veterinary Medicine, The Ohio State University, Columbus, OH, USA

Prosper Boyaka, Duncan Russell and Alicia L. Bertone
Department of Veterinary Biosciences, College of Veterinary Medicine, The Ohio State University, Columbus, OH, USA

Andrei Kochegarov and Larry F Lemanski
Department of Biological and Environmental Sciences, Texas A&M University-Commerce, Commerce, Texas, USA

Kenyon S. Tweedell
Department of Biological Sciences, University of Notre Dame, Notre Dame IN 46556 USA

Stoyan G Petkov
German Primate Center, Goettingen, Germany

Silke Glage
Hannover Medical School, Hannover, Germany

Heiner Niemann
Institute for Farm Animal Genetics (FLI), Neustadt, Germany

Baldeep Chani and Sanjeev Puri
Centre for Stem Cell & Tissue Engineering; University Institute of Engineering & Technology, Panjab University, Chandigarh, India

Veena Puri
Systems Biology & Bioinformatics;University Institute of Engineering & Technology, Panjab University, Chandigarh, India

Ranbir Chander Sobti
Biotechnology Department; Biotechnology branch, University Institute of Engineering & Technology, Panjab University, Chandigarh, India

Alexey Yu Lupatov and Konstantin N Yarygin
Institute of Biomedical Chemistry, Moscow, Russia

Rimma A Poltavtseva, Oxana A Bystrykh and Gennady T Sukhikh
Research Center of Obstetrics, Gynecology and Perinatology, Moscow, Russia

Ashu Bhasin, Rohit Bhatia and M V Padma Srivastava
Department of Neurology, All India Institute of Medical Sciences (AIIMS), New Delhi, India

Senthil S. Kumaran
Department of NMR, All India Institute of Medical Sciences (AIIMS), New Delhi, India

Sujata Mohanty
Stem Cell Facility, All India Institute of Medical Sciences (AIIMS), New Delhi, India

Alessandro Bertolo, David Pavlicek, Armin Gemperli and Jivko Stoyanov
Swiss Paraplegic Research, Nottwil, Switzerland

Armin Gemperli
Department of Health Sciences and Health Policy, University of Lucerne, Lucerne, Switzerland,

Martin Baur and Tobias Pötzel
Cantonal Hospital of Lucerne, Lucerne, Switzerland

Martin Baur
Swiss Paraplegic Centre, Nottwil, Switzerland

Jivko Stoyanov
Institute for Surgical Technology and Biomechanics, University of Bern, Bern, Switzerland,
Center for Applied Biotechnology and Molecular Medicine, University of Zurich, Zurich, Switzerland

José F. S. D. Lana, Eduardo F. Vicente and Stephany Cares Huber
Bone and Cartilage Institute – (IOC) Indaiatuba – Brazil

Steve E. Sampson
David Geffen School of Medicine at UCLA – USA

Adam Weglein
Regenerative Ortho Med Clinic – USA

José F. S. D. Lana, Clarissa V. Souza, William D. Belangero and Clarissa V. Souza
Institute of Orthopedics and Traumatology of University of Campinas (UNICAMP) - Brazil

Mary A. Ambach
Orthohealing Center – USA

Hunter Vincent
Department of Physical Medicine and Rehabilitation: UC Davis

Aline Urban-Paffaro, Stephany Cares Huber, Carolina M. K. Onodera and Joyce M. Annichino-Bizzacchi
Hemocentro of Campinas, University of Campinas (UNICAMP)- Brazil

Maria Helena A. Santana
School of Chemical Engineering University of Campinas (UNICAMP) – Brazil

Takumi Takeuchi, Akiko Tonooka, Yumiko Okuno, Mami Hattori-Kato and Koji Mikami
Department of Urology, Kanto Rosai Hospital, Kizukisumiyoshi-cho, Nakahara-ku, Kawasaki, Japan Department of Pathology, Kanto Rosai Hospital, Kizukisumiyoshi-cho, Nakahara-ku, Kawasaki, Japan

Tao Lihong
Wisconsin National Primate Research Center, University of Wisconsin, Madison, WI, USA

Togarrati Padma Priya
Cell Therapy Core, Blood Systems Research Institute, San Francisco, CA, U.S.A

Choi Kyung-Dal
Lillehei Heart Institute, Department of Medicine, University of Minnesota, Minneapolis, MN, USA

Suknuntha Kran
Department of Pharmacology, Faculty of Science, Mahidol University, Bangkok, Thailand

Swapan Kumar Maiti and Naveen Kumar
Principal Scientist, Surgery Division, Indian Veterinary Research Institute, Izatnagar, 243122, Uttar-Pradesh, India

Ajantha Ravindran Ninu, Palakkara Sangeetha, Dayamon D Mathew and Paramasivam Tamilmahan
Ph.D Scholars, Surgery Division, Indian Veterinary Research Institute, Izatnagar, 243122, Uttar-Pradesh, India

Deepika Kritaniya
Senior Research Fellow, Surgery Division, Indian Veterinary Research Institute, Izatnagar, 243122, Uttar-Pradesh, India

Jurgen Hescheler
Director, Institute of Neurophysiology, Universität zu Köln, Robert-Koch-Strasse 39, D-50931, Köln, Germany

Kathryn S. Jones and Bronwen J. Connor
Centre for Brain Research, Department of Pharmacology and Clinical Pharmacology, School of Medical Science, Faculty of Medical and Health Sciences, University of Auckland

Muhammad Mehdi Amirrasouli
Department of Cardiovascular Medicine, Institute of Genetic Medicine, International centre for life, School of Medicine, Newcastle University, UK

Muhammad Mehdi Amirrasouli and Mehdi Shamsara
National Institute of Genetic Engineering and Biotechnology (NIGEB), Shahrak-e- Pajoohesh, 15th Km, Tehran -Karaj Highway, Tehran, Iran

Muhammad Mehdi Amirrasouli
Molecular Genetics Department, Ghanoon Medial Laboratory, West Hakim highway, Tehran, Iran

Fatma M. Elhusseini
Pathology Department, Mansoura University, Mansoura, Egypt

Mohamed-Ahdy A.A. Saad
Pharmacology Department, Mansoura University, Mansoura, Egypt

Nahla Anber
Emergancy Hospital, Mansoura University, Mansoura, Egypt

Doaa Elghannam and Hassan Abdel-Ghaffar
Clinical Pathology, Mansoura University, Mansoura, Egypt

Mohamed-Ahmed Sobh
Zoology-Urology and Nephrology Center, Mansoura University, Mansoura, Egypt

Hussein Sheashaa and Mohamed Sobh
Urology and Nephrology Center, Mansoura University, Mansoura, Egypt

Aziza Alsayed and Sara El-dusoky
Medical Experimental Research Center (MERC), Faculty of Medicine, Mansoura University, Mansoura, Egypt

Samiksha Mahapatra, Dianna Martin and G. Ian Gallicano
Department of Biochemistry and Molecular Biology, Georgetown University Medical Center, 3900 Reservoir Rd, Washington, DC, USA

Jan Philipp Krüger, Sylvia Hondke and Michaela Endres
TransTissue Technologies GmbH, 10117 Berlin, Germany

Andreas Enz, Alice Wichelhaus and Thomas Mittlmeier
Department of Trauma, Hand and Reconstructive Surgery, Universitätsmedizin Rostock, 18057 Rostock, Germany

Naresh Kumar Tripathy, Syed Husain Mustafa Rizvi, Saurabh Pratap Singh, Venkata Naga Srikanth Garikipati and Soniya Nityanand
Stem Cell Research Facility, Department of Hematology, Sanjay Gandhi Post-Graduate Institute of Medical Sciences (SGPGIMS), Raebareli Road, Lucknow-226014, India

Rebecca Playne, Kathryn Jones and Bronwen Connor
Department of Pharmacology & Clinical Pharmacology, Centre for Brain Research, Faculty of Medical and Health Sciences, University of Auckland, Auckland, New Zealand

Index

A

Acute Kidney Injury, 137, 148-149

Adipogenic Lineage, 46, 51-52

Alkaline Phosphatase, 10-12, 14, 38, 44

Angiogenesis, 1, 7, 20-21, 63, 68, 95, 127, 129, 133-134, 152

B

Bladder Tissue, 92-93, 95

Bone Marrow, 9-10, 13-16, 18, 21-22, 24-27, 30, 33, 53, 55-57, 61, 63-64, 67-71, 80-81, 91-92, 98, 103-104, 113-115, 137, 147-148, 150, 163, 165, 173, 175, 179-180

Bone Marrow Stem, 14, 18, 21, 24, 103, 114, 150, 163

Bone Morphogenetic Protein, 25, 35, 103, 113-115

Bone Resorption, 9, 14-16

C

Cardiac Progenitors, 127, 129

Cardiogenesis, 20, 150, 180

Cardiomyocyte, 19-24, 41, 135, 150, 152-154, 163-165, 180

Cardiosphere, 21, 24-25, 127-128, 135

Cardiosphere-derived Cells, 21, 24-25, 127, 135

Cathepsin K, 9-10, 12, 14-16

Cell Recruitment, 116, 123, 127

Cell Therapy, 18, 21, 24, 55, 60, 63, 66-68, 80-81, 90, 127, 134-135, 137, 148, 163, 175, 180-181

Chondrocytes, 9-10, 12, 21, 69, 89, 135, 167, 172-174

Cisplatin, 96, 137, 139, 142-148

Clonal Subpopulations, 175, 179

Coronary Heart Disease, 127, 135

Cytokine, 7, 14, 27, 69-71, 73, 79-81, 90, 152

Cytokine Osteopontin, 27

D

Dendritic Cells, 14, 55, 58-59, 61-62

Doxycycline, 37, 44

E

Electro-resection, 92-93, 95-96

Embryoid Body, 39

Embryonic Stem Cell, 23-24, 31, 68, 98-99, 101, 151, 155, 164-165, 182

Epigallocatechin Gallate, 46, 53

Equine Bone, 9-10, 13-15

Excitotoxic Brain Injury, 116

Exogenous Thrombin, 2

Explant-derived Cell, 127

Extracellular Matrix, 10, 19, 26-27, 35, 82, 89, 169, 173

F

Fetal Bovine Serum, 38, 44, 53, 70, 81, 115, 138, 149, 175

Fibroblasts, 16, 20, 37-38, 43-44, 79, 90, 99, 114, 150, 155, 157-158, 164-165, 167, 182-191

G

Gel Formation, 1-2, 6-7

Gene Expression, 9-14, 20, 37-38, 41-42, 51-53, 60-61, 79, 81, 99, 116-117, 124, 132, 135, 150, 156-158, 162, 165, 169, 172-173, 179-180, 184-191

Glutathione, 137, 147, 149

Granulocyte, 27, 56, 58, 62, 69, 71, 73, 81, 99

Growth Factor, 1-4, 6-7, 19-20, 22-25, 27, 30, 35, 55-56, 62, 69-71, 89-91, 103, 113-114, 129, 133, 135, 151-152, 164, 166, 169, 173-174, 180, 192

H

Heart Failure, 18, 21, 163

Hematopoietic Cells, 21, 57, 98-99

Hematopoietic Progenitor, 98, 100-101

Hematopoietic Stem Cells, 21, 26, 33, 98, 101

Human Embryonic Stem Cell, 31, 98-99, 101, 151, 165, 182

Hyaluronic Acid, 82, 84-85, 89-91

Hypoxia, 127-135, 190-191

I

Immunocytochemistry, 38, 56, 130, 183, 186-187

Immunomodulation, 55, 61, 69-70, 79-80, 137

Immunomodulatory Mechanism, 69

Immunomodulatory Potential, 69-70, 79

Immunosuppression Therapy, 22

Inflammation, 1, 9, 15-16, 21, 52, 55, 73, 81, 84-85, 89, 118, 125, 135, 167

Interleukin, 69-71, 73, 80-81

J

Joint Pathology, 82

K

Karyotyping, 39-40, 190

L

Leukocytes, 1-2, 7, 84-85, 88-89

Lymphocytes, 16, 21, 29, 55, 79, 81, 93-95, 98, 101

M

Macrophage, 14, 16, 27, 56, 58, 62, 69, 71, 73, 81, 99

Mammary Gland, 31-34

Mesenchymal Stem Cell, 10, 16, 24, 46-48, 51-53, 63, 67, 73, 80, 103, 115, 140, 148, 163, 180-181

Monocyte Differentiation, 55-57

Monothioglycerol, 99

Myocardial Damage, 21-22

N

Neural Stem, 29-30, 33-35, 55, 57-62, 67, 117, 124, 183, 188-192

Neuregulin, 19-20, 23, 25, 150, 152, 166

Neuroblast, 29, 56, 67, 116-117, 119-120, 123-124

Neurodegenerative Diseases, 46, 53, 55

Neuroepithelium, 56, 164

O

Obesity, 46, 52-53

Oligodendrocyte Progenitor Cell, 116

Osteoarthritis, 9, 15, 82, 90-91, 167, 172-174

Osteoblast, 9, 14-16, 27, 29, 112, 114

Osteoclast, 9-10, 13, 15-16

Osteogenic Differentiation, 9-10, 14-15, 103, 112, 114, 138-141, 169, 177

Osteoporosis, 9, 15

Oxidative Stress, 18, 52, 137, 139, 142-143, 147-148

P

Peripheral Blood Mononuclear Cells, 69-70, 73, 79, 81

Plasticity, 26, 29-30, 32-33, 61, 63, 67, 116, 124, 137, 148, 162, 164

Platelet Rich Plasma, 1, 7, 82, 84, 91

Platelets, 1, 3-7, 18, 83-85, 89-90

Pluripotency, 22, 37-41, 43-44, 46, 52, 92, 95-96, 98, 141, 150, 152, 157, 164-165, 183, 189-190

Progenitor Cells, 9-10, 12-15, 19, 21-22, 25-27, 29-33, 35, 55, 57-62, 67, 98, 100-101, 103-104, 114, 123-125, 127, 134-135, 150, 152, 167-168, 170-174, 180, 190-191

Prostate Gland Stem Cells, 30

S

Scaffold, 23, 89-91, 103-104, 109, 111-114, 174

Somatic Stem Cells, 26, 33

Stem Cell Transplantation, 24, 63-64, 66-67, 69, 127

Subchondral Cancellous Bone, 167-168

Subventricular Zone, 29, 34, 116, 118, 124-125

T

Teratoma Formation, 39, 150, 152, 157

Thrombin, 1-7, 84, 128

Thrombinoscope, 2

Trypsinization, 10, 38-39, 138, 159, 176

Tumor Necrosis Factor, 14, 16, 22, 25, 56, 62, 69, 73, 81

www.ingramcontent.com/pod-product-compliance
Lightning Source LLC
Chambersburg PA
CBHW050448200326
41458CB00014B/5107